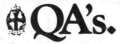

BAILLIÈRE'S
NURSES' DICTIONARY

PERSONAL INFORMATION

NAME RUTH J. MacFARLANE

ADDRESS_____ **Tel. No.**_____

Training School
  Date of entry 20-8-84 Date of completion_____

General Nursing Council Index No._____

State Examination_____

  Date passed_____

  State Registration No._____ Date_____

Additional training at_____

Examinations passed_____ **Date**

Appointments held_____ **From**____**To**

1._____

2._____

3._____

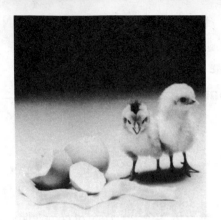
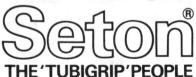

BAILLIÈRE'S NURSES' DICTIONARY

Nineteenth Edition

Revised by

PAMELA M. JEFFERIES

SRN, RSCN, RNT

Senior Nurse Tutor, Normanby College,
King's College Hospital, London

BAILLIÈRE TINDALL • LONDON

A BAILLIÈRE TINDALL book published by
Cassell Ltd,
1 St Anne's Road,
Eastbourne BN21 3UN

First published 1912
Eighteenth edition 1974
    Reprinted 1975, 1976, 1977, 1978
Nineteenth edition 1979
    Reprinted 1981
    Reprinted 1982
    Reprinted 1983
ISBN 0 7020 0743 9

Educational Low-priced Book Series edition 1979
Spanish edition (Elicien, Barcelona) 1977
Italian edition (Editorial Ermes, Milan) 1977
French edition (Librarie Maloine, Paris) 1978

Typeset by CCC, printed and bound in Great Britain by Bemrose
Specialist Print, Derby

British Library Cataloguing in Publication Data

Jefferies, Pamela M
    Baillières' nurses' dictionary.—19th ed.
    1. Nursing—Dictionaries
    I. Title
    610.73'03   RT21

ISBN 0–7020–0743–9

PREFACE

When I assumed responsibility for the revision of this well known dictionary, my first priority was to increase the size of the section devoted to word definitions; my second was to review and perhaps shorten the appendixes which make up the second part of the book. In fact, I have found it desirable to incorporate a considerable amount of new appendix material, so although some of the less useful appendices have been omitted and others pruned, the size of the section has not been reduced.

Keeping abreast of the constant changes in medical terminology and the rapid advance of knowledge is not easy, but I hope that the addition of a large number of new entries, coupled with the omission of those which are now infrequently used, will help to ensure that this well established work will remain as useful to nurses as it has always been. For the first time details have been included of the nationality and, where available, the dates of those people whose names are used to describe diseases and anatomical and physiological details. This is information which nurses often seek and which they frequently find difficult to obtain.

Many of the illustrations have been redrawn and some new ones have been added. The section of

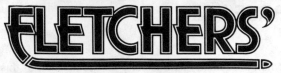

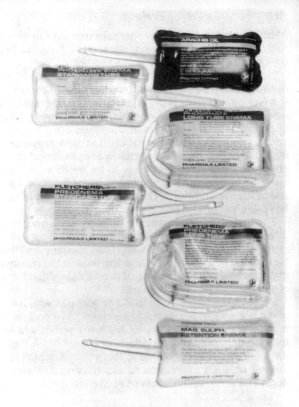

photographic plates has undergone revision in order to illustrate equipment and aspects of hospital life which are encountered by nurses today.

New material has been included in the appendices, dealing with nursing education, the reorganization of the National Health Service and the introduction and use of the SI System of weights and measures. A list of commonly used prefixes and suffixes has also been added. Some of the information that was previously included in this part of the book was considered to be obsolescent or to be less likely to be useful now than hitherto and has been excluded in order to create space for the additions. That which has been retained has been extensively revised and up-dated.

The book has been reset in a different style from that of earlier editions. The new setting provides room for rather more words on each page than formerly and this has helped to prevent any large increase in the number of pages in the book in spite of the increase in volume of the material that it contains.

I would like to thank all those colleagues who have given me suggestions and ideas during the course of my work. I would also like to thank the publishers for their advice, guidance and forbearance. I hope that I have managed to do justice to this volume, which has proved of such assistance to the nursing profession during its sixty-seven years of existence.

July 1979   PAMELA M. JEFFERIES

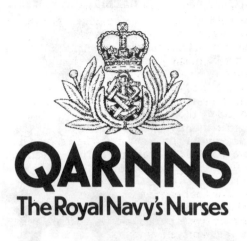

QARNNS
The Royal Navy's Nurses

They are a dedicated team of sisters and nurses who work together as a team caring for Naval personnel, their families and civilians.

Pay is good, and there is six weeks' annual leave. The Royal Navy also has first-class sports and social facilities.

If you would like further information call in at any Royal Navy and Royal Marines Careers Information Office.

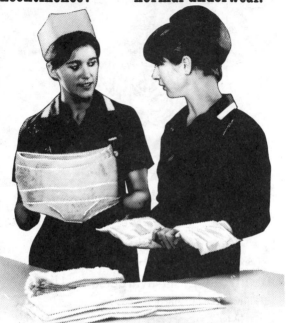

CONTENTS

LIST OF PLATES

between pp. 238 and 239

A

a- or **an-**. Prefix denoting 'lacking' or 'without'.

ab-. Prefix denoting 'from'.

abarticulation (*ab-ar-tik-u-la'-shun*). (1) Dislocation. (2) Diarthrosis (*q.v.*).

abdomen (*ab-do'-men*). The belly. The cavity between the diaphragm and the pelvis, lined by a serous membrane, the peritoneum, and containing the stomach, intestines, liver, gallbladder, spleen, pancreas, kidneys, suprarenal glands, ureters and bladder.

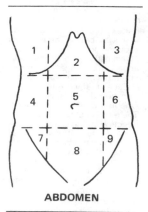

ABDOMEN

For descriptive purposes, its area can be divided into nine regions:

1. *Right hypochondriac.*
2. *Epigastric.*
3. *Left hypochondriac.*
4. *Right lumbar.*
5. *Umbilical.*
6. *Left lumbar.*
7. *Right iliac.*
8. *Hypogastric.*
9. *Left iliac.*

abdominal (*ab-dom'-in-al*). Pertaining to the abdomen. *A. aneurysm.* A dilatation of the abdominal aorta. *A. aorta.* That part of the aorta below the diaphragm. *A. bandage.* A many-tailed bandage. *A. breathing.* Deep breathing—hyperpnoea (*q.v.*). *A reflex.* Reflex contraction of abdominal wall muscles observed when skin is lightly stroked. *A. section.* Incision through the abdominal wall.

abdominoperineal excision (*ab-dom'-in-o-per-in-e'-al*). An operation for excision of the rectum by means of two incisions, an abdominal and a perineal. Often done as a combined synchronized operation by two surgeons, one working at each approach. A colostomy is performed.

abducent (*ab-du'-sent*). Abducting. (*Abducens.* Drawing away.) *A. muscle.* The external rectus muscle of the eye, which rotates it outward. *A. nerve.* The sixth cranial nerve, which supplies this muscle.

abduct (*ab-dukt'*). To draw away from the midline, e.g. of the body.

abductor muscle (*ab-duk'-tor*). One which abducts.

aberrant (*ab-er'-ant*). Taking an unusual course. Used of blood vessels and nerves that are not following their usual course.

aberration (*ab-er-a'-shun*). Deviation from the normal. In optics, failure to focus rays of light. *Mental a.* Mental disorder of an unspecified kind.

ability (*a-bil'-it-e*). The power to perform an act either mental or physical, with or without training. *Innate a.* The ability with which a person is born.

abiosis (*a-bi-o'-sis*). Lifelessness.

abiotrophy (*a-bi-ot'-tro-fe*). A nutritional defect, causing a loss of vitality and diminished resistance.

ablation (*ab-la'-shun*). Taking away from, as in amputation or excision of a growth or part of the body.

abnormal (*ab-nor'-mal*). Varying from what is regular or usual.

abort (*ab-ort'*). (1) To give birth to a fetus earlier than the 28th week of pregnancy. (2) To terminate a process or disease before it has run its normal course.

abortifacient (*ab-or-te-fa'-shent*). A drug which produces abortion.

abortion (*ab-or'-shun*). (1) Premature cessation of a normal process. (2) Emptying of the pregnant uterus before the end of the 28th week. *Complete a.* The contents of the uterus are expelled intact. *Criminal a.* The termination of pregnancy for reasons other than those stated in The Abortion Act 1967 (danger to mental or physical health of mother or child or family), carried out without the approval of two registered medical practitioners and by persons other than registered medical practitioners. *Incomplete a.* That in which some part of the fetus or placenta is retained in the uterus. *Induced a.* Term used when the uterus is emptied intentionally. *Inevitable a.* Abortion where bleeding is profuse and accompanied by pains, the cervix is dilated and the contents of the uterus can be felt. *Missed a.* One where all signs of pregnancy disappear and later the uterus discharges

a blood clot surrounding a shrivelled fetus, i.e. a carneous mole (*q.v.*). *Septic a.* Abortion associated with infection. *Therapeutic a.* One induced on medical advice because of danger to the mother's health. *Threatened a.* The appearance of signs of premature expulsion of the fetus; bleeding is slight, the cervix is closed.

abrasion (*ab-ra'-zhun*). A superficial injury, where the skin is rubbed or torn.

abreaction (*ab-re-ak'-shun*). A form of psychotherapy in which a patient relives a past painful experience, with the release of repressed emotion.

abscess (*ab'-ses*). A collection of pus in a cavity. This is termed suppuration and results from inflammation due to the presence of pyogenic microorganisms. It may rupture to a surface or require surgical incision and drainage. *Alveolar a.* One in a tooth socket. *Cold a.* The result of chronic tubercular infection and so called because there are few, if any, signs of inflammation. *Psoas a.* A cold abscess that has tracked down the psoas muscle from caries of the lumbar vertebrae. *Subphrenic a.* One situated under the diaphragm.

absorbent (*ab-sor'-bent*). Any agent that takes up by suction.

abulia (*a-bu'-le-ah*). Deficient will power.

acanthosis (*ak-an-tho'-sis*). A thickening of the lowest stratum of the epidermis.

acapnia (*a-kap'-ne-ah*). Deficient carbonic acid content of the blood.

acatalasia (*a-kat-al-a'-ze-ah*). A condition in which there is absence of the enzyme catalase in the patient's cells. Many of these patients may suffer from oral sepsis.

acatalepsy (*a-kat-al-ep'-se*). Lack of understanding.

acataphasia (*a-kat-a-fa'-ze-ah*). Lack of power to express connected thought. Associated with a cerebral lesion.

accidental haemorrhage. See Haemorrhage.

accommodation (*ak-kom-o-da'-shun*). The process which, on contraction of the ciliary muscles of the eye, renders the lens more convex, so enabling better focus of the rays of light for near vision, e.g. for reading.

accouchement (*ak-koosh-mon'*). Childbirth.

accoucheur (*ak-koosh-ur'*). An obstetrician.

accoucheuse (*ak-koosh-urz'*). A female obstetrician.

accretion (*ak-kre'-shun*). Accumulation of deposits, e.g. of salts to form a calculus in the bladder.

accumulator (*ak-ku'-mu-la-tor*). An apparatus for the collection and storage of electricity.

acephalous (*a-kef'-al-us*). Without a head.

acetabuloplasty (*as-et-ab'-u-lo-plas'-te*). An operation per-

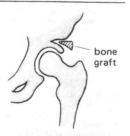

bone graft

ACETABULOPLASTY

formed to improve the depth and shape of the hip socket in correcting congenital dislocation of the hip or in treating osteo-arthritis of the hip.

acetabulum (*as-et-ab'-u-lum*). The cup-like socket in the innominate bone, receiving the head of the femur.

acetazolamide (*as-et-a-zol'-am-ide*). A sulphonamide compound which is an oral diuretic and has proved of great benefit in treating glaucoma by reducing the formation of aqueous humour and encouraging its drainage from the anterior chamber. Diamox is a proprietary preparation.

acetic acid (*as-e'-tik as'-id*). The acid of vinegar. It may be used as an antidote to alkaline poisons or as a reagent in urine testing. See Appendix 11.

aceto-acetic acid (*as-e'-to as-e'-tik as'-id*). Diacetic acid. A product of fat metabolism. It occurs in excessive amounts in diabetes and starvation giving rise to acetone bodies in the urine.

acetonaemia (*as-e-ton-e'-me-ah*). Acetone bodies in the blood.

acetone (*as'-e-tone*). A colourless inflammable liquid with a characteristic odour. Traces are found in the blood and in normal urine. A. bodies. Ketones, a result of incomplete breakdown of fatty acids causing acidosis. May occur in diabetes or starvation. Test for a. See Appendix 11.

acetonuria (*as-e-to-nu'-re-ah*). Acetone in the urine which gives it a peculiar sweet smell.

acetylcholine (*as-et-il-ko'-lin*). A chemical transmitter that is released by some nerve endings at the synapse between one neurone and the next or between a nerve ending and the effector organ it supplies. These nerves are said to be cholinergic, e.g. the parasympathetic nerves and the lower motor neurones to skeletal muscles. It is rapidly destroyed in the body by cholinesterase (*q.v.*).

acetylcoenzyme A (*as-et-il-ko-en'-zime*). Active form of acetic acid, to which carbohydrates, fats and amino acids not needed for protein synthesis are converted.

acetylsalicylic acid (*as-et-il-sal-e-sil'-ik as' id*). The same as aspirin (*q.v.*). An analgesic and antipyretic.

achalasia (*a-kal-a'-ze-ah*). Failure of relaxation of a muscle sphincter causing dilatation of the part above, e.g. of the oesophagus above the cardiac sphincter.

Achilles tendon (*ak-il'-eez*). That which inserts the gastrocnemius and soleus muscles into the calcaneum (os calcis).

achillorrhaphy (*ak-il-or'-raf-e*). Repair of the Achilles tendon after it has been torn.

achillotomy (*ak-il-ot'-o-me*). The subcutaneous division of the Achilles tendon.

achlorhydria (*a-klor-hi'-dre-ah*). Absence of hydrochloric acid in the stomach. A condition found in pernicious anaemia and gastric cancer.

acholia (*a-ko'-le-ah*). A lack of secretion of bile.

acholuria (*a-ko-lu'-re-ah*). Absence of bile from the urine.

acholuric jaundice (*a-ko-lu'-rik*). *See* Jaundice.

achondroplasia (*a-kon-dro-pla'-ze-ah*). An inherited condition in which there is early union of the epiphysis and diaphysis of long bones. Growth is arrested and dwarfism is the result.

achromasia (*a-kro-ma'-ze-ah*). (1) Loss of colour; pallor. (2) Loss of staining reaction in a cell.

achromatopsia (*a-kro-mat-op'-se-ah*). Colour blindness. It is most often a partial colour deficiency. The subject has cones that are sensitive to only two of the three primary colours (red, blue and green), and the missing colour is interpreted as a mixture of the other two.

achylia (*a-ki'-le-ah*). Literally, absence of chyle. *A. gastrica*. A condition in which gastric secretion is reduced or absent.

acid (*as'-id*). A substance which, when combined with an alkali, will form a salt. Any acid substance will turn blue litmus red. Individual acids may be found under their proper names.

acidaemia (*as-id-e'-me-ah*). Acidity of the blood. The normal reaction is just on the alkaline side of neutrality.

acid–base balance. The normal ratio between the acid ions and the basic or alkaline ions required to maintain the pH of the blood and body fluids. *See* Appendix 8.

acid-fast. A bacteriological term to describe those microorganisms not easily decolorized when once stained.

acid–alcohol-fast. Stained bacteria that are resistant to decolorization by both acid and alcohol.

acidity (*as-id'-it-e*). The quality of being acid.

acidosis (*as-id-o'-sis*). A condition in which the relation of alkalinity to acidity of the blood is very delicately balanced. A diminution of alkali content or increase of acid will cause this condition. It is characterized by vomiting, drowsiness, hyperpnoea, acetone odour of breath (of 'new-mown hay') and acetone bodies in the urine. It may occur in diabetes mellitus owing to incomplete metabolism of fat. May also be termed ketosis.

acidotic (*as-id-ot'-ik*). A term applied to one suffering from acidosis.

acid phosphatase (*as'-id fos'-fat-aze*). An enzyme secreted by the prostate gland. Higher levels than normal in the blood serum are indicative of carcinoma of the gland or of secondary deposits from the same cause.

acini (*as'-in-e*). Minute saccules or alveoli lined by secreting cells, e.g. the secreting portion of the mammary gland.

acme (*ak'-me*). The highest part of a fever when the symptoms are fully developed.

acne (*ak'-ne*). A term denoting an inflammatory condition of the sebaceous glands. *A. rosacea.* A redness of the forehead, nose and cheeks due to chronic dilatation of the subcutaneous capillaries, which becomes permanent with the formation of pustules in the affected areas. *A. vulgaris.* This occurs commonly in adolescents and young adults on the face, chest and back with the formation of comedones and then pustules. It is thought to be due to androgenic stimulation.

acousma (*a-koos'-mah*). The hearing of imaginary sounds.

acoustic (*a-koos'-tik*). Relating to sound or the sense of hearing.

acquired (*ak-wi'-rd*). Term applied to disease, habits or immunity developed after birth; not congenital.

acriflavine (*ak-re-fla'-veen*). A powerful antiseptic derived from coal tar used in an aqueous solution 1:1000.

acro- (*ak'-ro*). Prefix meaning extremity.

acrocentric (*ak-ro-sen'-trik*). Chromosomes which have the centromere (*q.v.*) near to one end.

acrocephalia (*ak-ro-kef-a'-le-ah*). Malformation of the head, in which the top is pointed.

acrocyanosis (*ak-ro-si-an-o'-sis*). A blue appearance of the hands and feet often associated with a vasomotor defect.

acrodynia (*ak-ro-din'-e-ah*). Neuritic pains in the fingers and toes with erythema.

acromegaly (*ak-ro-meg'-al-e*). Marked bony overgrowth especially of the jaw, hands and feet. Associated with overactivity of the anterior lobe of the pituitary gland in adults.

acromioclavicular (*ak-ro'-me-o-klav-ik'-u-lah*). Refers to the joint between the acromion process of the scapula and the lateral aspect of the clavicle.

acromion (*ak-ro'-me-on*). The outward projection of the spine of the scapula, forming the point of the shoulder.

acronyx (*ak'-ron-iks*). A toe or finger nail which becomes ingrown.

acroparaesthesia (*ak-ro-par-es-the'-ze-ah*). An orthopaedic condition in which pressure on the nerves of the brachial plexus causes numbness, pain and tingling of the hand and forearm.

acrophobia (*ak-ro-fo'-be-ah*). Morbid terror of being at a height.

acrosclerosis (*ak-ro-skler-o'-sis*). Scleroderma which affects the hands, feet, face or chest.

acrosome (*ak'-ro-sohm*). Part of the head of a spermatozoon.

acrylics (*ak-ril'-iks*). Synthetic plastic materials derived from acrylic acid, from which dental and medical prostheses may be made.

ACTH. Adrenocorticotrophic hormone. Corticotrophin (q.v.).

actinism (ak'-tin-izm). The chemical action of rays of light.

actinodermatitis (ak'-tin-o-der-mat-i'-tis). Inflammation of the skin, due to the action of Röntgen rays, sun rays or ultra-violet light.

Actinomyces (ak-tin-o-mī'-seez). A genus of branching, spore-forming, vegetable parasites, which may give rise to a chronic infective disease, actinomycosis, and from which many antibiotic drugs are produced, e.g. streptomycin.

actinomycin (ak-tin-o-mi'-sin). A group of cytotoxic drugs used in the treatment of malignant disease, e.g. Wilms' tumour.

actinotherapy (ak-tin-o-ther'-ap-e). Treatment of disease by rays of light, e.g. artificial sunlight.

action potential (ak'-shun po-ten'-shal). The electrical change which takes place when a nerve conducts an impulse or a muscle fibre contracts.

activate (ak'-ti-vate). To render active. (1) Yeast is the activator in the process by which sugar is converted into alcohol. (2) The digestive secretions are activated by hormones to carry out normal digestion. See Gastrin and Secretin.

activator (ak'-ti-va-tor). A substance, hormone or enzyme, that stimulates a chemical change though it may not take part in the change.

active immunity (ak'-tiv im-mu'-nit-e). An immunity in which the individual has been stimulated to produce his own antibodies.

active movements (ak'-tiv moov'-ments). Refers to movement or effort to move by the patient as distinct from 'passive movements' (q.v.).

active principle (ak'-tiv prin-sip-I). Applied to drugs it is the potent part of the drug responsible for its action. See Alkaloid.

actomyosin (ak-to-mi'-o-sin). Muscle protein complex; the myosin component acts as an enzyme which causes the release of energy.

acupuncture (ak'-u-punkt-chur). (1) Puncture of any part of the body by needles in order to carry off fluid. (2) Form of medical treatment used in China in which pain can be prevented by the insertion of needles through the skin at strategic body points.

acuity (ak-u'-it-e). Sharpness. *A. of hearing.* An acute perception of sound. *A. of vision.* Clear focusing ability.

acus (a'-kus). A needle. (Latin.)

acute (ak-ute'). A term applied to a disease in which the attack is sudden, severe and of short duration.

acute yellow atrophy (at'-ro-fe). Severe damage to the liver, caused by a toxic agent. See Atrophy.

acystia (a-sis'-te-ah). Absence of bladder.

ad-. Prefix meaning 'to'.

adactylia (a-dak-til'-e-ah). Congenital absence of fingers or toes.

Adam's apple (ad'-amz ap'-I). The prominentia laryngea, a protrusion of the front of the neck caused by the thyroid cartilage.

adaptation (ad-ap-ta'-shun). The ability to overcome difficulties and to adjust oneself to changing circumstances. Neuroses and psychoses are often associated with failures of adaptation.

addiction (*ad-ik'-shun*). The habitual taking of drugs or alcohol, for which a craving develops that is beyond the will of the person addicted to control. Excessive quantities are consumed. *See* Drug dependence.

Addison's anaemia (*T. Addison, British physician, 1793–1860*). Pernicious anaemia. *See* Anaemia.

Addison's disease. Deficiency disease of the suprarenal cortex; often tuberculous. There is wasting, brown pigmentation of the skin and extreme debility. Treated by deoxycortone acetate (DOCA), cortisone and sodium chloride.

adducens (*ad-du'-sens*). Leading toward the midline. *A. oculi.* The internal rectus muscle of the eye which turns it inward.

adduct (*ad-dukt'*). To draw towards the midline of the body.

adductor (*ad-dukt'-or*). Any muscle which adducts. The opposite of abductor.

adenectomy (*ad-en-ek'-to-me*). Excision of a gland.

adenine (*ad'-en-een*). One of the purine bases found in deoxyribonucleic acid. Necessary for the formation of nucleic acids.

adenitis (*ad-en-i'-tis*). Inflammation of a gland.

adenocarcinoma (*ad'-en-o-kar-sin-o'-mah*). A malignant new growth of glandular epithelial tissue.

adenoid (*ad'-en-oid*). Resembling a gland. Generally applied to abnormal lymphoid growth in the nasopharynx.

adenoidectomy (*ad-en-oid-ek'-to-me*). The removal of adenoid tissue from the nasopharynx by curettage.

adenoma (*ad-en-o'-mah*). A simple tumour of glandular tissue, often containing fibrous tissue when it is, strictly, a *fibroadenoma*, e.g. of the breast or thyroid.

adenomatome (*ad-en-o-mat-ohm*). An instrument for the removal of adenoids.

adenomyoma (*ad-en-o-mi-o'-mah*). An innocent new growth involving both glandular and muscle tissue, usually applied to benign growths of the uterus.

adenopathy (*ad-en-op'-ath-e*). Any disease of a gland, particularly of a lymphatic gland.

adenosclerosis (*ad-en-o-skler-o'-sis*). Hardening of a gland. Usually the result of calcification.

adenosine triphosphate (ATP) (*ad-en'-o-seen tri-fos'-fate*). Molecule in which heat is stored when not required immediately.

adenovirus (*ad-en-o-vi'-rus*). A variety of virus. Many types

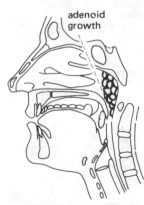

adenoid growth

ADENOID GROWTH

have been isolated, some of which cause respiratory tract infections, while other are associated with conjunctivitis or epidemic keratoconjunctivitis.

adeps (*ad'-eps*). Lard. (Latin.) A foundation fat for ointments. *A. lanae hydrosus* is lanolin (*q.v.*).

ADH. Antidiuretic hormone (*q.v.*).

adhesion (*ad-he'-zhun*). Union between two surfaces normally separated. Usually the result of inflammation when fibrous tissue forms, e.g. peritonitis may cause adhesions between organs. A possible cause of intestinal obstruction.

adiaphoresis (*a-di-af-or-e'-sis*). Deficiency in the secretion of sweat.

adiaphoretic (*a-di-af-or-et'-ik*). An anhidrotic agent. A drug that prevents the secretion of sweat.

adipocele (*ad'-ip-o-seel*). A hernia, with the sac containing fatty tissue. A lipocele.

adipocere (*ad'-ip-o-seer*). A waxy substance formed in dead bodies when decomposing in water.

adipose (*ad'-ip-ose*). Of the nature of fat. Fatty.

adiposuria (*ad-ip-o-su'-re-ah*). Fat in the urine. Lipuria.

aditus (*ad'-it-us*). An opening or passageway, often applied to that between the middle ear and the mastoid antrum.

adjustment (*ad-just'-ment*). In psychology the ability of a person to adapt to changing circumstances or environment.

adjuvant (*ad'-ju-vant*). A secondary remedy assisting the action of another.

Adler's theory (*A. Adler, Austrian psychiatrist, 1870–1937*). The theory that neuroses develop as a compensation for feelings of inferiority either social or physical.

adnexa (*ad-neks'-ah*). Appendages. *Uterine a.* The ovaries and fallopian tubes.

adolescence (*ad-o-les'-ense*). The period between puberty and maturity. In the male—14 to 25 years. In the female—12 to 21 years.

adrenal (*ad-re'-nal*). The suprarenal gland, and endocrine gland placed on top of each kidney.

adrenalectomy (*ad-ren-al-ek'-to-me*). Surgical removal of the adrenal glands. Replacement therapy by giving cortisone is essential.

adrenaline (*ad-ren'-al-in*). A hormone secreted by the medulla of the adrenal gland. Has an action similar to normal stimulation of the sympathetic nervous system: (1) Causing dilatation of the bronchioles. (2) Raising of the blood pressure by constriction of surface vessels and stimulation of the cardiac output. (3) Releasing glycogen from the liver. It is therefore used to treat such conditions as asthma, collapse and hypoglycaemia. It acts as a haemostat in local anaesthetics.

adrenergic (*ad-ren-er'-jik*). A term applied to nerves that release the chemical transmitter noradrenaline in order to stimulate the muscles and glands they supply.

adrenocorticotrophic hormone (*ad-ren'-o-kor'-tik-o troff'-ik hor'-mohn*). Corticotrophin (*q.v.*).

adrenogenital (*ad-ren-o-jen'-it-al*). Relating to both the adrenal glands and the gonads. *A. syndrome.* A condition of masculinization in women caused by over-activity of the adrenal cortex.

adrenolytic (*ad-ren-o-lit'-ik*). Drugs that inhibit the stimulation of the sympathetic nerves and the activity of adrenaline.

adsorbent (*ad-sorb'-ent*). A substance that has the power of attracting gas or fluid to itself.

adsorption (*ad-sorp'-shun*). The power of certain substances to attach other gases or substances in solution to their surface and so concentrate them there. This is made use of in chromatography (*q.v.*).

advancement (*ad-vans'-ment*). An operation to detach a tendon or muscle and reattach it further forward.

adventitia (*ad-ven-tish'-e-ah*). The outer coat of an artery or vein.

Aëdes aegypti mosquito (*ah-e'-des e-gip'-ti mos-ke'-to*). The intermediate host of the germ of yellow fever.

aegophony (*e-gof'-o-ne*). A sound heard in the chest on auscultation, when the patient speaks. Compared to the 'bleat of a goat'.

aeration (*air-a'-shun*). Supplying with air. Describes the oxygenation of blood which takes place in the lungs.

aerobe (*air'-obe*). An organism that can live and thrive only in the presence of oxygen.

aerogenous (*air-oj'-en-us*). Applied to micro-organisms that give rise to the formation of gas, usually by the fermentation of lactose or other carbohydrate.

aerophagy (*air-off'-aj-e*). Swallowing of air.

aerosol (*air'-o-sol*). Finely divided particles or droplets. *A. sprays*. Used in medicine to humidify air or oxygen, or for the administration of drugs by inhalation and as a local analgesic.

aetas (*e'-tas*). Age. (Latin.)

aetiology (*e-te-ol'-o-je*). The science of the cause of disease.

afebrile (*a-feb'-ril*). Without fever.

afibrinogenaemia (*a-fib-rin'-o-jen-e'-me-ah*). Absence of fibrinogen in the blood. The clotting mechanism of the blood is impaired as a result.

affect (*af-fekt'*). The feeling experienced in connection with an emotion or mood. A term used in psychiatry.

affective (*af-fekt'-if*). Pertaining to the emotions or moods. *A. psychoses*. Major mental disorders in which there is grave disturbance of the emotions. *See* Psychoses.

afferent (*af'-fer-rent*). Conveying towards the centre. *A. nerves*. The sensory nerve fibres which convey impulses from the periphery towards the brain. *A. paths or tracts*. The course of the sensory nerves up the spinal cord and through the brain. *A. vessels*. Arterioles entering the glomerulus of the kidney, or lymphatics entering a lymph gland. *See* Efferent.

affiliation (*af-fil-e-a'-shun*). The judicial decision of paternity of a child with a view to a maintenance order.

affinity (*af-fin'-it-te*). Chemically, the attraction of two substances to each other, e.g. carbon monoxide has a greater affinity with haemoglobin than has oxygen.

affusion (*af-fu'-zhun*). Treatment by pouring hot or cold water over the body.

African tick fever. Disease caused by a spirochaete, *Borrelia duttoni*. Transmitted by ticks. *See* Relapsing fevers.

after-birth (*ahf'-ter-berth*). The placenta, cord and membranes, expelled after childbirth.

after-care (*ahf'-ter-kare*). The term applied to social, medical or nursing care following a period of hospital treatment.

after-image (*ahf'-ter-im'-ij*). A visual impression that remains briefly following the cessation of sensory stimulation.

after-pains (*ahf'-ter-pa'-nz*). Pains due to uterine contraction after childbirth.

agalactia (*a-gal-ak'-te-ah*). Absence of the milk secretion after childbirth.

agammaglobulinaemia (*a-gam-mah-glob-u-lin-e'-me-ah*). A condition found in children in which there is no gamma-globulin (*q.v.*) in the blood. They are therefore susceptible to infections because of an inability to form antibodies.

agar-agar (*a'-gah a'-gah*). A gelatinous substance prepared from seaweed. Used as a culture-medium for bacteria and as a laxative because it absorbs liquid from the digestive tract and swells, so stimulating peristalsis.

agenesis (*a-jen-e'-sis*). Failure of a structure to develop properly.

agglutination (*ag-glu-tin-a'-shun*). The collecting into clumps. *Cross a.* A simple test to decide the group to which a given blood belongs. (*See* Blood grouping) A drop of serum of known classification is put on a microscope slide, to this is added a drop of the blood to be tested. An even admixture indicates compatibility. A flaky, spotted appearance shows incompatibility as the corpuscles have clumped together. *A. test.* A means of aiding diagnosis and identification of bacteria. If serum containing known agglutinins comes into contact with the specific bacteria clumping will take place. *See* Widal reaction.

agglutinative (*ag-glu'-tin-a-tiv*). (1) Adherent or glueing together. (2) A term applied to serum which causes clumping of bacteria, e.g. in Widal reaction.

agglutinins (*ag-glu'-tin-ins*). Antibodies formed in blood which cause clumping together of bacteria, so that they are more readily destroyed by phagocytes.

agglutinogen (*ag-glu-tin'-o-jen*). Any substance that, when present in the blood stream, can cause the production of specific antibodies or agglutinins.

aggressin (*ag-gres'-sin*). A substance said to be produced by some bacteria which increases their effect upon the host.

aggression (*ag-gresh'-un*). Animosity or hostility shown towards another person or object, as a response to opposition or frustration.

aglossia (*a-glos'-e-ah*). Absence of the tongue.

aglutition (*a-glu-tish'-un*). Difficulty in the act of swallowing. Dysphagia (*q.v.*).

agnathia (*ag-na'-the-ah*). Absence or defective development of the jaw.

agnosia (*ag-no'-se-ah*). An inability to recognize objects as the sensory stimulus cannot be interpreted in spite of a normal sense organ.

agoraphobia (*ag-or-af-fo'-be-ah*). A fear of open spaces.

agranulocyte (*a-gran'-u-lo-site*). A white blood cell without granules in the cytoplasm. Includes monocytes and lymphocytes.

agranulocytosis (*a-gran'-u-lo-si-to'-sis*). A condition in which there is a marked decrease or complete absence of granular leucocytes in the blood. May result from: (1) The use of drugs, e.g. gold salts, sulphonamides, thiouracil and benzol preparations. (2) Excessive irradiation of the bone marrow. Characterized by a sore throat, ulceration of the mouth and pyrexia. It may result in severe prostration and death.

agraphia (*a-graf'-e-ah*). Loss of the power of expressing thought in writing.

ague (*a'-gu*). Malaria. Intermittent fever, accompanied by recurring fits of shivering and sweating. *See* Malaria.

AHG. Antihaemophilic globulin (*q.v.*).

AID. Artificial insemination with donor semen.

AIH. Artificial insemination of a woman by her husband's semen.

air (*a-er*). A mixture of gases surrounding the earth. It consists of: non-active nitrogen 79 per cent, oxygen 21 per cent which supports life and combustion; traces of neon, argon, hydrogen, etc., and carbon dioxide 0·03 per cent except in expired air, when 6 per cent is exhaled, due to diffusion which has taken place in the lungs. Air has weight and exerts pressure. The latter aids in syphonage from body cavities. *Complemental a.* Additional air which can be inhaled with inspiratory effort. *Residual a.* Air remaining in the lungs after deep expiration. *Stationary a.* That retained in the lungs after normal expiration. *Supplemental a.* The extra air forced out of the lungs with expiratory effort. *Tidal a.* That which passes in and out of the lungs in normal respiratory action.

air-bed (*a-er bed*). A rubber mattress inflated with air.

air embolism (*a-er em'-bolizm*). An embolism caused by air entering the circulatory system. *See* Embolism.

air encephalogram (*a-er enkef'-al-o-gram*). An X-ray of the brain taken after the injection of air into the subarachnoid space.

air hunger (*a-er hung'-ger*). A form of dyspnoea in which there are deep sighing respirations, characteristic of severe haemorrhage or acidosis.

akinesia (*a-kin-e'-ze-ah*). Loss of muscle power. This may be the result of a brain or spinal cord lesion or temporarily due to anaesthesia.

akinetic (*a-kin-et'-ik*). An adjective applying to states or conditions where there is lack of movement.

alalia (*al-a'-le-ah*). Loss or impairment of the power of speech due to muscle paralysis or cerebral lesion.

alanine (*al'-an-een*). An amino acid formed by the ingestion of dietary protein.

alastrim (*a-las'-trim*). A contagious eruptive fever probably a mild form of smallpox. *See* Variola.

Albee's operation (*F. H. Albee, American surgeon, 1876–1945*). A bone graft from the tibia is placed along the affected vertebrae to secure immobilization. The spinous processes are split and the graft inserted.

Albers-Schönberg's disease (*H. E. Albers-Schönberg, German radiologist, 1865–1921*). A condition in which there is a great increase in bone density which can be seen radiographically. Also known as marble bone disease. There are three types: fetal, juvenile and adult.

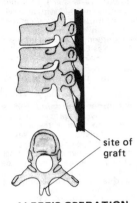

site of
graft

ALBEE'S OPERATION

---

albinism (*al'-bin-izm*). A condition in which there is congenital absence of pigment in the skin, hair and eyes. It may be partial or complete.

albino (*al-be'-no*). A person affected with albinism.

Albright's syndrome (*F. Albright, American physician, 1900–). Syndrome in which there is abnormal development of bone, excessive pigmentation of the skin and, in females, precocious sexual development.

albumin (*al-bu'-min*). A protein present in most animal tissues. It is soluble in water and coagulates on heating, e.g. white of egg. *Tests for a. See* Appendix 11.

albuminuria (*al-bu-min-u'-re-ah*). The presence of albumin in the urine, occurring, e.g. in renal disease, in most feverish conditions and sometimes in pregnancy. *Orthostatic* or *postural a.*

A non-pathological form which affects some individuals after prolonged standing.

albumose (*al'-bu-mose*). A substance formed during gastric digestion, intermediate between albumin and peptone.

alcohol (*al'-ko-hol*). C_3H_5OH. Ethyl hydroxide. A volatile liquid distilled from fermented saccharine liquids. Used: (1) As an antiseptic. (2) In the preparation of tinctures. (3) As a preservative for anatomical specimens. Taken internally, it acts as a temporary heart stimulant, and in large quantities as a depressant poison. It has some value as a food, 30 ml brandy producing about 400 J. *Absolute a.* Contains not more than 1 per cent by weight of water.

alcohol-fast (*al'-ko-hol fahst*). A term used of bacteria that having once been stained are resistant to decolorization by alcohol.

alcoholism (*al'-ko-hol-izm*). The state of poisoning by excessive consumption of alcohol.

alcoholic (*al-ko-hol'-ik*). A person addicted to excessive, uncontrolled alcohol consumption. This results in loss of appetite and vitamin B deficiency, leading to peripheral neuritis with eye changes and cirrhosis of the liver and to progressive deterioration in the personality. *A. delirium. See* Delirium.

alcoholuria (*al-ko-hol-u'-re-ah*). The presence of alcohol in the urine. This may be estimated when excess blood levels of alcohol are suspected.

aldosterone (*al-dos'-ter-ohn*). A hormone, isolated from the adrenal cortex, that aids the retention of sodium and the excretion of potassium in the body and by so doing aids in maintaining the electrolyte balance.

aldosteronism (*al-dos'-ter-on-izm*). An excess secretion of aldosterone caused by an adrenal neoplasm. The serum potassium is low and the patient has hypertension.

aleukaemia (*a-lu-ke'-me-ah*). Diminished numbers of white cells in the blood. Leucopenia (*q.v.*).

alexia (*a-leks'-e-ah*). A form of aphasia, when there is inability to recognize written or printed words. Word blindness.

algae (*al'-je*). Simple forms of plant life. These form a slimy film on sand filter beds and aid purification of water.

algesia (*al-je'-ze-ah*). Sensitiveness to pain.

algesimeter (*al-jes-im'-e-ter*). An instrument which indicates

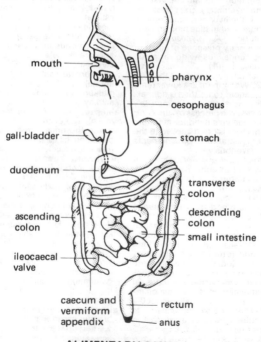

mouth

pharynx

oesophagus

gall-bladder

stomach

duodenum

transverse colon

ascending colon

descending colon

small intestine

ileocaecal valve

caecum and vermiform appendix

rectum

anus

ALIMENTARY CANAL

the degree of sensitiveness of the skin.

algid (*al'-jid*). Chilly and cold. *A. state.* One of severe collapse and prostration which may occur in certain types of malaria and in cholera.

aliment (*al'-e-ment*). Food or nourishment.

alimentary (*al-e-ment'-ar-e*). Relating to the system of nutrition. *A. canal.* The passage through which the food passes, from mouth to anus. *A. system.* The alimentary tract together with the liver and other organs concerned in digestion and adsorption. *A. glycosuria.* The temporary presence of sugar in the urine following a meal. Causes: (1) An excessive amount of this taken in the diet. (2) When there is a lower renal threshold (*q.v.*) than is normal.

alimentation (*al-e-men-ta'-shun*). The process of supplying the patient's need for nutrition. The term is often applied to the administration of nutrients intravenously.

aliquot (*al'-e-kwot*). One of a number of equal parts forming a compound or solution.

alkalaemia (*al-kal-e'-me-ah*). An increase in the alkali content of the blood. The pH is above 7·40. Alkalosis (*q.v.*).

alkali (*al'-kal-i*). A substance capable of uniting with acids to form salts, and with fats to form soaps. It turns red litmus paper blue. Sodium, potassium and ammonia are the chief ones used in medicine. *A. reserve.* An estimation of the plasma bicarbonate. The normal is about 0·2 per cent of carbon dioxide. In acidosis there is a fall and in alkalosis a rise in this figure.

alkaline phosphatase (*al'-kal-ine fos'-fat-aze*). An enzyme capable of splitting off phosphate groups from certain substrates, especially active in alkaline solution. Its level in blood plasma is a measure of osteoblastic activity. It is raised in hyperparathyroidism.

alkaloid (*al'-kal-oid*). The name given to active nitrogenous compounds that are alkaline in solution and have a bitter taste. Many found in medicinal plants can now be synthesized.

alkalosis (*al-kal-o'-sis*). An increase in the alkali reserve in the blood. It may be confirmed by estimation of the blood carbon dioxide content and treated by giving normal saline or ammonium chloride intravenously to encourage the excretion of bicarbonate by the kidneys.

alkapton (*al-kap'-ton*). An abnormal product of protein metabolism, from the amino acid, tyrosine.

alkaptonuria (*al-kap-ton-u'-re-ah*). The excretion of alkapton in the urine. On standing, oxidation takes place giving a dark-brown colour to the urine.

alkylating agents (*al'-ke-la-ting a-jents*). Drugs that damage the DNA molecule of the nucleus of malignant tumour cells. Many are nitrogen mustard preparations and may be termed chromosome poisons.

all-or-none law. Physiological law relating to irritable tissues. In nerves there are only two possible reactions to a stimulus: either there is no reaction at all or there is a full reaction with no graduation of response according to the strength of the stimulus.

allantois (*al-lan'-to-is*). A membranous sac projecting from the ventral surface of the fetus in its early stages. It eventually helps to form the placenta.

allelomorph (*al-e'-lo-morf*).

One of a pair of genes which occupy the same relative positions on homologous chromosomes and produce different effects on the same process of development.

allergen (*al'-er-jen*). A substance that stimulates an altered reaction in the body known as an allergy.

allergy (*al'-er-je*). A hypersensitiveness to some foreign protein, small doses of which produce a violent reaction in the patient. Asthma, hay fever, angioneurotic oedema, migraine, and some types of urticaria and eczema are allergic states. *See* Anaphylaxis.

allocheiria (*al-o-ki'-re-ah*). A response or sensation felt on (referred to) the opposite side from that to which a stimulus is applied.

allopurinol (*al-o-pu'-rin-ol*). A drug which reduces the formation of uric acid. Used in the long-term treatment of gout to lessen the frequency and severity of attacks. Zyloric is a proprietary preparation.

allograft (*al'-o-graft*). Tissue transplanted from one person to another. *Non-viable a*. Skin taken from a cadaver that cannot regenerate. *See* Lyophilized skin. *Viable a*. Living tissue transplanted.

almoner (*ah'-mon-er*). A medical social worker (*q.v.*).

aloes (*al'-oze*). Extract from the leaves of the aloe. An irritant purgative likely to cause griping. It is contraindicated in pregnancy.

alopecia (*al-o-pe'-she-ah*). Baldness.

alpha cells (*al'-fah sells*). Cells found in the islets of Langerhans in the pancreas. They produce the hormone, glucagon (*q.v.*).

alpha receptors (*al'-fah re-sep'-tors*). Tissue receptors associated with the stimulation (contraction) of smooth muscle.

Alport's syndrome (*A. C. Alport, South African physician, 1880– *). Familial deafness which is also associated with albuminuria and nephritis.

altitude sickness. Condition caused by hypoxia (*q.v.*) which occurs as a result of the decrease in the partial pressure of atmospheric oxygen in the alveoli of the lung at high altitudes.

alternating current. An electrical current that runs alternately from the negative and positive poles, as in the ordinary faradic coils.

altruism (*al'-tru-izm*). A regard for the well-being of other people.

alum (*al'-um*). A powerful astringent and styptic, composed of aluminium and potassium sulphate. *A. precipitated toxoid.* APT (*q.v.*).

aluminium (*al-u-min'-e-um*). A silver-white metal with a low specific gravity, compounds of which are astringent and antiseptic. *A. hydroxide.* Used in the treatment of gastric cases as an antacid. *A. paste.* Combined with zinc oxide and liquid paraffin it forms a good skin protective against ileostomy discharge. *A. silicate.* Kaolin used as a dusting powder or as a poultice. Refined kaolin may be given orally to check diarrhoea.

alveolar air. Air found in the alveoli or air sacs of the lungs.

alveoli (*al-ve-o'-li*). (1) The sockets of the teeth. (2) The air sacs of the lungs. (3) The acini of glands.

alveolitis (*al-ve-o-li'-tis*). Inflammation of the alveoli. *E trinsic allergic a.* Inflamma' of the alveoli of the lung caused by inhalation of an antigen such as pollen.

Alzheimer's disease (*A. Alzheimer, German neurologist, 1864–1915*). Presenile dementia with cerebral atrophy and characteristic histological changes.

amalgam (*am-al'-gam*). A compound of mercury and other metals. *Dental a.* Used for filling teeth.

amastia (*a-mas'-te-ah*). Congenital absence of breast tissue.

amaurosis (*am-aw-ro'-sis*). Blindness in which there are no discernible changes in the structures of the eye. Often temporary, it may be present in hysteria, nephritis, uraemia or may be due to a sudden change of posture.

amaurotic familial idiocy (*am-aw-rot'-ik*). Tay-Sachs disease. A familial metabolic disorder commencing in infancy or childhood. Characterized by progressive mental deterioration, blindness and spastic paralysis.

ambidextrous (*am-be-deks'-trus*). Equally skilful with either hand.

ambivalence (*am-biv'-al-ense*). The existence of contradictory emotional feelings towards an object, commonly of love and hate for another person. If these feelings occur to a marked degree they lead to psychological disturbance.

amblyopia (*am-ble-o'-pe-ah*). Dimness of vision.

amblyoscope (*am'-ble-o-skope*). An instrument used in orthoptic treatment to aid the correction of strabismus and develop binocular vision.

ambulant (*am'-bu-lant*). One who is able to walk.

ambulatory (*am-bu-la'-tor-e*). Having the capacity to walk.

amelia (*a-me'-le-ah*). The complete absence of an extremity at the shoulder or pelvic girdle.

amelioration (*am-me-le-or-a'-shun*). Improvement of symptoms; a lessening of the severity of a disease.

amenorrhoea (*a-men-or-e'-ah*). Absence of menstruation. *Primary a.* The non-occurrence of the menses. *Secondary a.* The cessation of the menses after they have been established owing to disease or pregnancy.

amentia (*a-men'-she-ah*). Mental subnormality. May be due to hereditary factors, failure of development of the embryo or birth trauma.

amethocaine (*a-meth'-o-kane*). A local anaesthetic for mucous membranes. *A. pastille.* This, slowly dissolved in the mouth, will aid the passage of a bronchoscope or gastroscope.

ametria (*a-me'-tre-ah*). Congenital absence of the uterus.

ametropia (*a-me-tro'-pe-ah*). Defective vision. A general word applied to incorrect refraction.

amidone (*am'-e-dohn*). Methadone, a powerful analgesic which is included in the Misuse of Drugs Act list. Physeptone is a proprietary preparation of the drug.

amino acids (*am'-in-o as'-ids*). Chemical compounds containing the radical NH_2. The end-products of protein digestion. *Essential a. a.* Those required for replacement and growth, which cannot be synthesized in the body in sufficient amounts. *Non-essential a. a.* Those necessary for proper growth but which can be synthesized in the body.

aminophylline (*am-in-off'-il-*

in). An alkaloid from camellia, it relaxes plain muscle spasm of the bronchioles and coronary arteries. It may be given by mouth, intravenously or as a suppository, and is useful in treating asthma and heart failure.

aminosalicyclic acid. *See* Para-aminosalicylic acid.

Aminosol (*am-in'-o-sol*). A proprietary preparation of protein substances which is given intravenously.

amino transferase (*am'-in-o trans'-fer-aze*). One of a group of enzymes found in the liver.

amiphenazole (*am-e-fen'-a-zol*). A drug that stimulates the central nervous system and respiratory centre. Daptazole is a proprietary preparation of it.

amitosis (*a-mi-to'-sis*). Multiplication of cells by simple division or fission.

amitriptyline (*am-e-trip'-til-een*). An antidepressant drug that is chemically related to chlorpromazine. It is useful in relieving tension and anxiety but may cause dizziness and hypotension.

ammonia (*am-mo'-ne-ah*). NH_3. A colourless pungent liquid. Used as a cardiac stimulant, a diuretic and an expectorant.

amnesia (*am-ne'-ze-ah*). Loss of memory for a circumscribed period of time. *Anterograde a.* Loss of memory for recent events, more common in old age and organic brain disease. *Retrograde a.* Loss of memory for events prior to an injury. It often applies to the time immediately preceding an accident.

amniocentesis (*am-ne-o-sente'-sis*). The withdrawal of fluid from the uterus through the abdominal wall by means of a

syringe and needle in cases of hydramnios.

amnion (*am'-ne-on*). The innermost membrane enveloping the fetus and enclosing the liquor amnii.

amnioscopy (*am-ne-os'-kope*). Inspection of the amniotic sac using an amnioscope.

amniotomy (*am-ne-ot'-o-me*). The surgical rupture of the amniotic sac via the cervical os. *A. forceps.* Forceps used.

Amoeba (*am-e'-bah*). A family of one-celled protozoan micro-

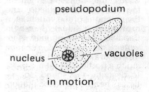

pseudopodium

nucleus — vacuoles

in motion

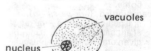

vacuoles

nucleus —

resting stage

AMOEBA

organisms. One type is the cause of dysentery. *See* Entamoeba histolytica.

amoebiasis (*am-e-bi'-as-is*). An ulcerative colitis due to the *Entamoeba histolytica*, with special tendency to formation of liver abscess.

amoeboid (*am-e'-boid*). Referring to structure or movement like that of the amoeba.

amorphous (*a-mor'-fus*). Without definite shape. The term may be applied to fine powdery particles, as opposed to crystals.

ampère (*am'-pair*). The unit of intensity of an electrical current.

amphetamine (*am-fet'-am-een*). A synthetic drug which stimulates the higher nerve centres, so increasing mental alertness and abolishing fatigue. It is a controlled drug and may give rise to addiction, so should be used with care.

amphiarthrosis (*am-fe-ar-thro'-sis*). A form of joint in which the bones are joined together by fibrocartilage, e.g. the junctions of the vertebrae.

amphibian (*am-fib'-e-an*). Capable of living on land or in water.

amphoric (*am-for'-ik*). Pertaining to a bottle. The term is used to describe the sound, sometimes heard on auscultation over cavities in the lungs. It resembles that produced by blowing across the mouth of a bottle.

ampicillin (*am-pe-sil'-in*). An oral penicillin with a wide range of antibacterial action. It may be given orally or by intramuscular injection.

ampoule (*am'-pool*). A small glass vessel in which drugs of specified dose for injection are sealed.

ampulla (*am-pull'-ah*). The dilated end of a canal, e.g. of a uterine tube.

amputation (*am-pu-ta'-shun*). Surgical removal of a limb or part of the body, e.g. the breast.

amputee (*am-pu-tee'*). A person who has had a limb amputated.

amyl (*am'-il*). C_5H_{11}. *A. nitrite.* Prescribed for inhalation in cases of angina pectoris. It is a vasodilator and heart stimulant.

Capsules can be broken into a handkerchief and the fumes inhaled.

amylase (*am'-il-ase*). An enzyme that reduces starch to maltose. Found in saliva (ptyalin) and pancreatic juice (amylopsin).

amylobarbitone (*am-il-o-bar'-be-tone*). A barbiturate hypnotic. Amytal is a proprietary preparation.

amyloid (*am'-il-oid*). Resembling starch. *A. degeneration.* A degenerative change in tissues, with formation of an abnormal, white, waxy substance.

amyloidosis (*am-il-oid-o'-sis*). Degenerative changes in the tissues in which amyloid tissue is formed. It may be a primary condition or secondary to prolonged infection.

amylopsin (*am-il-op'-sin*). Amylase (*q.v.*).

amylum (*am'-il-um*). Starch.

anabolic (*an-ab-ol'-ik*). Referring to a substance that aids in the repair of body tissue, particularly protein. Androgens may be used in this way.

anabolism (*an-ab'-ol-izm*). The building up or synthesis of cell structure from digested food materials. *See* Metabolism.

anacidity (*an-as-id'-it-e*). Decrease in normal acidity.

anacrotic (*an-ak-rot'-ik*). An abnormal curve in the ascending line of a pulse tracing by sphygmograph. Typical of aortic stenosis.

anaemia (*an-e'-me-ah*). Deficiency in either quality or quantity of red corpuscles in the blood, giving rise especially to symptoms of anoxaemia (*q.v.*). There is pallor, breathlessness on exertion with palpitations, slight oedema of ankles, lassitude, headache, giddiness, albuminuria, indigestion, constipation and amenorrhoea. Anaemia may be due to many different causes. *Addison's a.* or *pernicious a.* Due to the inability of the stomach to secrete the intrinsic factor necessary for the absorption of vitamin B_{12} from the diet. *Aplastic a.* The bone marrow is unable to produce red blood corpuscles. A rare condition of unknown cause in most cases, but it may arise from the administration of certain drugs or from their injudicious use, e.g. benzol preparations or chloramphenicol. *Deficiency a.* Any type which is due to the lack of the necessary factors for cell formation, e.g. hormones or vitamins. *Iron deficiency a.* The commonest anaemia in Great Britain, due to a lack of iron in the diet. It may also be due to excessive blood loss. *Haemolytic a.* A variety in which there is excessive destruction of red blood corpuscles caused by antibody formation in the blood (*see* Rhesus factor) by drugs or by severe toxaemia, as in extensive burns. *Macrocytic a.* A type in which the cells are larger than normal; present in pernicious anaemia (*q.v.*). *Microcytic a.* A variety in which the cells are smaller than normal, as in iron deficiency. *Splenic a.* A congenital, familial disease in which the red blood corpuscles are fragile and easily broken down.

anaerobe (*an'-er-obe*). Microorganisms which derive their oxygen from the media in which they grow and not from the air, e.g. the bacilli of tetanus and gas gangrene.

anaesthesia (*an-es-the'-ze-ah*). (1) Insensibility to touch or pain. Loss of sensation in a part or in the whole of the body, induced by drugs. (2) *Basal a.* Loss of consciousness, but supplemental drugs have to be given to ensure complete anaesthesia. (3) *Hysterical a.* A common symptom in hysteria, in which the insensibility to touch or pain has a local distribution unrelated to the nerve supply. (4) *Inhalation a.* The drugs or gas used are administered by a face mask or endotracheal tube to cause general anaesthesia. (5) *Intravenous a.* Unconsciousness is produced by the introduction of a drug, e.g. hexobarbitone, into a vein. (6) *Rectal a.* A barbiturate or paraldehyde given per rectum. (7) *Regional, block* or *local a.* Anaesthesia either by infiltration of the operation field with injections of procaine (*field block*); or by injecting it near main nerve trunks (*nerve block*). (8) *Spinal a.* Injection of procaine or Nupercaine into the spinal canal to anaesthetize the lower half of the body. (9) *Splanchnic a.* A cocaine preparation injected into the splanchnic ganglion which causes complete relaxation of abdominal viscera. A preliminary local skin anaesthesia is needed to make the incision.

anaesthetic (*an-es-thet'-ik*). A drug causing anaesthesia, either local or general.

anaesthetist (*an-ees'-thet-ist*). One who administers an anaesthetic.

anal (*a'-nal*). Pertaining to the anus. *A. eroticism.* Sexual pleasure derived from anal functions. *A. fissure.* Fissure in ano. *See* Fissure. *A. fistula.* Fistula in ano. *See* Fistula.

analeptic (*an-al-ep'-tik*). A drug that stimulates the central nervous system and is an antagonist to drugs causing depression.

analgesia (*an-al-je'-ze-ah*). Insensibility to pain.

analgesic (*an-al-je'-sik*). A remedy which relieves pain.

analogous (*an-al'-o-gus*). Having the same function but different in structure and origin.

analogue (*an'-al-og*). (1) An organ with different structure and origin but the same function. (2) A compound with similar structure but differs in respect of a particular element.

anamnestic reaction (*an-am-nes'-tik re-ak'-shun*). When antibodies from one type of an organism previously encountered are stimulated during the response to another type.

anaphylaxis (*an-ah-fil-ak'-sis*). Often termed anaphylactic shock. It is the name given to a severe reaction, often fatal, occurring when a second injection of a particular foreign protein is given, e.g. horse serum. The symptoms are severe dyspnoea, rapid pulse, profuse sweating and collapse. The condition may be avoided by giving a test dose before all serum injections. If the patient has any reaction he may be desensitized by giving repeated small doses.

anaplasia (*an-ah-pla'-se-ah*). Without form or a reversion of cells to a more primitive form.

anasarca (*an-ah-sar'-kah*). Fluid in the cellular tissues. Generalized oedema. *See* Ascites.

anastomosis (*an-as-to-mo'-sis*). In *surgery*, any artificial connection of two hollow structures, e.g. gastroenterostomy (*q.v.*). *Portacaval a.* The operation of choice in portal hypertension. The portal vein is joined to the inferior vena cava. In *anatomy*, the joining of the branches of two blood vessels.

anatomy (*an-at'-o-me*). The science of the structure of the body.

anconeus (*an-ko'-ne-us*). An extensor muscle of the forearm.

Ancylostoma duodenale (*an-si-lo-sto'-mah du-o-den-ah'-le*). A hookworm which may inhabit the duodenum and cause extreme anaemia.

androgens (*an'-dro-jens*). Hormones secreted by the testes and adrenal cortex. They are steroids which can be synthesized and produce the secondary male characteristics and the building up of protein tissue.

anencephalous (*an-en-kef'-al-us*). Having no brain. A form of congenital monstrosity.

anergic (*an-er'-jik*). Sluggish, inactive.

aneurine hydrochloride (*an'-u-reen hi-dro-klor'-ide*). Vitamin B_2; thiamine. *See* Appendix 10.

aneurysm (*an'-u-rizm*). A local dilatation of an artery. It may start as a congenital weakness, be due to chronic inflammation or be caused by trauma. The pressure of blood causes it to increase in size and rupture is likely. Sometimes excision of the aneurysm or ligation of the artery is possible. *Dissecting a.* A condition in which a tear occurs in the aortic lining where the middle coat is necrosed and blood gets between the layers stripping them apart. Death usually occurs from rupture of the vessel.

angiectasis (*an-je-ek'-tas-is*). Abnormal enlargement of capillaries.

angiitis (*an-je-i'-tis*). Inflammation of a blood or lymph vessel.

angina (*an-ji'-nah*). (1) A tight strangling sensation or pain. *A. of effort* or *a. pectoris.* Cardiac pain which occurs on exertion,

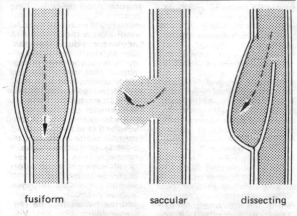

| fusiform | saccular | dissecting |

TYPES OF ANEURYSM

owing to insufficient blood supply to the heart muscle. It can be relieved by a vasodilator drug, glyceryl trinitrate. (2) An inflammation of the throat causing pain on swallowing. *Ludwig's a.* Acute pharyngitis with swelling and abscess formation. *Vincent's a.* Infection and ulceration of the gums, fauces and tonsils by a spirochaete, *Borrelia vincenti*, and a rod-like bacillus, *Fusiformis*.

angiocardiography (*an-je-o-kar-de-og'-raf-e*). The radiological examination of the heart and large blood vessels by means of cardiac catheterization and a radio-opaque dye.

angiogram (*an'-je-o-gram*). A radiological picture of blood vessels.

angioma (*an-je-o'-mah*). An innocent tumour composed of dilated blood vessels. *See* Lymphangioma.

angioneurotic oedema (*an-je-o-nu-rot'-ik e-de'-mah*). An allergic reaction causing increased permeability of the capillary walls, with often sudden marked oedema. There is danger of asphyxia if the larynx is involved. It may be treated by adrenaline, antihistamine drugs or corticosteroids.

angioplasty (*an'-je-o-plas-te*). Plastic surgery of a blood vessel.

angiosarcoma (*an-je-o-sar-ko'-mah*). A malignant vascular growth.

angiospasm (*an'-je-o-spazm*). A spasmodic contraction of an artery. This may be caused by a clot within the vessel, by trauma or by impairment to the nerve supply.

angiotensin (*an-je-o-ten'-sin*). A substance that raises the blood pressure. It is a polypeptide produced by the action of renin on plasma globulins.

Ångström unit (*A. J. Ångström, Swedish physicist, 1814–74*). A measure of wavelength. One unit is one ten-thousand millionth of a metre.

anhidrosis (*an-hi-dro'-sis*). Marked deficiency in the secretion of sweat.

anhidrotic (*an-hi-drot'-ik*). An agent that diminishes the secretion of sweat. An adiaphoretic.

anhydraemia (*an-hi-dre'-me-ah*). Deficiency of fluid in the blood.

anhydrous (*an-hi'-drus*). Containing no water.

aniline (*an'-il-een*). A chemical compound derived from coal tar, used for the making of dyes, e.g. methylene blue. It is a strong antiseptic.

anion (*an'-i-on*). An electro-negative ion which travels against (or up) the current towards the anode. *See* Cation.

aniridia (*an-i-rid'-e-ah*). Lack or defect of the iris.

anisocoria (*an-i-so-ko'-re-ah*). Inequality of diameter of the pupils.

anisocytosis (*an-i-so-si-to'-sis*). Inequality in the size of cells, especially applied to red blood cells.

anisomelia (*an-i-so-me'-le-ah*). A congenital condition in which one pair of limbs is longer than the other.

ankle (*an'-kl*). The joint between the leg and the foot formed by the tibia and fibula articulating with the talus (*astragalus*).

ankyloblepharon (*an-ki-lo-blef'-ar-on*). Adhesions and scar tissue on the ciliary borders of the eyelids, giving the eye a distorted appearance. This may result from burns or from chronic blepharitis (*q.v.*).

ankylosis (*an-ki-lo'-sis*). Abnormal consolidation and immobility of the bones of a joint.

annular (*an'-nu-lah*). Ring-shaped. *A. ligament.* That surrounding the wrist or ankle.

anoci-association (*an-o'-se as-so-se-a'-shun*). The exclusion of pain, fear and shock in surgical operations, brought about by means of local anaesthesia and basal narcosis (*q.v.*).

anode (*an'-ode*). The positive pole of an electric battery or accumulator.

anodyne (*an'-o-dine*). A drug which relieves pain.

anomaly (*a-nom'-al-e*). Considerable variation from the normal.

anomie (*an'-om-e*). A sociological term denoting a person who no longer identifies himself with other people. He is lonely and cannot project his own personality.

anonychia (*an-o-nik'-e-ah*). Having no nails.

Anopheles (*an-off'-el-eez*). A genus of mosquito. Many are carriers of the malarial parasite and by their bite infect human beings. Other species transmit filariasis (*q.v.*).

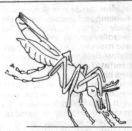

ANOPHELES

anorchism (*an-or'-kizm*). Absence of testicles.

anorexia (*an-or-rek'-se-ah*).

Loss of appetite. *A. nervosa*. A symptom occurring in hysteria, in which there is complete lack of appetite with extreme emaciation.

anosmia (*an-oz'-me-ah*). Loss of the sense of smell.

anovular (*an-ov'-u-lah*). Applied to the absence of ovulation, usually refers to uterine bleeding or the menstrual cycle when drugs have been taken to inhibit ovulation.

anoxaemia (*an-oks-e'-me-ah*). Lack of oxygen in the blood.

anoxia (*an-oks'-e-ah*). Lack of oxygen to an organ or tissue. *Cerebral a.* Insufficient oxygen to the brain. *See* Hypoxia.

antacid (*ant-as'-id*). A substance neutralizing acid.

antagonism (*an-tag'-on-izm*). Applied to drugs, the impairment of efficacy of one or of each drug in the presence of the other.

antagonist (*an-tag'-on-ist*). One that has an opposite action to another, e.g. the biceps muscle to the triceps or one drug neutralizing another.

ante-. Prefix meaning 'before'.

anteflexion (*an-te-flek'-shun*). A bending forward, as of the body of the uterus. *See* Retroflexion.

ante mortem (*an-te mort'-em*). Before death.

antenatal (*an-te-na'-tal*). Before birth.

antepartum (*an-te-par'-tum*). An event that occurs before birth. *A. haemorrhage*. Bleeding occurring before birth. *See* Placenta praevia.

anterior poliomyelitis (*anteer'-e-or po-le-o-mi-el-i'-tis*). *See* Poliomyelitis.

anteversion (*an-te-ver'-shun*). The state of tilting forward, e.g. the normal position of the uterus. *See* Retroversion.

anthelmintic (*an-thel-min'-tik*). Destructive to worms. A vermifuge.

anthracene purgatives (*an'-thrah-seen purg'-at-ivs*). Vegetable drugs which stimulate peristalsis and increase secretion, e.g. senna, rhubarb, cascara, etc.

anthracosis (*an-thrah-ko'-sis*). A disease of the lungs, caused by inhalation of coal dust. 'Miner's lung'.

anthrax (*an'-thraks*). A contagious disease of cattle, transmitted to man by direct contact or by wool or hide infected with the *Bacillus anthracis*, causing malignant pustules of the skin or wool-sorter's pneumonia if inhaled. It is treated by penicillin.

anthropoid (*an'-thro-poid*). (1) Resembling a man, e.g. a species of ape. (2) Applied to a pelvis that is narrowed from side to side. A form of contracted pelvis.

anti-. Prefix which means 'against'.

antibiotic (*an-te-bi-ot'-ic*). A drug derived from living matter, which prevents the growth of, or destroys bacteria, e.g. penicillin.

antibodies (*an'-te-bod-ees*). Specific protein substances or globulins formed in the body which counteract the effects of bacterial antigens or toxins.

anticholinergic (*an-te-ko-liner'-jik*). Drugs that inhibit the action of acetylcholine, the chemical transmitter by which the vagus nerve stimulates the stomach and intestines.

anticholinesterase (*an-te-kolin-est'-er-aze*). A substance that will inhibit cholinesterase and thereby block the nerve impulse transmitted by the latter.

anticoagulant (*an-te-ko-ag'-u-lant*). A substance which prevents blood from clotting, e.g. sodium citrate or heparin.

anticonvulsants (*an-te-kon-vuls'-ants*). A group of drugs which arrest or prevent convulsions and are used in epilepsy and other conditions in which convulsions occur. Such drugs include phenobarbitone and phenytoin (Epanutin).

antidepressants (*an-te-de-press'-ants*). Drugs that are used in the treatment of depression. There are three groups: (1) Stimulants such as amphetamine of only limited use; (2) Monoamine oxidase inhibitors (*q.v.*); (3) Imipramine, chemically related to chlorpromazine.

antidiabetic (*an-te-di-ah-bet'-ik*). Drugs that aid in controlling diabetes by lowering the blood sugar. *See* Tolbutamide. *A. hormone*. Insulin secreted by the pancreas.

antidiuretic (*an-te-di-u-ret'-ik*). Against diuresis, i.e. reducing the volume of urine. *A. hormone*. Secreted by the posterior pituitary gland, its function is to regulate the reabsorption of water by the kidney tubules.

antidote (*an'-te-dote*). An agent which counteracts the effect of a poison, e.g. alkalis neutralize acids.

antiemetic (*an-te-e-met'-ik*). Drugs that prevent or overcome nausea and vomiting.

antifibrinolytic (*an-te-fib-rin-o-lit'-ik*). Drugs that neutralize or block the action of the enzyme that causes fibrinolysis. Fibrinolysis may be a cause of haemorrhage.

antigen (*an'-te-jen*). Any substance, bacterial or otherwise, which stimulates the production of an antibody. *Pollen a.* Extract of the pollen of plants used for diagnosis and treatment in hay fever.

antihaemophilic globulin (*an-te-hem-o-fil'-ik glob'-u-lin*). One of the factors (Factor VIII) present in plasma, necessary for blood clotting. There is a deficiency of it in haemophilia (*q.v.*).

antihistamine (*an-te-hist'-am-een*). Any one of a group of drugs, which block the tissue receptors for histamine. They are used to treat allergic conditions, e.g. drug rashes, hay fever, serum sickness, etc. They include promethazine and mepyramine.

antihypertensive (*an-te-hi-per-ten'-siv*). A drug that lowers raised blood pressure.

antilymphocytic serum (*an-te-lim-fo-sit-ik se'-rum*). Serum used to suppress the activity of the lymphocytes and prevent rejection of a recently transplanted organ.

antimalarial (*an-te-mal-air'-e-al*). A drug that suppresses or cures malaria.

antimetabolites (*an-te-met-ab'-ol-ites*). Chemical compounds which prevent the effective utilization of the corresponding metabolite, so that the action is selective and interferes with normal growth or cell mitosis if the process requires that metabolite. They are used in treating malignant disease.

antimitotic (*an-te-mi-tot'-ik*). Preventing mitosis in the cells. *A. drugs*. Those drugs that prevent malignant cell multiplication. Cytotoxic drugs.

antimony (*an'-tim-on-e*). A metallic drug poisonous to protozoa now used mainly in the treatment of tropical parasitic infestation, e.g. schistosomiasis.

antimycotic (*an-te-mi-kot'-ik*). A preparation that is effective in treating fungal infections.

antineoplastic (*an-te-ne-o-plast'-ik*). A term applied to drugs that are effective against the multiplication of malignant cells. *See* Cytotoxic *and* Antimitotic.

antiperistalsis (*an-te-per-e-stal'-sis*). A movement reversing that of peristalsis (*q.v.*). It may cause vomiting.

antipruritic (*an-te-pru-rit'-ik*). An external application or drug that relieves itching.

antipyretic (*an-te-pi-ret'-ik*). An agent which reduces fever.

anti-rhesus serum (*an-te-re'-sus seer'-um*). A substance containing rhesus agglutinins produced in the blood of those who are rhesus-negative if the rhesus-positive antigen obtains access to it, e.g. by blood transfusion. Haemolysis and jaundice are the result. *See* Rhesus factor.

antisepsis (*an-te-sep'-sis*). The use of antiseptic methods.

antiseptic (*an-te-sep'-tik*). A chemical sterilizing substance for preventing infection. An agent which tends to prevent the growth of organisms causing sepsis in wounds.

antiserum (*an-te-seer'-um*). A serum prepared against a specific disease by immunizing an animal so that antibodies are formed. These can then be used to create a passive immunity in man or to treat the infection in man.

antisocial (*an-te-so'-shal*). Against society. *A. behaviour.* A term used in psychiatry to describe the refusal of an individual to accept the normal obligations and restraints imposed by the community upon its members.

antispasmodic (*an-te-spas-mod'-ik*). Preventing spasm: especially by drugs, such as atropine or chloroform. *A. enema. See* Enema.

antistatic (*an-te-stat'-ik*). A term applied to measures taken to prevent the build up of static electricity. *See* Appendix 4.

antitoxin (*an-te-toks'-in*). A substance produced by the body cells as a reaction to invasion by bacteria, which neutralizes their toxins. Serum from immunized animals contains these antitoxins, and is used in the treatment of specific diseases, e.g. diphtheria, tetanus, etc. *See* Immunity.

antivenin (*an-te-ven'-in*). An antitoxic serum to neutralize the poison injected by the bite of a snake or insect.

antrostomy (*an-tros'-to-me*). Opening the maxillary antrum, usually for drainage purposes.

antrum (*an'-trum*). A cavity in a bone. *A. of Highmore* or *maxillary a.* is the air-containing hollow in the upper jawbone (maxilla). *Mastoid a.* That in the mastoid bone.

anuria (*an-u'-re-ah*). Suppression of urine.

anus (*a'-nus*). The extremity of the alimentary canal, through which the faeces are discharged. *Imperforate a.* One which is not patent (*q.v.*). Usually due to congenital defect.

anxiety (*ang-zi'-et-e*). A chronic state of tension which affects both mind and body. *A. neurosis. See* Neurosis.

aorta (*a-ort'-ah*). The large artery rising out of the left ventricle of the heart. *Abdominal a.* That part of the vessel in the abdomen. *Arch of the a.* The curve of the tube over the heart. *Thoracic a.* That part which passes through the chest.

aortic (*a-or'-tik*). Pertaining to

the aorta. *A. incompetence.* This is due to previous inflammation where the aortic valve has become fibrosed and unable to close completely, thus allowing backward flow of blood (*a. regurgitation*) into the left ventricle during diastole. *A. stenosis.* Scar tissue causing narrowing of the aortic valve. *A. valve.* The valve between the left ventricle and the ascending aorta.

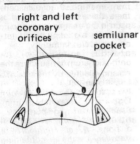

right and left coronary orifices

semilunar pocket

AORTIC VALVE

aortitis (*a-or-ti-tis*). Inflammation of the aorta.

aortography (*a-or-tog'-raf-e*). A radio-opaque dye inserted into the aorta to render visible lesions of the aorta or its main branches. The insertion may be translumbar or by passing a catheter up the femoral or brachial artery.

apathy (*ap'-ath-e*). An appearance of indifference, with no response to stimuli or display of emotion.

apepsia (*a-pep'-se-ah*). Impairment or absence of gastric digestion.

aperient (*ap-peer'-e-ent*). A drug which produces an action of the bowels.

aperistalsis (*a-per-e-stal'-sis*).

Lack of peristaltic movement of the intestines.

Apert's syndrome (*E. Apert, French paediatrician, 1868–1940*). A congenital abnormality in which there is fusion at birth of all the cranial sutures in addition to syndactyly (webbed fingers).

apex (*a'-peks*). The top or pointed end of a cone-shaped structure. *A. of the heart.* The blunt end enclosing the left ventricle. *A. beat.* The beat of the heart against the chest wall which can be felt during systole. *A. of lung.* The extreme upper part of the organ.

Apgar score (*V. Apgar, American anaesthetist, 1909– *). A numerical expression used in the assessment of the newborn; values are given for heart rate, respiratory effort, muscle tone, reflex irritability and colour.

APH. Antepartum haemorrhage (*q.v.*).

aphagia (*a-fa'-je-ah*). Loss of the power to swallow.

aphasia (*a-fa'-ze-ah*). Loss of the power of speech or of understanding the written or spoken word. The cause may be disease or haemorrhage affecting the speech centre in the brain. *Motor a.* Inability to speak. *Sensory a.* Inability to understand the written or spoken word.

aphonia (*a-fo'-ne-ah*). Inability to produce sound. The cause may be organic disease of the larynx or be purely functional.

aphrodisiac (*af-ro-dis'-e-ak*). A drug which excites sexual desire.

aphthae (*af'-the*). Thrush. Small greyish-white vesicles, which form ulcers on the tongue and inside the mouth (*aphthous stomatitis*). It is likely to occur in infants with fever or digestive disorders, but can be prevented by careful regard to mouth hygiene.

apicectomy (*ap-e-sek'-to-me*). Excision of the root of a tooth.

apicolysis (*ap-e-kol'-is-is*). A treatment to ensure collapse of the apex of a tuberculous lung by stripping off the parietal pleura.

aplasia (*a-pla'-ze-ah*). Defective development of tissue.

aplastic (*a-plas'-tik*). Without power of development. *A. anaemia. See* Anaemia.

apnoea (*ap-ne'-ah*). Cessation of respiration due to temporary reduction of the CO_2 content in the blood. *See* Cheyne–Stokes respiration.

apocrine (*ap'-o-krine*). Sweat glands that develop in hair follicles, mainly found in the axilla and pubic and perineal areas.

apomorphine (*ap-o-mor'-feen*). A derivative of morphine which produces vomiting.

aponeurosis (*ap-o-nu-ro'-sis*). A tendinous expansion on broad muscles to give attachment usually to bone.

apophysis (*ap-off'-is-is*). A bony prominence or excrescence.

apoplexy (*ap'-o-pleks-e*). A sudden fit of insensibility, usually caused by rupture of a cerebral blood vessel. The symptoms are coma, accompanied by stertorous breathing, and a varying degree of paralysis of the opposite side of the body to the lesion. *Embolic a.* The blocking of a blood vessel in the brain; e.g. by a fragment of clot carried by the blood from a diseased heart valve.

apothecaries' weight and fluid measure (*ap-oth'-e-kair-eez*). The English system of weights and measures. Now replaced by the metric system.

apothecary (*ap-oth'-e-kair-e*). One who prepares and sells drugs.

appendectomy (*ap-pen-dek'-to-me*). *See* Appendicectomy.

appendicectomy (*ap-pen-de-sek'-to-me*). Removal of the appendix vermiformis (*q.v.*).

appendices epiploicae (*ap-pen'-de-seez ep-e-ploi'-see*). Small taglike structures of peritoneum containing fat which are scattered over the surface of the large intestine, especially the transverse colon.

appendicitis (*ap-pen-de-si'-tis*). Inflammation of the appendix vermiformis.

appendix vermiformis (*ap-pen'-diks ver-me-for'-mis*). A worm-like tube with a blind end, projecting from the caecum in the right iliac region. It may be from 2·5 to 15 cm long.

apperception (*ap-per-sep'-shun*). Conscious reception and recognition of a sensory stimulus.

applicator (*ap'-lik-a-tor*). An instrument for setting in place such local remedies as radium.

apposition (*ap-po-sish'-un*). Fixing together correctly, e.g. fragments of bone in setting a fracture.

apprehension (*ap-pre-hen'-shun*). A feeling of dread or fear.

apraxia (*a-praks'-e-ah*). The inability to perform correct movements because of a brain lesion and not because of sensory impairment or loss of muscle power in the limbs. It may result from cerebral arteriosclerosis.

APT (alum precipitated toxoid). A special preparation used for diphtheria immunization. *See* Toxoid.

aptitude (*ap'-te-tude*). The natural ability or capacity to acquire mental and physical skills.

apyrexia (*a-pi-reks'-e-ah*). The absence of fever.

aqua (*ak'-wah*). Water. *A. bulliens* (*aq. bull.*) = boiling water. *A. destillata* (*aq. dest.*) = distilled water. *A. fontana* (*aq. font.*) = tap water. *A. fortis* (*aq. fort.*) = nitric acid. *A. marina* (*aq. mar.*) = seawater.

aqueduct (*ak'-we-dukt*). A canal for the passage of fluid. *A. of Sylvius.* The canal connecting the third and fourth ventricles of the brain.

aqueous humour (*a'-kwe-us hu'-mor*). The fluid filling the anterior and posterior chambers of the eye.

arachis oil (*ar'-ak-is*). Peanut oil; used as a substitute for olive oil.

arachnodactyly (*ar-ak-no-dakt'-il-e*). Spider fingers. A congenital condition.

arachnoid (*ar-ak'-noid*). A web-like membrane covering the central nervous system between the dura and pia mater.

arborization (*ar-bor-i-za'-shun*). The branching terminations of many nerve fibres and processes.

arboviruses (*ar-bo-vi'-rus-ez*). Viruses transmitted by insect vectors (arthropod-borne), e.g. mosquitoes, sandflies or ticks. The diseases caused include many types of encephalitis, also yellow, dengue, sandfly and Rift Valley fevers.

arcus senilis (*ar'-kus sen-il'-is*). An opaque circle appearing round the edge of the cornea in old age.

areola (*a-re-o'-lah*). A ring of pigmentation, e.g. that surrounding the nipple.

areolar tissue (*a-re-o'-lah tis'-u*). See Tissue.

argentum (*ar-jen'-tum*). Silver.

arginine (*ar'-jin-een*). A basic amino acid which is necessary for urea formation and creatine synthesis.

argon (*ar'-gon*). An inert gaseous element in the atmosphere.

Argyll Robertson pupil (*D. Argyll Robertson, Scottish ophthalmologist, 1837–1909*). See Pupil.

Arnold–Chiari deformity (*J. Arnold, German pathologist, 1835–1915: H. Chiari, German pathologist, 1851–1916*). Herniation of the cerebellum and elongation of the medulla oblongata, associated with spina bifida (*q.v.*).

arrector pili (*ar-rek'-tor pi'-li*). *Pl.* Arrectores pilorum. Small muscle attached to the hair follicle of the skin. When contracted causes the hair follicle to become more erect.

arrhenoblastoma (*ar-ren-o-blast-o'-mah*). A rare ovarian tumour which causes masculinization in the woman, with male distribution of hair and coarsening of the skin.

arrhythmia (*ar-rith'-me-ah*). Lack of rhythm, e.g. in the heart's action. *Sinus a.* An abnormal pulse rhythm due to disturbance of the sino-atrial node (*see* Node), causing quickening of the heart on inspiration and slowing on expiration. It seems to be normal in some children.

arsenic (*ar'-sen-ik*). A soft grey metal, organic preparations of which are used in medicine.

artefact (*ar'-te-fakt*). Something that is man-made or introduced artificially.

arteriectomy (*ar-te-re-ek'-to-me*). The removal of a portion of artery wall usually followed by anastomosis or a replacement graft. See Arterioplasty.

arteriography (*ar-te-re-og'-raf-e*). Radiography of arteries.

arteriole (*ar-te'-re-ole*). A small artery.

arterioplasty (*ar-te-re-o-plas'-te*). The reconstruction of an artery by means of replacement surgery. Now most often achieved by using a portion of vein from the patient or a tube made from plastic.

arteriorrhaphy (*ar-te-re-or'-raf-e*). Ligature of an artery.

arteriosclerosis (*ar-te'-re-o-skler-o'-sis*). A gradual loss of elasticity in the walls of arteries due to thickening and calcification. It is accompanied by high blood pressure, and precedes the degeneration of internal organs associated with old age or chronic disease.

arteriotomy (*ar-te-re-ot'-o-me*). An incision into an artery. This may be done for removal of an embolus.

arteritis (*ar-ter-i'-tis*). Inflammation of an artery. *Giant-cell a.* A variety of polyarteritis resulting in partial or complete occlusion of a number of arteries. The carotid arteries are often involved. Corticosteroids may result in complete resolution.

artery (*ar'-ter-e*). A tube of muscle and elastic fibres lined with endothelium which distributes blood from the heart to the capillaries.

arthralgia (*ar-thral'-je-ah*). Neuralgic pains in a joint.

arthrectomy (*ar-threk'-to-me*). Excision of a joint.

arthritis (*ar-thri'-tis*). Inflammation of a joint. *Osteo-a.* A degenerative condition attacking the articular cartilage and aggravated by an impaired blood supply, previous injury or overweight. *Pyogenic a.* An infection of a joint by pyogenic organisms. These may be gonococci, staphylococci, or streptococci. *Rheumatoid a.* A

chronic inflammation, usually of unknown origin. The disease is progressive and incapacitating, owing to the resulting ankylosis.

arthro- (*ar'-thro-*). A prefix meaning relating to a joint.

arthroclasia (*ar-thro-kla'-ze-ah*). The breaking down of adhesions in a joint to produce freer movement.

arthrodesis (*ar-thro-de'-sis*). The fixation of a movable joint by surgical operation. *Compression a.* Two bone ends held together by clamps. *See* Charnley.

arthrodynia (*ar-thro-din'-e-ah*). Painful joints. *See* Arthralgia.

arthrogram (*ar'-thro-gram*). An X-ray film taken after a joint has been injected with a radio-opaque substance to outline the bone and cartilage.

arthrography (*ar-throg'-raf-e*). The examination of a joint by means of X-rays. A contrast or opaque medium may be used.

arthrogryposis (*ar-thro-gri-po'-sis*). A congenital abnormality in which fibrous ankylosis of some or all of the joints in the limbs occurs.

arthroplasty (*ar'-thro-plas-te*). Plastic surgery for the reorganization of a joint, frequently the hip joint. *Cup a.* The articular surface reconstructed and covered by a vitallium cup. *Replacement a.* The head of the femur partially removed and replaced by a metal prosthesis. *Excision a.* The affected joint surfaces excised. The gap then fills with fibrous tissue or muscle. *Girdlestone a.* An excision arthroplasty of the hip. *McKee Farrar a.* Replacement of both the head of the femur and the socket, the latter being cemented into the prepared acetabulum.

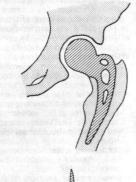

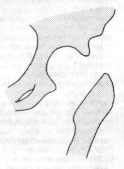

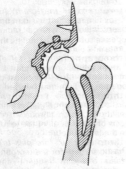

McKEE FARRAR ARTHROPLASTY
The stainless steel ball and cup are embedded in plastic cement. A screw is driven into the bone, through the cement, above the joint

---

arthrotomy (*ar-throt'-o-me*). An incision into a joint.

Arthus phenomenon (*N. M. Arthus, French physiologist, 1862–1945*). Damage to tissue which occurs after repeated exposure to antigens.

articulation (*ar-tik-u-la'-shun*). (1) A junction point of two or more bones. (2) The enunciation of words.

articulo mortis (*ar-tik'-u-lo mor'-tis*). In the act of dying.

artificial feeding. The giving of food by orifices other than the mouth. (1) *Nasal route*, by introducing nutritive fluids into the stomach, through a fine tube via the nostril. (2) *Via the mouth*, by means of an oesophageal or Ryle's tube. (3) *Rectal route*, by catheter and funnel. Only suitable for substances ready for absorption, e.g. water, salt, and glucose. (4) *Gastrostomy*, by direct introduction of nutritive fluids into the stomach through an abdominal opening, in cases of oesophageal obstruction.

artificial insemination (*ar-tif-ish'-al in-sem-in-a'-shun*). The insertion of sperm into the uterus by means of syringe and cannula instead of by coitus. Husband's or donor semen may be used.

artificial lung (*ar-tif-ish'-al lung*). Iron lung. A mechanical device to aid respiration. *See* Respirator.

artificial pneumothorax (*ar-tif-ish'-al nu-mo-thor'-aks*). *See* Pneumothorax.

artificial respiration (*ar-tif-ish'-al res-pir-a'-shun*). A means of resuscitation from asphyxia. *See* Appendix 2.

arytenoid (*ar-e-tee'-noid*). Resembling the mouth of a pitcher. *A. cartilages*. Two cartilages of the larynx, whose function is to regulate the tension of the vocal cords attached to them.

asbestos (*as-bes'-tos*). A fibrous non-combustible silicate of magnesium and calcium.

asbestosis (*as-bes-to'-sis*). A form of pneumoconiosis (*q.v.*) caused by the inhalation of asbestos dust.

ascariasis (*as-kar-i'-as-is*). The condition in which round- or thread-worms are found in the alimentary tract.

Ascaris (*as'-kar-is*). A genus of roundworm. Some types may infest the human intestine. *See* Lumbricus *and* Oxyuris.

Aschheim–Zondek test (*S. Aschheim, German gynaecologist, 1878– : B. Zondek, German gynaecologist, 1891–). To determine pregnancy after one period has been missed. Similar to Friedman's test (*q.v.*) but using mice instead of rabbits

and 100 hours are necessary for its completion.

Aschoff's nodules or **bodies** (*K. A. L. Aschoff, German pathologist, 1866–1942*). The nodules present in heart muscle in rheumatic myocarditis.

ascites (*as-si'-teez*). Free fluid in the peritoneal cavity. It may be the result of local inflammation, of venous obstruction, or part of a generalized oedema.

ascorbic acid (*as-kor'-bik*). Vitamin C. This acid promotes healing and should therefore be given pre- and postoperatively especially when nutrition is below normal, e.g. in gastric disease. *See* Appendix 10.

asemia (*a-se'-me-ah*). Inability to understand or to use speech or signs. A symptom of cerebral lesion.

asepsis (*a-sep'-sis*). Freedom from pathogenic microorganisms.

aseptic technique (*a-sep'-tik tek-neek'*). A method of carrying out sterile procedures so that there is the minimum risk of introducing infection. Achieved by the sterility of equipment and a non-touch method. *See* Appendix 5.

asexual (*a-seks'-u-al*). Without sex. *A. reproduction*. The production of new individuals without sexual union, e.g. by cell division or budding.

aspergillosis (*as-per-jil-o'-sis*). A bronchopulmonary disease in which the mucous membrane is attacked by the fungus, *Aspergillus*. Most likely to occur in patients with leukaemia or those being treated with corticosteroids or cytotoxic drugs.

Aspergillus (*as-per-jil'-us*). A genus of moulds. *A. fumigatus* may infect the nose, antrum, etc.

asphyxia (*as-fiks'-e-ah*). Suffocation. Treatment is by artificial respiration. *See* Appendix 2.

aspiration (*as-pi-ra'-shun*). The drawing off of fluid from a cavity by means of suction.

aspirator (*as'-pi-ra-tor*). Any apparatus for withdrawing air or fluid from a cavity of the body.

aspirin (*as'-pi-rin*). A compound of acetylsalicyclic acid which reduces temperature and relieves pain. *A. in mucilage.* Prescribed for tonsillitis, following tonsillectomy, and for other conditions when the throat is painful. *Soluble a.* Combined with citric acid and calcium carbonate it becomes less of an irritant to the gastric mucosa.

assimilation (*as-sim-il-a'-shun*). The process of transforming food, so that it can be absorbed into the circulatory system and utilized as nourishment for the tissues of the body.

association (*as-so-se-a'-shun*). Co-ordination of function of similar parts. *A. fibres.* Nerve fibres linking different areas of the brain. *A. of ideas.* In which a thought or any sensory impulse will call to mind another object or idea connected in some way with the former. *Free a.* A method employed in psychoanalysis in which the patient is encouraged to express freely whatever comes into his mind. By this method material that is in the unconscious can be recalled. *See* Psychoanalysis.

astasia (*as-ta'-ze-ah*). Inability to stand or walk normally, due to incoordination of muscles.

asteatosis (*a-ste-at-o'-sis*). Lack of sebaceous secretion. There is a dry and scaly skin in which fissures may occur.

astereognosis (*a-ster-e-og-no'-sis*). Inability to recognize

the shape of objects by feeling or touch.

asthenia (*as-the'-ne-ah*). Want of strength. Loss of tone.

asthenopia (*as-then-o'-pe-ah*). Eye strain giving rise to an aching, burning sensation, and headache. Likely to arise in long-sighted people when continual effort of accommodation is required for close work in artificial light.

asthenic (*as-then'-ik*). A term used to describe a type of body build. A pale, lean, narrowly built person with poor muscle development.

asthma (*asth'-mah*). Paroxysmal dyspnoea. *Bronchial a.* Attacks of dyspnoea in which there is wheezing and difficulty in expiration due to muscular spasm of the bronchi. The attacks may be precipitated by hypersensitivity to foreign substances or associated with emotional upsets. There is often a family history of asthma or other allergic condition. Attacks may accompany chronic bronchitis. They can be relieved by adrenaline or isoprenaline and between attacks the cause should be sought and removed if possible and breathing exercises instituted. *Cardiac a.* Attacks of dyspnoea and palpitation arising most often at night, associated with left-sided heart failure and pulmonary congestion. *Renal a.* Dyspnoea occurring in kidney disease, which may be a sign of developing uraemia (*q.v.*).

astigmatism (*as-tig'-mat-izm*). Inequality of the refractive power of an eye, due to defective curvature of its corneal meridians. The curve across the front of the eye from side to side is not quite the same as the curve from above downwards.

The focus on the retina is then not a point, but a diffuse and indistinct area.

astragalus (*as-trag'-al-us*). The talus or ankle-bone which articulates with the tibia.

astringent (*as-trin'-jent*). An agent causing contraction of organic tissues, so checking secretions, e.g. silver nitrate, tannic acid.

astrocytoma (*as-tro-si-to'-mah*). A slow growing infiltrating cerebral or cerebellar tumour, relatively benign. A glioma.

asymmetry (*a-sim'-et-re*). Inequality in size or shape of two structures normally the same.

asymptomatic (*a-simp-to-mat'-ik*). Without symptoms.

atavism (*at'-av-izm*). The reappearance of some hereditary peculiarity which has missed a few generations.

ataxia, ataxy (*a-taks'-e-ah, a-taks'-e*). Failure of muscle coordination. *Locomotor a.* or *tabes dorsalis*. A degenerative disease of the spinal cord; a manifestation of tertiary syphilis allied to general paralysis of the insane (*q.v.*). Among signs and symptoms are: incoordinated movements of the legs in walking, absence of reflexes, and loss of sphincter control. The disease is chronic and progressive, but can be controlled by antisyphilitic treatment.

atelectasis (*at-el-ek'-tas-is*). Partial collapse of the air vesicles of the lungs: (1) From imperfect expansion at birth. (2) As the result of disease when small air passages are constricted and air cannot reach the alveoli. *See* Emphysema.

atherogenic (*ath-er-o-jen'-ik*). Predisposing to the formation of atheroma. Animal fat and mental stress have been named as possible causative factors.

atheroma (*ath-er-o'-mah*). (1) A sebaceous cyst. (2) Patchy degeneration of the walls of large arteries in which fat-like plaques appear.

atherosclerosis (*ath-er-o-skler-o'-sis*). A condition in which the fatty degenerative plaques of atheroma are accompanied by arteriosclerosis, a narrowing and hardening of the vessels.

athetoid cerebral palsy (*ath'-e-toid ser'-e-bral pawl'-ze*). *See* Cerebral palsy.

athetosis (*ath-et-o'-sis*). A recurring series of abnormal movements of the hands and feet usually due to a cerebral lesion, and most often seen in children.

athlete's foot (*ath'-leetz fut*). A fungal infection between the toes which is easily transmitted to others. *See* Tinea.

atlas (*at'-las*). The first cervical vertebra, articulating with the occipital bone of the skull.

atmosphere (*at'-mos-feer*). *See* Air.

atmospheric pressure (*at-mos-fer'-ik presh'-er*). The term given to the pressure exerted by the air in all directions. At sea level it is about 101 kN/m^2 (15 lbf/in^2), depending on the humidity. Dry air exerts more pressure than moist air.

atom (*at'-om*). A minute particle of matter made up of a central nucleus positively charged and, moving around it in an orbit, negatively charged electrons.

atomizer (*at'-om-i-zer*). An instrument by which a liquid is very finely divided to form a spray.

atony (*at'-o-ne*). Lack of tone.

atopen (*at'-o-pen*). An antigen responsible for causing atopy.

atopic (*a-top'-ik*). Out of place or misplaced.

atopy (*at'-o-pe*). A state of hypersensitivity to certain antigens. There is an inherited tendency and it includes asthma, eczema and hay-fever.

atresia (*a-tre'-ze-ah*). Absence of a natural opening, e.g. of the anus or vagina, usually a congenital malformation.

atrial (*a'-tre-al*). Relating to the atrium or auricle. *A. fibrillation.* Over-stimulation of the atrial walls so that many areas of excitation arise and the atrioventricular node is bombarded with impulses, many of which it cannot transmit. *A. flutter.* Rapid regular action of atria, the atrioventricular node transmits alternate impulses or one in three or four. *A. septal defect.* The non-closure of the foramen ovale at the time of birth giving rise to a congenital heart defect.

atrioventricular (*a'-tre-o-ventrik'-u-lah*). Pertaining to the atrium and ventricle. *A. bundle.* See Bundle of His. *A. node.* A node of neurogenic tissue situated between the two and transmitting impulses. *A. shunts.* (1) Vascular connections between arteries and veins. When the body temperature rises these shunts open and blood flow to that part of the body increases greatly, e.g. the reddening of the skin after a hot bath. (2) Artificial communications between arteries and veins which are created surgically before starting haemodialysis. *A. valves.* The bicuspid and tricuspid valve on the left and right sides of the heart respectively.

atrium (*a'-tre-um*). One of the two upper chambers of the heart. *Pl.* atria. Also called auricle.

atrophy (*at'-ro-fe*). Wasting of any part of the body, due to degeneration of the cells from disuse, lack of nourishment, or of nerve supply. *Acute yellow a.* Massive necrosis of liver cells. A rare condition that may follow acute hepatitis or eclampsia or be precipitated by certain drugs, e.g. cinchophen, mepacrine, or phosphorus. *Muscular a.* Wasting of muscle tissue. Myopathy (*q.v.*).

atropine (*at'-ro-pin*). The active principle of belladonna. An alkaloid which inhibits respiratory and gastric secretions, relaxes muscle spasm and dilates the pupil. Used preoperatively, and to relieve renal and biliary colic and as drops to aid examination of the eye.

attenuation (*at-ten-u-a'-shun*). A bacteriological process by which organisms are rendered less virulent by culture in artificial media through many generations, exposure to light, air, etc. Used for vaccine preparations.

atypical (*a-tip'-ik-al*). Not conforming to type, e.g. *a. pneumonia.*

audiogram (*aw'-de-o-gram*). A tracing of the intensity of hearing which is helpful in deciding the type of deafness present.

audiometer (*aw-de-om'-e-ter*). An instrument for measuring hearing.

auditory (*aw'-de-tor-e*). Pertaining to the sense of hearing.

Auerbach's plexus (*L. Auerbach, German anatomist, 1828–97*). The ganglionic neurones of the vagus nerve that supply the muscle fibres of the intestine.

aura (*aw'-rah*). The premonition peculiar to individuals which often precedes an epileptic fit.

aural (*aw'-ral*). Referring to the ear.

auricle (*aw'-rik-l*). (1) Appendage to the cardiac atrium. (2) The external portion of the ear.

auricular (*aw-rik'-u-lar*). Relating to the auricle or atrium. *A. fibrillation. See* Atrial fibrillation. *A. flutter. See* Atrial flutter.

auriculoventricular bundle (*aw-rik'-u-lo ven-trik'-u-lar bun'-dl*). Atrioventricular bundle. *See* Bundle of His.

auriscope (*aw'-ris-kope*). An instrument for examining the drum of the ear.

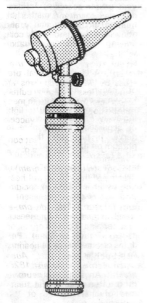

AURISCOPE

auscultation (*aws-kul-ta'-shun*). A method of examining the internal organs by listening to the sounds which they give out. *Immediate a.* The ear is placed directly against the body. *Mediate a.* A stethoscope is used.

Australia antigen (*an'-te-jen*). Antigen found in the blood of patients with serum hepatitis (*q.v.*). Originally discovered in Australian aborigines.

autism (*aw'-tizm*). Self-absorption.

autistic (*aw-tis'-tik*). A term used to describe a withdrawn personality; the patient is apathetic and appears absorbed in his own thoughts or daydreams, showing little awareness of his surroundings. A condition occurring in schizophrenia.

autoclave (*aw'-to-klave*). A steam-heated sterilizing apparatus in which the temperature is raised by reducing the atmospheric pressure and then injecting steam under pressure, so bringing about efficient sterilization. The aim of newer patterns is to raise the pressure and shorten the time, so that the capacity of the machines is increased and they can be used to replace water boilers for many articles.

auto-eroticism (*aw-to-e-rot'-is-izm*). Sexual pleasure derived from self-stimulation of erogenous zones, the mouth, the anus, the genitals and the skin.

autogenous (*aw-toj'-en-us*). Generated within the body and not acquired from external sources. *A. vaccine.* Vaccine made from the patient's serum.

autograft (*aw'-to-graft*). The transfer of skin or other tissue from one part of the body to another to repair some deficiency.

autoimmune disease (*aw-to-im-mune'*). Condition in which the body develops antibodies to its own tissues. Usually one organ is involved. Degeneration and malfunction occur as a result.

autoimmunization (*aw-to-im-mu-ni-za'-shun*). The formation of antibodies against the individual's own tissue proteins.

autoinfection (*aw-to-in-fek'-shun*). Self-infection, i.e. transferred from one part of the body to another by fingers, towels, etc.

autointoxication (*aw-to-in-toks-ik-a'-shun*). Poisoning by toxins generated within the body itself.

autolysis (*aw-tol'-is-is*). A breaking up or digestion of living tissues as may occur, e.g. if pancreatic ferments escape into surrounding tissues.

automatic (*aw-to-mat'-ik*). Performed without the influence of the will.

automatism (*aw-tom'-at-izm*). Performance of acts without apparent volition, and of which there is no memory afterwards. *Post-epileptic a.* Automatic acts following an epileptic fit of which the patient has no knowledge.

autonomic (*aw-to-nom'-ik*). Self-governing. *A. nervous system.* This consists of the sympathetic and parasympathetic nerves which control involuntary muscles and glandular secretion over which there is no conscious control.

autoplasty (*aw'-to-plas-te*). Replacement of missing tissue by grafting a healthy section from another part of the body.

autopsy (*aw'-top-se*). Post-mortem examination.

autosomal trait (*aw-to-so'-mal tra'*). The presence of a particular gene on a chromosome other than the sex chromosomes.

autosome (*aw'-to-sohm*). Any chromosome other than the sex chromosomes. In man there are 22 pairs of autosomes and 1 pair of sex chromosomes.

autotransfusion (*aw-to-trans-fu'-zhum*). The reinjection of blood taken from one part of the body into another.

avascular (*a-vas'-ku-lah*). Not vascular. Bloodless. *A. necrosis.* Death of bone owing to deficient blood supply, usually following an injury.

aversion (*av-er'-shun*). Intense dislike. *A. therapy.* A method of treating alcoholism and other addictions by associating the craving for what is addictive with painful or unpleasant stimuli.

avitaminosis (*a-vit-a-min-o'-sis*). The result of insufficiency of vitamins in the diet. Also known as *deficiency disease*.

avulsion (*av-vul'-shun*). Tearing away. *Phrenic a.* A crushing or separation of the phrenic nerve. It paralyses the diaphragm on the affected side.

axilla (*aks-il'-ah*). The armpit.

axis (*aks'-is*). The second cervical vertebra.

axis cylinder (*aks'-is sil'-in-der*). See Axon.

axon (*aks'-on*). The nerve fibre which extends from a nerve cell to its termination in an organ, or its arborization with the dendrites of other nerve cells. *Syn.,* Axis cylinder.

azathioprine (*az-ah-thi''-o-preen*). An immunosupressive drug, often used in the treatment of renal failure.

azoospermia (*a-zo-o-sperm'-e-ah*). Absence of spermatozoa in the semen. Tests for this are carried out following vasectomy.

azotaemia (*az-o-te'-me-ah*).

37   BAC

The accumulation of urea in the blood.

azote (*az'ote*). Nitrogen gas.

azoturia (*az-o-tu'-re-ah*). Increase of urea in the urine.

azygos (*az'-e-gos*). An unpaired vein that ascends the posterior mediastinum and enters the superior vena cava.

B

Babinski's reflex *or* **sign** (*J. F. Babinski, French neurologist, 1857–1937*). Present in disease or injury to the upper motor neurone. On stroking the sole of the foot, the great toe bends upwards instead of downwards (*dorsal* instead of *plantar* flexion). Babies who have not walked react in the same way, but normal flexion develops later.

bacillaemia (*bas-il-e'-me-ah*). The presence of bacilli in the blood.

Bacille Calmette–Guérin (*A. L. C. Calmette, French bacteriologist, 1863–1933: C. Guérin, French bacteriologist 1872– *). A vaccine prepared from living tubercle bacilli which through prolonged culture have lost their virulence. It is used to produce active immunity against tuberculosis in children and young adults, particularly those liable to become infected. Also called BCG vaccine.

bacilluria (*bas-il-u'-re-ah*). The presence of bacilli in the urine.

bacillus (*bas-il'-us*). *Pl.* bacilli. A rod-shaped bacterium. Bacilli may be divided into: (1) Those which form spores (*q.v.*) and require oxygen (*aerobic*), e.g. *B. anthracis*, the cause of anthrax. (2) Those that form spores and need the exclusion

of oxygen (*anaerobic*), e.g. *Clostridium botulinum*, the cause of botulism; *Cl. tetani*, the cause of tetanus and *Cl. welchii* (*Cl. perfringens*) a cause of gas gangrene. (3) Non-spore-bearing bacilli, e.g. *Escherichia coli*. A normal inhabitant of the bowel but a common cause of urinary infection. *Klebs-Löffler b.* (*Corynebacterium diphtheriae*). The cause of diphtheria. *Döderlein's b.* A lactic-acid-forming organism normally found in the vagina, which destroys other bacteria. *Flexner, Shiga and Sonne b.* The causative organisms of bacillary dysentery. The salmonellas are a food-poisoning group which includes *Salmonella typhimurium* and *S. enteritidis* (*Gärtner's bacillus*). *Bordet-Gengou b.* (*Haemophilus pertussis*). The cause of whooping cough or pertussis. *Smegma b.* A type found in urine, closely resembling the tubercle bacillus, which makes diagnosis by identification unreliable.

bacitracin (*bas-e-tra'-sin*). An antibiotic drug derived from *Bacillus subtilis*. Used for surface application.

back pressure (*bak presh'-er*). Describes the damming back of the blood through the pulmonary circulation and into the veins as the result of organic heart disease. A cause of many of the symptoms in advanced mitral stenosis.

bacteraemia (*bak-ter-e'-me-ah*). The presence of bacteria in the blood stream.

bacteria (*bak-te'-re-ah*). *Sing.* bacterium. A general name given to minute vegetable organisms which live on organic matter. Each consists of a single cell and, given favourable conditions, multiplies by subdivi-

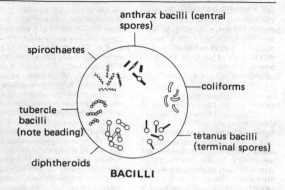

anthrax bacilli (central spores)

spirochaetes

coliforms

tubercle bacilli (note beading)

tetanus bacilli (terminal spores)

diphtheroids

BACILLI

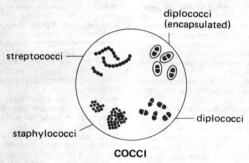

diplococci (encapsulated)

streptococci

diplococci

staphylococci

COCCI

sion. Bacteria are classified according to their shape into: (1) *Bacilli*, rod-shaped. (2) *Cocci*, spherical: (*a*) streptococci—in chains; (*b*) staphylococci—in groups; (*c*) diplococci—in pairs. (3) *Spirilla*, spiral-shaped. *Pathogenic b.* Those whose growth in the body gives rise to disease, either by destruction of tissue, or by formation of toxins which circulate in the blood. They thrive on organic matter in the presence of warmth and moisture.

bactericidal (*bak-te-re-si'-dal*). Capable of killing bacteria, e.g. disinfectants, great heat, intense cold or sunlight.

bactericide (*bak-te'-re-side*). An agent that kills bacteria.

bacteriologist (*bak-te-re-ol'-oj-ist*). One who has studied and is skilled in the science of bacteriology.

bacteriology (*bak-te-re-ol'-o-*

je). The science which studies the behaviour of bacteria.

bacteriolysin (*bak-te-re-ol'-is-in*). An antibody (*q.v.*) produced in blood to assist in the destruction of bacteria. The action is specific.

bacteriolysis (*bak-te-re-ol'-is-is*). The dissolution of bacteria by a bacteriolytic agent.

bacteriolytic (*bak-te-re-o-lit'-ik*). Capable of destroying or dissolving bacteria.

bacteriophage (*bak-te'-re-o-faj*). A virus parasite on bacteria. Many strains exist, some of which are used for typing staphylococci and organisms of the typhoid group.

bacteriostatic (*bak-te-re-o-stat'-ik*). Inhibiting the growth of bacteria.

bacteriotherapy (*bak-te-re-o-ther'-ap-e*). Treatment of disease by the injection of bacteria into the blood, e.g. malaria therapy in the treatment of neurosyphilis.

bacteriuria (*bak-te-re-u'-re-ah*). The presence of bacteria in urine.

Bainbridge reflex (*F. A. Bainbridge, English physiologist, 1874–1921*). The inhibition of vagal impulses caused by an increase in right atrial pressure.

baker's itch *or* **eczema**. *See* Itch.

balanitis (*bal-an-i'-tis*). Balanoposthitis. Inflammation of the glans penis and of the prepuce.

Balkan frame. A framework fitted over a bed to carry pulleys and slings or splints for the support of a limb undergoing surgical treatment. Used chiefly in fracture or osteo-arthritic cases or to aid physiotherapy.

ballotement (*bal-ot-mon'*). A method of testing pregnancy from the fourth month. The uterus is pushed upward by a finger in the vagina, and if a fetus is present it will fall back again like a heavy body in water.

balsam (*bawl'-sam*). An aromatic vegetable juice. *Friar's b.* A compound containing tincture of benzoin. Used for steam inhalations and as an antiseptic for ulcers. *Peru b.* Used externally as an antiseptic ointment or in *tulle gras* (*q.v.*). *B. of Tolu.* Used as an expectorant.

bandage (*band-'aj*). A binder to give support or apply pressure to a part or for fixing a dressing in position.

banding (*band'-ing*). Pulmonary arterial banding. A palliative operation used in treating infants with ventricular septal defects.

Bandl's ring (*L. Bandl, German*

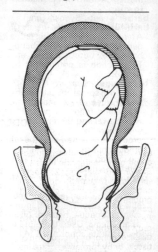

BANDL'S RING

obstetrician, 1842–92). A ridge appearing between the upper retracted segment of the uterus and the lower dilated segment, occurring during an obstructed labour. It suggests that rupture of the uterus is likely.

Bankhart's operation (*A. S. B. Bankhart, English orthopaedic surgeon, 1879–*). An operation carried out to repair the defect in the glenoid cavity when there is repeated dislocation of the shoulder joint.

Banti's disease (*G. Banti, Italian pathologist, 1852–1925*). A clinical syndrome characterized by splenomegaly, cirrhosis of liver, anaemia, leucopenia and gastrointestinal bleeding.

Barbados leg (*bar-ba´-doze*). Swelling and enlargement of the leg. A form of elephantisis (*q.v.*).

barber's rash. Sycosis (*q.v.*).

barbiturates (*bar-bit´-u-rates*). A large group of hypnotic drugs derived from urea, e.g. phenobarbitone, butobarbitone, etc. Their action is potentiated by alcohol.

barbotage (*bar-bo-taj´*). A method of spinal anaesthesia by which some of the anaesthetic is injected followed by partial withdrawal and then reinjected with more of the drug. This process is repeated until the full amount has been given, allowing dilution and mixing with the cerebrospinal fluid.

barium sulphate (*bair´-e-um sul´-fate*). A heavy mineral salt that is comparatively impermeable to X-rays. The chief ingredient of opaque meals or given as an enema. Used therefore to demonstrate abnormality in the stomach or intestines, and to show peristaltic movement. Bismuth is used similarly.

barium sulphide (*bair´-e-um*

sul´-fide). The chief constituent of depilatory preparations, i.e. those which remove hair.

Barlow's disease (*Sir T. Barlow, British physician, 1845–1945*). Infantile scurvy. A deficiency disease due to lack of vitamin C.

baroreceptor nerves (*bar-o-re-sep´-tor*). The sensory branches of the glosso-pharyngeal and vagus nerves that influence the blood pressure. The receptors are situated in the walls of the carotid vessels and aortic arch.

Barr body (*M. L. Barr, Canadian anatomist, 1908–*). Small dark-staining area underneath the nuclear membrane of female cells. Represents an inactive X chromosome. When sex is being determined the necessary cells are frequently obtained from the mucosa of the mouth.

barrier-nursing. A method of bed isolation which enables a patient suffering from an infectious disease to be nursed amongst those not so infected.

Bartholin's glands (*C. T. Bartholin, Danish anatomist, 1655–1738*). Two glands situated in the labia majora, with ducts opening inside the vulva.

basal ganglia (*ba´-sal gang´-le-ah*). The collections of nerve cells or grey matter in the base of the cerebrum. They consist of the caudate nucleus and putamen forming the corpus striatum and the globus pallidus. Parkinson's disease is associated with degenerative changes in these structures.

basal metabolic rate (BMR) (*ba´-sal met-ah-bol´-ik*). An indirect method of estimating the rate of metabolism in the body by measuring the O_2 intake and CO_2 output on breathing. For this to be done, the patient must be quiet in bed and have had no food for 12 hours. The age, weight and size of the patient have to be taken into account.

basal narcosis (*ba'-sal nar-ko'-sis*). See Narcosis.

base (*base*). (1) The lowest part or foundation. (2) An alkali or substance which can unite with an acid to form a salt.

base units. The seven units which have been adopted as the basis for the Système International d'Unités (SI). See Appendix 6.

basement membrane. A thin layer of modified connective tissue supporting layers of cells, found at the base of the epidermis and underlying mucous membranes.

basilar (*bas'-il'-ar*). Situated at the base. *B. artery.* Midline artery at the base of the skull, formed by the junction of the vertebral arteries.

basilic (*bas-il'-ik*). Prominent. *B. vein.* A large vein on the inner side of the arm.

basophile (*ba'-zo-fil*). Leucocytes or white cells of the blood having an affinity for basic dyes.

basophilia (*ba-zo-fil'-e-ah*). Increase of basophiles in the blood.

Batchelor plaster (*J. S. Batchelor, contemporary English surgeon*). A plaster of Paris splint which corrects congenital dislocation of the hip. See Plaster.

Bateman's needle (*T. Bateman, English physician, 1778–1821*). A special type used for intravenous injection in infants. It has two cannulas which fit into each other.

bath. Used for cleansing and to stimulate the circulation. Suggested temperatures for a *cold b.* 18°C (65°F); *tepid b.* 29°C (85°F); *warm b.* 38°C (100°F); *hot b.* 40°C (105°F). Baths containing bran, oatmeal, starch or sodium bicarbonate are soothing for e.g. skin diseases. *Electric b.* One in which a current is passed through the water. Can be used in the treatment of peripheral nerve or vascular conditions of the limbs. *Saline b.* Used in the treatment of burns. *Wax b.* Used to increase the circulation to the small joints of the hands and feet and relax the muscles.

battered baby syndrome. A clinical condition in which an infant or young child is found to have soft tissue injuries, e.g. bruises, and radiological evidence of fractures either new or at different stages of healing. It usually results from serious physical abuse by parents or foster parents, who may admit injuring the child or whose explanation of the injury may be at variance with the medical evidence.

battery (*bat'-ter-e*). An apparatus for generating electricity by chemical means. *Faradic b.* One which produces a faradic or induced current. *Galvanic b.* A battery which produces a continuous electric current from chemicals.

battledore placenta (*bat'-tl-dor plas-en'-tah*). A condition

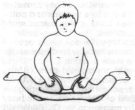

BATCHELOR PLASTER

in which the umbilical cord is attached to the margin of the placenta and not the centre.

BBA. Born before arrival (with nursing or medical help).

BCG. Bacille (Bacillus) Calmette–Guérin (*q.v.*).

'bearing down' (1) The expulsive pains in the second stage of labour. (2) A feeling of heaviness and downward strain in the pelvis present with some uterine growths or displacements.

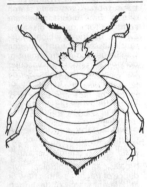

BED-BUG

bed-bug (*bed'-bug*). *Cimex lectularius.* A blood-sucking parasite which lives in cracks of woodwork and furniture and can survive for up to 12 months without food.

bed-sore (*bed'-sore*). Better termed a pressure sore. Decubitus ulcer. A wound caused by constant pressure of the bed on any part of the body and a consequently diminished blood supply. The chief pressure points are the buttocks, shoulders, hips, heels and elbows. The best preventive measures are cleanliness of the part, a good diet with ample fluid and vitamins, and a frequent change of position.

Beer's knife (*G. J. Beer, German ophthalmologist, 1763–1821*). One with a triangular blade used in cataract operations, for incising the cornea preparatory to removal of the lens.

beeswax (*beez'-waks*). Yellow wax secreted by bees, and used in the manufacture of ointments.

behaviour (*be-ha'-vyor*). The way in which an organism reacts to an internal or external stimulus. *Incongruous b.* Behaviour that is out of keeping with the person's normal reaction or has the opposite effect to that consciously desired. *B. disorders* may take many forms, such as truancy, stealing, temper-tantrums, bed wetting, or thumb sucking. For example, they may occur when a child is put under stress in his home or school environment.

behaviourism (*be-ha'-vyor-izm*). A psychological term describing the purely objective study and observation of the behaviour of individuals.

bejel (*be'-jel*). A non-venereal but infectious skin disease caused by a treponema indistinguishable from that causing syphilis.

Belcroy feeder (*bel'-croy*). A bottle for baby feeding whereby a weak sucking action may be assisted by light pressure on a rubber bulb at the opposite end from the teat.

Bell's palsy (*Sir C. Bell, British physiologist, 1774–1842*). Facial paralysis.

belladonna (*bel-ah-don'-ah*).

A drug from the deadly nightshade plant. Used as an antispasmodic in colic, and to check secretions. Atropine is its active principle.

belle indifference (*bel in-dif'-er-ance*). A sign in conversion hysteria. The patient describes his symptoms, appearing not to be distressed by them.

Bellocq's sound or **cannula** (*J. J. Bellocq, French surgeon, 1732–1807*). A curved tube for the arrest of nasal bleeding by passing it, with plugging attached, into the nose.

bellringer's wrist. Tendinitis or tenosynovitis of the wrist which may result from chronic mechanical strain or from trauma.

Bence-Jones's protein (*H. Bence-Jones, British physician, 1813–73*). That present in the urine in cases of bone-marrow diseases—particularly if malignant. It coagulates at a lower temperature than does albumin, and is redissolved on boiling.

bendrofluazide (*ben-dro-flu'-az-ide*). An oral diuretic of the thiazide group. Apinox and Neo-Naclex are proprietary preparations.

bends. A colloquial term for caisson disease in which there is severe abdominal cramp. Decompression sickness.

Benedict's solution (*S. R. Benedict, American biochemist, 1884–1936*). A solution of copper sulphate used as a test for sugar in urine. See Appendix 11.

benethamine penicillin (*beneth'-am-een*). An antibiotic. See Penicillin.

benign (*be-nine'*). The opposite to malignant (*q.v.*). B. tumour. See Tumour. B. tertian fever. Fever due to a malarial parasite, more tractable to treatment than that which causes malignant tertian fever.

benzathine penicillin (*benz'-ath-een*). A long-acting antibiotic. See Penicillin.

benzene (*ben-zeen'*). Benzol. A coal-tar derivative used externally as a parasiticide.

benzhexol (*benz'-hex-ol*). An antispasmodic drug which helps to overcome the tremors and rigidity of Parkinson's disease. Artane and Pipanol are proprietary preparations.

benzoin (*ben'-zo-in*). An aromatic resin. Compound Tincture of B. See Friar's balsam under Balsam.

benzyl benzoate (*ben'-zil ben'-zo-ate*). An emulsion used in the treatment of scabies. A hot bath is taken and then a 25 per cent emulsion is applied carefully over the whole body except the face and scalp and left on for 24 hours. In 99 per cent of cases one application is sufficient and it must never be applied more than twice.

benzylpenicillin (*benz-il-pen-e-sill'-in*). A soluble penicillin, quickly absorbed, by which high blood levels can be obtained. See Penicillin

beri beri (*ber'-e ber'-e*). A deficiency disease due to insufficiency of vitamin B_1 in the diet. It is a form of neuritis, with pain, paralysis and oedema of the extremities.

berylliosis (*ber-il-e-o'-sis*). An industrial lung disease in which the inhalant is beryllium. Interstitial fibrosis arises impairing lung function. Steroids may improve the condition.

Besnier's prurigo (*E. Besnier, French dermatologist, 1831–1909*). An inherited neurodermatitis with impaired peripheral circulation and dry, thickened epidermis with outbreaks of eczema. The atopic syndrome.

beta (*be'-tah*). The second letter in the Greek alphabet—β.

beta blockers (*be'-tah*). Drugs used to block the action of adrenaline on receptors in cardiac muscle.

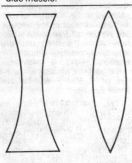

BICONCAVE   BICONVEX

beta cells. Insulin-producing cells found in the islets of Langerhans in the pancreas.

beta receptors. Receptors associated with the inhibition (relaxation) of smooth muscle. They also bring an increase in the force of contraction and rate of the heart.

betamethasone (*be-tah-meth'-az-one*). A derivative of prednisolone but seven times more active. It may be used in eye drops, creams, ointments or as tablets. It is the chief ingredient in Betnovate.

Betz cells (*V. A. Betz, Russian anatomist, 1834–94*). The pyramidal cells in the pre-Rolandic area of the cerebrum.

bi-. A prefix meaning 'two'.

bicarbonate (*bi-kar'-bon-ate*). A compound containing two equivalents of carbonic acid with one of an alkali or base.

biceps (*bi'-seps*). Having two heads. *B. muscles.* (*a*) A flexor of the arm. (*b*) One of the hamstring muscles of the thigh.

biconcave (*bi-kon'-kave*). A lens or structure with a hollow or depression on each surface.

biconvex (*bi-kon'-veks*). A lens or structure that protrudes on both surfaces.

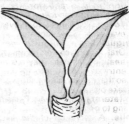

BICORNUATE UTERUS

bicornuate (*bi-korn'-u-ate*). Having two horns. *B. uterus.* A congenital malformation in which there is a partial or complete vertical division of the body of the uterus.

bicuspid (*bi-kus'-pid*). Having two cusps. *B. teeth.* The premolars. *B. valve.* The mitral valve of the heart, between the left atrium and ventricle.

bidet (*be'-da*). A low broad basin for washing the perineum and genitalia. It can also be used for vaginal and rectal injections.

bifid (*bi'-fid*). Divided or cleft into two parts.

bifocal spectacles (*bi-fo'-kal*). Those in which the lens has two different foci, the lower for close work and the upper for distant vision.

bifurcate (*bi'-fur-kate*). To divide into two; arteries bifurcate frequently, thereby getting smaller.

bifurcation (bi-fur-ka'-shun). The junction where a vessel divides into two halves, e.g. where the aorta divides into the right and left iliac vessels.

bigeminus (bi-jem'-in-us). Double. *Pulsus b.* Two pulse beats which occur together, regular in time and force—the third beat being missed. A regular irregularity.

Bigelow's evacuator (*H. J. Bigelow, American surgeon, 1818–90*). Similar to Freyer's evacuator. See Evacuator.

biguanides (bi-gwan'-ides). Oral hypoglycaemic drugs for treating diabetes. They aid the entry of glucose into the cells so that metabolism of sugar can take place.

bilateral (bi-lat'-er-al). Pertaining to both sides.

bile. A secretion of the liver, golden-brown in colour, which has a bitter taste and is slightly antiseptic. It passes into the intestine, where it assists digestion by emulsifying fats and stimulates peristalsis. *B. pigments.* Bilirubin and biliverdin produced by haemolysis in the spleen. Normally these colour the faeces, but in jaundice cause the coloration of the skin and urine. *B. salts.* Sodium taurocholate and sodium glycocholate which cause the emulsification of fats. They are the constituents responsible for irritation of the skin and the slow pulse in jaundice. *Urine tests for b.* See Appendix 11.

Bilharzia (bil-har'-ze-ah). The type of fluke, now called *Schistosoma*, which causes schistosomiasis (*q.v.*).

bilharziasis (bil-har-zi'-a-sis). A parasitic infection of the intestinal or urinary tract, now termed schistosomiasis (q.v.).

biliary (bil'-e-ar-e). Pertaining to bile. *B. ducts.* The tubes through which the bile passes from the liver and gall-bladder to the intestine. *B. colic.* Spasm of muscle walls of the duct causing excruciating pain when gall-stones are blocking the tube. Pain is in the right upper quadrant of the abdomen and referred to the shoulder. *B. fistula.* An abnormal opening between the gall-bladder and the surface of the body or some internal portion of the gastrointestinal tract. It may be a complication of operation on the gall-bladder, especially if there has been drainage of the ducts.

bilious (bil'-e-us). A condition caused by an excessive secretion of bile, and its regurgitation into the stomach with catarrh of that organ.

bilirubin (bil-e-ru'-bin). A bile pigment. See Bile.

biliuria (bil-e-u'-re-ah). Bile or bile salts in the urine.

biliverdin (bil-e-ver'-din). A bile pigment, derived from haemolysis of red blood cells and quickly converted to bilirubin. See Bile.

Billroth's operation (*C. A. T. Billroth, Austrian surgeon, 1829–94*). See Gastrectomy.

bimanual (bi-man'-u-al). Using both hands. *B. examination.* Examination with both hands. Used chiefly in gynaecology, when the internal genital organs are examined between one hand on the abdomen, and the other hand or finger within the vagina.

binary fission (bi'-nar-e). The multiplication of cells by division into two equal parts.

binaural (bin-aw'-ral). Pertaining to both ears. *B. stethoscope.* See Stethoscope.

binder (bine'-der). An abd

nal bandage which can be used:
(1) For support after childbirth
or abdominal operation; (2) For
support when ascitic fluid is
removed by tapping.

Binet's test (*A. Binet, French
physiologist, 1857–1911*). A
method of ascertaining the
mental age of children or young
persons by using a series of
questions standardized on the
capacity of normal children at
various ages.

biniodide of mercury (*bin-i'-
o-dide*). Mercuric iodide. A
little-used mercurial antiseptic.

binocular (*bin-ok'-u-lar*). Relating to both eyes.

binovular (*bin-o'-vu-lar*). Derived from two ova. *B. twins.*
Twins, but may be of different
sexes. *See* Uniovular.

biochemistry (*bi-o-kem'-is-
tre*). Chemistry of living matter.
Physiological chemistry.

biogenesis (*bi-o-jen'-es-is*).
The reproduction of living
beings from those already living.

biology (*bi-ol'-o-je*). The science of living forms, dealing
with their structure, function
and organization.

biomicroscopy(*bi-o-mi-cros'-
ko-pe*). A microscopic examination of the structures of the
anterior of the eye during life.
See Slit lamp.

bioplasm (*bi'-o-plazm*). Protoplasm. The active principle in
matter which produces living
organisms.

biopsy (*bi-op'-se*). Observation
of the living. Used to describe
the removal of some tissue or
organ of the body, e.g. a lymph
gland, for examination to establish a diagnosis.

Biot's respiration (*C. Biot,
19th century French physician*). Periods of hyperpnoea
occurring in normal respiration.
It is sometimes seen in menin-

gitis. Also called grouped
breathing.

biotin (*bi'-ot-in*). Formerly
termed vitamin H, now part of
vitamin B complex and present
in all normal diets.

biparous (*bip'-ar-us*). Giving
birth to twins or two at a time.

bipolar (*bi-po'-lah*). With two
poles. *B. nerve cells.* Cells having two nerve fibres, e.g. ganglionic cells.

BIPP. An antiseptic paste composed of bismuth, iodoform and
paraffin.

birth (*berth*). The act of being
born. *B. control.* Limiting the
size of the family by abstention
or the use of contraceptives. *B.
mark.* A haemangioma (*q.v.*)
present from birth. *Premature b.*
One taking place after 28 weeks
of pregnancy but before term.
Now all infants under 2500 g
weight are considered premature.

bisacodyl (*bis-a-ko'-dil*). A laxative that acts directly on the
rectum. Used most frequently in
the form of suppositories.

bisexual (*bi-seks'-u-al*). Possessing characteristics of both
sexes; hermaphroditic.

bismuth (*biz'-muth*). A greyish
metal. Used in medicine as a
gastric sedative; by injection for
the treatment of syphilis; and as
an antiseptic in skin diseases.
Taken internally it causes a
greyish-black coloration of the
stools.

bistoury (*bis'-too-re*). A slender
surgical knife: sometimes
curved.

Bitot's spots (*P. A. Bitot,
French physician, 1822–88*).
Collections of dried epithelium,
micro-organisms, etc., forming
shiny, greyish spots on the cornea. A sign of vitamin A deficiency. *See* Appendix 10.

bitters. Drugs characterized by

bitter taste; used to stimulate the appetite.

bivalve (*bi'-valv*). Consisting of two halves. Cutting a plaster cast into an anterior and posterior section. *B. speculum.* A vaginal one having two blades that can be adjusted for easy insertion.

blackhead (*blak'-hed*). See Comedone.

blackwater fever. A rare complication of malaria in which severe haemolysis causes a dark discoloration of the urine.

bladder. A membraneous sac. *B. worm.* A cysticercus (*q.v.*). *Atonic b.* Lack of tone in the bladder wall, which may be the result of over dilatation. *Gall-b.* The reservoir for bile. *Irritable b.* Frequent desire to micturate. *Urinary b.* The reservoir for urine.

Blalock–Taussig operation (*A. Blalock, American surgeon, 1899–1964: H. B. Taussig, American paediatrician, 1898– *). Operation in which the subclavian artery is anastomosed to the pulmonary artery. Performed in cases of congenital pulmonary stenosis, i.e. Fallot's tetralogy.

bland fluids. Mild and non-irritating fluids such as barley water and milk.

blastocyst (*blas'-to-sist*). Blastula (*q.v.*).

blastocyte (*blas'-to-site*). An embryonic cell that has not yet become differentiated into its specific type.

blastoderm (*blas'-to-derm*). The germinal cells of the embryo consisting of three layers, the ectoderm, mesoderm and entoderm.

blastomycosis (*blas-to-mi-ko'-sis*). A fungal infection which after invasion of the skin may cause granulomatous le-

sions in the mouth, pharynx and lungs.

blastolysis (*blas-tol'-is-is*). The destruction of germ substance.

blastula (*blas'-tu-lah*). Blastocyst. An early stage in the development of the fertilized ovum when the morula becomes cystic and later infolds to become the gastrula.

bleaching powder. Chlorinated lime, which is a powerful disinfectant.

bleb. A blister (*q.v.*).

bleeders. A popular name for those who suffer from haemophilia (*q.v.*).

'bleeding time'. The time taken for oozing to cease from a sharp finger prick. The normal is 3 to 4 min. It is influenced by the retraction of the blood vessel wall as well as by the clotting power of blood. See Clotting time.

blennophthalmia (*blen-off-thal'-me-ah*). Catarrhal conjunctivitis.

blennorrhagia (*blen-or-raj'-e-ah*). An excessive discharge of mucus, e.g. leucorrhoea (*q.v.*).

blepharitis (*blef-ar-i'-tis*). Inflammation of the eyelids.

blepharon (*blef'-ar-on*). The eyelid.

blepharoptosis (*blef-ar-op-to'-sis*). Drooping of the upper eyelid.

blepharospasm (*blef'-ar-o-spazm*). Prolonged spasm of both orbicularis muscles.

blind. Without sight. *B. spot.* The point where the optic nerve leaves the retina, which is insensitive to light.

blind loop syndrome. A condition of stasis in the small intestine which aids bacterial multiplication leading to diarrhoea and salt deficiencies. The cause may be intestinal obstruction or surgical anastomosis.

blister. A bleb or vesicle. A collection of serum between the epidermis and the true skin.

blood. The fluid that circulates through the heart and blood vessels, supplying nutritive material to all parts of the body, and carrying off waste products.

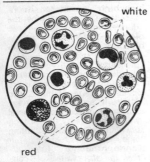

white

red

BLOOD CELLS — MICROSCOPICAL APPEARANCE

It is a colourless fluid (*plasma*) in which float myriads of minute bodies (*corpuscles*). These are of three kinds; *red* and *white* (in the proportion of about 500:1), and *platelets*. (1) The red corpuscles or *erythrocytes* contain haemoglobin which combines with oxygen in passing through the lungs. This oxygen is released into the tissues from the capillaries and oxidation (*q.v.*) takes place. (2) The white corpuscles or *leucocytes* defend against invading micro-organisms, which they have power to destroy. (3) Blood platelets or *thrombocytes* are concerned with the clotting of blood. *See*

Normal values, Appendix 9. Injury to the wall of a blood vessel activates the formation of a clot, which is nature's method of sealing a wound, so preventing prolonged haemorrhage. *See* Thrombin.

blood–brain barrier. A hypothetical bar dividing the blood from the parenchyma of the central nervous system. Some substances will pass from the blood stream into the cerebrospinal fluid and some will not do so; streptomycin, for instance, will not pass this barrier.

blood casts. Minute filaments of coagulated blood found in the urine in some cases of kidney disease.

blood count. Calculation of the number of red and white corpuscles in one cubic millimetre of blood, as seen through the microscope. *Differential b.c.* One which gives the relative number of the different types of white cells. *See* Leucocytes *and* Appendix 9.

blood culture. The cultivation of bacteria present in blood in order that a disease may be diagnosed or sensitivity tests carried out.

blood grouping. All human blood belongs to one of four groups. If two which are incompatible are mixed, agglutination of corpuscles results. Therefore in blood transfusion the donor's and recipient's blood must be of the same or a compatible group. Introduction of incompatible blood produces a severe reaction which may be fatal. Theoretically, Group O (universal donors) can give to anyone but this is not invariably so and it is imperative that direct cross-matching should precede blood transfusion. *See* Rhesus factor *and* Appendix 8.

blood plasma. The fluid portion of blood that contains proteins, salts, hormones, and the end products of digestion, together with waste and toxic substances for excretion.

blood pressure. The pressure exerted on the arteries by the blood as it flows through them. It can be measured in milligrams of mercury using a sphygmomanometer or Doppler apparatus. Two readings are made. One records the pressure whilst the heart is in systole and is the higher or *systolic pressure*. The other records the pressure whilst the heart is in diastole and is the lower or *diastolic pressure*. The range of normal readings varies according to age but in a young adult is approximately 100–120/70–80.

blood serum (*seer'-um*). Plasma without the clotting agents. It may be used: (1) For intravenous infusion. (2) As a bacteriological culture medium.

blood sugar. The amount of glucose present in the blood. The normal range is 2·5–4·7 mmol/litre. When the amount exceeds 10 mmol/litre glucose is executed in the urine, as in diabetes mellitus.

blood transfusion (*trans-fu'-zhun*). Introduction of blood from the vein of one person (*donor*) to the vein of another (*recipient*). Clotting must be prevented in the transition stage. This is usually done by admixture with sodium citrate (1 g to 450 ml of blood). Too much sodium citrate tends to produce a reaction, and rigor and shock may occur. Transfusion of fresh blood has been largely replaced by the use of stored blood or plasma. *See* Appendix 8. Used as treatment: (1) In severe loss of blood from

any cause. (2) For the treatment or prevention of shock. (3) In severe infections, to supply healthy blood to fight the infection.

blood urea. Excretory product of protein present in the blood. The normal range is 3–7 mmol/litre. This increases in renal failure when the kidneys cease to function normally.

'blue baby'. A child born with a very blue colour. It may be due to a defect in the heart, in consequence of which arterial and venous blood become mixed. *See* Fallot's tetralogy.

blue paint. An antiseptic made from aniline dyes. It consists of 1 per cent *brilliant green* and 1 per cent *gentian violet* in 25 per cent *spirit*. Both skin and linen are badly stained by it. Bonney's blue.

blue stone. Copper sulphate.

BMR. Basal metabolic rate. *See* Basal.

Boeck's disease (*C. P. M. Boeck, Norwegian dermatologist, 1845–1917*). A form of sarcoidosis (*q.v.*).

Böhler's plaster (*L. Böhler, Austrian orthopaedic surgeon, 1885–*). *See* Plaster.

boil. An acute staphylococcal inflammation of the skin and subcutaneous tissues round a hair follicle. It causes a painful swelling with a central core of dead tissue (*slough*), which is eventually discharged. A furuncle.

bolus (*bo'-lus*). (1) A large pill. (2) A rounded mass of masticated food immediately before being swallowed.

bone. The dense connective tissue forming the skeleton. It is composed of cartilage or membrane impregnated with mineral salts, chiefly calcium phosphate and calcium carbonate. This i

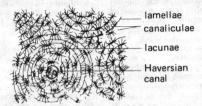

lamellae
canaliculae
lacunae
Haversian
canal

BONE

arranged as an outer hard *compact* tissue and an inner network of cells as *cancellous* tissue, in the spaces of which is red bone marrow. In the shaft of long bones is a medullary cavity containing white marrow. Microscopically, the bone tissue is perforated with minute (Haversian) canals containing blood vessels and lymphatics for the maintenance and repair of the cells. Bone is covered by a fibrous membrane—the *periosteum*—containing blood vessels and by which the bone grows in girth.

bone-graft. Transplantation of healthy bone to replace missing or defective bone.

boracic acid (*bor-as'-ik as'-id*). Boric acid. A mild antiseptic prepared from borax and used mainly for the irrigation of mucous or delicate surfaces, e.g. the eyes.

borax (*bor'-aks*). A compound of soda and boric acid. Used as a mild antiseptic and to allay irritation of the mouth and skin.

borborygmus (*bor-bor-ig'-mus*). A rumbling sound caused by gas in the intestines.

Bordet–Gengou bacillus (*J. J. B. V. Bordet, Belgian bacteriologist, 1870–1961: O. Gengou, French bacteriologist,* 1875–1957). *Bordetella pertussis,* the causal agent of whooping cough (*q.v.*). See Bacillus.

Bornholm disease (*born'-holm*). An epidemic myalgia with pleural pain due to Coxsackie virus infection. It receives its name from the Danish island of Bornholm.

Bothriocephalus (*both-re-o-kef'-al-us*). See Diphyllobothrium.

botulism (*bot'-u-lizm*). A rare form of food poisoning in which the central nervous system is affected by the toxins from the *Clostridium botulinum.* It is an anaerobic spore-forming organism from the soil and survives in imperfectly canned vegetables and in meat and fish preparations. These may be normal in taste and appearance.

bougie (*boo'-je*). A flexible instrument used to dilate a stricture, as in the oesophagus or urethra. *Medicated b.* A soluble form impregnated with a medicinal substance. Used for urethral treatment. *Whip b.* This has a fine whip-like commencement, but gradually enlarges.

Bourneville's disease (*D. M. Bourneville, French neurologist, 1840–1909*). Tuberous sclerosis. See Epiloia.

bovine (*bo'-vine*). Relating to the cow or ox. *B. tuberculosis.* That caused by infection from infected cow's milk, usually affecting glands and bones.

bowel (*bow'-el*). The intestine (*q.v.*).

Bowman's capsule (*Sir W. P. Bowman, British physician, 1816–92*). The commencement of the kidney tubule, which surrounds a tuft of renal capillaries—the *glomerulus.* Filtration takes place from the blood into the tubule.

Boyle's anaesthetic machine (*H. E. G. Boyle, English surgeon, 1875–1941*). Apparatus by which chloroform, ether, nitrous oxide gas and now cyclopropane may be administered.

Boyle's law (*R. Boyle, English physicist, 1627–91*). Law stating that at any determined temperature a known mass of gas varies in volume inversely as the pressure.

Bozeman's catheter (*M. Bozeman, American surgeon, 1825–1905*). For uterine irrigation, grooved on one side to allow back flow, and to avoid danger of forcing fluid into the fallopian tubes.

brachial (*bra'-ke-al*). Relating to the arm. *B. artery.* The continuation of the axillary artery along the inner side of the upper arm. *B. plexus.* A network of nerves, at the root of the neck, supplying the upper limb.

brachium (*bra'-ke-um*). The arm, from shoulder to elbow.

brachycephaly (*brak-e-kef'-al-e*). Name given to a head shape in which the antero-posterior diameter is relatively short.

Bradford's frame (*E. H. Bradford, American surgeon, 1848–1926*). A metal and canvas

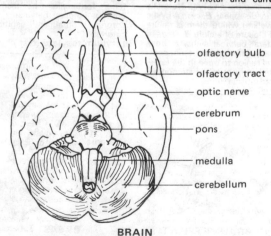

olfactory bulb

olfactory tract

optic nerve

cerebrum

pons

medulla

cerebellum

BRAIN

frame which immobilizes the bones, and is used in the treatment of spinal tuberculosis.

bradycardia (*brad-e-kar'-de-ah*). Abnormally low rate of heart contractions and consequent slow pulse.

bradykinin (*brad-e-ki'-nin*). Peptide formed from the degradation of protein by enzymes.

brain. That part of the central nervous system contained in the skull. It consists of the cerebrum, cerebellum, medulla oblongata and pons varolii.

bran. The husk of grain. The coarse outer coat of cereals. High in roughage and vitamins of the B complex. Frequently recommended as a dietary component both for those with alimentary disorders and for those in normal health.

branchial (*bran'-ke-al*). Relating to the clefts that are present in the neck and pharynx in the developing embryo. Normally they disappear. *B. cyst.* A cystic swelling where there is failure of closure of a cleft. *B. sinus* or lateral cervical sinus. A track leading from the posterior cervical region to open in the lower neck in front of the sternomastoid muscle.

Braun's splint (*H. F. W. Braun, German surgeon, 1862–1934*). A metal splint which incorporates one or more pulleys and is used chiefly to elevate the lower limb and to apply skeletal traction for a compound fracture of tibia and fibula.

breast. (1) The anterior or front region of the chest. (2) The mammary gland. *B. abscess.* Formation of pus in the mammary gland, a possible complication from infection in nursing mothers. *B. bone.* The sternum. *B. feeding.* Suckling of an infant by its mother. *Pigeon b.* Prominent sternum, a deformity resulting from rickets. *B. pump.* An apparatus for removal of milk from the breast.

breech. The buttocks. *B. presentation.* The position of the fetus in the uterus is such that the buttocks present.

bregma (*breg'-mah*). The anterior fontanelle. The membranous junction between coronal, frontal and sagittal sutures.

bretylium tosylate (*bret-il'-e-*

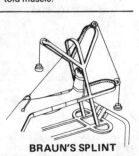

BRAUN'S SPLINT

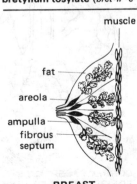

muscle

fat

areola

ampulla

fibrous septum

BREAST

um tos'-il-ate). A vasodilator drug that affects the peripheral blood vessels supplied by the sympathetic nervous system. It is used in the treatment of hypertension. Darenthin is a proprietary preparation of it.

Bright's disease (*B. Bright, British physician, 1789–1858*). An inflammation of the kidneys. *See* Nephritis.

brilliant green. An aniline dye used as an antiseptic.

British Pharmacopoeia (*far-mah-ko-pe'-ah*). List of 'official' drugs which is published by H.M. Stationery Office on behalf of the Health Minister. The drugs are listed on the recommendations of the Medicines Commission in accordance with the Medicines Act 1968.

brittle (*brit'-tl*). A term applied to diabetes when the patient's blood sugar and glycosuria appear to vary from day to day or hour to hour, and so make his diabetes difficult to control.

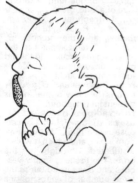

CORRECT POSITION FOR BREAST FEEDING

broad ligaments. Folds of peritoneum extending from the uterus to the sides of the pelvis, and supporting the blood vessels to the uterus and uterine tubes.

Broca's area of speech (*P. P. Broca, French surgeon, 1824–80*). Nerve cells in the left cerebral hemisphere which have some control over speech.

Brodie's abscess (*Sir B. C. Brodie, British surgeon, 1783–1862*). Abscess of the head of the tibia or other long bone. A form of chronic tuberculosis or staphylococcal osteomyelitis.

bromide (*bro'-mide*). A compound of bromine. *Potassium b., sodium b.* and *ammonium b.* can be prescribed as hypnotics that are strongly depressant and cumulative in action.

bromidrosis (*brom-id-ro'-sis*). Offensive and foetid sweat, especially associated with the feet.

bromsulphthalein (*brom-sulf-thal'-een*). Agent used in certain tests for liver function.

bronchi (*brong'-ki*). The two branches into which the trachea divides before entering the lungs. *Sing.* bronchus.

bronchial tubes (*brong'-ke-al*). Subdivisions of the bronchi within the lungs.

bronchiectasis (*brong-ke-ek'-tas-is*). Dilatation of the bronchial tubes, associated with the formation of fibrous tissue. The dilated bronchi become infected resulting in a copious secretion of pus. Treatment is unsatisfactory, but lobectomy, pneumonectomy or segmental resection offer the best chance of cure when the disease is localized.

bronchiole (*brong'-ke-ole*). The smallest bronchial tubes.

bronchiolitis (*brong-ke-o-li'-*

tis). Inflammation of the bronchioles.

bronchitis (*brong-ki'-tis*). Inflammation of the bronchi. *Acute b.* Common in young children and the elderly. It is a descending infection from the common cold, influenza, measles or other upper respiratory condition. *Chronic b.* (winter cough), common in older people, is particularly troublesome in cold and foggy weather, and in time causes organic change in the lungs. Heart failure may result from prolonged strain.

broncho-adenitis (*brong'-ko ad-en-i'-tis*). Inflammation of bronchial glands.

bronchodilator (*brong-ko-di-la'-tor*). A drug that relaxes the plain muscle of the bronchi and bronchioles and so increases the lumen.

bronchogram (*brong'-ko-gram*). The X-ray film of the lungs after radio-opaque dye has been inserted.

bronchography (*brong-kog'-raf-e*). X-ray photography of the bronchial tree after introduction of an iodized oil opaque to the rays.

bronchomycosis (*brong-ko-mi-ko'-sis*). An industrial disease affecting agricultural workers, stablemen, etc., and due to inhalation of microfungi which infect the air-passages. Causes can be the *Actinomyces* or *Aspergillus* species. Symptoms are similar to those of pulmonary tuberculosis.

bronchophony (*brong-koff'-on-e*). Resonance of the voice as heard in the chest over the bronchi on auscultation.

bronchopleural fistula (*brong-ko-plu'-ral*). An opening between the pleural space and one of the bronchi.

bronchopneumonia (*brong-*

ko-nu-mo'-ne-ah). *See* Pneumonia.

bronchopulmonary (*brong-ko-pul'-mon-ar-e*). Relating to the lungs, bronchi and bronchioles.

bronchorrhoea (*brong-kor-re'-ah*). Copious expectoration from the bronchi.

bronchoscope (*brong'-ko-skope*). An instrument which enables the operator to see inside the bronchi; to remove foreign bodies or to take a biopsy.

bronchoscopy (*brong-kos'-ko-pe*). Examination of the bronchi by means of a bronchoscope.

bronchospasm (*brong'-ko-spazm*). Difficulty in breathing caused by the sudden constriction of plain muscle in the walls of the bronchi. This may arise in asthma, whooping cough or pneumoconiosis.

bronchospirometer (*brong-ko-spi-rom'-e-ter*). An instrument used to measure the capacity of one lung or of one lobe of a lung.

bronchotracheal (*brong-ko-trak'-e-al*). Relating to both the trachea and the bronchi. *B. suction.* A term applied to the removing of mucus with the aid of suction, using an electrical or foot operated sucker.

brow. The forehead. *B. presentation.* The brow of the child is present first in labour.

brown adipose tissue (*ad'-ip-ose tis'-u*). Special type of adipose tissue found in the newborn infant, and which is widely distributed throughout the body. The tissue is highly vascular and owes its colour to the large number of mitochondria organelles found in the cytoplasm of its cells. It allows the infant to increase its metabolic rate and thus its heat production when subjected to cold. At the same time the fat itself is used up. *See* Adipose.

Brown-Séquard syndrome (*C. E. Brown-Séquard, French physiologist, 1818–94*). Lesion of the spinal cord occurring laterally which causes paralysis on the same side and sensory loss on the other. Frequently caused by a tumour.

Brucella (*bru-sel'-ah*). A genus of bacteria primarily pathogenic in animals but which may affect man. *B. abortus* produces abortion in cattle and undulant fever in man. *B. melitensis* in infected goats' milk causes brucellosis or Malta fever in man.

brucellosis (*bru-sel-o'-sis*). Undulant fever. An intermittent fever caused by organisms transmitted in infected milk from cattle or goats. Malta fever.

Brudzinski's sign (*J. Brudzinski, Polish physician, 1874–1917*). (1) When passive flexion of one thigh causes spontaneous flexion of the opposite thigh. (2) When flexion of the neck causes bilateral flexion of the hips and knees. These signs are indicative of meningeal irritation.

bruise (*brooz*). A superficial injury to tissues produced by sudden impact, in which the skin is unbroken. A contusion.

bruit (*bru'-e*). An abnormal sound or murmur heard on auscultation of the heart and large vessels. It occurs in disease of the heart and in anaemia.

Brunner's glands (*J. C. Brunner, Swiss anatomist, 1653–1727*). Small compound tubular glands in the mucous membrane of the duodenum.

bruxism (*bruks'-izm*). Teeth clenching. This occurs in persons under tension and due to muscle fatigue may cause headaches.

bubo (*bu'-bo*). A term applied to inflammation of the lymphatic glands of the axilla or groin. Typical of bubonic plague (*see* Plague) and venereal infections.

bubonocele (*bu-bon'-o-seel*). An early stage of inguinal hernia resembling a bubo.

buccal (*buk'-kal*). (1) Pertaining to the cheek. (2) Pertaining to the mouth.

buccinator (*buk'-sin-a-tor*). A muscle of the cheek.

Budd–Chiari syndrome (*G. Budd, British physician, 1808–82: H. Chiari, Austrian pathologist, 1851–1916*). A condition in which thrombosis of the hepatic vein causes vomiting, jaundice, enlargement of the liver and ascites.

Buerger's disease (*L. Buerger, American physician, 1879–1943*). Thrombo-angeitis obliterans (*q.v.*).

buffer (*buff'-er*). A chemical substance which, when present in a solution, will allow only a very slight change in reaction when an acid (or alkali) is added to it. Sodium bicarbonate is the chief buffer of the blood and tissue fluids.

bulbar (*bul'-bar*). Pertaining to the medulla oblongata. *B. paralysis. See* Paralysis.

bulbo-urethral glands (*bulbo-u-re'-thral*). Small glands opening into the male urethra. Cowper's glands.

bulimia (*bu-lim'-e-ah*). Excessive appetite.

bulla (*bul'-lah*). A large blister. *Pl.* bullae.

Buller's shield (*F. Buller, Canadian ophthalmologist, 1844–1905*). A type of protection placed over one eye when the other is infected. A watch glass placed over the eye and fixed with adhesive strapping or Sellotape is a simple substitute.

bundle branch block. Term used to describe the delay in conduction along either branch of the atrioventricular bundle of the heart. The abnormality is detected by an ECG recording.

bundle of His (*L. His (Jr.), German physiologist, 1863–1934*). The special band of neuromuscular fibres which passing through the septum of the heart divides at the apex into two parts, these being distributed into the wall of the ventricles. The impulse of contraction is conducted through this structure. Disease of it causes heart block (*q.v.*).

bunion (*bun'-yon*). A prominence on the head of the metatarsal bone at its junction with the great toe, caused by inflammation and swelling of the bursa at that joint. Usually due to shoes which distort the natural shape of the foot. The bone itself is much enlarged from chronic irritation.

burr hole. Circular hole drilled in the cranium to permit access to the brain or to release raised intercranial pressure.

Burkitt's tumour (*D. P. Burkitt, contemporary Irish surgeon*). African lymphoma. A lymphosarcoma occurring almost exclusively in children living in low-lying moist areas of Central Africa. It may attack the jaw, lymph nodes, kidneys or thyroid gland.

burn. An injury to tissues caused by: (1) Physical agent, the sun, excess heat or cold. (2) Chemical agents, acids or caustic alkalis. (3) Electrical current in which part of the body is placed in the circuit and the damage to tissue may be more extensive than is immediately apparent. Burns are now divided into partial thickness or full thickness according to the depth of skin destroyed. The former will heal from the germinal cells below but the latter require grafting. The treatment of shock and prevention of infection need special attention. For First Aid treatment, see Appendix 1.

bursa (*bur'-sah*). A small sac of fibrous tissue, lined with synovial membrane and containing synovial fluid. It is situated between parts that move upon one another at a joint to reduce friction.

bursitis (*bur-si'-tis*). Inflammation of a bursa. *Prepatellar b.* Housemaid's knee (*q.v.*).

busulphan (*bu-sul'-fan*). A cytotoxic drug that depresses the bone marrow and may be used to treat myeloid leukaemia. A proprietary name is Myleran.

butacaine (*bu'-ta-kane*). A local anaesthetic used in ophthalmology. Butyn is a proprietary preparation.

Butazolidin (*bu-tah-zol'-id-in*). A proprietary preparation of phenylbutazone (*q.v.*), an analgesic and antiseptic drug.

butobarbitone (*bu-to-bar'-bit-ohn*). A widely used barbiturate drug whose sedative actions lasts 4–8 hours and is unlikely to cause drowsiness on the following morning. Soneryl is a proprietary preparation of it.

buttock (*but'-ok*). The flesh-covered gluteal muscles at either side of the lower spine.

byssinosis (*bis-in-o'-sis*). An industrial disease caused by inhalation of cotton dust in factories. A type of pneumoconiosis (*q.v.*).

C

C. (1) The chemical symbol for *carbon.* (2) The abbreviation of *centigrade* or *Celsius.*

Ca. The chemical symbol for calcium.

cacao butter (*kak-a'-o*). A solid fat obtained from the seeds of *Theobroma cacao*, used as a base for suppositories.

cachet (*kash'-a*). Two pieces of wafer, joined in the form of a capsule to contain an unpalatable medicine.

cachexia (*kak-eks'-e-ah*). A condition of extreme debility. The patient is emaciated, the skin loose and wrinkled from rapid wasting, but shiny and tense over bone. The eyes are sunken, the skin yellowish, and there is a grey 'muddy' complexion. The mucous membranes are pale and anaemia is extreme. The condition is typical of the late stages of cancer.

cadaver (*kad-av'-er*). A corpse. The dead body used for dissection.

caecostomy (*se-kos'-to-me*). The making of an opening into the caecum by incision through the abdominal wall.

caecum (*se'-kum*). The commencement of the large intestine, to which the vermiform appendix is attached.

caesarean section (*se-zair'-e-an sek'-shun*). Delivery of a fetus by an incision through the abdominal wall and uterus. Tradition has it that Julius Caesar was born in this way.

caesium 137 (*se'-se-um*). Radioactive c. An element that is a fission product from uranium. Sealed in a suitable container it can be used for beam therapy instead of cobalt, or sealed in needles or tubes it can be used for local application instead of radium.

café au lait pallor (*kaf-eh-o-lá pal'-or*). Pallor characteristic of subacute bacterial endocarditis in which the skin resembles milky coffee.

caffeine (*kaf'-een*). An alkaloid of tea and coffee, used as a nerve stimulant and diuretic.

caisson disease (*ka'-son*). Decompression sickness (*q.v.*).

Calabar bean (*kal'-ab-ah*). The seed of the *Physostigma venenosum*. The alkaloid (*eserine* or *physostigmine*) is stimulative to involuntary muscle and is used as a miotic.

calamine (*kal'-am-ine*). Prepared from zinc carbonate. It is an astringent and antipruritic used in lotion or ointment form for skin diseases.

calcaneum (*kal-ka'-ne-um*). The heel-bone.

calcaneus (*kal-ka'-ne-us*). The

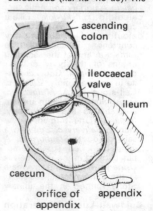

ascending colon

ileocaecal valve

ileum

caecum

orifice of appendix

appendix

CAECUM

heel. *Talipes c.* Clubfoot, in which only the heel touches the ground.

calcareous (*kal-kar'-e-us*). Chalky.

calciferol (*kal-sif'-er-ol*). The chemical name for vitamin D. It is formed in irradiated ergosterol. *See* Appendix 10.

calcification (*kal-sif-ik-a'-shun*). The deposit of lime in any tissue, e.g. in the formation of callus (*q.v.*).

calcitonin (*kal-se-to'-nin*). Hormone produced by the thyroid gland which regulates blood calcium levels.

calcium (*kal'-se-um*). A silver-white metal, the base of lime. *C. carbonate.* Chalk. *C. chloride.* Disinfectant. *C. gluconate.* Easily absorbed and can be given by intramuscular or intravenous route to raise the blood calcium *C. hydroxide.* Slaked lime. *C. lactate.* This increases coagulability of blood. *C. mandelate.* A urinary antiseptic.

calculoid (*kal'-ku-loid*). Like a calculus.

calculus (*kal'-ku-lus*). A stony concretion which may be formed in any of the secreting organs of the body or their ducts. *Arthritic c.* Gouty deposits in or near joints. *Biliary c.* Gall-stone (*q.v.*). *Mulberry c.* One made of calcium oxalate and shaped like a mulberry. *Renal c.* One formed in the kidney. *Salivary c.* Stone in a salivary duct. *Staghorn c.* A many-branched stone sometimes found in the renal pelvis. *Urinary c.* One found anywhere in the urinary tract. *Vesical c.* Stone formed in the urinary bladder.

Caldwell–Luc operation (*G. W. Caldwell, American otolaryngologist, 1834–1918: H. Luc, French laryngologist,* *1855–1925*). An antrostomy operation to drain the maxillary sinus. The incision is made above the upper canine tooth.

calibrator (*kal'-e-bra-tor*). An instrument for measuring the size of openings.

caliper (*kal'-ip-er*). (1) A two-pronged instrument that may be used to exert traction on a part. *Walking c.* An appliance fitted to a boot or shoe to give support to the lower limb. It may be used when the muscles are paralysed or in the repair stage of fractures. (2) Compasses for measuring diameters and curved surfaces. *See* Pelvimeter.

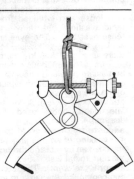

SKULL CALIPER FOR TRACTION

callisthenics (*kal-is-then'-iks*). Mild gymnastics for developing the muscles and producing a graceful carriage.

callosity (*kal-os'-it-e*). The plaques of thickened skin often seen on the soles of the feet or the palms of the hand.

callous (*kal'-us*). Hard and thickened.

callus (*kal'-us*). The tissue which grows round fractured ends of bone and develops into new bone to repair the injury.

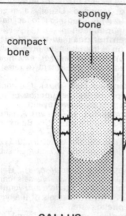

spongy bone

compact bone

CALLUS

caloric test (*kal-or'-ik*). A method of estimating vestibular disease of the ear by using warm or cool irrigations.

calorie (*kal'-or-e*). A standard unit of heat. Used to denote physiological values of various food substances, estimated according to the amount of heat they produce on being oxidized in the body. *See* Oxidation. A *Calorie* represents the heat required in raising 1 kg (1000 g or 2·2 lb) by 1°C. A *small calorie*=the heat produced in raising 1 g of water 1°C. In the SI system the calorie is replaced by the joule (1 Cal = 4·18 kJ). For calorie value of foods, *see* Appendix 10.

calorific (*kal-or-if'ik*). Heat producing.

calorimeter (*kal-or-im'-e-ter*). An apparatus for measuring the heat that is produced by combustion.

calvities (*kal-vish'-e-ez*). Baldness.

calx (*kalks*). Calcium oxide or lime. The basis of slaked lime, bleaching powder, and quick lime. Used in making eusol (*q.v.*).

calyx (*ka'-lix*). Any cup-shaped vessel or part. *C. of kidney.* The cup-like terminations of the ureter in the renal pelvis surrounding the pyramids of the kidney. *Pl.* Calyces.

camphor (*kam'-for*). A crystalline substance prepared from the camphor laurel. It is used internally as a carminative. *Camphorated oil* is 1 part camphor to 4 parts oil prepared for external application as a rubefacient.

canaliculus (*kan-al-ik'-ul-us*). A small channel or canal. *See* Bone.

cancellous (*kan-sel'-us*). The spongy or honeycomb type of bone tissue in the ends of long bones and in flat and irregular bones. *See* Tissue.

cancer (*kan'-ser*). A general term to describe malignant growths in tissues, of which *carcinoma* (*q.v.*) is of epithelial, and *sarcoma* (*q.v.*) of connective tissue origin, as in bone and muscle. A cancerous growth is one which is not encapsulated, but infiltrates into surrounding tissues, the cells of which it replaces by its own. It is spread by the lymph and blood vessels and causes metastases (*q.v.*) in other parts of the body. Death is caused by destruction of organs to a degree incompatible with life; to extreme debility and anaemia; or to haemorrhage. The importance of early recognition and treatment cannot be over-emphasized. *Anaplastic c.* One in which the cells are so lacking in form that it is not possible to differentiate them or tell from which type of tissue they have arisen.

cancroid (*kan'-kroid*). (1) A skin tumour of some malignancy. (2) Resembling cancer.

cancrum oris (*kan'-krum aw'-ris*). Gangrenous stomatitis. An ulceration of the mouth, which is a rare complication of measles in debilitated children. Penicillin lessens the severity of this condition. *Syn.*, Noma.

candela (*kan-de'-lah, kan'-del-ah*). (1) Unit of luminous intensity used in the Système International d'Unités (SI unit system). (2) A medicinal candle used in fumigation.

Candida (*kan'-did-ah*). A genus of small fungi, formerly called Monilia. *C. albicans.* The variety which causes moniliasis.

canine teeth (*kan'-ine*). Four in number. Two in each jaw between the incisors and molars, commonly known as 'eye teeth'.

canker (*kan'-ker*). Ulceration, usually of the mouth.

Cannabis indica (*kan'-ab-is in'-dik-ah*). An Indian hemp (*hashish*), antispasmodic and narcotic. Large doses cause intoxication and delirium. A drug

of addiction controlled by the Misuse of Drugs Act.

cannula (*kan'-u-lah*). A metal tube for insertion into the body by which fluids are introduced or removed. Usually a trocar (*q.v.*) is fitted into it to facilitate introduction.

cantharides (*kan-thar'-id-eez*). An extract from the body of the Spanish fly, applied externally as a counter-irritant to raise a blister.

canthus (*kan'-thus*). The angle formed by the junction of the upper and lower eyelids.

capeline (*cap'-el-een*). A bandage for the head. *See* Bandage.

capillarity (*kap-il-lar'-it-e*). The action by which a liquid will rise upwards in a fibrous substance or in a fine tube.

capillary (*kap-il'-ar-e*). Hairlike. (1) Minute vessels connecting an arteriole and venule. (2) Minute vessels of the lymphatic system.

capitellum (*kap-it-el'-um*). (1) The small rounded head at the elbow end of the humerus. (2) The bulb of a hair.

capsular ligaments (*kap'-su-lah lig'-a-ments*). The ligaments which completely envelop a joint. This capsule loosely encloses the bones and is lined with synovial membrane which secretes a fluid for lubrication of

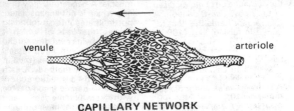

CAPILLARY NETWORK

the articular surfaces. Known also as *articular capsule*.

capsule (*kap'-sule*). (1) A fibrous or membranous sac enclosing an organ. (2) A small soluble case of gelatin in which a nauseous medicine may be enclosed. (3) The gelatinous envelope which surrounds and protects some bacteria.

capsulotomy (*kap-sul-ot'-o-me*). The tearing of a hole in the remaining lens capsule after an extracapsular cataract extraction. Needling.

caput (*kap'-ut*). Head. *C. succedaneum*. A soft swelling on an infant's head due to pressure during labour.

carbachol (*karb'-ak-ol*). A drug related to and acting like acetylcholine (*q.v.*), but more stable. It causes contraction of plain muscle and relaxation of the voluntary sphincter, so relieving postoperative retention of urine.

carbamino (*karb'-am-in-o*). A neutral compound formed by carbon dioxide and haemoglobin.

carbaminohaemoglobin (*karbam'-in-o-he-mo-glo'-bin*). The combination of carbon dioxide with haemoglobin. This takes place most readily with reduced haemoglobin.

carbenoxolone (*karb-en-oks'-o-lone*). A derivative of liquorice that increases the healing rate of gastric ulcers. Biogastrone is a proprietary preparation.

carbimazole (*kar-bim'-az-ol*). An antithyroid drug that is used to stabilize a patient with thyrotoxicosis.

carbohydrate (*karb-o-hi'-drate*). That class of food represented by the starches and sugars—they are energy- and heat-producing substances. *See* Appendix 10.

carbol fuchsin (*karb'-ol fook'-sin*). A mixture of carbolic acid and fuchsin used for staining purposes in bacteriology.

carbolic acid (*karb-ol'-ik*). Phenol. A powerful disinfectant and poison derived from coal tar. In its pure form it can be used as a caustic. Diluted, used to disinfect linen and excreta. Lotion containing 1 per cent has an anaesthetic action.

carbo ligni. Wood charcoal. Used for the relief of digestive disorders and diarrhoea.

carbon dioxide (CO_2) (*karb'-on di-oks-ide*). A gas which, dissolved in water, forms weak carbonic acid. As a product of metabolism by the oxidation of carbon, it leaves the body by the lungs. It can be compressed till it freezes, and then forms a solid—*carbon dioxide* snow, used to destroy superficial naevi. Inhalations of CO_2 (5 per cent) are useful to stimulate the depth of respiration.

carbon monoxide (CO) (*karb'-on mon-oks'-ide*). A colourless gas produced by incomplete combustion of coal. It is a major constituent of coal gas. In poisoning there is vertigo, flushed face with very red lips, loss of consciousness, and convulsions. The blood is bright red, from carboxyhaemoglobin.

carbon tetrachloride (*karb'-on tet-rah-klor'-ide*). A powerful anthelmintic used in treating hookworm and whipworm but in certain individuals can lead to severe necrosis of liver cells. A high carbohydrate and high protein diet are good preventive measures. The drug must not be given to alcoholics.

carbonic anhydrase (*karbon'-ik an-hi'-draze*). An enzyme important in the carriage of carbon dioxide in the blood.

carboxyhaemoglobin (*kar-boks'-e-he-mo-glo'-bin*). The combination of carbon monoxide with haemoglobin in the blood in carbon monoxide poisoning.

carboxyhaemoglobinaemia (*kar-boks'-e-he-mo-glo-bin-e'-me-ah*). The condition of carbon monoxide in the blood.

carbromal (*kar'-brom-al*). A drug of the barbiturate group combined with bromine. A useful sedative with no unpleasant after effects.

carbuncle (*kar'-bung-kl*). An acute staphylococcal inflammation of subcutaneous tissues, which causes local thrombosis in the veins and death of tissue. In appearance it resembles a collection of boils.

carcinogen (*kar'-sin-o-jen*). Any substance which can produce a cancer.

carcinogenic (*kar-sin-o-jen'-ik*). A term applied to agents which produce or predispose to cancer. Crude oils are said to contain a *c. factor*.

carcinoma (*kar-sin-o'-mah*). A malignant growth of epithelial tissue. Microscopically the cells resemble those of the tissue in which the growth has arisen. (1) Squamous-celled, like the outer layers of the skin (*epithe-lioma*). (2) Spheroidal-celled arising from glandular tissue, e.g. the breast. (3) Columnar-celled, e.g. from the intestinal tract.

carcinomatosis (*kar-sin-o-mat-o'-sis*). The condition when a carcinoma has given rise to widespread metastasis.

cardia (*kar'-de-ah*). (1) The cardiac orifice of the stomach. (2) The heart.

cardiac (*kar'-de-ak*). Pertaining to the heart. *C. asthma. See* Asthma. *C. atrophy*. Fatty degeneration of the heart muscle. *C. bed*. One which can be manipulated to form a chair shape for those heart cases who are comfortable only when sitting up. The head can be raised to form a back rest, and the foot lowered. An angle to flex the knees prevents slipping. *C. catheterization*. A radio-opaque catheter is passed from an arm vein to the heart. Its passage through the heart can be watched on a screen. Also blood pressure readings and specimens can be taken, thus aiding diagnosis of heart abnormalities. *C. compensation*. Hypertrophy of the muscle of the heart by which valvular defects are compensated, and the circulation is effectively maintained. *C. cycle*. The sequence of events lasting about 0·8 seconds dur-

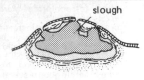

slough

before separation   after separation

CARBUNCLE

ing which the heart completes one contraction.

cardialgia (*kar-de-al'-je-ah*). Pain in the region of the heart.

cardinal ligaments (*kar-din-al lig'-a-ments*). Fan-shaped ligaments which pass from the cervix and vault of the vagina to the pelvic wall and which form part of the support of the uterus and vagina.

cardiogenic (*kar-de-o-jen'-ik*). Originating in the heart. *C. shock.* A term applied to shock caused by disease or failure of heart action.

cardiogram (*kar'-de-o-gram*). A tracing made by the cardiograph.

cardiograph (*kar'-de-o-graf*). An instrument for registering the movements of the heart.

cardiologist (*kar-de-ol'-o-jist*). One who has made a particular study of the diagnosis and treatment of heart disease.

cardiology (*kar-de-ol'-o-je*). The study of the heart and how it works.

cardiolysis (*kar-de-ol'-is-is*). The breaking down of adhesions between the pericardium and chest wall, by operation.

cardiomyopathy (*kar-de-o-mi-op'-ath-e*). A myocarditis that may accompany an acute fever and require prolonged rest even after the original condition is cured.

cardiomyotomy (*kar-de-o-mi-ot'-o-me*). An operation to divide the circular muscle fibres at the cardiac end of the stomach to relieve cardiospasm.

cardiopathy (*kar-de-op'-ath-e*). Any disease of the heart.

cardiopulmonary (*kar-de-o-pul'-mon-ar-e*). Relating to the heart and lungs. *C. bypass.* The use of the heart lung machine to oxygenate and pump the blood round the body while the surgeon operates on the heart.

cardiospasm (*kar'-de-o-spazm*). Spasm of the sphincter muscle at the cardiac end of the stomach, it may result in dilatation of the oesophagus.

cardiotocography (*kar-de-o-to-kog'-raf-e*). The instantaneous recording of the fetal heart rate, fetal movements and the uterine contractions in order to discover possible lack of oxygen (hypoxia) to the fetus. Fetal monitoring.

cardiotomy syndrome (*kar-de-ot'-o-me sin'-drome*). An inflammatory reaction following heart surgery. There is pyrexia, pericarditis, and pleural effusion.

cardiovascular (*kar-de-o-vas'-ku-lar*). Concerning the heart and blood vessels.

cardioversion (*kar-de-o-ver'-shun*). A method of terminating abnormal heart rhythm as in atrial fibrillation by means of electrodes and an electrical discharge.

carditis (*kar-di'-tis*). Inflammation of the heart.

caries (*kair'-re-eez*). Suppuration and subsequent decay of bone, corresponding to ulceration in soft tissues. In *caries*, the bone dissolves; in *necrosis* it separates in large pieces and is thrown off. *Dental c.* Decay of the teeth due to penetration of bacteria through the enamel to the dentine. *Spinal c.* Pott's disease (*q.v.*).

carina (*kar'-een-ah*). The term applied to the bifurcation of the trachea into the bronchi as the terminal cartilage is keel-shaped.

carminative (*kar'-min-a-tiv*). An aromatic drug which relieves flatulence. Cloves, ginger, cardamon, and peppermint are examples.

carneous mole (*kar'-ne-us*). A tumour of organized blood clot surrounding a dead fetus in the uterus. *See* Abortion.

carotene (*kar'-ot-een*). The colouring matter in carrots, tomatoes, and other yellow foods and fats. It is a provitamin capable of conversion into vitamin A in the liver. *See* Appendix 10.

carotid (*kar-ot'-id*). The principal artery on each side of the neck

carpal tunnel syndrome (*kar'-pal tun'-nel sin'-drome*). Condition in which compression of the median nerve at the wrist causes numbing and tingling in the fingers.

carphology (*kar-fol'-o-je*). Constant picking at the bedclothes, occurring in cases of serious illness, especially in the typhoid state (*q.v.*).

carpopedal spasm (*kar'-po-pe'-dal*). Spasm of the hands and feet as occurs in tetany.

carpus (*kar'-pus*). The eight bones forming the wrist and arranged in two rows: (1) Scaphoid, lunate, triquetral, pisiform. (2) Trapezium, trapezoid, capitate, hamate.

carrier. A person who harbours the micro-organisms of a disease, but is not necessarily affected by it; e.g. *meningococci*

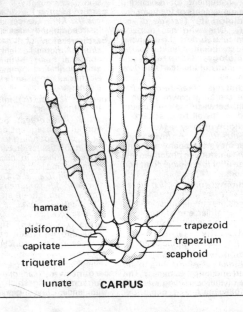

hamate
pisiform
capitate
triquetral
lunate
trapezoid
trapezium
scaphoid

CARPUS

and *diphtheria bacilli* can be harboured in the throat of a healthy person who may infect others by direct contact. *Typhoid c.* One who harbours the organism, as a rule in the gallbladder, by which the faeces are infected. This may be the origin of an epidemic, especially if the water supply be contaminated from such a source.

cartilage (*kar'-til-aj*). Gristle. A tough connective tissue of three varieties: (1) *Hyaline c.* A dense groundwork containing cartilaginous cells, forming the embryonic bones before ossification and covering the articular surfaces of bone. (2) *Fibro-c.* Cartilage in which bundles of white fibres predominate, forming the intervertebral discs and costal cartilages. (3) *Elastic c.* Cartilage containing elastic fibres and forming the pinna of the ear, the epiglottis and part of the nasal septum. *Costal c.* Joins the ribs to the sternum. *Ensiform c.* (xiphoid process). The cartilaginous termination to the sternum.

cartilaginous (*kar-til-aj'-in-us*). Of the nature of cartilage.

caruncle (*kar-ung'-kl*). (1) A small reddish body situated at the medial junction of the eyelids. (2) A small fleshy growth, occurring chiefly at the urinary orifice in females, and giving rise to great pain on micturition.

cascara (*kas-kar'-ah*). A laxative prepared from the bark of the Californian buckthorn. It may be prepared as an elixir or as tablets.

caseation (*ka-se-a'-shun*). Degeneration in tuberculous infection, forming a cheesy mass.

casein (*ka'-se-in*). The chief protein of milk. It forms a curd from which cheese is made. *C. hydrolysate.* A predigested con-

centrated protein; a useful supplement for a high protein diet.

caseinogen (*ka-se-in'-o-jen*). The precursor of casein—activated by rennin.

Casilan (*kas'-e-lan*). A proprietary preparation of calcium caseinate. A fine powder containing 90 per cent protein. A useful aid where a high protein diet is required.

castor oil (*kah'-stor*). Internally it is a purgative. Least nauseous when given with lemon or brandy. Externally it is protective and soothing and may be used in ointments or in eye drops.

castration (*kas-tra'-shun*). Removal of the testicles or, in a female, the ovaries.

casts (*kahsts*). Plastic material thrown off in various diseases, and moulded to the shape of that part in which it has accumulated. *Renal c.* or *hyaline c.* are degenerating cells cast off into the urine in some cases of chronic kidney disease.

catabolism (*kat-ab'-ol-izm*). Katabolism. The breaking down process in tissue structure. *See* Metabolism.

catalase (*kat'-al-aze*). An enzyme found in many body cells.

catalepsy (*kat'-a-lep-se*). (1) A nervous state characterized by a trance-like sleep with passive rigidity of the muscles. During an attack the limbs will remain in any position in which they are placed. (2) A stage of hypnosis where the limbs remain rigid and in any position suggested.

catalyst (*kat'-a-list*). A substance which hastens or brings about a chemical change without itself undergoing alteration; e.g. enzyme action during digestion.

catamenia (*kat-a-me'-ne-ah*).

The menses or monthly discharge of blood from the uterus.

cataphoresis (*kat-a-for-e'-sis*). A method of introducing drugs through the skin. *See* Ionization.

cataplasm (*kat'-a-plazm*). A poultice. It acts as a counter-irritant. Materials of which it can be made are: *linseed*, *bread* and *bran*. Kaolin is more frequently used.

cataract (*kat'-a-rakt*). Opacity of the crystalline lens of the eye causing blindness. It may be congenital, senile or due to diabetes.

catarrh (*kat-ar'*). Simple inflammation of a mucous membrane accompanied by an excessive discharge of mucus. It is usually a chronic condition of the nose or nasopharynx with few signs of inflammation.

catatonia (*kat-a-to'-ne-ah*). A symptom occurring in schizophrenia, but less commonly in organic cerebral disease, characterized by stupor (*q.v.*), the adoption of strange postures and outbursts of excitement and hyperactivity. The patient may change suddenly from one of these states to another.

catecholamines (*kat-e-kol-am'-eens*). A group of compounds that have the effect of sympathetic nerve stimulation. They have an aromatic and an amine portion and include dopamine, adrenaline and noradrenaline.

catechu (*kat'-e-choo*). A powerfully astringent extract of the leaves and young shoots of Acacia. It may be given to check diarrhoea but refined kaolin is more effective.

catgut (*kat'-gut*). A substance prepared from the intestines of sheep and used in surgery for sutures and ligatures. It be-

comes gradually absorbed in the body. Careful and thorough sterilization is needed, as it cannot be subjected to high temperatures.

catharsis (*kath-ar'-sis*). (1) Purgation. (2) Abreaction (*q.v.*).

cathartic (*kath-ar'-tik*). Purgative.

catheter (*kath'-e-ter*). A fine hollow tube for removing or inserting fluid into a body cavity or viscus. Most commonly associated with the urinary bladder and made of plastic material or rubber. *Cardiac c.* A plastic one used in investigation of heart abnormalities. *See* Cardiac. *Eustachian c.* A silver one used to open up the pharyngotympanic tube. *Self-retaining c.* A catheter made in such a way that after introduction the blind end expands so that it can remain in the bladder. Useful for continuous or intermittent drainage or where frequent specimens are required. *Ureteric c.* A fine catheter passed up the ureter to the renal pelvis and used to insert a dye in retrograde pyelography.

catherization (*kath'-et-er-i-za'-shun*). The use of a catheter.

cathode (*kath'-ode*). The negative electrode which is joined to the negative pole of a battery.

cation (*kat'-i-on*). A positively charged ion which moves towards the cathode when an electric current is passed through an electrolytic solution. *See* Anion.

cauda (*kaw'-dah*). A tail. *C. equina.* The bundle of sacral and lumbar nerves with which the spinal cord terminates.

caudal (*kaw'-dal*). Referring to the cauda. *C. block.* An anaesthetic agent injected into the sacral canal, so that operations may be carried out in the perineal area without the risk of a general anaesthetic.

caul (*kawl*). The amnion, which occasionally does not rupture, but envelops the infant's head at birth.

causalgia (*kaws-al'-je-ah*). An intense burning pain which persists after nerve injuries.

caustic (*kaws'-tik*). A substance capable of burning organic tissue. Silver nitrate (*lunar c.*), carbolic acid, and carbon dioxide snow are those most commonly used in surgery.

cautery (*kaw'-ter-e*). The means of applying a caustic substance. *Actual c.* Cauterizing by direct heat. *Electric c.* A wire heated to red or white heat by means of electricity.

cavernous (*kav'-er-nus*). Having caverns or hollows. *C. breathing.* Sounds heard on auscultation over a pulmonary cavity. *C. sinus.* A venous channel lying on either side of the body of the sphenoid bone through which pass the internal carotid artery and several nerves. *C. sinus thrombosis.* A very serious complication of any infection of the face, the veins from the orbit draining into this and carrying the infection into the cranium.

cavitation (*kav-e-ta'-shun*). The formation of cavities, e.g. in the lung in tuberculosis.

cavity (*kav'-et-e*). A confined space or hollow with containing walls.

cells (*sels*). Microscopic masses of protoplasm of which all organic tissues are made.

cellulitis (*sel-u-lī'-tis*). Streptococcal inflammation of cellular tissue which causes a typical brawny, oedematous appearance of the part, but local abscess formation is not common.

cellulose (*sel'-u-loze*). (1) A carbohydrate forming the covering of vegetable cells, i.e. vegetable fibres. Not digestible in the alimentary tract of man, but gives bulk, and as 'roughage' stimulates peristalsis. (2) Specially prepared cellulose tissue is a cheap form of absorbent dressing for wounds.

Celsius scale (*A. Celsius, Swedish astronomer, 1701–44*). Name now frequently applied to the centigrade temperature scale.

censor (*sen'-sor*). According to Freud, the psychic phenomenon which normally prevents impressions from the unconscious mind reaching the consciousness.

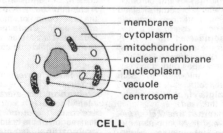

membrane
cytoplasm
mitochondrion
nuclear membrane
nucleoplasm
vacuole
centrosome

CELL

centi-. A prefix meaning a hundredth part of. Used in the metric system of weights and measures. *See* Appendix 6.

centigrade (*sen'-te-grade*). The scale of heat measurement used in those countries where the metric system is employed. It is now usually called the Celsius scale. The thermometer registers 100°, as the boiling-point of water, and 0° (zero) as the freezing-point. *See* Fahrenheit.

central venous pressure. The pressure recorded by the introduction of a catheter into the right atrium, in order to monitor the condition of a patient after major operative procedures such as heart surgery.

centrifugal (*sen-trif'-u-gal*). Conveying away from a centre, such as from the brain to the periphery. Efferent.

centrifuge (*sen'-trif-uj*). An apparatus which will hold a test-tube, and permits rotation at great speed. If the tube is filled with fluid, e.g. blood or urine, any bacteria, cells, or other solids in it are precipitated by such rotation.

centripetal (*sen-trip'-et-al*). The reverse of centrifugal. Conveying from the periphery to the centre. Afferent.

centromere (*sen'-tro-meer*). The region(s) of the chromosomes which become(s) allied with the spindle fibres at mitosis (*q.v.*) and meiosis(*q.v.*).

centrosome (*sen'-tro-som*). A body in the cytoplasm of most animal cells, close to the nucleus. It divides during mitosis, and half migrates to each daughter cell.

cephalalgia (*kef-al-al'-je-ah*). Pain in the head.

cephalhaematoma (*kef-al-he-mat-o'-mah*). A subcutaneous swelling containing blood, which may be present on the head of a newborn infant.

cephalic version (*kef-al'-ik ver'-shun*). The method used to convert a transverse into a head presentation to facilitate labour, i.e. turning an abnormal presentation.

cephalocele (*kef'-al-o-seel*). Cerebral hernia. *See* Hernia.

cephalometry (*kef-al-om'-et-re*). The measurement of the fetal head by radiography.

cephaloridine (*kef-al-or'-id-een*). An antibiotic that is effective against a wide range of organisms and useful against penicillin-resistant strains and for urinary infection.

cerebellum (*ser-e-bel'-um*). The portion of the brain below the cerebrum and above the medulla oblongata. The hind-brain.

cerebral (*ser'-e-bral*). Relating to the cerebrum. *C. haemorrhage.* Rupture of a cerebral blood vessel. Likely causes are aneurysm and hypertension. *See* Apoplexy. *C. hernia. See* Hernia. *C. irritation.* A condition of general nervous irritability and abnormality, often with photophobia, which may be an early sign of meningitis, tumour of the brain, etc. It is also associated with trauma, as concussion or contusion. *C. palsy.* A condition caused by injury to the brain during or immediately after birth. Coordination of movement is affected, and may cause the child to be flaccid or athetoid, in which condition he has constant random and uncontrolled movement. *See* Spastics.

cerebration (*ser-e-bra'-shun*). Mental activity.

cerebritis (*ser-e-bri'-tis*). Inflammation of the brain.

cerebrospinal (*ser'-e-bro-spi'-*

nal). Relating to the brain and spinal cord. *C. fever.* A meningitis caused by the meningococcus. *C. fluid.* The fluid made in the choroid plexus of the ventricles of the brain and circulating from them into the subarachnoid space around the brain and spinal cord.

cerebrovascular accident (*ser'-e-bro-vas'-ku-lah*). General term used to describe a cerebral embolism, thrombosis or haemorrhage.

cerebrum (*ser'-e-brum*). The largest part of the brain, occupying the greater portion of the

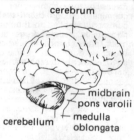

cerebrum

midbrain
pons varolii
cerebellum   medulla
oblongata

CEREBRUM

cranium and consisting of the right and left hemispheres. The centre of the higher functions of the brain.

cerumen (*ser-u'-men*). A waxy substance secreted by the ceruminous glands of the auditory canal.

cervical (*sur-vi'-kal*). Pertaining to the neck. *C. rib.* A short, extra rib, often bilateral, which sometimes occurs on the seventh cervical vertebra and may cause pressure on an artery or nerve.

cervix (*sur'-viks*). A constricted portion or neck. *C. uteri.* The neck of the uterus; it is about 2 cm long and opens into the vagina.

cestode (*ses'-tode*). Tapeworm (*q.v.*).

cetrimide (*set'-re-mide*). Cetyltrimethylammonium bromide (CTAB). A detergent and antiseptic widely used for preoperative skin preparation and the cleansing of wounds. Strength 1 per cent. Cetavlon is a proprietary preparation of it.

cevitamic acid (*se-vit-am'-ik*). Ascorbic acid (*q.v.*).

chalazion (*kal-a'-ze-on*). A Meibomian or tarsal cyst. A sebaceous cyst in the eyelid.

chalicosis (*kal-ik-o'-sis*). A condition resembling silicosis (*q.v.*), but found mainly among stone-cutters, and due to the inhalation of stone dust.

chancre (*shan'-ker*). The initial lesion of syphilis (*q.v.*) developing at the site of inoculation.

chancroid (*shang'-kroid*). Soft chancre. A venereal ulceration, due to Ducrey's bacillus, accompanied by inflammation and suppuration of the local glands.

charcoal (*char'-kole*). Carbon, obtained by burning animal or vegetable tissue. Vegetable charcoal is sometimes given in the form of biscuits or tabloids, in cases of dyspepsia.

Charcot's joint (*J. M. Charcot, French neurologist, 1825–93*). A disease of the head of bones with effusion of fluid into the joints, occurring in locomotor ataxia.

Charcot's triad (*J. M. Charcot, French neurologist, 1825–93*). Nystagmus, intention tremor and scanning speech. An early sign of disseminated sclerosis.

Charnley's clamps (*Sir J. Charnley, contemporary British orthopaedic surgeon*). These consist of two horizontal bars connected by two screw clamps and are used to exert tension on two bone ends following arthrodesis.

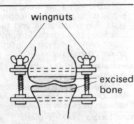

CHARNLEY'S CLAMPS

cheilitis (*ki-li'-tis*). Inflammation of the lip.

cheiloplasty (*ki'-lo-plas-te*). Any plastic operation on the lip.

cheilorrhaphy (*ki-lor'-raf-e*). A suturing or repair of a hare-lip.

cheiloschisis (*ki-los'-kis-is*). Hare-lip (*q.v.*).

cheiropompholyx (*ki-ro-pom'-fo-liks*). A skin disease characterized by vesicles on the palms and soles.

chelate (*kel'-ate*). A chemical organized into a fixed ring structure.

chelating agent (*kel'-at-ing*). A drug that has the power of combining with certain metals and so aiding excretion to prevent or overcome poisoning. *See* Dimercaprol *and* Penicillamine.

chemopallidectomy (*ke-mo-pal-le-dek'-to-me*). The insertion of a chemical to limit activity of the globus pallidum. A treatment for paralysis agitans.

chemoreceptor (*ke-mo-re-sep'-tor*). A sensory nerve ending or group of cells that are excited by chemical stimuli, often those present in the blood stream.

chemosis (*ke-mo'-sis*). Swelling of the conjunctiva, due to the presence of fluid—an oedema of the conjunctiva.

chemotaxis (*kem-o-tak'-sis*). The reaction of living cells to chemical stimuli. These are either attracted (*positive c.*) or repelled (*negative c.*) by acids, alkalis or other substances.

chemotherapy (*ke-mo-ther'-ap-e*). The specific treatment of disease by the administration of chemical compounds. A term commonly applied to the sulphonamide group of drugs.

chest leads. Leads applied to the chest during the course of an electrocardiographical recording.

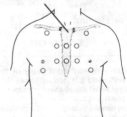

CHEST LEADS FOR ECG

Cheyne–Stokes respiration (*J. Cheyne, British physician, 1776–1836; W. Stokes, British physician, 1804–78*). Tidal respiration. A form of irregular but rhythmic breathing caused by increase in acidity in the blood (e.g. of carbonic acid). There are alternating periods of *hyperpnoea* and *apnoea*. It is likely to be present in advanced cases of arteriosclerosis, uraemia, etc.

chickenpox (*chik'-en-poks*). Varicella (*q.v.*).

chilblain (*chil'-blain*). A condition resulting from defective circulation when exposure to cold causes localized swelling and inflammation of the hands or feet, with severe itching and burning sensations.

chiniofon (*kin'-e-o-fon*). A quinine compound used in treating amoebic dysentery. Quinoxyl is a proprietary preparation.

chiropodist (*ki-rop'-o-dist*). One who treats the feet, particularly regarding corns and conditions of the nails.

chiropody (*ki-rop'-o-de*). The treatment of corns, callosities, and other foot conditions.

chloasma (*klo-az'-mah*). A condition in which there is brown, blotchy discolouration of the skin, appearing on the face, especially during pregnancy.

chloral hydrate (*klor'-al hi'-drate*). A drug used as a hypnotic which does not cause respiratory depression and is well tolerated by children.

chlorambucil (*klor-am'-bu-sil*). A nitrogen mustard preparation used in treating chronic myeloid leukaemia. A cytoxic drug. Leukeran is a proprietary preparation.

chloramine (*klor'-a-min*). An antiseptic which owes its power to its chlorine content (used in 3 per cent solution). A special preparation of it is *chloramine T.*

chloramphenicol (*klor-am-fen'-e-kol*). An oral antibiotic which may give rise to agranu-

locytosis. The drug of choice for treating typhoid fever. Used in drops and ointment for eye infections. Chloromycetin is a proprietary preparation of it.

chlorbutol (*klor-bu'-tol*). Chloretone. A mild sedative; used to prevent sea-sickness or overcome vomiting due to radiotherapy.

chlordiazepoxide (*klor-di-az-e-poks'-ide*). A drug that depresses the central nervous system and so relieves anxiety and tension. Librium is a proprietary preparation.

chlorhexidine (*klor-heks'-e-din*). An antiseptic derived from coal tar that has a wide antibacterial action and is used as a skin antiseptic and as a disinfectant solution for instruments. Hibitane is a proprietary preparation of it.

chloride of lime (*klor'-ide*). A powerful disinfectant and bleaching agent, composed of lime and chlorine.

chlorine (*klor'-een*). A yellow, irritating poisonous gas. A well-known poison gas. The chief element in Dakin's solution and eusol (*q.v.*).

chloro-acetone (*klor'-o as'-e-tone*). Tear gas.

chlorocresol (*klor-o-kre'-sol*). A coal tar product with a bacteriocidal action more powerful than phenol and a lower toxicity. Used as an antiseptic and as a preservative in injection fluids.

chlorodyne (*klor'-o-deen*). A carminative mixture used for treating diarrhoea containing chloroform and morphine.

chloroform (*klor'-o-form*). A colourless volatile liquid, administered through inhalation as a general anaesthetic. *C. liniment.* Equal parts of chloroform and camphor liniment. *C. water.* Used in pharmacy to disguise the taste of nauseous drugs.

chloroma (*klor-o'-mah*). A sarcoma having a greenish colour, usually found in skull bones. It is accompanied by symptoms resembling leukaemia.

chlorophyll (*klor'-o-fil*). The green pigment of plants, closely related to the pigment in haemoglobin. An ingredient in many deodorants.

chloroquine (*klor'-o-kwin*). An antimalarial drug that has a strong suppressant action and may also be used in the treatment of amoebic hepatitis and rheumatoid arthritis.

chlorothiazide (*klor-o-thi'-azide*). An oral diuretic which is rapidly excreted. If used for long periods potassium chloride should be administered as there is a loss of chloride and potassium in the diuresis. This may be supplied as chlorothiazide K. Saluric is a proprietary preparation of it.

chloroxylenol (*klor-ok-zi'-lenol*). An antiseptic which is less irritating to the skin and mucous membranes than cresol and has a powerful disinfectant action. Roxenol is a proprietary preparation of it and Dettol is very similar.

chlorpheniramine maleate (*klor-fen-ir'-a-meen mal'-e-ate*). An antihistamine drug that has no sedative action but is useful in combating or preventing allergic reactions to blood transfusions and to other drugs. Piriton is a propietary preparation of it.

chlorpromazine (*klor-pro'-maz-een*). A sedative antiemetic drug used in psychiatry. It is also hypotensive and enhances the effect of analgesics and anaesthetics. It may cause skin sensitization, jaundice and Parkinsonism. Largactil is a proprietary preparation of it.

chlorpropamide (*klor-pro'-pam-ide*). An hypoglycaemic agent used in the treatment of mild diabetes. Diabinese is a proprietary preparation.

chlortetracycline (*klor-tet-rah-si'-kleen*). A wide-range antibiotic effective in treating many pathogenic infections that do not respond to penicillin. Aureomycin.

chocolate cyst. *See* Cyst.

cholaemia (*ko-le'-me-ah*). The presence of bile in the blood, causing jaundice.

cholagogue (*ko'-la-gog*). A drug which increases the flow of bile, e.g. magnesium sulphate.

cholangiogram (*ko-lan'-je-o-gram*). A radiological film of the hepatic, cystic and bile ducts after the insertion of a dye.

cholangitis (*ko-lan-ji'-tis*). Inflammation of the bile ducts.

cholecystangiogram (*ko-le-sis-tan'-je-o-gram*). A radiological film of the gall-bladder, and the cystic and common bile ducts.

cholecystduodenostomy (*ko-le-sist-du-o-den-os'-to-me*). An anastomosis between the gall-bladder and the duodenum.

cholecystectomy (*ko-le-sis-tek'-to-me*). Excision of the gall-bladder.

cholecystenterostomy (*ko-le-sis-ten-ter-os'-to-me*). The formation of an artificial opening from the gall-bladder into the intestine. An operation performed in cases of obstruction of the bile duct, e.g. due to a growth of the head of the pancreas.

cholecystitis (*ko-le-sis-ti'-tis*). Inflammation of the gall-bladder.

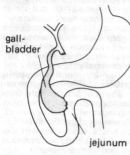

**CHOLECYST—
ENTEROSTOMY**

cholecystogastrostomy (*ko-le-sis-to-gas-tros'-to-me*). An operation by which the gall-bladder is made to open into the stomach.

cholecystography (*ko-le-sis-tog'-raf-e*). X-ray photography of the gall-bladder after it has been made opaque by administration of a radio-opaque dye.

cholecystokinin (*ko-le-sis-to-kin'-in*). A hormone released by the presence of fat in the duodenum which causes contraction of the gall-bladder.

cholecystolithiasis (*ko-le-sis-to-lith-ī'-as-is*). Stones in the gall-bladder.

cholecystotomy (*ko-le-sis-tot'-o-me*). An incision into the gall-bladder.

choledocholithotomy (*ko-le-dok-o-lith-ot'-o-me*). Incision into the bile ducts to remove stones.

choledochostomy (*ko-le-dok-os'-to-me*). Opening and draining the common bile duct.

cholelithiasis (*ko-le-lith-ī'-as-is*). Presence of gall-stones in the gall-bladder or bile ducts.

cholera (*kol'-er-ah*). An acute infectious disease caused by *Vibrio cholerae* from infected water. It is marked by profuse diarrhoea, muscle cramp, suppression of urine and severe prostration.

cholestasis (*ko-le-sta'-sis*). Arrest of the flow of bile.

cholesteatoma (*ko-les-te-at-o'-mah*). (1) A small tumour of dermal tissue which may occur in the middle ear. (2) A type of cerebral tumour.

cholesterol (*ko-les'-ter-ol*). A sterol found in nervous tissue, red blood corpuscles, animal fat and bile. Excess in the bile can lead to gall-stone formation.

cholesterolosis (*ko-les-ter-ol-o'-sis*). A condition of the gall-bladder when the mucosa is studded with deposits of cholesterol.

choline (*ko'-leen*). A vitamin of the B group that exists in the colon and in many plants. It aids fat metabolism and deficiency leads to fatty degeneration and cirrhosis of the liver. *C. theophyllinate*. An antispasmodic drug used in respiratory conditions. Choledyl is a proprietary preparation.

cholinergic (*ko-lin-er'-jik*). Applied to nerves that release acetylcholine at their nerve endings as the chemical stimulator. *C. drugs*. These inhibit cholinesterase and so prevent the destruction of acetylcholine.

cholinesterase (*ko-lin-est'-er-ase*). An enzyme which rapidly destroys the chemical transmitter acetylcholine (*q.v.*).

choluria (*ko-lu'-re-ah*). The presence of bile in the urine.

chondritis (*kon-dri'-tis*). Inflammation of cartilage.

chondroblast (*kon'-dro-blast*).

CHO 74

An embryonic cell which forms cartilage.

chondrocyte (*kon'-dro-site*). A cartilage cell.

chondroma (*kon-dro'-mah*). An innocent new growth arising in cartilage.

chondromalacia (*kon'-dro-mal-a'-she-ah*). A condition of abnormal softening of cartilage.

chondrosarcoma (*kon'-dro-sar-ko'-mah*). A malignant new growth arising from cartilaginous tissue.

chordee (*kor-de'*). Painful erection of the penis, usually due to gonorrhoeal inflammation.

chorditis (*kor-di'-tis*). Inflammation of a vocal cord.

chordotomy (*kor-dot'-o-me*). An operation on the spinal cord to divide the anterolateral nerve pathways for relief of intractable pain. Also cordotomy.

chorea (*ko-re'-ah*). St Vitus' dance. A nervous disease of rheumatic origin characterized by irregular and involuntary contraction of muscles. *Huntington's c.* The adult form, with cerebral degenerative changes, leading to dementia. A familial disease. *Sydenham's c.* Usually acute chorea.

choreic (*ko'-re-ik*). Involuntary movements of an irregular jerky nature.

choreo-athetotic (*ko'-re-o-ath-e-tot'-ik*). A combination of the jerky movements with the writhing action of athetosis. Seen in some cerebral lesions, most often in children.

chorion (*kor'-e-on*). The outer membrane enveloping the fetus. The placenta (*q.v.*).

choriocarcinoma (*kor-e-o-kar-sin-o'-mah*). A malignant growth originating from chorionic tissue. *See* Chorion epithelioma.

chorion epithelioma (*kor'-e-on ep-e-the-le-o'-mah*). A malignant growth of the uterus which may develop after an abortion or evacuation of a hydatidiform mole, when the uterus was not completely emptied. Metastases usually develop rapidly.

chorionic gonadotrophin (HCG) (*kor-e-on'-ik gon-ad-o-tro-fin'*). *See* Human chorionic gonadotrophin.

chorionic villi (*kor-e-on'-ik*). Structures of the chorion which give it a shaggy appearance, and from which the placenta is formed. They are in close association with the maternal blood, and by diffusion interchange of nutriment, oxygen, and waste matters is effected between it and the fetal blood.

chorioretinitis (*kor'-e-o-ret-in-i'-tis*). Inflammation affecting both the choroid coat and the retina of the eye.

choroid (*kor'-oid*). The pigmented and vascular coat of the eyeball, continuous with the iris and situated between the sclera and retina. *C. plexus.* Specialized cells in the ventricles of the brain which produce cerebrospinal fluid. There is one choroid plexus in each ventricle.

choroiditis (*kor-oid-i'-tis*). Inflammation of the choroid.

choroidocyclitis (*kor-oid-o-si-kli'-tis*). Inflammation of the choroid and ciliary body.

choroidoretinitis (*kor-oid-o-ret-in-i'-tis*). An inflammatory condition of both the choroid and retina of the eye. May be termed chorioretinitis.

Christmas disease (*krist'-mas*). A form of haemophilia in which the blood is defective in clotting Factor IX. Name devised from the first patient to be studied.

chromatogram (*kro'-mat-o-*

gram). The tracing produced by chromatography.

chromatography (*kro-mat-og'-raf-e*). A method of chemical analysis by which substances in solution can be separated as they percolate down a column of powdered absorbent or ascend an absorbent paper by capillary traction. A definite pattern is produced and substances may be recognized by the use of appropriate colour reagents. Amino acids can be separated in this way and the antianaemic factor isolated from liver extract.

chromatolysis (*kro-mat-ol'-is-sis*). The disintegration and disappearance of the Nissl granules of a neurone if the axon is severed.

chromatosis (*kro-mat-o'-sis*). A condition of abnormal pigmentation of the skin. *See* Addison's disease.

chromic acid (*kro'-mik as'-id*). A strong caustic sometimes used for the removal of warts.

chromicize (*kro'-mis-ize*). To impregnate with chromic acid, e.g. chromicized catgut.

chromophil adenoma (*kro'-mo-fil ad-en-o'-mah*). The tumour of the pituitary gland that gives rise to gigantism and acromegaly.

chromophobe adenoma (*kro'-mo-fobe*). The commonest of the pituitary tumours giving rise to hypopituitarism.

chromosomes (*kro'-mo-somes*). The filaments into which the nucleus of a cell divides during mitosis (*q.v.*). Each chromosome consists of hundreds of molecules of nucleoprotein called genes (*q.v.*).

chronic (*kron'-ik*). Of long duration, the opposite to acute.

Chvostek's sign (*F. Chvostek, Austrian surgeon, 1835–84*). A spasm of the facial muscles which occurs in tetany. It can be elicited by tapping the facial nerve.

chrysarobin (*kris-ar-o'-bin*). A derivative of Goa powder, used in ointment form, especially in the treatment of psoriasis. As it is irritant to the eyes, it must be used with care and not applied to the face. It stains linen a yellow colour, therefore special sheets should be kept for these cases. Benzole will remove the stains. *See* Dithranol.

chyle (*kile*). Digested fats which, as a milky fluid, are absorbed into the lymphatic capillaries (*lacteals*) in the villi of the small intestine.

chyluria (*ki-lu'-re-ah*). The presence of chyle in the urine. Possibly due to a lymphatic vessel communicating with the urinary tract, as may occur in filariasis.

chyme (*kime*). The semi-liquid, acid mass of food which passes from the stomach to the intestines.

chymotrypsin (*ki-mo-trip'-sin*). An enzyme from the pancreatic secretion. It is activated by trypsin and aids in the breakdown of proteins.

cicatrix (*sik'-a-triks*). The scar of a healed wound.

cilia (*sil'-e-ah*). (1) Eyelashes. (2) Slender microscopic filaments projecting from some epithelial cells, e.g. in the bronchi, which wave the secretion upwards.

ciliary (*sil'-e-ar-e*). Hair-like. *C. body.* Structure just behind the corneo-scleral margin composed of the ciliary muscle and processes. *C. muscle.* The circular muscle surrounding the lens of the eye. *C. processes.* The fringed part of the choroid coat arranged in a circle in front of the lens.

Cimex (*sī'-meks*). A genus of blood-sucking bugs. *C. lectularius.* The common bed-bug.

cinchocaine (*sin'-ko-kane*). A local anaesthetic agent. It may be used in the form of a solution, eye drops, lozenges or rectal suppositories.

cinchona (*sin-ko'-nah*). Peruvian bark, from which quinine is obtained.

cinchonism (*sin'-ko-nizm*). Poisonous effect of cinchona and its alkaloids, i.e. tinnitus, deafness, headache and giddiness, and weakness of heart muscle. Quininism.

cineangiocardiography (*sin-e-an-je-o-kar-de-og'-raf-e*). The photographic record of fluoroscopic images of the heart and blood vessels, by which the movements of the organs may be seen.

cinnamon (*sin'-am-on*). An extract from the bark of an East Indian laurel, used in medicine as a digestive and carminative.

circinate (*sur'-sin-ate*). Having a circular outline. Ringworm of the body is *tinea circinata.*

circle of Willis (*T. Willis, British physician and anatomist, 1621–75*). An anastomosis of arteries at the base of the brain, formed by the branches of the internal carotids and the branches of the basilar artery.

circulation (*sur-ku-la'-shun*). Movement in a circular course, as of the blood. *Collateral c.* Enlargement of small vessels, establishing adequate blood supply when the main vessel to the part has been occluded. *Coronary c.* The system of vessels which supply the heart muscle itself. *Extracorporeal c.* The blood is removed by intravenous cannulae, passed through a machine to oxygenate it and then pumped back into circulation. Termed the 'heart-lung' machine or pump respirator, it is used in cardiac surgery. *Lymph c.* The flow of lymph through lymph vessels and glands. *Portal c.* The passage of the blood from the alimentary tract, pancreas, and spleen, via the portal vein and its branches through the liver and into the hepatic veins. *Pulmonary c.* Passage of the blood from the right ventricle via the pulmonary artery through the lungs and back to the heart by the pulmonary veins. *Systemic c.* That of the blood throughout the body. The direction of flow is from the left atrium to the left ventricle and through the aorta with its branches and capillaries. Veins then carry it back to the right atrium, and so into the right ventricle.

circumcision (*sur-kum-siz'-shun*). Excision of a circular portion of the prepuce. An operation usually performed on young boys to allow the prepuce to be drawn back over the glans penis to facilitate urination and cleansing of the penis.

circumduction (*sur-kum-duk'-shun*). Moving in a circle, e.g. the circular movement of the upper limb.

circumoral (*sur-kum-or'-al*). Around the mouth. *C. pallor.* A pale area around the mouth contrasting with the flushed cheeks in scarlet fever.

circumvallate (*sur-kum-val'-ate*). Surrounded by a wall. *C. papilla. See* Papilla.

cirrhosis (*sir-o'-sis*). A degenerative change which can occur in any organ, but especially in the liver, caused by various poisons bacterial or otherwise. Fibrosis results, and this interferes with the working of the organ. In the liver it causes portal obstruction, with consequent ascites. *Alcoholic c.* A result of chronic alcoholism and nutritional deficiency which affects the liver.

cisterna (*sis-ter' nah*). A space or cavity containing fluid. *C. chyli.* The dilated portion of the thoracic duct containing chyle. *C. magna.* The subarachnoid space between the cerebellum and medulla oblongata.

cisternal (*sis-ter'-nal*). Concerning the cisterna. *C. puncture.* Insertion of a hollow needle into the cisterna magna to withdraw cerebrospinal fluid as an alternative to lumbar puncture.

citric acid (*sit'-rik as'-id*). The juice of lemons, limes, etc. An antiscorbutic.

clamp. A metal surgical instrument used to compress any part of the body, e.g. to prevent or arrest haemorrhage.

claudication (*klaw-dik-a'-shun*). Lameness. *Intermittent c.* Limping, accompanied by severe pain in the legs on walking, which disappears with rest. Associated with spasm of arteries

claustrophobia (*klaw-stro-fo'-be-ah*). Fear of confined spaces like small rooms.

clavicle (*klav'-ikl*). The collarbone.

clavus (*kla'-vus*). A corn. *C. hystericus.* A pain near the midline on top of the skull associated with hysteria.

cleft palate. A congenital defect in the roof of the mouth, due to failure of the medial plates of the palate to meet. Speech is indistinct, words being slurred. A plastic operation may be performed, or a plate fitted over the gap. Hare-

lip is often present at the same time.

climacteric (*kli-mak'-ter-ik*). The period of the menopause in women. *C. psychoses.* Mental disorders occurring at this time.

clinical (*klin'-ik-al*). Relating to bedside observation and treatment of patients.

clinicopathological (*klin-e-ko-path-o-loj'-ik-al*). Relating to both the symptoms and pathology of disease.

clinicoradiological (*klin-e-ko-ra-de-o-loj'-ik-al*). Relating the bedside observations to the results of radiological investigations.

clitoridectomy (*klit-or-id-ek'-to-me*). Excision of the clitoris.

clitoris (*klit'-or-is*). A small organ, formed of erectile tissue, in front of the urethra in the female. The homologue of the penis.

cloaca (*klo-a'-kah*). An opening to the exterior for the purpose of discharge of waste: (1) An anus; (2) Opening through newly formed bone from a diseased area so that pus may escape. *See* Involucrum.

clofibrate (*klo-fib'-rate*). A drug used to lower the blood cholesterol. Atromid-S is a proprietary preparation.

clonic (*klon'-ik*). Having the character of clonus.

clonus (*klo'-nus*). Muscle rigidity and relaxation which occurs spasmodically. *Ankle c.* Spasmodic movements of the calf muscles when the foot is suddenly pushed upwards, the leg being extended. A reaction which may be an indication of spinal cord disease.

Clostridium (*klos-trid'-e-um*). A genus of anaerobic spore-forming bacilli, found as commensals of the gut of animals and man and as saprophytes of the soil. Pathogenic species include *Cl. tetani* (tetanus), *Cl. welchii* (gas gangrene), *Cl. botulinum* (botulism).

clotting or coagulation time. The length of time taken for shed blood to coagulate. The normal is 4 to 8 min.

clove hitch. A knot. A simple sling formed by making two similar loops with a length of bandage and placing the first behind the second.

cloxacillin (*kloks-a-sil'-in*). A form of penicillin effective against penicillin - resistant staphylococci for the treatment of which it should be reserved. Orbenin is a proprietary name.

clubbed fingers. Broadening and thickening of the tips of the fingers (and toes), due to bad circulation. It occurs in chronic diseases of the heart and respiratory system, e.g. congenital cardiac defect, tuberculosis, etc.

clubfoot. Talipes (*q.v.*).

clumping. Describes the action of bacteria and blood cells when agglutination (*q.v.*) occurs.

Clutton's joint (*H. H. Clutton, British surgeon, 1850–1909*). A painless synovial swelling of joints, which may occur in congenital syphilis.

coagulase (*ko-ag'-u-laze*). An enzyme formed by pathogenic staphylococci that causes coagulation of plasma. Such bacteria are termed *C. positive*.

coagulum (*ko-ag-u-lum*). The mass of fibrin and cells when blood clots or the mass formed when other substances coagulate, e.g. milk curd.

coalesce (*ko-al-ess'*). To come together or to converge.

coal tar. A viscid fluid obtained from coal and petroleum, from which many germicides are derived, e.g. benzole, phenol, aniline dyes, etc.

coarctation (*ko-ark-ta'-shun*). A condition of contraction or

COARCTATION OF AORTA

stricture. *C. of aorta.* Usually a congenital defect which may be incompatible with life, but in many cases a compensating collateral circulation is established. Surgical resection of the stricture may be performed.

cobalt (*ko-balt*). A hard metal. *Radioactive c.* Cobalt 60 used as a source of gamma irradiation in radiotherapy.

cocaine (*ko-kane'*). A colourless alkaloid obtained from coca leaves, used as a local anaesthetic applied to mucous membranes for nose and throat treatments. For local anaesthesia it is increasingly being replaced by less toxic synthetic preparations like procaine, lignocaine and amethocaine. Cocaine is a drug of addiction.

cocainism (*ko-kane'-izm*). The condition following continued use of cocaine, when the initial stimulation and feeling of well-being is followed by mental and physical deterioration. Danger of cardiac failure.

coccus (*kok'-us*). A micro-organism of spheroidal shape.

coccydynia (*koks-e-din'-e-ah*). Persistent pain in the region of the coccyx usually following trauma.

coccygodynia (*koks-e-go-din'-e-ah*). Coccydynia (*q.v.*).

coccyx (*koks'-iks*). The terminal bone of the spinal column, in which four rudimentary vertebrae are fused together.

cochlea (*kok'-le-ah*). The spiral canal of the internal ear.

codeine (*ko'-deen*). An alkaloid of opium said to be less depressant to the respiratory centre than other forms, and particularly favoured for persistent cough in bronchitis, etc. An analgesic and hypnotic.

cod-liver oil. Purified oil from the liver of the cod-fish, partic-

ularly valuable for its vitamin A and D content.

coeliac disease (*se'-le-ak*). A condition of early childhood characterized by steatorrhoea (*q.v.*), distended abdomen and failure to grow. The failure of carbohydrate and fat metabolism appears to be due to the gluten in wheat flour. It is treated by giving a gluten-free diet. *See* Appendix 10.

co-enzyme (*ko-en'-zime*). Small non-protein molecules that are accessory to the larger protein enzyme and necessary for its function.

coffee ground vomit. Vomit which contains blood which has been partly digested.

cognition (*kog-nish'-un*). Action of knowing. Cognitive function of the conscious mind in contrast to the affective (feeling) and conative (willing).

coitus (*ko'-it-us*). Sexual intercourse. Copulation.

colchicum (*kol'-chik-um*). A drug obtained from the seeds of *Colchicum autumnale.* Used in treating gout.

colectomy (*ko-lek'-to-me*). The excision of a portion or all of the colon.

colic (*kol'-ik*). Severe pain due to spasmodic contraction of the involuntary muscle of tubes. *Biliary c.* Due to presence of a gall-stone in a bile duct. *Intestinal c.* Severe griping abdominal pain which may be a symptom of food poisoning or of intestinal obstruction. *Painter's c.* A sign of chronic lead poisoning to which painters are especially prone. *Renal c.* Presence of a stone in the ureter. *Uterine c.* Dysmenorrhoea (*q.v.*).

coliform (*ko'-li-form*). Resembling the bacillus *Escherichia coli.*

colitis (*ko-li'-tis*). A condition

of inflammation of the colon. It may be due to a specific organism, as in dysentery, but the term *ulcerative c.* denotes a chronic disease often of unknown cause in which there are attacks of diarrhoea with the passage of blood and mucus.

collagen (*kol'-a-jen*). A protein constituent of fibrous tissue. *C. diseases.* Those in which there is a typical fibrinoid degeneration of collagen, e.g. rheumatic fever, rheumatoid arthritis and scleroderma (*q.v.*).

collapse (*kol-laps'*). (1) A state of extreme prostration due to defective action of the heart, severe shock or haemorrhage. (2) Falling in of a structure. *C. of lung.* A condition due to alteration of air pressure between the inside of the lung and the pleural cavity. *See* Pneumothorax. *Lobar c.* One or more lobes of the lung collapse due to blockage of a bronchus.

collateral (*kol-lat'-er-al*). Accessory to. *C. circulation.* An alternative to the direct route.

Colles's fracture (*A. Colles, Irish surgeon, 1773–1843*). Fracture of the lower end of the radius at the wrist. It is usually impacted and the styloid process of the ulna may be torn off. Typically, it produces the 'dinner fork' deformity.

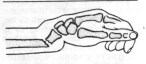

COLLES'S FRACTURE

collodion (*kol-lo'-de-on*). A solution of *pyroxylin* (gun-cotton) in alcohol and ether, which, when exposed to the air, becomes solid by evaporation of the solvents. It is used in surgery as a protective covering for small clean wounds. *C. flexile.* Solution which contains oils to prevent cracking.

colloid (*kol'-loid*). A gelatinous fluid made by substances suspended in a medium but not forming a sediment.

colloidal gold test (*kol-loid'-al*). *See* Test.

coloboma (*kol-o-bo'-mah*). A congenital fissure of the eye affecting the choroid coat and the retina.

colon (*ko'-lon*). The large intestine from the caecum to the rectum. *Ascending c.* That part to the right of the abdomen to the liver. *Descending c.* From the spleen to the rectum. *Giant c.* Megalon (*q.v.*). *Irritable c.* A nervous type, associated with abdominal pain and distension. *Pelvic c.* That part in the pelvis. *Transverse c.* That across the upper abdomen connecting the ascending and descending portions.

colonic lavage (*ko-lon'-ik lav'-aj*). *See* Lavage.

colony (*kol'-on-e*). A mass of bacteria formed by multiplication of cells when bacteria are incubated under favourable conditions.

colostomy (*ko-los'-to-me*). The surgical formation of a permanent opening into the colon. This acts as an abdominal artificial anus.

colostrum (*kol-os'-trum*). The first fluid from the mother's breasts after childbirth. It contains more protein but less fat and sugar than true milk.

colour blindness. Achromatopsia (*q.v.*).

colour index. Estimated in examination of the blood by finding the ratio between the per-

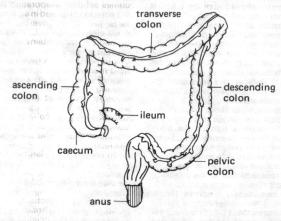

transverse colon

ascending colon

descending colon

ileum

caecum

pelvic colon

anus

COLON

centage of haemoglobin present to the number of red blood cells. Normal is taken to = 1. *See* Blood.

colpitis (*kol-pi'-tis*). Inflammation of the vagina.

colpocele (*kol'-po-seel*). A hernia into the vagina.

colpocleisis (*kol-po-kli'-sis*). Closure of the vagina by surgical means.

colpohysterectomy (*kol-po-his-ter-ek'-to-me*). Removal of the uterus through the vagina, usually for prolapse of uterus.

colpoperineorrhaphy (*kol-po-per-in-e-or'-af-e*). The repair by suturing of an injured vagina and torn perineum.

colporrhaphy (*kol-por'-af-e*). Repair of the vagina. *Anterior c.* Repair for cystocele (*q.v.*). *Posterior c.* Repair for rectocele (*q.v.*).

colpos (*kol'-pos*). The vaginal

canal leading from the vulva to the cervix.

colposcope (*kol'-po-skope*). A binocular instrument with magnification, used to study the vagina and cervix uteri. Benign and malignant changes may be seen and selective biopsy taken, so aiding early diagnosis of malignant disease.

colpotomy (*kol-pot'-o-me*). Incision of the vaginal wall. *Posterior c.* Incision to drain a pelvic or parametric abscess.

coma (*ko'-mah*). Complete unconsciousness, in which all reflexes are absent. *Diabetic c.* Due to ketosis which occurs in diabetes mellitus. Treated by immediate administration of insulin and intravenous saline. *Hypoglycaemic c.* (*insulin c.*) results from too much insulin or too little food taken. Treated by giving sugar. *Uraemic c. See* Uraemia.

comatose (*ko'-ma-toze*). In the condition of coma.

comedone (*kom'-e-done*). A blackhead. Formed of epithelial cells enclosing dried sebum blocking the entrance to the sebaceous gland. Caused by hyperkeratosis of the neck of the follicle and blackened by melanin. Common during adolescence.

commensal (*kom-en'-sal*). An organism which normally lives in or on a part of the body without detriment to it. Some are potentially pathogenic.

communicable disease (*kom-mu'-nik-abl*). One that can be transmitted from one person to another.

comminuted fracture (*kom'-in-u-ted*). See Fracture.

commutator (*kom'-mu-ta-tor*). A device by which the direction of an electrical current can be interrupted or reversed.

compact tissue. See Bone.

compatibility (*kom-pat-ib-il'-it-e*). Mixing together of two substances without chemical change, or loss of power. See Blood grouping.

compensation (*kom-pen-sa'-shun*). (1) Making good a functional or structural defect. (2) Mental mechanism (unconscious) by which a person covers up a weakness by exaggerating a lesser or more desirable characteristic. *Cardiac c.* See Cardiac.

Complan (*kom'-plan*). A proprietary hydrolysed preparation containing protein, carbohydrate and fat and all the necessary mineral salts and vitamins for maintaining health, useful for tube feeds and to supplement the diet, particularly where a high protein diet is required.

complement (*kom'-ple-ment*). In bacteriology, a substance present in blood which aids the destruction of bacteria invading the body.

complemental air (*kom-ple-men'-tal*). See Air.

complementary feed. Feed given to infants to complement breast feeding when the mother has insufficient milk of her own.

complex (*kom'-pleks*). A grouping of ideas of emotional origin which are completely or partially repressed in the unconscious mind. A possible cause of mental illness. *Inferiority c.* A compensation by assertiveness or aggression to cover a feeling of inadequacy. See Electra *and* Oedipus.

complicated fracture. See Fracture.

complication (*kom-ple-ka'-shun*). Another disease process arising during the course of or following the primary condition. Many diseases have their particular hazards and close observation should be kept for early signs.

compos mentis (*kom'-pos men'-tis*). Of sound mind.

compound fracture. See Fracture.

comprehension (*kom-pre-hen'-shun*). Mental grasp of the meaning of a situation.

compress (*kom'-press*). Folded material, e.g. lint, wet or dry, applied to a part of the body. (1) For the relief of swelling and pain. (2) To produce localized pressure. *Lead lotion c.* Applied to bruised areas, or to relieve pain in a strained muscle.

compression (*kom-presh'-un*). Pressing together. *C. bandage,* One in which there are alternate layers of wool and bandage to exert a firm pressure without constriction of the blood supply. *C. of brain.* May be due to pressure of tumour, blood clot, etc.

compulsion (*kom-pul'-shun*). An urge to perform some action that the patient recognizes to be irrational but resistance leads to mounting anxiety which is only relieved by the performance of the act. The term may also be applied to compulsive words, thoughts and fears.

conation (*ko-na'-shun*). A striving in a certain direction.

concept (*kon'-sept*). A group of abstract ideas.

conception (*kon-sep'-shun*). The act of becoming pregnant by the fertilization of an ovum.

concha (*kon'-shah*). A shell. Applied in anatomy to shell-like structures; e.g. *c. auriculae*, the hollow part of the external ear.

concordance (*kon-kord'-ance*). Running a parallel course. In medicine may be applied to twins developing the same disease, e.g. diabetes.

concretion (*kon-kre'-shun*). A calculus or other hardened material. *Faecal c.* One of faecal material, a faecalith (*q.v.*).

concussion (*kon-kush'-un*). A violent jarring shock. *C. of the brain.* This is produced by a fall or blow on the head, and is characterized by unconsciousness, prostration, pallor, feeble pulse and shallow breathing. Return of consciousness is often heralded by sudden drawing up of the knees and by vomiting. Rest, quietness, and protection of the eyes from light, aid recovery.

condenser (*kon-den'-ser*). (1) An apparatus for collecting charges of electricity in which two conducting surfaces are separated by some insulating material, such as glass. (2) An arrangement for condensing light on to a microscope slide.

conditioning (*kon-dish'-un-ing*). The process by which a response is obtained by a stimulus by repetition of a situation until it becomes automatic.

condom (*kon'-dom*). A contraceptive sheath worn by the male.

conductor (*kon-duk'-tor*). (1) The portion of an electric battery which transmits the current. (2) Any part of the nervous system which conveys impulses. (3) A means of transmitting heat: *good c.*—copper, silver, cotton materials; *bad c.*—a vacuum, air, wool, etc.

condyle (*kon'-dile*). A rounded eminence occurring at the end of some bones.

condyloma (*kon-dil-o'-mah*). A wart-like growth of syphilitic origin occurring during the secondary stage, at the junction of skin and mucous membrane, e.g. the anal or vulval margins. It is covered with a moist epithelium and the discharge teems with spirochaetes, so is highly infectious.

cones (*kones*). Receptor end organs in the retina of the eye, used for the most acute and colour vision.

confabulation (*kon-fab-u-la'-shun*). The production of fictitious memories, and the relating of experiences which have no relation to truth to fill in the gaps due to loss of memory. A symptom of Korsakoff's syndrome (*q.v.*).

confection (*kon-fek'-shun*). A preparation of sugar or honey containing drugs, e.g. senna.

conflict (*kon'-flict*). When two opposing wishes or impulses cause emotional tension and often cannot be resolved without repressing one of the impulses into the unconscious. Conflict situations may be associated with an anxiety neurosis (q.v.).

confluent (kon'-flu-ent). Running together. *C. smallpox.* A variety in which the pustules coalesce.

confusion (kon-fu'-zhun). A clouding of consciousness so that the capacity to think is impaired, perception is dulled and response to stimuli is less acute.

congenital (kon-jen'-it-al). Applied to conditions existing at or before birth. *C. dislocation of hip.* Failure in position of the head of the femur and development of the acetabulum. *C. heart disease.* Abnormalities in development or failure to adjust to extra-uterine life. *See* Fallot's tetralogy.

congestion (kon-jest'-shun). Hyperaemia (q.v.). *C. of lungs.* Pneumonia.

conization (ko-ni-za'-shun). A method of treating erosion of the cervix by removing a cone-shaped piece of tissue by diathermy.

conjugate (kon'-ju-gate). (1) United in pairs or couples. (2) The distance between two parts. *True c.* The distance between the symphysis pubis and the sacral prominence.

conjugation (kon-ju-ga'-shun). In biochemistry, inactivation by a change in solubility.

conjunctiva (kon-junk-ti'-vah). The mucous membrane covering the eyeball and lining the eyelids.

conjunctivitis (kon-junk-tiv-i'-tis). Inflammation of the conjunctiva. Ophthalmia (q.v.). *Catarrhal c.* A mild form, usually due to cold or irritation. *Granular c.* Trachoma (q.v.). *Phlyctenular c.* Marked by small vesicles or ulcers on the membrane. *Purulent c.* Caused by virulent

organisms, with discharge of pus.

connective (kon-ek'-tiv). Joining together. *C. tissues.* Those that develop from the mesenchyme and are formed of a matrix containing fibres and cells. Areolar tissue, cartilage, and bone are examples.

Conn's syndrome (W.J. Conn, American physician, 1907–). Also known as primary hyper-aldosteronism. A disease characterized by attacks of muscle weakness, tetany, paraesthesia, hypertension and impaired renal function. Often the result of an adenoma of the adrenal cortex which causes an overproduction of aldosterone.

consanguinity (kon-sanguin'-it-e). Blood relationship.

conservative treatment. See Treatment.

consolidation (kon-sol-e-da'-shun). A state of becoming solid. *C. of lung.* In pneumococcal pneumonia the infected lobe becomes solid and congested with blood—known as red hepatization (q.v.).

constipation (kon-stip-a'-shun). Incomplete or infrequent action of the bowels. *Atonic c.* Due to lack of muscle tone in the bowel wall. *Spastic c.* A form of constipation where spasm of part of the bowel wall narrows the canal.

consumption (kon-sump'-shun). The popular name for phthisis (q.v.) or advanced pulmonary tuberculosis.

contact (kon'-tact). A person who has been exposed to a contagious disease. *C. lens.* A glass or plastic lens worn under the eyelids close to the cornea. It may be worn for therapeutic or cosmetic reasons.

contagion (kon-ta'-jun). Communication of disease from one person to another by direct contact.

contraceptive (*kon-trah-sep'-tiv*). An agent used to prevent conception, e.g. male sheath, cap that occludes the cervix, spermicidal pessary or cream, intra-uterine device, i.e. IUD (*q.v.*) and the oral pill (steroid hormones).

contracted pelvis. See Pelvis.

contraction (*kon-trak'-shun*). A shortening or drawing together. Applied to muscle action and the healing process in scar tissue.

contracture (*kon-trak'-chur*). Fibrosis causing deformity, *Dupuytren's c.* One of the palmar fascia. *Volkmann's ischaemic c.* One of the hand and forearm due to lack of blood to the muscles.

contrecoup (*kon'-tre-coo*). An injury occurring on the opposite side or at a distance from the site of the blow, e.g. fracture or haemorrhage on the opposite side of the skull.

controlled drugs. Drugs which are defined in the Misuse of Drugs Act 1971. They include those drugs which are habit-forming and certain other narcotics which have a profound effect on the central nervous system.

contusion (*kon-tu'-zhun*). A bruise.

convection (*kon-vek'-shun*). A method of transmission of heat by the circulation of warmed molecules of a liquid or a gas.

conversion (*kon-ver'-shun*). In psychology, the mechanism whereby repressed mental conflicts manifest themselves by physical symptoms.

convolutions (*kon-vo-lu'-shuns*). Folds or coils, e.g. of the cerebrum or renal tubules.

convulsions (*kon-vul'-shuns*).

Spasmodic contractions of muscles. They may herald the onset of an infectious disease but may be a symptom of a more serious underlying cause. All cases should be fully investigated. *See* Fits *and* Epilepsy. *Localized c.* Tetany (*q.v.*) is an example of this type.

Cooley's anaemia (*T. B. Cooley, American paediatrician, 1871–1945*). A rare progressive anaemia confined to children of the Mediterranean races. *See* Thalassaemia.

Coombs' test (*R. R. A. Coombs, British immunologist, 1921– *). A quantitative test carried out on the mother's blood for the formation of antibodies to the Rhesus factor where there is likelihood of incompatibility.

copper (*kop'-per*). Cuprum. An irritant poison. *C. sulphate.* In solid form (*blue stone*) it is used as a caustic for granulating surfaces. It is also the reagent in tests for the presence of sugar in urine. *See* Appendix 11.

coprolalia (*kop-ro-la'-le-ah*). Uncontrolled obscene speech.

coprolith (*kop'-ro-lith*) A faecalith (*q.v.*).

coprostasia (*kop-ro-sta'-se-ah*). The accumulation of faecal matter in the intestines, causing obstruction.

copulation (*kop-u-la'-shun*). Coitus. Sexual intercourse.

coracoid (*kor'-ak-oid*). (1) Shaped like a raven's beak. (2) The coracoid process of the scapula.

cord. A rope, a long flexible body. *Spermatic c.* That which suspends the testicle in the scrotum, and contains the spermatic artery and vein, and vas deferens. *Spinal c.* The part of the central nervous system enclosed in the spinal column. *Umbilical c.* The connection

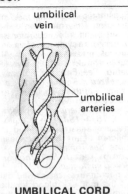

umbilical
vein

umbilical
arteries

UMBILICAL CORD

between the fetus and its mother by which it receives nourishment. *Vocal c.* Structures in the larynx which vibrate to produce the voice.

cordotomy (*kord-ot'-o-me*). See Chordotomy.

corium (*kor'-e-um*). The true skin. *See* Dermis.

corn. A local hardening and thickening of the skin from pressure or friction occurring usually on the toes.

cornea (*kor'-ne-ah*). The transparent portion of the anterior surface of the eyeball continuous with the sclerotic coat.

corneal graft. A means of restoring sight by grafting healthy transparent cornea in place of tissue opaque from scarring, following corneal ulceration.

corneoscleral(*kor-ne-o-skler'-al*). Relating to both the cornea and sclera. *C. junction.* Where these two join the limbus.

cornify (*kor-ne'-fi*). To harden. To lay down keratin.

cornu (*kor'-nu*). Hornlike. *C. of uterus.* The area where the fal-

lopian tubes join the uterus at the upper pole on either side.

corona (*ko-ro'-nah*). A crown. *C. dentis.* The crown of a tooth.

coronal suture (*kor'-o-nal su'-chur*). The junction of the frontal and parietal bones.

coronary (*kor'-on-ar-e*). Encircling. *C. arteries.* The vessels which supply the heart. *C. circulation. See* Circulation. *C. embolism.* Obstruction of a coronary artery—usually by a clot. *C. sinus. See* Sinus. *C. thrombosis. See* Thrombosis.

coronoid (*kor'-o-noid*). Shaped like a crow's beak. A bony process of the mandible and ulna.

cor pulmonale (*kor pul-mon-ah'-le*). Heart failure secondary to disease of the lungs or pulmonary circulation.

corpus (*kor'-pus*). Body. *C. callosum.* The mass of white matter which joins the two cerebral hemispheres together. *C. luteum.* The yellow body left on the surface of the ovary and formed from the remains of the Graafian follicle after the discharge of the ovum. If it retrogresses menstruation occurs, but it persists for several months if pregnancy supervenes. *C. striatum.* A mass of grey and white matter in the base of each cerebral hemisphere.

corpuscle (*kor-pus'-l*). A small protoplasmic body or cell, as of blood or connective tissue. *See* Blood cells.

correctives (*kor-rek'-tivs*). Drugs which modify the action of other drugs.

Corrigan's pulse (*Sir D. J. Corrigan, Irish physician, 1802-80*). Water-hammer pulse. *See* Pulse.

corrosive (*kor-o'-siv*). Destroying, eating into. *C. sublimate.*

Perchloride of mercury. An antiseptic.

cortex (*kor'-teks*). The external layer of an organ, e.g. of the cerebrum.

corticospinal tract (*kor'te ko-spi'-nal*). Also known as the pyramidal tract. Pathway for rapid voluntary movement.

corticosteroids (*kor-te-ko-ster'-oids*). Hormones produced by the adrenal cortex or their synthetic substitutes.

corticotrophin (*kor-te-ko-tro'-fin*). ACTH. Adrenocorticotrophic hormone, secreted by the anterior lobe of the pituitary body. Stimulates the adrenal cortex to produce cortisol. If lacking, it can be given by injection.

cortisol (*kor'-te-zol*). The naturally occurring hormone of the adrenal cortex. Hydrocortisone (*q.v.*).

cortisone (*kor'-te-zone*). A synthetic preparation of cortisol. It is of most value and least likely to cause side effects if given where there is lack of secretion, e.g. in Addison's disease and following adrenalectomy or hypophysectomy.

Corynebacterium (*kor-i'-ne-bak-ter'-e-um*). A genus of slender, rod-shaped. Gram-positive and non-motile bacteria. *C. diphtheriae*. Cause of diphtheria.

coryza (*ko-ri'-zah*). Cold in the head, with headache, nasal catarrh, and purulent discharge.

costal (*kos'-tal*). Relating to the ribs. *C. cartilages*. Those which connect the ribs to the sternum directly or indirectly.

cotyledon (*kot-e-le'-don*). A cup-shaped depression. A term applied to the subdivisions of the placenta.

counterextension (*kown'-ter-ex-ten'-shun*). (1) Holding back the upper fragment of a fractured bone while the lower is pulled into position. (2) Raising the foot of the bed in such a way that the weight of the body counteracts the pull of the

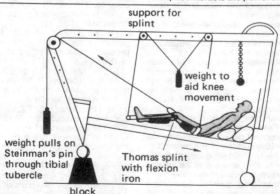

support for splint

weight to aid knee movement

weight pulls on Steinman's pin through tibial tubercle

Thomas splint with flexion iron

block

COUNTEREXTENSION

extension apparatus on the lower part of the limb. Used especially for fracture of the femur.

counter-irritants (*kown'-ter ir'-rit-ants*). Applications to the skin which relieve deep-seated pain. Now applied in the form of heat.

counting chamber. A specially designed microscope slide which is divided into squares 0·05 mm square. It allows for the accurate counting of blood cells.

Cowper's glands (*W. Cowper, English surgeon and anatomist, 1666–1709*). Two small glands situated close to the bulb of the urethra in the male.

cowpox (*kow'-poks*). An eruption occurring on the cow, considered to correspond to smallpox in man.

coxa (*koks'-ah*). The hip. *C. valga*. A deformity of the hip causing increased abduction of the femur and marked external rotation. *C. vara*. Less acute angle of the neck and shaft of the femur.

coxalgia (*koks-al'-je-ah*). Pain in the hip joint.

coxitis (*koks-i'-tis*). Inflammation of the hip joint.

Coxsackie viruses (*koks'-sak-e*). A group of enteroviruses that may give rise to a variety of illnesses including meningitis, pleurodynia and the common cold.

crab louse. *Pediculus pubis. See* Louse.

cracked nipples. A split on the outer surface of the nipple. Organisms entering are a common cause of abscess of the breast.

cramp. Involuntary, slow, forcible, and painful contraction of a muscle. Associated with muscle fatigue, salt loss through dehydration and poisons of various kinds affecting either the muscles or the nerves which control them.

craniopharyngioma (*kra'-ne-o-far-in-je-o'-mah*). A cerebral tumour arising in the craniopharyngeal pouch just above the sella turcica.

craniostenosis (*kra-ne-o-sten-o'-sis*). Premature closure of the suture lines of the skull in an infant. If this leads to raised intracranial pressure surgery is indicated.

craniotabes (*kra-ne-o-ta'-beez*). A patchy thinning of the bones of the vault of the skull. Seen in rickets (*q.v.*).

craniotomy (*kra-ne-ot'-o-me*). A surgical opening of the skull made to relieve pressure, arrest haemorrhage or remove a tumour.

cranium (*kra'-ne-um*). The bony cavity which contains the brain.

creatine (*kre'-at-in*). A nitrogenous compound found in muscle and present in urine in conditions in which muscle is rapidly broken down, e.g. acute fevers, starvation, etc.

creatinine (*kre-at'-in-een*). A normal constituent of urine—a product of protein metabolism.

creatorrhoea (*kre-at-or-re'-ah*). The presence of muscle fibres in the faeces. It occurs if trypsin is absent from the intestine or in acute diarrhoea.

Credé's method (*K. S. F. Credé, German gynaecologist, 1819–92*). The expulsion of the placenta by exerting pressure on the uterus through the abdominal wall.

crepitation (*krep-it-a'-shun*). (1) The grating sound caused by friction of the two ends of a fractured bone. (2) The sound produced on pressure when there is air in the subcutaneous tissues as in surgical emphysema (q.v.).

cresol (kre'-sol). A coal-tar phenol from which a number of commonly used disinfectants are derived. Modern derivatives are chlorocresol or parachlorometacresol; chloroxylenol of which Roxenol and Dettol are proprietary preparations.

cretinism (kret'-in-izm). A congenital disease due to lack of thyroid secretion, characterized by thickness of neck, stunted growth, and impaired mental development. Myxoedema (q.v.) is the acquired form. Usually called hypothyroidism.

cri du chat syndrome (kre'-du-sha'). Congenital abnormalities which cause an infant to be mentally retarded and to utter a cry which sounds like the mewing of a cat.

cribriform (krib'-rif-orm). Perforated like a sieve. *C. plate.* Part of the ethmoid bone.

cricoid cartilage (kri'-koid). The ring-shaped cartilage at the lower end of the larynx.

crises (kri'-seez). Plural of crisis. Especially recurrent attacks of the varieties listed below.

crisis (kri'-sis). A decisive point in acute disease; the turning-point towards (a) recovery; (b) death. *Cf.* Lysis. Sudden, violent attacks of pain affecting certain of the viscera. *Dietl's c.* Attack of severe pain in the loins, with nausea and vomiting, and the passing of a small amount of blood-stained urine. Probably due to kinking of a ureter in the condition of 'movable kidney'. *Gastric c.* of the stomach and *renal c.* of the kidney occur in locomotor ataxia. *Gastrointestinal c.* Intense upper abdominal pain. Occurs in some cases of untreated pernicious anaemia. *Thyroid c.* Sudden exacerbation

of symptoms in a patient with exophthalmic goitre. *See* Thyrotoxicosis.

Crohn's disease (B. B. Crohn, American physician, 1884–). Regional ileitis (q.v.).

Crosby capsule. Capsule used for obtaining tissue biopsies from the intestine.

cross infection. *See* Infection.

cross resistance. *See* Resistance.

croup (kroop). A group of symptoms associated with inflammation or spasm of the larynx. There is spasmodic dyspnoea, a harsh cough, and stridor. *See* Laryngismus stridulus. *Membranous c.* Laryngeal diphtheria.

Crouzon's disease (O. Crouzon, French neurologist, 1874–1938). Condition in which all the cranial sutures are fused at birth.

cruciate (kru'-shate). Resembling a cross. *C. ligament. See* Ligament.

crural (kru'-ral). Relating to the thigh.

'crush' syndrome (krush' sin'-drohm). Occurs when large areas of muscle tissue are damaged by crushing accidents. There is severe shock with local necrosis and oedema and scanty output of urine leading to acute uraemia.

cryoextractor (kri-o-eks-trak'-tor). An instrument in which intense cold coagulates the lens to the needle for removal in cataract extraction.

crutch palsy. *See* Palsy.

cryptogenic (krip-to-jen'-ik). Of unknown or obscure origin.

cryptomenorrhoea (krip-to-men-o-re'-ah). Menstruation occurs but the loss fails to escape from the vagina due to an obstruction such as imperforate hymen or vaginal atresia. *Syn.* Haematocolpos.

cryptorchism (kript-or'-kizm). Failure of the testicles to descend into the scrotum.

crypts of Lieberkühn (J. N. Lieberkühn, German anatomist, 1711–56). Glands secreting intestinal juice which are found in the mucous membrane of the small intestine.

crystalline lens (kris'-tal-line lens). The lens of the eye. See Lens.

cubitis (ku'-bit-us). The forearm.

cuirass respirator (kui-rass'). A mechanical device that fits round the chest to aid respiration.

culdocentesis (kul-do-sen-te'-sis). The aspiration of fluid from the pouch of Douglas via the posterior fornix of the vagina.

culdoscope (kul'-do-skope). An instrument consisting of a trocar, cannula and lighted telescope for viewing the pelvic cavity by passing it through the posterior vaginal wall.

culture (kul-chur). The development of micro-organisms on artificial media.

cumulative action (ku'-mu-la-tiv). The toxic effects produced by prolonged use of a drug, given in comparatively small doses.

cuneiform (ku'-ne-form). Three of the tarsal bones of the feet.

cuprum (ku'-prum). Copper (q.v.).

curare (ku-rah'-re). Arrow poison. An extract from a South American plant. Now used in surgery to produce complete muscle relaxation. It is given intravenously as Intocostrin or tubocurarine.

curettage (ku-ret-ahj'). Treatment by the use of a curette.

curette (ku-ret'). A spoon-shaped instrument used for the removal of unhealthy tissues by scraping. Curetting may be performed on membranous surfaces, e.g. of the uterus; on tuberculous and other chronic ulcers or to remove dead bone.

Cushing's disease (H. W. Cushing, American surgeon, 1869–1939). A condition of oversecretion of the adrenal cortex due to an adenoma of the pituitary gland. Symptoms include abnormal distribution of hair, and atrophy of the genital organs.

cusp. (1) The projections on the crown of a molar tooth. (2) One of the sections of the heart valves, formed of fibrous tissue and endocardium.

cutaneous (ku-ta'-ne-us). Pertaining to the skin. C. ureterostomy. Transplantation of the ureters to open on to the skin of the abdominal wall.

cuticle (ku'-tikl). The epidermis or external layer of skin.

cutis (ku'-tis). The derma or true skin.

cyanocobalamin (si-an-o-ko-bal'-am-een). A preparation of vitamin B_{12} administered by injection in the treatment of pernicious anaemia. Cytamen is a proprietary preparation.

cyanosis (si-an-o'-sis). A bluish appearance of the skin and mucous membranes, caused by imperfect oxygenation of the blood. It indicates circulatory failure and is also common in respiratory diseases. Constriction of veins from any cause will result in localized blueness.

cyclic AMP (si'-klik). Cyclic adenosine monophosphate. Enzyme activator found in cells. A deficiency in its production has been thought to be connected with certain forms of depressive illness.

cyclical syndrome (si'-klik-

al). Applied to the emotional and physical changes occurring in women, not only in the premenstrual period, but also before puberty and after the menopause. During the menstrual cycle referred to as premenstrual syndrome or tension.

cyclical vomiting (*si'-klik-al*). See Vomiting.

cyclitis (*si-kli'-tis*). Inflammation of the ciliary body of the eye.

cyclizine (*si'-kli-zeen*). An antihistamine drug and mild sedative. Useful to prevent travel sickness. Marzine is a proprietary preparation.

cyclobarbitone (*si-klo-bar'-be-tone*). A short-acting barbiturate drug. Phanodorm is a proprietary preparation of it.

cyclodialysis (*si-klo-di-al'-is-is*). An operation to improve drainage from the anterior chamber of the eye at the corneoscleral junction.

cyclodiathermy (*si-klo-di-a-ther'-me*). A treatment for glaucoma without opening the eye. Diathermy is applied to the sclera to cause fibrosis around the ciliary body, so decreasing the amount of aqueous humour made.

cyclopenthiazide (*si-klo-pen-thi'-az-ide*). A thiazide diuretic. Navidrex is a proprietary preparation.

cyclopentolate (*si-klo-pent'-o-late*). Mydriatic eye drops that dilate the pupil. Cyclogyl is a proprietary preparation.

cyclophosphamide (*si-klo-fos'-fam-ide*). A cytotoxic drug that can be given by mouth or intravenously. Endoxana is a proprietary preparation.

cycloplegia (*si-klo-ple'-je-ah*). Paralysis of the ciliary muscle of the eye.

cyclopropane (*si-klo-pro'-*

pane). A gas used for general anaesthesia. It is not irritating to the respiratory tract but must be used with a high oxygen concentration and is therefore potentially dangerous. Diathermy must not be used in the theatre at the same time.

cyclothymia (*si-klo-thi'-me-ah*). A term used to describe the mood swings in manic-depressive psychosis (*q.v.*).

cyclotomy (*si-klot'-o-me*). An operation to relieve glaucoma by incision of the ciliary muscle.

cyclotron (*si'-klo-tron*). A machine, for imparting high velocities to atomic particles, by means of which radioactive isotopes can be prepared.

cyesis (*si-e'-sis*). Pregnancy. *Pseudo-c.* Signs and symptoms suggestive of pregnancy arising when no fertilization has taken place.

cyst (*sist*). A tumour with membranous capsule and containing fluid. *Branchial c.* One formed in the neck due to non-closure of the branchial cleft during development. *Chocolate c.* Cyst of the ovary. Endometrial cells are present so bleeding occurs during each menstrual period, causing enlargement and congestion. It is associated with endometriosis (*q.v.*). *Corpus luteal c.* One which develops from a corpus luteum. *Daughter c.* A small one which develops from a larger. *Dermoid c.* A congenital type containing skin, hair, teeth, etc. It is due to abnormal development of embryonic tissue. *Hydatid c.* Contains the larval form of the tapeworm. *Meibomian c.* A chalazion (*q.v.*). *Multilocular c.* Cyst of the ovary. Divided into compartments or locules. *Papilliferous c.* Cyst of the ovary. It is lined with papillae which may grow through the cyst wall and on to the peritoneum and other organs, giving rise to ascites. *Pseudomucinous c.* Ovarian cyst containing fluid similar to mucin. *Retention c.* One caused by blockage of a duct, e.g. ranula (*q.v.*). *Sebaceous c.* Due to blockage of a duct from a sebaceous gland so that the sebum collects. *Thyroglossal c.* One in the thyroglossal tract near the hyoid bone at the base of the tongue. *Unilocular c.* One containing only one cavity.

cystadenoma (*sist-ad-en-o'-mah*). An innocent new growth of glandular tissue, e.g. *c. of breast.*

cystalgia (*sist-al'-je-ah*). Pain in the bladder.

cystectomy (*sist-ek'-to-me*). Usually refers to complete or partial removal of the urinary bladder.

cysteine (*sis'-te-een*). An amino acid formed by the ingestion of dietary proteins.

cystic disease of lung (*sist'-ik*). A congenital condition in which there is an abnormal amount of thick viscid secretion starting in the pancreas and later involving the lung with widespread bronchiectasis and emphysema. Now more usually known as cystic fibrosis. *See* Fibrocystic disease of pancreas.

cysticercus (*sist-e-ser'-kus*). The cystic or larval form of the tapeworm, causing hydatid cysts. *See* Echinococcus and Hydatid.

cystine (*sist'-in*). An amino acid. Sometimes excreted in urine in the form of minute crystals.

cystitis (*sist-i'-tis*). Inflammation of the bladder.

cystitome (*sist'-e-tome*). A surgical knife used in cataract operations.

cysto- (*sist'-o*). A prefix relating to the bladder.

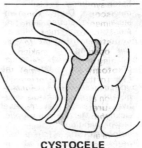

CYSTOCELE

cystocele (*sist'-o-seel*). A hernia of the bladder, usually into the vagina, as the result of overstretching of the wall during childbirth. *See* Colporraphy.

cystodiathermy (*sist-o-di-a-ther'-me*). The application of a high-frequency electric current to the bladder mucosa, usually for the removal of papilloma.

cystogram (*sist'-o-gram*). A radiological film demonstrating the urinary bladder. *Micturating c.* One taken during the act of passing urine.

cystography (*sist-og'-raf-e*). The X-ray examination of the bladder by the introduction of a radio-opaque dye.

cystolithiasis (*sist-o-lith-i'-as-is*). Stone in the urinary bladder.

cystoma (*sist-o'-mah*). A term applied to a tumour containing cysts. Most usual in the ovary.

cystometry (*sist-om'-e-tre*). A method of ascertaining the tone of the urinary bladder wall.

cystonephrosis (*sist-o-nef-ro'-sis*). A cystic condition of the kidney.

cystopexy (*sist'-o-peks-e*). An operation for stress incontinence in which the bladder neck is slung to the fascia at the back of the symphysis pubis.

cystoscope (*sist'-o-skope*). An instrument for examining the interior of the bladder.

cystostomy (*sist-os'-to-me*). The operation of making an opening into the bladder.

cystotomy (*sist-ot'-o-me*). Incision of the bladder for removal of calculi, etc. *Supra-pubic c.* Incision above the pubes.

cysto-urethroscope (*sist'-o-u-re'-thro-skope*). A telescopic instrument for examining the urethra and bladder.

cytogenetics (*si-to-jen-et'-iks*). The study of cells during mitosis to examine the chromosomes and the relationship between chromosome abnormality and disease.

cytology (*si-tol'-o-je*). The microscopic study of the form and functions of the cells of the body. *Exfoliative c.* An aid to the early diagnosis of malignant disease. Secretions or surface cells are examined for pre-malignant changes. *See* Papanicolaou *under* Test.

cytolysis (*si-tol'-is-is*). The property of certain substances to dissolve cells. *See* Bacteriolysin *and* Haemolysin.

cytomegalovirus (*si'-to-meg'-al-o vi'-rus*). Virus belonging to the same group as the herpes simplex virus. It may cause symptomless infection and is excreted in the saliva and urine. If contracted as an intrauterine infection it may cause severe congenital abnormality.

cytoplasm (*si'-to-plazm*). The protoplasmic part of the cell surrounding the nucleus.

cytosine (*si'-to-seen*). One of the pyramidine bases found in deoxyribonucleic acid. *See* DNA.

cytotoxic (*si-to-toks'-ik*). Damaging to cell structure and division. *C. drugs.* Those that influence the course of malignant disease by their action on cells, the aim being the destruction of malignant cells without harming normal tissues.

cytotoxin (*si-to-toks'-in*). A toxin or antibody that prevents the normal function of a cell.

D

Dacron (*dak'-ron*). A synthetic fibre used widely in replacement surgery of the heart and blood vessels.

dacryo-adenectomy (*dak-re-o-ad-en-ek'-to-me*). Removal of the lacrimal gland.

dacryo-adenitis (*dak-re-o-ad-en-i'-tis*). Inflammation of a lacrimal gland.

dacryo-adenotomy (*dak-re-o-ad-en-ot'-o-me*). An incision into a lacrimal gland to drain pus.

dacryocystitis (*dak-re-o-sist-i'-tis*). Inflammation of a lacrimal sac.

dacryocystorrhinostomy (*dak'-re-o-sis-to-ri-nos'-to-me*). An operation to establish drainage from the lacrimal sac to the middle meatus of the nasal cavity.

dacryocystotomy (*dak-re-o-sist-ot'-o-me*). Incision of a lacrimal sac to remove pus from an abscess.

dacryolith (*dak'-re-o-lith*). Calculus in a lacrimal duct.

dacryoma (*dak-re-o'-mah*). A benign tumour which arises from the lacrimal epithelium.

dactyl (*dak'-til*). A finger or toe. A digit.

dactylion (*dak-til'-e-on*).

Webbed fingers. *See* Syn-dactylism.

dactylitis (*dak-til-i'-tis*). In-flammation of one or more fingers or toes. The bone and subcutaneous tissue are affected.

dactylology (*dak-til-ol'-o-je*). Deaf and dumb language. Talk-ing by signs made with the fingers and hands.

Dakin's solution (*H. D. Dakin, American biochemist, 1880–1952*). An antiseptic (*sodium hypochlorite*) which liberates chlorine gas in the presence of septic material.

Dalton's law (*J. Dalton, English chemist, 1766–1844*). Also Henry's law. It relates to respir-atory gases and states that: (1) The pressure exerted by a mix-ture of gases is equal to the sum of the pressures which each would exert if it alone occupied the space. (2) The pressure exerted by a saturated vapour depends only upon the temper-ature and the particular liquid considered.

daltonism (*dawl'-ton-izm*). Colour blindness.

dandruff (*dan'-druff*). White scales shed from the scalp. If moist from serous exudate they have a greasy appearance. Scurf.

dapsone (*dap'-zone*). A sul-phone drug used in the treat-ment of leprosy.

darwinism (*C. R. Darwin, Eng-lish naturalist, 1809–82*). The theory of evolution as described by Darwin.

daughter cyst. *See* Cyst.

day dreams. Ideas drifting through the mind that do not lead to action.

DDT (dichlor-diphenyltrichlor-ethane). Dicophane. A syn-thetic insecticide formerly widely used, but now banned in many countries owing to its deposition in body tissues.

dead space. The area of the respiratory passages in which there is no exchange of gases.

deafness (*def'-ness*). The in-ability to hear. *Conduction* or *middle ear d.* Obstruction to the sound waves reaching the cochlea. *Nerve d.* Disease of the cochlea or auditory nerve.

deamination (*de-am-in-a'-shun*). A process of hydrolysis taking place in the liver by which amino acids are broken down and urea formed.

debility (*de-bil'-it-e*). A condi-tion of feebleness, weakness and lack of physical tone.

débridement (*da-breed-mon'*). The removal of foreign sub-stances and injured tissues from a traumatic wound. Part of the immediate treatment to pro-mote healing.

decalcification (*de-kal-sif-ik-a'-shun*). Removal of lime salts, e.g. from bone in some disorders of calcium metabolism.

decapitation (*de-kap-it-a'-shun*). Severing the head from the body.

decapsulation (*de-kaps-u-la'-shun*). Removal of a fibrous capsule. *Renal d.* Freeing and removing the capsule of the kidney.

decidua (*de-sid'-u-ah*). The thickened lining of the uterus for the reception of the fertilized ovum to protect the developing embryo. It is shed when preg-nancy terminates. *D. basalis.* That part which becomes the maternal placenta. *D. capsu-laris.* That part which covers the embryo. *D. parietalis.* The de-cidua that lines the rest of the uterine cavity.

deciduoma malignum (*de-sid-u-o'-mah mal-ig'-num*). Chorion epithelioma (*q.v.*).

decannulation (*de-kan-u-la'-shun*). A term applied to the introduction of decreasingly smaller tubes to wean an infant after a tracheotomy and still ensure adequate lung ventilation.

decompensation (*de-kom-pen-sa'-shun*). Failure of the heart to overcome disability or increased work load.

decomposition (*de-komp-o-zish'-un*). (1) The state of resolving into original elements, as decomposition of water into hydrogen and oxygen by electrolysis. (2) Decay or putrefaction (*q.v.*).

decompression (*de-kom-presh'-un*). Removal of internal pressure. *D. of brain.* A trephining operation to relieve pressure, e.g. of fluid on the brain. *D. chamber.* One to bring about a gradual lowering of atmospheric pressure to normal. *D. sickness.* A condition caused by too-rapid return from high to normal pressure environments, affecting caisson workers, deep sea divers, high altitude fliers, etc. Symptoms include severe abdominal and joint pain, cramps, vomiting and asphyxia. Treatment is to recompress the patient urgently, and return him slowly to normal environmental pressure.

decongestion (*de-kon-jest'-shun*). The overcoming of congestion, e.g. the use of ephedrine for inflammation and swelling of the nasal mucosa.

decortication (*de-kort-e-ka'-shun*). Removal of the cortex. (1) *D. of lung.* Removal of fibrosed pleura surrounding the lung, following chronic empyema, to allow expansion of the lung. (2) *Renal d.* Removal of the capsule of the kidney.

decubitus (*de-ku'-bit-us*). In a recumbent position. *D. ulcer.* A bed-sore.

decussation (*de-kus-a'-shun*). A crossing. *Pyramidal d.* The crossing of the pyramidal nerve fibres in the medulla oblongata.

defaecation (*de-fe-ka'-shun*). Evacuation of the bowels.

defence mechanism (*de-fense' mek'-an-izm*). The means by which the body resists invasion by pathogenic organisms.

defervescence (*de-fer-ves'-ense*). The period involved in the falling of a raised temperature to normal.

defibrillation (*de-fib-ril-a'-shun*). The restoration of normal rhythm to the heart in ventricular fibrillation by means of a high voltage electric shock applied to the heart or the chest wall.

defibrillator (*de-fib-ril-a'-tor*). An instrument by which normal rhythm is restored in ventricular fibrillation.

defibrinate (*de-fib'-rin-ate*). To remove fibrin from blood plasma. Used in the preparation of sera.

deficiency disease (*de-fish'-en-se dis-eez'*). See Disease.

degeneration (*de-jen-er-a'-shun*). A structural change which lowers the vitality of the tissue in which it takes place. *Amyloid d.* A waxy starch-like substance occurring in tissues in chronic wasting diseases. *Calcareous d.* Tissues which become impregnated with lime salts. *Fatty d.* Fat deposited in the tissues. *Fibroid d.* The change into fibrous tissue. See Fibrosis. *Red d.* See Necrobiosis. *Subacute combined d.* of the spinal cord. A complication of untreated pernicious anaemia due to vitamin B_{12} deficiency.

deglutition (*de-gloo-tish'-un*). The act of swallowing.

dehydration (*de-hi-dra'-shun*). Excessive loss of fluid from the body by persistent vomiting, diarrhoea or sweating or from the lack of intake. A cause of the loss of weight in diabetes mellitus owing to polyuria.

déjà vu (*da'-jah voo*). A disturbance of memory where a new experience or situation is experienced as if it has happened before.

deleterious (*de-le-te'-re-us*). Harmful; injurious.

deliquency (*de-lin'-kwen-se*). Usually applied to asocial and antisocial acts committed during youth, e.g. stealing and truancy.

delirium (*de-lir'-e-um*). Mental excitement. A common condition in high fever. It is marked by an irregular expenditure of nervous energy, incoherent talk, and delusions. *Chronic alcoholic d.* Korsakoff's syndrome (*q.v.*). *D. tremens.* A form common in alcoholics. *Traumatic d.* This may occur after severe head injury. There is much confusion and disorientation.

delivery (*de-liv'-er-e*). Childbirth. See Parturition.

delouse (*de-lows'*). To free from lice.

deltoid (*del'-toid*). Triangular. *D. muscle.* The triangular muscle of the shoulder arising from the calvicle and scapula, with insertion into the humerus. Frequently the site for intramuscular injections.

delusion (*de-lu'-zhun*). A false idea or belief held by the patient which cannot be corrected by reasoning. *D. of grandeur.* The patient has an erroneous belief in his own greatness, wealth or position.

demand pace-maker. See Pace-maker.

demarcation (*de-mar-ka'-shun*). Definition of the bounds of. *Line of d.* The limit of a gangrenous area shown by a red or black line.

dementia (*de-men'-she-ah*). A condition of permanent mental deterioration as a result of organic cerebral disease. *Arteriosclerotic d.* Dementia due to insufficient blood supply to the brain caused by arteriosclerosis. *D. praecox.* The old term for schizophrenia, implying the early onset of dementia. *Organic d.* Dementia occurring in the course of damage to the brain produced by infections, neoplasms or senile changes, etc. *Presenile d.* A group of conditions which produce dementia before the age of sixty. These show cerebral atrophy and histological changes of a distinct nature. *Senile d.* Dementia occurring after the age of sixty-five due to cerebral atrophy of unknown cause.

demography (*de-mog'-raf-e*). The social study of people viewed collectively in regard to race, occupation or conditions. Concerned with vital statistics.

demulcents (*de-mul'-sents*). Agents which soothe and allay irritation, especially of sensitive mucous membranes.

demyelinization (*de-mi-el-in-i-za'-shun*). Destruction of the medullary or myelin sheaths of nerve fibres as occurs in disseminated sclerosis (*q.v.*).

dendrite (*den'-drite*). One of the protoplasmic filaments of a nerve cell by which impulses are transmitted from one neurone to another. *Syn.,* dendron.

dendritic ulcer (*den-drit'-ik*). A corneal ulcer caused by the virus of herpes simplex during the course of a febrile illness. It has a branching appearance on straining.

denervation (*de - nerv - a' - shun*). Severing or removing of the nerve supply to a part.

dengue (*deng'-ga*). A mild infectious fever lasting about seven days, occurring in the tropics and conveyed by mosquitoes. The symptoms are headache, an eruptive rash and pains in the muscles and joints—especially the knee-joints—causing a peculiar or 'dandy' gait.

denitrify (*de-ni'-tre-fi*). To remove nitrogen.

Denis Browne splints (*Sir J. W. Browne, English orthopaedic surgeon, 1892-1967*). Metal splints for the treatment of club foot in infancy, so designed that the more the baby kicks the more he corrects the deformity.

dentalgia (*den-tal'-je-ah*). Toothache.

dentine (*den'-teen*). The substance forming the bulk of a tooth beneath the enamel.

dentition (*den-tish'-un*). The process of teething. *Primary d.* Cutting of the temporary or milk teeth, beginning at the age of six or seven months and continuing until the end of the second year. A full set consists of eight incisors, four canines, and eight pre-molars; twenty in all. *Secondary d.* or appearance of the permanent tooth, begins in the sixth or seventh year, and is complete by the twelfth to fifteenth year except for the posterior molars or 'wisdom teeth'. There are thirty-two permanent teeth—eight incisors, four canines, eight premolars or bicuspids and twelve molars.

dentoid (*den'-toid*). Tooth-like.

denture (*dent'-chur*). A set of artificial teeth.

deodorant (*de-o'-dor-ant*). A substance which destroys an odour.

deoxycorticosterone (*de-oks-e-kor-te-kos'-ter-one*). A naturally occurring adrenal steroid.

deoxycortone acetate (*de-oks-e-kor'-tone as'-e-tate*). A synthetic preparation of cortisol (*q.v.*), used mainly in the treatment of Addison's disease. DOCA and Percorten are proprietary preparations of it.

deoxygenated (*de-oks'-e-jen-a-ted*). Deprived of oxygen. *D. blood.* That which has lost much

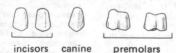

incisors   canine   premolars

TEMPORARY TEETH

incisors   canine   premolars   molars

PERMANENT TEETH

of its oxygen in the tissues and returns to the lungs for a fresh supply.

deoxyribonucleic acid (*de-oks'-e-ri-bo-nu'-kle-ik*). DNA. The nucleic acid molecule consists of long chains of atoms in a particular order. Variation in the structure may lead to congenital defects.

depersonalization (*de-per-son-al-iz-a'-shun*). A condition in which the patient feels his personality to have changed. It may occur in almost any mental illness.

depilatory (*de-pil'-at-or-e*). An agent which will destroy hair.

depolarization (*de-po-lar-i-za'-shun*). The neutralization of an electrical charge at the neuromuscular junction.

depression (*de-pres'-shun*). A lowering of psycho-physical activity. A mood change experienced as sadness, melancholy or suicidal thoughts. *Endogenous d.* This occurs in the course of manic-depressive psychosis. The mood change is associated with slowing of thought and action and feelings of guilt. *Involutional d.* Occurs for the first time between 45 and 64 years of age. *Reactive d.* Depression occurring as a result of some event, such as illness, loss of money, bereavement.

depressant (*de-pres'-ant*). A drug which reduces functional activity of an organ.

Derbyshire neck (*dar'-be-sher*). Goitre (*q.v.*).

derealization (*de-re-al-iz-a'-shun*). A symptom in which the surroundings appear to have lost their reality.

dermatitis (*der-mat-i'-tis*). Inflammation of the skin. *Contact d.* That arising from touching a substance to which the person is sensitive. *Secondary exfolia-*

tive d. This may arise during treatment by drugs, e.g. arsenic, bismuth, gold and mercury. *Sensitization d.* Dermatitis due to contact or it may be endogenous from the ingestion of certain foods to which there is sensitivity. *Traumatic d.* Inflammation due to exposure to irritants or physical agents, e.g. the sun or X-rays. *Varicose d.* Dermatitis usually of the lower portion of the leg due to varicosities of the smaller veins.

dermatology (*der-mat-ol'-o-je*). The science of skin diseases.

dermatome (*der'-mat-ome*). An instrument for cutting thin slices of skin for skin grafting.

dermatosis (*der-mat-o'-sis*). Any skin disease.

dermatographia (*der-mat-o-graf'-e-ah*). A condition in which urticarial weals occur on the skin if a blunt instrument or finger-nail is lightly drawn over it.

dermatomycosis (*der-mat-o-mi-ko'-sis*). A fungal infection of the skin.

dermatomyositis (*der'-mat-o-mi-o-si'-tis*). An inflammation of the voluntary muscles and skin with oedema.

dermis (*der'-mis*). The skin, especially the layer under the epidermis.

dermoid cyst (*der'-moid sist*). *See* Cyst.

Descemet's membrane (*J. Descemet, French anatomist and surgeon, 1732–1810*). The elastic membrane lining the posterior surface of the cornea.

desensitization (*de-sen-sit-i-za'-shun*). Lessening of sensitivity to foreign protein. This process is used to prevent reaction in those likely to be susceptible, by frequent small doses of the protein. *See* Anaphylaxis.

desoxycorticosterone (*des-oks-e-kor-te-kos'-ter-one*). Deoxycortone acetate (*q.v.*).

desquamation (*des-kwa-ma'-shun*). The peeling of the superficial layer of the skin either in flakes or in powdery form.

detergent (*de-ter'-jent*). A cleansing and antiseptic agent. It is present in many domestic cleansers and skin applications.

deterioration (*de-te-re-or-a'-shun*). Progressive impairment of function. Worsening.

detoxication (*de-toks-e-ka'-shun*). The process of neutralizing toxic substances. A function of the liver.

detritus (*de-tri'-tus*). Débris; material which has disintegrated or died.

detumescence (*de-tu-mes'-ense*). The subsidence of a swelling.

devitalized (*de-vi'-tal-ized*). Without vitality. Used especially to describe tissues which are deprived of their nerve supply and therefore of their recuperative powers.

dexamphetamine (*deks-am-fet'-a-meen*). A stimulant to the central nervous system. Used in depressive states, narcolepsy, post-encephalitic Parkinsonism and to control appetite in obesity. Dexedrine is a proprietary preparation of it.

dexter (*deks'-ter*). Upon the right side.

dextran (*deks'-tran*). A plasma substitute formed of large glucose molecules which given intravenously increase the osmotic pressure of blood and can be used to treat shock.

dextrin (*deks'-trin*). A soluble carbohydrate which is the first stage in the breakdown of starch and glycogen to sugar.

dextrocardia (*deks-tro-kar'-de-ah*). Situation of the heart in the right side of the thorax.

dextrose (*deks'-troze*). Grape sugar or glucose ($C_6H_{12}O_6$). The chief end-product of carbohydrate digestion.

dhobie itch (*do'-be*). A term used for tropical ringworm. (Hindu 'laundryman'). See Tinea cruris.

diabetes (*di-a-be'-teez*). A disease characterized by excessive excretion of urine. (1) *D. insipidus*. Marked by an increased flow of urine of low specific gravity, accompanied by great thirst. This disease is rare and some cases can be controlled by daily injections of pituitary extract. (2) *D. mellitus*. This is due to deficiency or ineffectiveness of the endocrine secretion of the pancreas—*insulin*. There is polyuria and sugar present in the urine, which makes it of high specific gravity. (For urine tests, see Appendix 11.) Other signs are lassitude and debility, loss of weight, pruritis and a lowered resistance to infection. It is especially serious in young people, coma and death resulting from acidosis in untreated or inefficiently treated cases. Treatment is by: (1) A properly regulated diet to maintain the nutrition of the patient. (2) To keep the blood sugar normal by injections of insulin if an adequate carbohydrate intake cannot be taken without. (For diet, see Appendix 10.) *Bronze d.* A special type marked by pigmentation of the skin and in which there is liver and pancreatic disease.

diabetic (*di-a-bet'-ik*). Relating to diabetes. *D. coma*. A severe acidosis (*q.v.*) occurring in diabetes mellitus. It is treated by immediate administration of insulin and intravenous fluids. *D.*

gangrene and *d. cataract* are complications of diabetes mellitus.

diabetogenic (*di-a-bet-o-jen'-ik*). Inducing diabetes. Some drugs precipitate the symptoms of diabetes in those prone to the disease.

diacetic acid (*di-a-se'-tik*). Aceto-acetic acid (*q.v.*).

diagnosis (*di-ag-no'-sis*). Determination of the nature of a disease. *Clinical d.* Diagnosis is made by the study of actual symptoms. *Differential d.* The patient's symptoms are compared and contrasted with those of other diseases. *Tentative d.* A provisional one—judged by apparent facts and observations.

dialyser (*di'-al-i-zer*). (1) The membrane used in dialysis. (2) The machine or 'artificial kidney' used to remove waste products from the blood in cases of renal failure.

dialysis (*di-al'-is-is*). The process by which crystalline substances will pass through animal membrane, while colloids cannot.

diameter (*di-am'-e-ter*). The chord passing through the centre of a circle. *D. of pelvis.* The measurements between the bones and joints of the pelvis made in women so as to determine whether or not the fetus can pass through at the time of childbirth. *D. of skull.* The measurements made of the fetal head at term. If these are abnormal delivery through the vagina may not be possible.

diamorphine hydrochloride (*di-a-mor'-feen hi-dro-klor'-ide*). Heroin. A powerful analgesic and drug of addiction. *See* Appendix 13.

diapedesis (*di-ap-e-de'-sis*). The passage of white blood cells through the walls of blood capillaries.

diaphoresis (*di-af-o-re'-sis*). Visible perspiration.

diaphoretics (*di-af-or-et'-iks*). Agents which increase perspiration.

diaphragm (*di'-af-ram*). The muscular dome-shaped partition separating the thorax from the abdomen. *D. needle.* One that can be left in a vein for further injections through a rubber seal. Gordh needle.

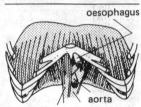

right crus   left crus

DIAPHRAGM

diaphragmatocele (*di-af-rag-mat'-o-seel*). Hernia of the diaphragm.

diaphysis (*di-af'-is-is*). The shaft of a long bone.

diarrhoea (*di-ar-e'-ah*). Frequent discharge of loose faecal matter from the bowels. Some of the causes are: (1) Incorrect diet. (2) Bacterial infections. (3) Poisons, e.g. arsenic. (4) Nervous influences. *Summer d.* Gastroenteritis (*q.v.*) of infants.

diarthrosis (*di-ar-thro'-sis*). A freely moving articulation, e.g. ball and socket joint.

diastase (*di'-as-tase*). (1) An enzyme formed during germination of seeds, which converts starch into sugar. (2) One of the pancreatic enzymes excreted in the urine. *D. test.* Used to estimate the excretion of diastase and therefore the pancreatic function in pancreatitis.

diastole (*di-as'-tol-e*). The resting stage of heart muscle, during which the chambers fill with blood, followed by systole or contraction. These stages occur simultaneously in both atria, and then in both ventricles, followed by a period during which all chambers rest, thus completing the cardiac cycle.

diastolic blood pressure (*di-as-tol'-ik*). *See* Blood pressure.

diastolic murmur (*di-as-tol'-ik*). An abnormal sound produced during diastole and occurring in valvular disease of the heart.

diathermy (*di-a-ther'-me*). Production of heat by a high frequency electric current. *Medical d.* Sufficient heat is used to warm the tissues but not to harm them. *Short wave d.* Used in physiotherapy to relieve pain or treat infection. *Surgical d.* Of very high frequency, used to coagulate blood vessels or to dissect tissues.

diathesis (*di-ath'-es-is*). A constitutional predisposition to certain diseases.

dichloralphenazone (*di-klor-al-fen'-a-zone*). A mild hypnotic drug, well suited to the elderly. Welldorm is a proprietary preparation.

dichlorophen (*di-klor'-o-fen*). An anthelminthic against tapeworms. There is no preliminary starvation and one dose can cause the worm to disintegrate. Anthiphen is a proprietary preparation.

dichotomy (*di-kot'-o-me*). Division into two parts.

dichromatic (*di-kro-mat'-ik*). A term applied to colour blind-

ness when there is ability to see only two of the three primary colours.

Dick test (*G. F. and Gladys Dick, American physicians, 1881–*). A test to determine the need for immunization against scarlet fever. This test is not now used.

dicrotic (*di-krot'-ik*). Having a double beat. *D. pulse.* A small wave of distension following the normal pulse beat; occurring at the closure of the aortic valve. It occurs when the output from the heart is forceful and the tension of the pulse is low as in fever.

didymitis (*did-e-mi'-tis*). Orchitis. Inflammation of the testicle.

diet (*di'-et*). A regularly ordered system of nourishment, according to the requirements of the body. Hospital diets are usually graded as: (1) *Full or ordinary d.* (2) *Light, or convalescent d.* of especially nutritive but easily digested foods of good calorie value. (3) *Fluid or milk d.* which may mean milk only, or include other fluids. Special diets usually consist of a reduction of, or increased quantities of, one or more of the food factors. *Diabetic d. See* Appendix 10. *High-calorie d.* A diet of 4000 calories (16 750 J) daily for those underweight. *Low-calorie d.* A diet reduced to 1000 calories (4200 J) daily for weight reduction. *Lawrence's Line Ration d.* A diabetic diet. *Low-fat d.* A diet used in conditions of the gall-bladder and jaundice. *High-protein d.* Used in all cases where there has been much protein loss or excess breakdown as in severe burns. *Low-protein d.* Suitable for cases of acute nephritis, hypertension and uraemia. *High-res-*

idue d. One containing much roughage for the treatment of constipation. *Low-residue d.* One with a restricted fibre or roughage content, suitable for inflammation of, or operations on, the intestinal tract. *Low-salt d.* May consist of no table salt and salt-free cooking or may require special low-salt bread and butter. Used particularly where there is tissue oedema.

dietetics (*di-et-et'-iks*). The science of regulating diet.

dietitian (*di-et-ish'-an*). One who specializes in dietetics.

Dietl's crisis (*J. Dietl, Polish physician, 1804–78*). See Crisis.

differential (*dif-er-en'-she-al*). Making a difference. *D. blood count.* Comparison of the numbers of the different cells present in the blood. *See* Blood count. *D. diagnosis. See* Diagnosis.

diffuse (*dif-fu'z*). Scattered or widespread, as opposed to localized.

diffusion (*di-fu'-shun*). The intermixing of molecules of liquid or gas so they are equally distributed in the containing structure or vessel.

digestion (*di-jest'-shun*). The process performed in the alimentary system, by which food is broken up, for the purpose of absorption and use by the body tissues.

digit (*dij'-it*). A finger or toe.

digitalis (*dij-it-a'-lis*). Comprises a group of drugs used extensively for their action on the heart. They strengthen the heart beat and slow down the conducting power of the bundle of His, thereby enabling the ventricles to beat more slowly and more effectively. Particularly valuable in treating atrial fibrillation (*q.v.*). Prepared digitalis tablets are formed from the powdered leaves of the purple foxglove. Its chief glycosides are *digitalin* and *digitoxin*. *Digoxin* is the chief glycoside from the white foxglove. The effects of digitalis are cumulative, indicated by a very slow pulse and coupling of the beats.

digitalization (*dij-it-al-i-za'-shun*). Large doses of digitalis are given within a short period of time, so that a powerful effect is produced quickly. Sometimes called *rapid* or *intensive d.*

diguanides (*di-gwan'-ides*). Hypoglycaemic drugs. Biguanides (*q.v.*).

dihydrocodeine bitartrate (*di-hi-dro-ko'-deen bi-tar'-trate*). An analgesic derived from codeine. It has greater analgesic powers but also greater risk of addition. DF 118 is a proprietary preparation.

dihydromorphinone (*di-hi-dro-mor'-fe-none*). An analgesic derived from morphine. Dilaudid is a proprietary preparation.

dihydrotachysterol (*di-hi-dro-tak-e-ster'-ol*). A preparation closely related to vitamin D that promotes calcium absorption.

dilatation (*di-la-ta'-shun*). (1) The operation of stretching a constricted passage, as in stricture of the urethra. (2) Stretching of a hollow organ. *D. of heart* when the muscle is overstrained; *d. of stomach* may be; (*a*) acute, following an anaesthetic when vomiting is persistent: (*b*) chronic, from scar tissue or growth obstructing the pylorus. Profuse vomiting at intervals is typical.

dilator (*di-la'-tor*). An instrument used for enlarging an opening, such as the rectum, cervix etc., by dilatation.

dill water. A weak carminative given for flatulence in infants.

dimenhydrinate (*di-men-hi'-drin-ate*). An antihistamine drug, useful for motion sickness. Dramamine is a proprietary preparation.

dimercaprol (*di-mer-kap'-rol*). A drug which combines with heavy metals to form a stable compound, which is rapidly excreted. Used when adverse effects are felt during treatment with gold or mercurial salts, or poisoning by arsenic, antimony or bismuth. Also called British anti-Lewisite or BAL.

dimethylphthalate (*di-meth-il-thal'-ate*). DIMP. An insecticide in liquid or ointment form that is effective for several hours when applied to the skin.

diodone (*di'-o-done*). A contrast medium similar to iodoxyl used in radiology, especially for arthrography.

diodoquin (*di-od'-o-kwin*). A quinoline preparation used in treatment of amoebic dysentery, especially useful for ambulant cases.

dioptre (*di-op'-ter*). The unit used in measuring lenses for spectacles. Normally parallel light entering a lens, focuses at a distance of 1 metre, i.e. the refractive power of the lens is one dioptre, and from this basis abnormalities are reckoned.

diphenhydramine (*di-fen-hi'-dram-een*). An antihistamine drug, used in treating hay fever and urticaria. Benadryl is a proprietary preparation of this substance.

diphtheria (*dif-the'-re-ah*). A specific infectious disease, caused by the *Corynebacterium diphtheriae* or Klebs-Löffler bacillus, which most often infects the fauces and tonsils, causing a greyish white membrane to form. Powerful exotoxins are produced that cause severe toxaemia and attack the heart muscle. It is a preventable disease by using a toxoid (*q.v.*). *D. immunization* should be carried out in infancy and booster doses given at intervals.

diphtheroid (*dif'-ther-oid*). Resembling diphtheria. A general term applied to organisms or membranes apparently similar to true diphtheria types.

Diphyllobothrium (*di-fi-lo-both'-ri-um*). A genus of tapeworm (*q.v.*). *D. latum*, the broad tapeworm, grows up to 10 m long and may infest man.

diplegia (*di-plee'-je-ah*). Paralysis of similar parts on either side of the body. *Spastic d.* Little's disease (*q.v.*).

diplococci (*dip-lo-kok'-i*). Cocci found always in pairs. They may be encapsulated, e.g. pneumococci. *See* Bacteria.

diploë (*dip'-lo-e*). The cancellous tissue between the outer and inner surfaces of the skull.

diplopia (*di-plo'-pe-ah*). Double vision in which two images are seen in place of one, due to lack of co-ordination of the external muscles of the eye.

dipsomania (*dip-so-ma'-ne-ah*). A morbid craving for alcohol which occurs in bouts.

director (*di-rek'-tor*). The grooved instrument for directing the knife in surgical operations.

Disablement Resettlement Officer. One appointed by the Ministry of Health and Social Security to advise and organize the retraining and placing of handicapped persons in suitable employment.

disaccharide (*di-sak'-ar-ide*). A sugar yielding two monosaccharides on hydrolysis. *D. intolerance.* The inability to absorb disaccharides owing to an enzyme deficiency.

disarticulation (*dis-ar-tik-u-la'-shun*). Amputation at a joint.

disc (*disk*). A flattened circular structure. *Intervertebral d.* A fibrocartilaginous pad that separates the bodies of two adjacent vertebrae. *Optic d.* A white spot in the retina. It is the point of entrance of the optic nerve.

discission (*dis-sis'-shun*). Dividing. In cataract operations, the cutting of the capsule of the lens.

discography (*dis-kog'-raf-e*). X-ray following the injection of a radio-opaque dye into an intervertebral disc. Degenerative changes or herniation may be seen

discrete (*dis-kreet'*). The opposite of confluent (*q.v.*). Separate.

disease (*dis-eez'*). Any departure from normal health. It may be congenital (that which has been present from birth) or acquired, and it may come under one of the following headings. *Degenerative d.* Regression of the tissues, commoner in older people. *Deficiency d.* Due to lack of vitamins or glandular secretion. *Functional d.* One which affects the working of an organ but in which no structural change can be found. *Infectious d.* One due to a specific organism which can be transmitted to others. *Malignant d.* One which is severe, progressive and likely to prove fatal. *Metabolic d.* One in which there is improper digestion and absorption of food or improper cell function. *Secondary d.* A condition resulting from another, e.g. bronchopneumonia consequent upon measles. (For separate diseases, see under individual names.)

disimpaction (*dis-im-pak'-shun*). Reduction of an impacted fracture.

disinfectant (*dis-in-fek'-tant*). An agent which is capable of destroying germs of disease, such as sunlight, heat and various chemicals.

disinfection (*dis-in-fek'-shun*). The destruction of microorganisms or their reduction to a level not normally harmful to health.

disinfestation (*dis-in-fest-a'-shun*). Getting rid of animal parasites and pests.

dislocation (*dis-lo-ka'-shun*). The displacement of a bone from its natural position.

disobliteration (*dis-ob-lit-er-a'-shun*). A method of recanalizing a blocked blood vessel by coring out the obstruction with the inner wall.

disorientation (*dis-or-e-en-ta'-shun*). Inability to appreciate surroundings, time or personal identity.

dissect (*dis-ekt'*). To cut carefully in the study of anatomy. (2) During operation to separate according to natural lines of structure.

disseminated (*dis-sem'-in-a-ted*). Scattered or dispersed. *D. sclerosis. See* Sclerosis.

dissociation (*dis-so-se-a'-shun*). Separation. The splitting up of molecules of matter into their component parts, e.g. by heat or electrolysis. *Medically.* Anaesthesia to pain and other sensations as may occur in spinal cord lesions. *Psychologically.* The separation of ideas, emotions or experiences from the rest of the mind, giving rise to a lack of unity of which the patient is not aware.

distal (*dis'-tal*). Situated away from the centre of the body or point of origin. *See* Proximal.

distension (*dis-ten'-shun*). Enlargement. *Abdominal d.* Distension of the abdomen by gas in the intestines or fluid in the abdominal cavity.

distichiasis (*dis-tik-i'-as-is*). A double row of eyelashes, the inner one causing irritation to the globe of the eye.

distillation (*dis-til-a'-shun*). Evaporation by heat of the volatile parts of a compound and subsequent condensation of the vapour.

dithranol (*dith'-ran-ol*). A synthetic preparation used as a substitute for chrysarobin in the treatment of psoriasis. It is more effective and less dangerous and only stains the linen slightly.

diuresis (*di-u-re'-sis*). Increased secretion of urine.

diuretic (*di-u-ret'-ik*). An agent which increases the flow of urine. Most act by preventing reabsorption in the renal tubule.

diverticulitis (*di-ver-tik-u-li'-tis*). Inflammation of a diverticulum. It is commonest in the colon and signs and symptoms similar to those of appendicitis may occur. With the formation of scar tissue there is narrowing of the tube. Colostomy is sometimes necessary.

diverticulosis (*di-ver-tik-u-lo'-sis*). The condition when many diverticula are present in the colon. They can be seen on barium X-ray.

diverticulum (*di-ver-tik'-u-lum*). A pouch or pocket in the lining of a hollow organ, as in the bladder, oesophagus or large intestine.

dizziness (*diz'-e-ness*). A feeling of unsteadiness or haziness, accompanied by anxiety.

DNA. Deoxyribonucleic acid, a complex molecule, part of the chromosome which is thought to be the carrier of the genetic code to the offspring.

Döderlein's bacillus (*A. S. G. Döderlein, German obstetrician and gynaecologist, 1860–1941*). A lactobacillus occurring normally in vaginal secretions.

dolichocephaly (*dol'-ik-o-kef'-al-e*). An abnormal shape of the head, which is unusually long.

dolor (*dol'-or*). Pain.

dominant genes (*dom'-in-ant jeenz*). Factors present in the chromosomes. *See* Genes.

donor (*do'-nor*). One who gives (1) Blood to another. *See* Blood grouping. (2) An organ, e.g. kidney, to another.

dopamine (*do-pam-een*). A compound that is an intermediate product in the synthesis of noradrenaline.

dorsal (*dor'-sal*). Relating to the back or posterior part of an organ.

dorsal root (*dor'-sal root*). Sensory nerve pathway. Route along which sensory impulses travel to the spinal cord from the periphery.

dorsalis pedis pulse (*dor-sa'-lis ped'-is puls*). The pulse which may be felt on the dorsum of the foot. It can be impalpable if the foot is cold. The dorsalis pedis artery is a continuation of the anterior tibial artery.

dorsiflexion (*dor-se-flek'-shun*). Bending backwards. In the foot and toes upwards. *See* Plantar flexion.

dorsum (*dor'-sum*). The upper or posterior surface.

douche (*doosh*). A stream of water directed to flush out a cavity of the body.

Douglas's pouch (*J. Douglas, Scottish anatomist, 1675–1742*). *See* Pouch.

Douglas bag (*C. G. Douglas,*

*English physiologist, 1882–
). A bag which is used to collect expired air in physiological experiments.

Down's syndrome (*J. L. H. Down, English physician, 1828–96*). Mongolism (q.v.).

Drager incubator (*dra'-ger in'-ku-ba-tor*). An incubator which allows intensive care of a sick infant to be carried out with minimal disturbance as the monitoring apparatus is inbuilt. Called after the German company who manufacture it. *See* Incubator.

drawsheet. A narrow sheet placed under a patient to prevent soiling of the main sheet.

Drinker respirator (*P. Drinker, American public health engineer, 1894–). See* Respirator.

droplet infection (*drop'-let in-fek'-shun*). *See* Infection.

dropsy (*drop'-se*). A popular term used to describe excess fluid in the tissues (*oedema*) or in the peritoneal cavity (*ascites*).

drug. Any substance used as a medicine.

drug dependence (*drug depend'-ense*). When drugs are taken repeatedly and the patient is unable to do without them either emotionally or physically. *D. d.* is now used in preference to the term drug addiction.

Duchenne dystrophy (*G. B. A. Duchenne, French neurologist, 1806–75*). A genetically determined disease in which the shoulder and hip girdles are affected first. Progressive muscle wasting leads to death in the second or third decade of life. *See* Muscular dystrophies.

duck bill speculum. Sims's speculum.

Ducrey's bacillus (*A. Ducrey, Italian dermatologist, 1860–*

1940). The organism causing soft chancre. *See* Chancroid.

duct (*dukt*). A tube or channel for conveying away the secretion of a gland.

ductless glands (*dukt'-less*). The endocrine glands, the secretion passes directly into the blood stream, e.g. the thyroid gland.

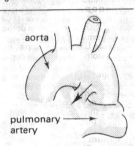

aorta

pulmonary
artery

DUCTUS ARTERIOSUS

ductus arteriosus (*duk'-tus ar-ter-e-o'-sus*). A passage connecting the pulmonary artery and aorta in intrauterine life, which normally closes at birth. In some cases it remains patent, and seems to predispose to the development of septic endocarditis. An operation to close the duct has benefited many cases.

Dulcolax (*dul-co-laks*). A proprietary aperient administered either orally or by suppository.

'dumping syndrome'. This may occur after meals following the operation of subtotal gastrectomy. The symptoms are: a feeling of fullness, weakness, sweating, dizziness and palpitations.

duodenal (*du-o-de'-nal*). Pertaining to the duodenum. *D.*

intubation. The use of a special tube having a metal end which is passed via the mouth and stomach into the duodenum. Used for withdrawal of duodenal contents for pathological examination. *D. ulcer.* One in the first 2·5 cm of the small intestine.

duodenitis (*du-o-den-i'-tis*). Inflammation of the duodenum.

duodenopancreatectomy (*du-o-den-o-pan-kre-a-tek'-to-me*). Surgical removal of the duodenum and much of the pancreas. Usually accompanied by anastomosis of the bile ducts and tail of the pancreas to the jejunum.

duodenostomy (*du-o-den-os'-to-me*). The formation of an artificial opening into the duodenum, through the abdominal wall, for purposes of feeding in cases of gastric disease.

duodenum (*du-o-de'-num*). The first 23 or 25 cm of the small intestine, from the pyloric opening of the stomach to the jejunum. The pancreatic and common bile ducts open to it.

Dupuytren's contraction or contracture (*Baron G. Dupuytren, French surgeon, 1777–1835*). Contracture of the palmar fascia, causing permanent bending and fixation of one or more fingers.

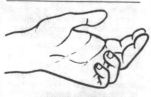

DUPUYTREN'S CONTRACTURE

dura mater (*du'-rah ma'-ter*). A strong fibrous membrane, forming the outer covering of the brain and spinal cord. It lines the inner surface of the protecting bones.

dwarfism (*dwarf'-izm*). Arrest of growth, e.g. due to renal rickets, cretinism or deficient pituitary function.

dynamometer (*di-nam-om'-e-ter*). An instrument by which the strength of the drip can be measured.

dys-. Greek prefix meaning 'difficult'.

dysaesthesia (*dis-es-the'-ze-ah*). Impaired sense of touch.

dysarthrosis (*dis-ar-thro'-sis*). Deformed, dislocated or false joint.

dyschezia (*dis-ke'-ze-ah*). Difficult defaecation. A form of constipation due to delay in the passage of faeces from the pelvic colon into the rectum for evacuation.

dyschondroplasia (*dis-kon-dro-pla'-ze-ah*). A condition in which cartilage is deposited in the shaft of some bones. The affected bones become shortened and deformed.

dyschromatopsia (*dis-kro-mat-op'-se-ah*). Partial loss of colour vision.

dyscoria (*dis-kor'-e-ah*). Abnormal formation of the pupil.

dyscrasia (*dis-kra'-ze-ah*). Disorder of development. *Blood d.* A developmental disorder of the blood.

dysdiadochokinesis (*dis-di'-ad-o-ko-kin-e'-sis*). A sign of cerebellar disease in which the ability to perform rapid alternating movements, such as rotating the hands, is lost.

dysentery (*dis'-en-ter-e*). A tropical or subtropical infectious disease, characterized by inflammation and ulceration of the large intestine, with frequent blood-stained evacuations. Specific forms are: (1) *Amoebic d.* Caused by the *Entamoeba histolytica*—treated by administration of emetine, which is specific for the organism. (2) *Bacillary d.* Due to the Shiga, Flexner or Sonne bacillus. Treatment by maintenance of the salt and water intake and the giving of neomycin or tetracycline.

dysfunction (*dis-funk'-shun*). Impairment of function.

dysgenesis (*dis-jen'-e-sis*). Defective development or loss of fertility.

dysgerminoma (*dis-jer-min-o'-mah*). A solid embryological tumour derived from germinal cells that have not been differentiated to either sex, occurring in either the ovary or testis.

dyshidrosis (*dis-hi-dro'-sis*). A disturbance of the sweat mechanism, in which an itching vesicular rash may be present.

dyskinesia (*dis-kin-e'-se-ah*). Impairment of voluntary movement.

dyslalia (*dis-la'-le-ah*). Impairment of articulation.

dyslexia (*dis-leks'-e-ah*). Difficulty in reading or learning to read; accompanied by difficulty in writing and spelling correctly.

dysmelia (*dis-me'-le-ah*). Malformation in the development of the limbs. There may be excessive or impaired growth. *See Amelia.*

dysmenorrhoea (*dis-men-or-re'-ah*). Painful menstruation. *Primary d. (spasmodic).* Painful contractions of the uterus arise just prior to or at the time of menstruation for the first few hours and then subside. *Secondary d. (congestive).* Most often owing to endometriosis (*q.v.*) and gets progressively worse as the local congestion increases.

dysostosis (*dis-os-to'-sis*). Abnormal development of bone.

dyspareunia (*dis-par-yu'-ne-ah*). Painful coitus.

dyspepsia (*dis-pep'-se-ah*). A term used to describe symptoms associated with the upper digestive tract. A feeling of fullness, discomfort, nausea and anorexia. *Nervous d.* Anxiety and tension aggravate the symptoms.

dysphagia (*dis-fa'-je-ah*). Difficulty in swallowing.

dysphasia (*dis-fa'-ze-ah*). Difficulty in speaking, due to a brain lesion.

dysplasia (*dis-pla'-ze-ah*). Abnormal development of tissue.

dyspnoea (*disp-ne'-ah*). Difficult or laboured breathing. *Inspiratory d.* Difficulty in intake of air. *Expiratory d.* Difficulty in expelling air.

dysrhythmia (*dis-rith'-me-ah*). Disturbance of a regular occurring pattern. Often applied to abnormality of rhythm of the cardiac cycle of the brain waves as shown on the electroencephalogram (*q.v.*).

dystaxia (*dis-taks'-e-ah*). Difficulty in controlling movements.

dystocia (*dis-to'-se-ah*). Difficult or slow labour. *Maternal d.* Difficult labour when the cause is with the mother, e.g. contracted pelvis. *Fetal d.* Difficult labour due to abnormal size or position of the child.

dystonia (*dis-to'-ne-ah*). A lack of tonicity in a tissue often referring to the muscles.

dystrophia (*dis-tro'-fe-ah*). Abnormal growth or deposition of tissue due to defective nutrition. *D. myotonica.* An hereditary disease of early adult life in which there is progressive muscle wasting and gonodal atrophy. *See* Frölich's syndrome.

dystrophy (*dis'-tro-fe*). Muscular weakness. *Muscular d.* A group of hereditary diseases in which there is progressive muscular weakness.

dysuria (*dis-u'-re-ah*). Difficult or painful micturition.

E

ear. The organ of hearing. It consists of three parts: (1) The *external e.* made up of the expanded portion, or pinna, and the auditory canal separated from the middle ear by the drum or tympanum. (2) The *middle e.,* an irregular cavity containing three small bones of the ear (*incus, malleus* and *stapes*) which link the tympanic membrane to the internal ear. It also communicates with the eustachian tube and the mastoid cells. (3) The *internal e.* which consists of a bony and a mem-

branous labyrinth (the *cochlea* and *semicircular canals*). *E. syringe.* A special metal type.

Eberth's bacillus (*K. J. Eberth, German pathologist, 1835–1926*). *Salmonella typhi.* The causative agent of typhoid fever (*q.v.*).

Ebstein's disease (*W. Ebstein, German physician, 1836–1912*). A congenital abnormality of the heart, in which there is downward displacement of the posterior and septal leaflets of the tricuspid valve. There is also a small right ventricle and large dilated right atrium.

eburnation (*e-burn-a'-shun*). Increased density of bone, following inflammation.

ecbolic (*ek-bol'-ik*). A type of drug which stimulates uterine contractions and so may be used to induce abortion.

ecchondroma (*ek-kon-dro'-mah*). An innocent cartilaginous tumour arising as an outgrowth to cartilage or bone.

ecchymosis (*ek-ke-mo'-sis*). A

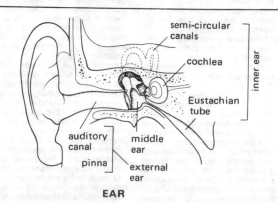

EAR

bruise. An effusion of blood under the skin, causing discoloration, e.g. a black eye.

eccrine (*ek'-krin*). Applied to sweat glands that are generally distributed over the body but densest on the palms and soles of the feet.

ECG. Electrocardiogram (*q.v.*).

Echinococcus (*ek-in-o-kok'-us*). A genus of tapeworms. *E. granulosus* infests dogs and may also infect man if the ova are swallowed with contaminated food. The larval form develops into cysts (*hydatids*), which may occur in the liver, lung, brain or other organ, being carried by the blood or lymph stream from the intestine.

echo-encephalography (*ek'-ko-en-kef-al-og'-raf-e*). A simple method of brain investigation by means of reflecting sound waves, using a probe fitted to a portable apparatus and mains electricity.

echolalia (*ek-o-la'-le-ah*). The repetition of phrases or words overheard.

echophony (*e-kof'-on-e*). The echo of the voice heard in the chest on auscultation.

echopraxia (*ek-o-praks'-e-ah*). The automatic repetition by a patient of acts he has seen performed by others. These are carried out without expression or emotion.

echovirus (*ek-o-vi'-rus*). Enteropathic cytopathic human orphan virus. Has the ability to cause benign lymphocytic meningitis and epidemic myalgia. *See* Bornholm disease.

eclampsia (*ek-lamp'-se-ah*). Fits which may occur in untreated cases of toxaemia of pregnancy. Now considered preventable as toxaemia should be diagnosed early by good antenatal care. This includes regular weighing, recording of the blood pressure and testing of the urine for albumin. *See* Toxaemia.

ecmnesia (*ek-ne'-ze-ah*). A gap in memory.

ecraseur (*a-krah'-zer*). An instrument having a wire loop that is tightened round the stalk of a projecting growth, such as a polyp to sever it.

ecstasy (*eks'-tas-e*). A feeling of exaltation. It may be accompanied by sensory impairment and lack of activity but with an expression of rapture.

ECT. Electroconvulsive therapy (*q.v.*).

ectasia (*ek-ta'-ze-ah*). Dilation of a canal or organ. *Alveolar e.* Distension of the air sacs of the lung. *Corneal e.* Bulging and thinning of the cornea due to disease or raised intraocular pressure.

ectasis (*ek'-tas-is*). A dilatation or over-stretching. *See* Bronchiectasis.

ecthyma (*ek-thi'-mah*). An inflammatory skin disease, with an eruption of pustules, usually with a hardened base. A pigmented scar remains after healing takes place.

ecto- (*ek'-to*). A prefix meaning 'outside'.

ectoderm (*ek'-to-derm*). The outer germinal layer of the developing embryo from which the skin and nervous system are derived.

ectogenous (*ek-toj'-en-us*). Produced outside the organism. *See* Endogenous.

-ectomy (*ek'-to-me*). A suffix denoting excision. *See* '-stomy'.

ectoparasite (*ek-to-par'-ah-site*). One that lives on the external surface of its host.

ectopia (*ek-to'-pe-ah*). Displacement or abnormal position of any part. *E. vesicae.* A congenital defect of the abdominal wall in which the bladder is exposed.

ectopic gestation (ek-top'-ik jes-ta'-shun). *See* Gestation.

ectozoon (ek-to-zo'-on). An external animal parasite.

ectrodactylia (ek-tro-dak-til'-e-ah). Congenital absence of one or more fingers or toes.

ectropion (ek-tro'-pe-on). Eversion of an eyelid, often due to contraction of the skin or to paralysis.

eczema (ek'-ze-mah). An acute or chronic inflammatory condition of the skin, non-contagious although secondary infection is common. The eruption appears first as papules which become moist and finally form scabs. There is great irritation of the affected part and constitutional disturbances may also be present. Many forms are allergic in origin. *Baker's e.* A type due to the irritating effect of flour. *Dry e.* Eczema where the affected area is dry and scaly. *Infantile e.* An allergic form commoner in babies fed on cow's milk. *Washer-woman's e.* Due to the irritation of soda in soaps. *Weeping e.* A serous exudation from the affected area, which precedes drying up and healing.

eczematous (ek-zem'-at-us). Affected with or resembling eczema.

EDTA. Ethylenediamine tetraacetic acid. A chelating agent used in the treatment of lead poisoning.

edentulous (e-dent'-ul-us). Without teeth, especially applied to the elderly.

EEG. Electro-encephalogram (q.v.).

effector (e-fek'-tor). A motor or sensory nerve ending in a muscle, gland or organ.

efferent (ef'-er-ent). Convey-

ing from the centre to the periphery. *E. nerves.* Motor nerves coming from the brain to supply the muscles and glands. *E. tracts.* The pathway of the motor nerves from the cerebral cortex and descending the spinal cord. *See* Afferent.

effervescent (ef-er-ves'-sent). Foaming or giving off gas bubbles.

effluent (ef'-lu-ent). The fluid portion of sewage. The sludge or more solid portion may have been separated from it.

effluvium (ef-flu'-ve-um). The subtle odour which may be given off by a substance or person, usually unpleasant.

effort syndrome (ef'-fort sin'-drome). A condition characterized by breathlessness, palpitations, chest pain and fatigue, a form of anxiety neurosis.

effusion (e-fu'-zhun). The escape of blood or serum into surrounding tissues or cavities.

ego (eg'-o). A term used in psychology of that part of the mind that the individual experiences as his 'self' and is concerned with satisfying the unconscious primitive demands of the 'id' in a socially acceptable form.

Ehrlich's side-chain theory (P. Ehrlich, German bacteriologist, 1854–1915). An explanation of the phenomena of immunity, in which protoplasmic cells are said to possess certain chemical attachments or side chains, which are capable of uniting with bacterial toxins and in so doing render them harmless.

Eisenmenger's complex (V. Eisenmenger, German physician, 1864–1932). A congenital heart defect in which a ventricular septal defect is associated with increased pulmonary vascular resistance. The resulting symptoms are similar to those of Fallot's tetralogy.

ejaculation (*e-jak-u-la'-shun*). The act of ejecting semen.

elastic (*e-las'-tik*). Capable of stretching. *E. bandage.* One that will stretch lengthways. *E. stocking.* A woven rubber stocking usually worn for varicose veins. *E. tissue.* Connective tissue containing yellow elastic fibres.

Elastoplast (*e-las'-to-plast*). A proprietary brand of adhesive elastic bandage useful to give support to a part or as a fixative for small dressings. *Extension E.* This stretches crossways instead of lengthwise and so moulds easily to the limb and allows a steady pull.

elation (*e-la'-shun*). In psychiatry a feeling of well-being or a state of excitement which may vary considerably in degree. A lesser degree may be termed euphoria, while it occurs in marked degree in hypomania and in intense degree in mania.

elbow (*el'-boh*). The joint between the upper arm and the forearm. It is formed by the humerus above and the radius and ulna below.

Electra complex (*e-lek'-trah*). From Greek mythology. The excessive attachment of a daughter for her father, with antagonism towards the mother.

electric (*e-lek'-trik*). Pertaining to electricity. *E. cautery.* See Cautery.

electricity (*e-lek-tris'-it-e*). A natural force and fundamental form of energy. *Static e.* The building up of an electric charge by friction between two different surfaces. *See* Appendix 4.

electrocardiogram (*e-lek-tro-kar'-de-o-gram*). A tracing made of the various phases of

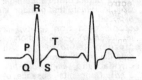

ELECTROCARDIOGRAM

the heart's action by means of an electrocardiograph.

electrocardiograph (*e-lek'-tro-kar'-de-o-graf*). A machine for recording the potential of electrical currents that traverse the heart muscle and initiate contraction.

electrocardiophonography (*e-lek'-tro-kar-de-o-fon-og'-raf-e*). The recording of the heart sounds by means of a phonocardiogram.

electrocoagulation (*e-lek-tro-ko-ag-u-la'-shun*). A method of coagulation using a high frequency current. A form of surgical diathermy (*q.v.*).

electroconvulsive therapy (*e-lek-tro-kon-vul'-siv ther'-a-pe*). The passage of an electric current through the frontal lobes of the brain in the treatment of mental disease. ECT. With the aid of relaxant drugs this no longer causes a convulsion and is now termed electroplexy.

electrocorticography (*e-lek-tro-kor-te-kog'-raf-e*). Electroencephalography with the electrodes applied directly to the cortex of the brain. Performed in the operating theatre to locate a small lesion, e.g. a scar.

electrode (*e-lek'-trode*). The terminal of the conducting coils of a battery, through which electricity is applied to the body.

113

EMB

electro-encephalogram (*e-lek'-tro en-kef'-al-o-gram*). A tracing of the electrical activity of the brain. Abnormal rhythm is an aid to diagnosis in epilepsy and cerebral tumour.

electro-encephalograph (*e-lek'-tro en-kef'-al-og-raf*). A machine for recording the electrical activity of the cortex of the brain.

electrolysis (*e-lek-trol'-is-is*). Chemical decomposition by means of electricity, e.g. an electric current passed through water decomposes it into oxygen and hydrogen.

electrolyte (*e-lek'-tro-lite*). A substance which can be decomposed by electrolysis. *E. balance*. The maintenance of the correct balance between the different elements in the body tissues and fluids. *See* Appendix 8.

electromotive force (EMF) (*e-lek-tro-mo'-tiv fors*). The measure of the force by which the current of electricity will flow from one point to another. The unit of EMF is the volt.

electromyography (*e-lek-tro-mi-og'-raf-e*). Recording of electrical currents generated in active muscle.

electron (*e-lek'-tron*). The unit of negative electricity revolving round a nucleus of positive electricity, of which the atom consists. *E. microscope*. A type of microscope which allows very small particles such as viruses to be identified.

electronarcosis (*e-lek-tro-nar-ko'-sis*). A state of sleep or unconsciousness induced by placing electrodes on the temple and passing an electric current through the brain.

electro-ocularography. *See* Electroretinography.

electroplexy (*e-lek'-tro-pleks-e*). Electroconvulsive therapy (*q.v.*).

electroretinogram (*e-lek-tro-re-tin'-o-gram*). A record of the tracings produced by electroretinography.

electroretinography (*e-lek-tro-re-tin-og'-raf-e*). A method of examining the retina of the eye by means of electrodes and light stimulation for assessment of retinal damage.

electrotherapy (*e-lek-tro-ther'-ap-e*). The treatment of disease by use of electricity.

element (*el'-e-ment*). The simplest form into which matter can be divided. It must consist of identical atoms. Iron oxide consists of the elements iron and oxygen.

elephantiasis (*el-ef-an-ti'-as-is*). A chronic disease of the lymphatics producing excessive thickening of the skin and swelling of the parts affected, usually the lower limbs. It may be due to filariasis.

elevator (*el'-e-va-tor*). An instrument used as a lever for raising bone, etc. *Tooth e.* Instrument used in dentistry. *Periosteal e.* Instrument that strips the periosteum in bone surgery.

elimination (*e-lim-in-a'-shun*). The removal of waste matter.

elixir (*e-liks'-er*). A sweetened spirituous liquid, used largely as a flavouring agent.

emaciation (*e-ma-she-a'-shun*). Excessive wasting of body tissues.

emanation (*em-an-a'-shun*). The act of giving out, e.g. the gamma rays from radium.

emasculation (*e-mas-ku-la'-shun*). Castration (*q.v.*).

Embden–Meyerhof pathway (*G. G. Embden, German biochemist, 1874–1933: O. F.*

Meyerhof, German physiologist, 1884–1951). The chemical processes which take place during the conversion of muscle glycogen to glucose phosphate and then pyruvic acid. Energy is released and then stored as molecules of adenosine triphosphate (ATP) (*q.v.*).

embolectomy (*em-bol-ek'-to-me*). An operation to remove an embolus. It has been performed for pulmonary embolism, but more frequently for arterial emboli that are cutting off the blood supply to the limbs.

embolism (*em'-bol-izm*). Obstruction of a blood vessel by a travelling blood clot or particle of matter. *Air e.* The presence of gas or air bubbles usually sucked into the large veins from a wound in the neck or chest. *Cerebral e.* Obstruction of a vessel in the brain. *Coronary e.* The blockage of a coronary vessel with a clot. *Fat e.* Globules of fat released into the blood from a fractured bone. *Infective e.* Detached particles of infected blood clot from an area of inflammation which, obstructing small vessels, result in abscess formation, i.e. pyaemia (*q.v.*). *Pulmonary e.* Blocking of the pulmonary artery or one of its branches by detached clot, usually due to thrombosis in the femoral or iliac veins. A complication of abdominal operations, occurring about the tenth day. Smaller clots cause infarction (*q.v.*).

embolus (*em'-bo-lus*). *Pl.* emboli. A substance carried by the blood stream until it causes obstruction by blocking a blood vessel. *See* Embolism.

embrocation (*em-bro-ka'-shun*). A liquid applied to the body by rubbing.

embryo (*em'-bre-o*). A name given to the fertilized ovum in its earliest stages until it shows human characteristics during the second month.

embryology (*em-bre-ol'-o-je*). The study of growth and development from the unicellular stage.

emesis (*em'-es-is*). Vomiting.

emetic (*em-et'-ik*). An agent which has power to induce vomiting, e.g. *salt* or *mustard* and water by mouth; or *apomorphine* hypodermically.

emetine (*em'-et-een*). An alkaloid prepared from ipecacuanha. Used widely in amoebic dysentery, for which it is the specific cure.

EMI scanner (*skan'-er*). A machine with which deep tissues may be scanned electronically and abnormalities detected without the use of X-ray opaque substances. Named after the firm that manufactures it.

emission (*e-mish'-un*). Involuntary ejection (of semen).

emmetropic (*em-me-tro'-pik*). Applied to normal vision that is neither long nor short sighted.

emollient (*e-mol'-e-ent*). Any substance used to soothe or soften the skin.

emotion (*e-mo'-shun*). A physical and psychological excitement in response to certain stimuli, e.g. happiness and sadness.

empathy (*em'-path-e*). The power of projecting oneself into the feelings of another person or situation.

emphysema (*em-fi-se'-mah*). The abnormal presence of air in tissues or cavities of the body. *Surgical e.* The presence of air, or any other gas, in the subcutaneous tissues introduced through a wound, and evidenced by crepitation on pressure. It may occur, e.g. from the lungs, owing to perforation by a fractured rib, or in tissues around a tracheostomy incision. The bacteria of gas-gangrene (*q.v.*) cause such a condition. *Pulmonary e.* A chronic disease of the lungs, in which there is abnormal distension of alveoli, so great in some cases that intervening walls are broken down and bullae form on the lung surface. An accompaniment of chronic respiratory diseases, in which narrowing of the tubes occurs so that expiration is difficult. *See* Atelectasis.

empiric (*em-pir'-ik*). Describes treatment based on experience and not on scientific reasoning.

empyema (*em-pi-e'-mah*). A collection of pus in a cavity, most commonly referring to the pleural cavity.

emulsion (*e-mul'-shun*). A mixture in which an oil is suspended in water, by the addition of a mucilage.

enamel (*en-am'-el*). The hard outer covering of the crown of a tooth.

encanthis (*en-kan'-this*). A small fleshy growth at the inner canthus of the eye.

encapsulated (*en-kap'-su-la-ted*). Enclosed in a capsule.

encephalitis (*en-kef-al-i'-tis*). Inflammation of the brain. *E. lethargica* (epidemic e.). An inflammation of the brain due to a virus. Typical signs are increasing languor and lethargy, deepening to stupor, and accompanied by muscle weaknesses and paralyses. After-effects may be serious, and include mental deficiency, paralysis agitans and deterioration of moral sense. *Post-vaccinal e.* An occasional complication of vaccination.

encephalocele (*en-kef'-al-o-seel*). Hernia of the brain through the skull.

encephalography (*en-kef-al-og'-raf-e*). An X-ray of the ventricles of the brain following the insertion of air via a lumbar or cisternal puncture.

encephaloma (*en-kef-al-o'-mah*). Tumour of the brain.

encephalomalacia (*en-kef-al-o-mal-a'-she-ah*). Softening of the brain.

encephalomyelitis (*en-kef-al-o-mi-el-i'-tis*). Inflammation of the brain and spinal cord.

encephalomyelopathy (*en-kef-al-o-mi-el-op'-ath-e*). Any disease condition of the brain and spinal cord.

encephalon (*en-kef'-al-on*). The brain.

encephalopathy (*en-kef-al-op'-ath-e*). Cerebral dysfunction. *Hypertensive e.* A transient disturbance of function associated with hypertension. Disorientation, excitability, and abnormal behaviour that may be reversed if the pressure is reduced.

enchondroma (*en-kon-dro'-mah*). A tumour of cartilage within the shaft of the bone.

encopresis (*en-ko-pre'-sis*). Incontinence of faeces.

encysted (*en-sis'-ted*). Enclosed in a cyst.

endarterectomy (*end-ar-ter-ek-to'-me*). The surgical removal of the lining of an artery usually for narrowing of the vessel by artheromatous plaques. *Thrombo-e.* Removal of a clot with the lining.

endarteritis (*end-ar-ter-i'-tis*). Inflammation of the innermost coat of an artery. *E. obliterans.* A type which causes collapse and obstruction in small arteries.

endaural (*end-aw'-ral*). Within the ear, usually referring to the auditory canal.

endemic (*en-dem'-ik*). A term applied to any disease prevalent in a particular locality.

endemiology (*en-dem-e-ol'-o-je*). The study of all the factors pertaining to endemic disease.

endo-. Prefix meaning 'within'.

endocarditis (*en-do-kard-i'-tis*). Inflammation of the endocardium. *Acute simple e.* This may be part of a general carditis complicating rheumatic fever. *Acute ulcerative* or *malignant e.* An acute illness resulting from infection of healthy heart valves by a blood-borne infection from another source, possibly the haemolytic streptococcus. *Subacute bacterial e.* Infection of the valves, already rendered abnormal by valvular heart disease or congenital deformity, by the *Streptococcus viridans.* As this organism is released into the blood stream during dental extraction, prophylactic penicillin should be given to patients with valvular heart disease before extractions are undertaken.

endocardium (*en-do-kar'-de-um*). The membrane lining the heart.

endocervicitis (*en-do-ser-vis-i'-tis*). Inflammation of the membrane lining the cervix uteri.

endocrine (*en'-do-krine*). Secreting within. Applied to those glands whose secretions (*hormones*) flow directly into the blood or lymph and greatly modify bodily development. The chief endocrine glands are the thyroid, parathyroids, suprarenals and pituitary. The pancreas, stomach, liver, ovaries and testicles also produce internal secretions.

endocrinology (*en-do-krin-ol'-o-je*). The science of the endocrine organs and their secretions.

endocrinopathy (*en-do-krin-op'-ath-e*). Any disease conditions of the endocrine glands.

endoderm (*en-do-derm*). Entoderm (*q.v.*).

endogenous (*en-doj'-en-us*). Produced within. *E. depression.* One in which the disease derives from an innate predisposition. *E. protein.* That derived from the body tissues and not ingested.

endolymph (*en'-do-limf*). The fluid inside the membranous labyrinth of the ear.

endolysin (*en-do-li'-sin*). A factor or enzyme present in cells that can cause dissolution of the cytoplasm.

endometriosis (*en-do-me-tre-o'-sis*). Endometrium in an abnormal situation. Chocolate cyst of the ovary contains some endometrial material.

endometritis (*en-do-me-tri'-tis*). Inflammation of the endometrium.

endometrium (*en-do-me'-tre-um*). The mucous membrane lining the uterus.

endoparasite (*en-do-par'-ah-site*). A parasite that lives within its host.

end-organ. An encapsulated sensory nerve ending.

endorrhachis (*en-do-rak'-is*). The spinal dura mater.

endoscope (*en'-do-skope*). An instrument fitted with a light, used to inspect a hollow organ or cavity.

endoscopic resection (*en-do-skop'-ik re-sek'-shun*). A method of removing part of an enlarged prostate gland by the transurethral route. Sections are excised by a cutting instrument or diathermy passed up the cystoscope.

endosteitis (*end-os-te-i'-tis*). Inflammation of endosteum.

endosteoma (*end-os-te-o'-*

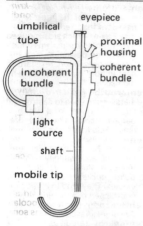

umbilical tube

eyepiece

proximal housing

coherent bundle

incoherent bundle

light source

shaft

mobile tip

ENDOSCOPE

mah). A new growth in the medullary cavity of a bone.

endosteum (end-os'-te-um). The lining membrane of bone cavities, a function of which is to enlarge the medullary cavity as the bone grows by the action of osteoclasts (q.v.).

endothelioma (en-do-the-le-o'-mah). A malignant growth originating in endothelium.

endothelium (en-do-the'-le-um). The membranous lining of serous, synovial and other internal surfaces.

endotoxin (en-do-toks'-in). A poison produced and retained within the micro-organism. See Exotoxin.

endotracheal (en-do-trak-e'-al). Within the trachea. E. anaesthesia. See Anaesthesia. E. tube. A tube which is inserted into the trachea when a patient requires ventilatory support.

enema (en'-e-mah). A liquid for injection into the rectum, which is either absorbed or ejected. Evacuant e. One to relieve constipation or to empty the bowel (600 to 1000 ml warm tap water or soap and water). Magnesium sulphate e. One to relieve intracranial pressure (60 g in 200 ml of water). Retention e. One to be retained, to increase body fluids (water or dextrose saline) or as a sedative (bromide, chloral or paraldehyde).

enervation (en-er-va'-shun). (1) General weakness and loss of strength. (2) Removal of a nerve.

enophthalmos (en-of-thal'-mos). Retracted eyeball in its orbit.

enostosis (en-os-to'-sis). A tumour or bony growth within the medullary canal of a bone.

ensiform cartilage (en'-se-form). The xyphoid process at the lower end of the sternum.

Entamoeba histolytica (en-ta-me'-bah his-to-lit'-ik-ah). The micro-organism of amoebic dysentery.

enteralgia (en-ter-al'-je-ah). Pain in the intestines.

enterectomy (en-ter-ek'-to-me). Excision of a portion of the intestine.

enteric fever (en-ter'-ik). See Typhoid fever.

enteritis (en-ter-i'-tis). Inflammation of the intestine.

enterobacteria (en-ter-o-bak-te'-re-ah). A family of bacteria, many of which are normally found in the human intestine. Included amongst them are the genera Escherichia, Klebsiella, Salmonella, Shigella and Proteus.

enterobiasis (en-ter-o-bi'-as-is). Infestation by threadworms (q.v.).

enterocele (en'-ter-o-seel). A

hernia of the intestine. *See* Hernia.

enterococcus (*en-ter-o-kok'-us*). Any streptococcus of the human intestine. An example is *Streptococcus faecalis*, only harmful out of its normal habitat when it may cause a urinary infection or endocarditis.

enterocolitis (*en-ter-o-ko'-li-tis*). Inflammation of both the large and small intestine. *Necrotizing e.* Disease of small preterm babies in which air in the intestinal wall may give rise to pneumoperitoneum and paralytic ileus. It may be caused by exchange transfusion, respiratory distress or infection of the amniotic sac.

enterokinase (*en-ter-o-ki'-naze*). The activator of trypsinogen into trypsin, found in succus entericus.

enterolith (*en'-ter-o-lith*). A hard faecal concretion, sometimes found in the intestines.

enteromegaly (*en-ter-o-meg'-al-e*). An unusually large intestine. For example megaduodenum (*q.v.*).

enteron (*en'-ter-on*). The intestine.

enteropexy (*en-ter-o-peks'-e*). Fixation of a part of the intestine to the abdominal wall.

enteroptosis (*en-ter-op-to'-sis*). A prolapse of the intestines, due to weakening of the mesenteric attachments or of the abdominal wall.

enterospasm (*en'-ter-o-spasm*). Intestinal colic.

enterostomy (*en-ter-os'-to-me*). An opening into the small intestine. It may be: (1) Temporary, to relieve obstruction. (2) Permanent, in the form of an ileostomy in cases of total colectomy.

enterotome (*en'-ter-o-tome*). Enterotribe (*q.v.*).

enterotomy (*en-ter-ot'-o-me*). Any incision of the intestine.

enterotoxins (*en-ter-o-toks'-ins*). Toxins which are produced by many of the organisms which cause food poisoning, and frequently prove more resistant to destruction than the bacteria themselves.

enterotribe (*en'-ter-o-tribe*). A metal clamp used to destroy the spur of tissue in a double-barrelled colostomy as a preliminary to its closure.

enteroviruses (*en-ter-o-vi'-rus-es*). Minute spherical particles that are normally parasitic in the intestines and include the polio, cocksackie and ECHO viruses. They tend to invade the central nervous system.

enterozoon (*en-ter-o-zo'-on*). Any intestinal parasite.

entoderm (*en'-to-derm*). The innermost of the three germ layers of the embryo. It gives rise to the lining of most of the respiratory tract, the intestinal tract and its glands.

entropion (*en-tro'-pe-on*). Inversion of an eyelid, so that the lashes rub against the globe of the eye.

enucleation (*en-u-kle-a'-shun*). The removal of a tumour or gland by shelling it out whole and free from other tissues.

enuresis (*en-u-re'-sis*). Involuntary passing of urine. *Nocturnal e.* That occurring during sleep. *E. alarm.* An apparatus used in the treatment of enuresis in children. It consists of two sheets of aluminium foil, which are separated by a bed sheet on which the child lies. When a few drops of urine wet the sheets, a circuit is closed and an alarm bell rings to waken the patient.

environment (*en-vi'-ron-ment*). The surroundings. This

may apply to objects or the habitat of living matter.

enzyme (*en'-zime*). *See* Catalyst.

enzymology (*en-zi-mol'-o-je*). The scientific study of enzymes and their action.

eosinophil (*e-o-sin'-o-fil*). Cell having an affinity for acid stains, e.g. some white blood cells.

eosinophilia (*e-o-sin-o-fil'-e-ah*). Excessive numbers of eosinophils present in the blood.

ependyma (*ep-en'-de-mah*). The membrane lining the cerebral ventricles and the central canal of the spinal cord.

ependymoma (*ep-en-de-mo'-mah*). A new growth arising from the lining cells of the ventricles or central canal of the spinal cord. It gives rise to signs of hydrocephalus and is treated by surgery and radiotherapy.

ephedrine (*ef'-ed-reen*). A drug that relieves spasm of the bronchi, having a similar action to adrenaline but it can be taken orally. May be used in asthma and chronic bronchitis.

ephidrosis (*ef-id-ro'-sis*). Profuse sweating.

epi-. Prefix meaning 'upon'.

epiblepharon (*ep-e-blef'-ar-on*). A congenital condition in which an excess of skin of the eyelid folds over the lid margin.

epicanthus (*ep-e-kan'-thus*). A fold of skin sometimes present over the inner canthus of the eye.

epicranium (*ep-e-kra'-ne-um*). Structures covering the cranium.

epicritic (*ep-e-krit'-ik*). Term applied to sensory nerve fibres in the skin which give the appreciation of touch and temperature.

epidemic (*ep-e-dem'-ik*). Any disease attacking a large number of people at the same time.

epidemiology (*ep-e-dem-e-ol'-o-je*). Scientific study of the distribution of diseases.

epidermis (*ep-e-der'-mis*). The non-vascular outer layer or cuticle of the skin. It consists of layers of cells which protect the dermis.

Epidermophyton (*ep-e-der-mo-fi'-ton*). A form of ringworm in which there is a fungus infection of the nails and adjoining skin.

epidiascope (*ep-e-di'-a-skope*). A projector to throw an image on a screen from a picture or a solid body such as a pathological specimen.

epididymis (*ep-e-did'-e-mis*). The convoluted tube which lies above the testicle and receives the ducts from that gland. It is prolonged into the vas deferens and conveys the semen.

epididymitis (*ep-e-did-e-mi'-tis*). Inflammation of the epididymis.

epididymo-orchitis (*ep-e-did-e-mo-or-ki'-tis*). Inflammation of the epididymis and the testis.

epidural (*ep-e-du'-ral*). Outside the dura mater. If a spinal anaesthetic is inserted here there is less risk to the spinal cord.

epigastrium (*ep-e-gas'-tre-um*). That region of the abdomen which is situated over the stomach.

epiglottis (*ep-e-glot'-tis*). A cartilaginous structure, which covers the opening from the pharynx into the larynx, and so prevents food from passing into the windpipe in the act of swallowing.

epilation (*ep-il-a'-shun*). Removal of hairs with their roots. It may be effected by X-rays or by electrolysis.

epilepsy (*ep'-e-lep-se*). Convulsive attacks due to excessive electrical discharges by brain cells. In a major attack or *'grand mal'* the patient falls to the ground unconscious, following an aura or unpleasant sensation. There are first tonic and then clonic contractions, from which stage the patient passes into a deep sleep. A minor attack or *'petit mal'* is a momentary loss of consciousness only. *Jacksonian e.* A symptom of a cerebral lesion. The convulsive movements are often localized and close observation of the onset and course of the attack may greatly assist diagnosis.

epileptiform (*ep-e-lep'-te-form*). Resembling an epileptic fit.

epiloia (*ep-e-loy'-ah*). Tuberous sclerosis. A congenital disorder with areas of hardening in the cerebral cortex and other organs, characterized clinically by mental deficiency and epilepsy.

epimenorrhoea (*ep-e-men-or-re'-ah*). Menstruation occurring at abnormally short intervals.

epinephrine (*ep-e-nef'-reen*). Adrenaline (*q.v.*).

epineurium (*ep-e-nu'-re-um*). The sheath of tissue surrounding a nerve.

epiphora (*ep-if'-or-ah*). Persistent overflow of tears, e.g. due to obstruction in the lacrimal passages.

epiphysis (*ep-if'-is-is*). The end of a long bone developed separately but attached by cartilage to the diaphysis, with which it eventually unites. From the line of junction growth in length takes place.

epiplocele (*ep-ip'-lo-seel*). A hernia containing omentum.

epiploon (*ep-ip'-lo-on*). The greater omentum (*q.v.*).

episcleritis (*ep-e-skler-i'-tis*).
Inflammation of the outer coat of the eyeball.

episiorrhaphy (*e-pis-e-or'-raf-e*). The repair of a laceration of perineum.

episiotomy (*e-pis-e-ot'-o-me*). An incision made in the perineum when it will not stretch sufficiently during the second stage of labour.

epispadias (*ep-e-spa'-de-as*). A condition in which there is an abnormal opening on the dorsal surface of the penis. *See* Hypospadias.

epistaxis (*ep-e-staks'-is*). Bleeding from the nose.

epithelioma (*ep-e-the-le-o'-mah*). Carcinoma originating in epithelium.

epithelium (*ep-e-the'-le-um*). The surface layer of cells either of the skin or lining tissues.

epithelization (*ep-e-the-li-za'-shun*). Development of epithelium. The final stage in the healing of a surface wound.

epizoon (*ep-e-zo'-on*). Any external parasite.

eponym (*ep'-on-im*). In medicine an anatomical part, disease or structure bearing a person's name, usually that of the man who first described it.

eponymous (*ep-on'-e-mus*). Named after a particular person.

Epstein-Barr virus (*M. A. Epstein-Barr, contemporary British pathologist*). A virus which is thought to be the causative organism of infectious mononucleosis or glandular fever (*q.v.*).

epulis (*ep-u'-lis*). A fibroid tumour of the gums.

Erb's palsy (*W. H. Erb, German physician, 1840–1921*). A paralysis of the arm, often due to birth injury causing pressure on the brachial plexus or lower cervical nerve roots.

erectile (*e-rek'-tile*). Having the

power of becoming erect. *E. tissue.* Vascular tissue which, under stimulus, becomes congested and swollen, causing erection of that part.

erepsin (*er-ep'-sin*). The enzyme of succus entericus which splits peptones into amino acids.

ergography (*er-gog'-raf-e*). A method of measuring the resistance to fatigue in a muscle by noting the output of effort to an electrical stimulus.

ergometrine (*er-go-met'-reen*). An alkaloid of ergot. It stimulates contraction of the uteric muscle.

ergonomics (*er-go-nom'-iks*). The scientific study of man in relation to his work and the effective use of human energy.

ergosterol (*er-gos'-ter-ol*). A substance present in subcutaneous fat which under the influence of ultra-violet light forms vitamin D. Hence the use of artificial sunlight for rickets. Also found in plant and animal foodstuffs, which produce the vitamin when irradiated with ultra-violet light.

ergot (*er'-got*). A drug from a fungus which grows on rye. It causes prolonged contraction of muscle fibres, especially those of blood vessels and of the uterus. Used chiefly to contract the uterus and check haemorrhage at childbirth.

ergotamine (*er-got'-a-meen*). An alkaloid of ergot used in the treatment of migraine.

ergotism (*er'-got-izm*). The effects of poisoning from ergot or of eating diseased rye, in which constriction of the arterioles may lead to gangrene.

erisiphake (*er-is'-e-fake*). A cup-shaped device attached to a suction motor used in intracapsular cataract extraction to remove the lens.

erosion (*e-ro'-zhun*). The breaking down of tissue, usually by ulceration.

eroticism (*e-rot'-is-izm*). A condition of sexual excitement.

eructation (*e-ruk-ta'-shun*). Belching. The escape of gas from the stomach, through the mouth.

erysipelas (*er-e-sip'-e-las*). An acute contagious disease, caused by the haemolytic streptococcus and characterized by localized inflammation of the skin, with pain and fever. The inflammation always commences round a wound, which is sometimes too small to be apparent, and is in the form of a raised red rash with small blebs, spreading gradually away from the centre, and having a well-defined margin. Considerable oedema occurs if near loose tissues, e.g. eyelids or scrotum. Seldom seen because sulphonamides and penicillin have so effectively treated all forms of streptococcal infection.

erythema (*er-e-the'-mah*). A superficial redness of the skin. *E. induratum.* A manifestation of vasculitis (*q.v.*). *E. multiforme.* An acute eruption of the skin, which may be due to an allergy or to drug sensitivity. *E. nodosum.* A painful disease in which bright red, tender nodes occur below the knee or on the forearm; it may be associated with tuberculosis. *Punctate e.* Erythema scarlatiniforme.

erythrasma (*er-e-thraz'-mah*). A skin disease due to a microsporon infection, attacking the armpits or groins. It causes no irritation, but is contagious.

erythroblast (*er-ith'-ro-blast*). Elementary red blood cell.

erythroblastosis fetalis (*er-ith-ro-blas-to'-sis fe-tal'-is*). Extensive production of erythroblasts in the newly born due to excessive destruction of red blood cells. Due to rhesus incompatibility between the child's and the mother's blood.

erythrocyte (*er-ith'-ro-site*). Red blood cells, which are developed in the red bone marrow found in the cancellous tissue of all bones. The *haemopoietic factor* vitamin B_{12} is essential

Deficiency in numbers of red blood cells.

erythrocytosis (*er-ith-ro-si-to'-sis*). Erythrocythaemia (*q.v.*).

erythroedema polyneuritis (*er-ith-re-de'-mah pol-e-nu-ri'-tis*). Infantile acrodynia. A rare disease of infants with redness and swelling of the hands, feet, and face; tachycardia, marked irritability, and photophobia. Cause unknown. 'Pink' disease.

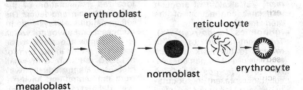

erythroblast

reticulocyte

megaloblast

normoblast

erythrocyte

ERYTHROCYTE DEVELOPMENT IN BONE MARROW

for the change from megaloblast to normoblast, and iron, thyroxin, and vitamin C are also necessary for its perfect structure. *See* diagram. *E. sedimentation rate.* ESR. The rate at which the cells of citrated blood form a deposit in a graduated 200-mm tube (*Westergren method*). The normal is less than 10 mm of clear plasma in 1 h. This is much increased in severe infection, acute rheumatism and tuberculosis.

erythrocythaemia (*er-ith-ro-si-the'-me-ah*). Polycythaemia. Increase in numbers of red blood cells due to over-activity of the bone marrow. *Syn.* Vaquez's disease, polycythaemia vera (*q.v.*).

erythrocytopenia (*er-ith-ro-si-to-pe'-ne-ah*). Erythropenia.

erythromycin (*er-ith-ro-mi'-sin*). An antibiotic drug with a wide range of activity but resistance quickly develops. Best used for staphylococcal infections resistant to other antibiotics.

erythropoiesis (*er-ith-ro-poye'-sis*). The manufacture of red blood corpuscles.

erythropoietin (*er-ith-ro-poye'-tin*). A hormone produced by the kidney that stimulates the production of red blood cells in the bone marrow.

erythropsia (*er-e-throp'-se-ah*). A defect of vision, in which all objects appear red.

Esbach's albuminometer (*G. H. Esbach, French physician, 1843–90*). A graduated glass tube for estimating the amount of albumen in urine. *See* Appendix 11.

eschar (*es'-kar*). A slough, as results from the destruction of living tissue by gangrene or burning.

Escherichia (*esh-er-ik'-e-ah*). A genus of Enterobacteriaceae. *E. coli.* An organism normally present in the intestines of man and vertebrate animals. Although not generally pathogenic it may set up infections of the gall-bladder, bile ducts and the urinary tract. It was formerly called *Bacterium coli.*

eserine (*es'-er-een*). Physostigmine (*q.v.*).

Esmarch's tourniquet (*J. F. A. von Esmarch, German surgeon, 1823–1908*). A rubber bandage used in surgery to express blood from a limb and render it less vascular.

esotropia (*es-o-tro'-pe-ah*). Convergent strabismus.

ESR. Erythrocyte sedimentation rate. *See* Erythrocyte.

essence (*es'-ens*). A volatile oil dissolved in alcohol.

essential amino acids (*e-sen'-shal am'-in-o as'-ids*). Those amino acids necessary for the maintenance of tissue growth and repair. Eight amino acids are essential for adults and ten for children. *See* Appendix 10.

ester (*es'-ter*). A compound ether formed by the combination of an organic acid and alcohol.

ethanolamine oleate (*eth-an-ol-a-meen o'-le-ate*). An intravenous sclerosing agent used to inject varicose veins.

ether (*e'-ther*). A subtle fluid said to fill all space and to penetrate all bodies and to be the medium of transmission of light, heat, X-rays, radio waves, magnetism and electricity. *Anaesthetic e.* A volatile liquid

used as a general anaesthetic agent. *E. solvens.* A skin antiseptic.

ethics (*eth'-iks*). A code of moral principles. *Nursing e.* The moral code governing a nurse's behaviour with her patients, their relatives and her colleagues.

ethmoid (*eth'-moid*). A sievelike bone, separating the cavity of the nose from the brain. The olfactory nerves pass through its perforations.

ethmoidectomy (*eth-moid-ek'-to-me*). Surgical removal of a portion of the ethmoid bone.

ethoheptazine (*eth-o-hep'-ta-zeen*). An analgesic related to pethidine. It relieves pain and muscle spasm. A proprietary preparation is Zactirin.

ethosuximide (*eth-o-suks'-im-ide*). An anticonvulsant used in the treatment of '*petit mal*' epilepsy. One proprietary preparation is known as Zarontin.

ethyl biscoumacetate (*eth'-il bi-coum-as'-e-tate*). An anticoagulant of the coumarin group. Tromexan is a proprietary preparation.

ethyl chloride (*eth'-il klor'-ide*). A volatile liquid used: (1) as a local anaesthetic. When sprayed on any part of the body it causes local insensitivity, through freezing. (2) A general anaesthetic by inhalation.

ethylene oxide (*eth'-il-een oks'-ide*). A gas which is capable of penetrating relatively inaccessible sites in apparatus during sterilization. It is also used for such equipment which is too delicate to be sterilized by other methods.

ethyloestrenol (*eth-il-e'-stren-ol*). An anabolic steroid that may be used to treat severe weight loss, debility and osteoporosis.

etiology (*e-te-ol'-o-je*). *See* Aetiology.

eu-. Greek prefix meaning 'good'.

eugenics (*u-jen'-iks*). The study of measures which may be taken to improve future generations both physically and mentally.

eugenol (*u'-jen-ol*). A local anaesthetic and antiseptic, derived from oil of cloves and cinnamon, used in dentistry.

eunuch (*u'-nuk*). A castrated male.

eupepsia (*u-pep'-se-ah*). A good digestion with normal function of the digestive juices. It is particularly applied to the stomach.

euphoria (*u-for'-e-ah*). An exaggerated feeling of well-being often not justified by circumstances.

euplastic (*u-plas'-tik*). Capable of being transformed into healthy tissue.

eusol (*u'-sol*). A chlorine antiseptic containing hypochlorous and boric acids. The name is coined from the initials of Edinburgh University Solution of Lime.

eustachian tube (*B. Eustachio, Italian anatomist, 1520–74*). The pharyngotympanic tube (*q.v.*).

eustachian valve (*B. Eustachio, Italian anatomist, 1520–74*). A fold in the lining membrane of the right atrium of the heart.

euthanasia (*u-than-a'-ze-ah*). The process of dying easily and painlessly, and the bringing of it about, as an act of mercy, in cases of incurable and distressing disease.

euthyroid (*u-thi'-roid*). Having a normally functioning thyroid gland. A term used after successful treatment of thyrotoxicosis (*q.v.*).

eutocia (*u-to'-se-ah*). Easy childbirth.

evacuant (*e-vak'-u-ant*). An aperient. Any drug or washout that empties the colon.

evacuation (*e-vak-u-a'-shun*). Emptying out. Usually referring to that of the rectum and lower bowel.

evacuator (*e-vak-u-a'-tor*). An instrument which produces evacuation. *Bigelow's e., Freyer's e.* Pattern designed to wash out small particles of stone from the bladder after these have been crushed by a lithotrite (*q.v.*).

evaporating lotion (*e-vap'-or-a-ting lo'-shun*). One which, used as a compress, produces local coldness and so relieves inflammation, e.g. lead lotion and eau de cologne. As these are applied in order to evaporate, they should not be covered in any way.

eventration (*e-ven-tra'-shun*). Protrusion of the intestines through the abdominal wall.

eversion (*e-ver'-shun*). Turning outwards.

evisceration (*e-vis-er-a'-shun*). Removal of internal organs. *E. of eye.* Removal of the contents of the eyeball, but not the sclera. *E. of orbit.* Removal of the eye and all structures in the orbit.

evulsion (*e-vul'-shun*). Plucking out. *See* Avulsion.

Ewing's tumour (*J. Ewing, American pathologist, 1866–1943*). A form of sarcoma usually affecting the shaft of a long bone.

ex-. Prefix meaning 'out' or 'away from'.

exacerbation (*eks-as-er-ba'-shun*). An increase in the severity of the symptoms of a disease.

exanthematous (*eks-an-*

them'-at-us). Any disease associated with a skin eruption.

exchange transfusion (*ex-cha'-ng trans-fu'-zhun*). *See* Transfusion.

excision (*eks-siz'-shun*). The cutting out of a part.

excitation (*eks-si-ta'-shun*). The act of stimulating.

excitement (*eks-site'-ment*). A physiological and emotional response to a stimulus.

excoriation (*eks-kor-e-a'-shun*). An abrasion of the skin.

excrement (*eks'-kre-ment*). Waste matter from the body.

excrescence (*eks-kres'-ense*). Abnormal overgrowth of tissue.

excreta (*eks-kre'-tah*). The natural discharges of the excretory system: faeces, urine, sweat, and sputum.

excretion (*eks-kre'-shun*). The discharge of waste from the body.

exenteration (*eks-en-ter-a'-shun*). Evisceration. The removal of an organ. *Pelvic e.* The removal of the pelvic contents. An extensive operation for malignant growth.

exfoliation (*eks-fo-le-a'-shun*). The separation of dead tissue in thin flaky layers.

exfoliative cytology (*eks-fo'-le-a-tiv si-tol'-o-je*). *See* Cytology.

exfoliative dermatitis (*ex-fo'-le-a-tiv der-mat-i'-tis*). *See* Dermatitis.

exhibitionism (*eks-hib-ish'-un-izm*). (1) Showing off. A desire to attract attention. (2) Exposing the genitals in order to provoke a response in one or more people.

exocrine (*eks'-o-krine*). A term applied to those glands which discharge their secretion by means of a duct, e.g. salivary glands. *See* Endocrine.

exogenous (*eks-oj'-en-us*). Of external origin. A condition arising due to environmental factors.

exomphalos (*eks-om'-fal-os*). Umbilical hernia.

exophthalmos (*eks-off-thal'-mos*). Abnormal protrusion of the eyeballs. *See* Goitre.

exostosis (*eks-os-to'-sis*). A bony outgrowth from the surface of a bone. May be due to chronic inflammation, constant pressure on the bone or tumour formation.

exotoxin (*eks-o-toks'-in*). Toxin secreted by micro-organisms into the surrounding media. *See* Endotoxin.

expectorant (*eks-pek'-tor-ant*). A remedy which promotes and facilitates expectoration.

expectoration (*eks-pek-tor-a'-shun*). Sputum (*q.v.*). Secretions coughed up from the air-passages. Its characteristics a valuable aid in diagnosis and note should be taken of the quantity ejected, its colour, and the amount of effort required. *Frothiness* denotes that it comes from an air-containing cavity, *fluidity* indicates oedema of the lung.

expiration (*eks-pi-ra'-shun*). The act of breathing out.

exploration. The operation of surgically investigating any part of the body.

expression (*eks-pres'-shun*). Pressing out. (1) Pressure on the uterus to facilitate the expulsion of the placenta or child. (2) Artificial extraction of milk from the breast.

exsanguination (*eks-san-gwin-a'-shun*). Making bloodless. *See* Esmarch's tourniquet.

extension (*eks-ten'-shun*). (1) The act of extending a joint as in the hip and knee when standing. (2) A weight applied at the end of a limb in such a way that tension is exerted, which first pulls it into normal position and then keeps it thus. The apparatus used can be strips of adhesive strapping or Elastoplast, attached to the leg on either side. The ends are fixed to a wooden stirrup perforated by a cord, which passes over a pulley at the foot of the bed and to which the weight is attached. This is also known as *skin traction*. *See* Counter extension.

extensor (*eks-ten'-sor*). A muscle which extends a part. *Quadriceps e.* That of the front of the thigh.

extirpation (*eks-ter-pa'-shun*). Complete removal.

extra (*eks'-trah*). A prefix meaning 'outside'.

extracapsular (*eks-trah-cap-su'-lah*). Outside the capsule. May refer to a fracture occurring at the end of the bone, but outside the joint capsule, or to cataract extraction.

extracellular (*eks-trah-sel'-u-lah*). Outside the cell. *E. fluid.* Tissue fluid that surrounds the cells.

extract (*eks'-tract*). A preparation made by extracting the soluble principles of a drug, by steeping in water or alcohol and then evaporating the fluid.

extradural (*eks-trah-du'-ral*). Outside the dura mater. *E. haemorrhage. See* Haemorrhage.

extragenital (*eks-trah-jen'-it-al*). Not related to the genitals. *E. syphilis.* Acquired but not venereal in origin; e.g. by infection of finger.

extrahepatic (*eks-trah-hep-at'-ik*). Outside the liver. Relating to a condition affecting the liver in which the cause is outside liver.

extrapleural (*eks-trah-plu'-ral*). Between the chest wall and

parietal layer of pleura. *See* Pneumothorax.

extrapyramidal tract (*eks-trah-pir-am'-id-al trakt*). The nerve fibres which exert some control over the anterior horn cells and originate in the higher centres of the brain.

extrasystole (*eks-trah-sis'-tol-e*). Premature contraction of atria or ventricles. *See* Systole.

extrauterine pregnancy (*eks-trah-u'-ter-ine*). Ectopic gestation. Development of a fetus outside the uterus.

extravasation (*eks-trah-vas-a'-shun*). Effusion or escape of fluid from its normal course into surrounding tissues. *E. of blood.* A bruise. *E. of urine* into the pelvic tissues may complicate a fracture of the pelvis if the bladder is injured.

extrinsic factor (*eks-trin'-sik*). First described by Castle, it is now considered to be vitamin B_{12}, which is necessary for the manufacture of red blood cells. The intrinsic factor produced in the stomach is necessary for the absorption of vitamin B_{12}.

extroversion (*eks-tro-ver'-shun*). Turning inside out, e.g. of the uterus, as sometimes occurs after labour.

extrovert (*eks'-tro-vert*). A person who is sociable, a good mixer and interested in what goes on around him. A personality type first described by Jung. *See* Introvert.

exudation (*eks-u-da'-shun*). Oozing.

eye. The organ of sight. A globular structure with three coats. The nerve tissue of the retina receives impressions of images via the pupil and lens. From this the optic nerve conveys the impressions to the visual area of the cerebrum.

eyelids. The protective cover-

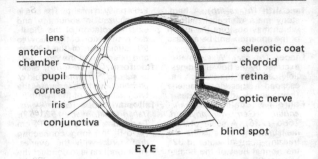

lens
anterior chamber
pupil
cornea
iris
conjunctiva

sclerotic coat
choroid
retina
optic nerve
blind spot

EYE

ings of the eye, composed of muscle and dense connective tissue covered with skin, lined with conjunctiva and fringed with eyelashes.

eye-teeth. The upper canine teeth.

F

F. Abbreviation for Fahrenheit (*q.v.*).

fabrication (*fab-re-ka'-shun*). *See* Confabulation.

Fabricius, bursa of (*H. Fabricius, Italian anatomist, 1533–1619*). The lymphoid organ in birds, which has a similar function to Peyer's patches and the appendix in man.

face presentation (*fase presen-ta'-shun*). Where the face presents first during labour.

facet (*fas'-et*). A smooth, level surface made by movement of one part on another. Gall-stones are faceted when many are present in the gall-bladder.

facet syndrome (*fas'-et sin'-drome*). A slight dislocation of the small facet joints of the vertebrae giving rise to pain and muscle spasm.

facial (*fa'-shal*). Pertaining to the face or lower anterior portion of the head. *F. nerve.* The seventh cranial nerve supplying the salivary glands and superficial face muscles. *F. paralysis. See* Paralysis. *F. pulse.* The pulse which can be detected on the chin near the angle of the jaw.

facies (*fa-she-eez*). Facial expression. *Abdominal f.* Seen in peritonitis. The face is cold and livid, eyes and cheeks sunken, and tongue and lips dry. *Adenoid f.* The open mouth and vacant expression associated with mouth breathing and nasal obstruction. *Hippocratic f.* The drawn, anxious expression seen in patients with extreme prostration; with the pinched, pointed nostrils and the cyanotic appearance of the lips and nose. *Parkinson f.* A characteristic fixed expression, due to paucity of movement of facial muscles. Characteristic of paralysis agitans.

facultative (*fak'-ul-ta-tiv*). Optional. *F. bacteria.* Those which, although normally *aerobes*, are also capable of being *anaerobes*.

faecalith (*fe'-ka-lith*). A hard, stony mass of faecal material which may obstruct the lumen of the appendix and be a cause of inflammation.

faeces (*fe'-sez*). Waste matter excreted by the bowel: indigestible cellulose; food which has escaped digestion; bacteria (living and dead); and water.

Fahrenheit scale. (*G. D. Fahrenheit, German physicist, 1686–1736*). A scale of heat measurement. It registers the freezing-point of water at 32°, the normal heat of the human body at 98·4°, and the boiling-point of water at 212°.

fainting. *See* Syncope.

Fairbank's splint (*T. J. Fairbank, contemporary British orthopaedic surgeon*). An appliance used for the treatment of Erb's palsy in infants. The arm is immobilized in abduction and external rotation of the shoulder, with flexion of the elbow to 90°, supination of the forearm and extension of the wrist.

falciform (*fal'-se-form*). Sickle-shaped. *F. ligament.* A fold of peritoneum which separates the two main lobes of the liver.

fallopian tubes (*G. Fallopius, Italian anatomist, 1523–63*). Two tubes about 10 to 14 cm (4 to 5½ in.) long, connecting the uterus with the ovaries. Their function is to conduct the ova from the ovaries to the interior of the uterus and spermatozoa from the uterus to the ovaries.

Fallot's tetralogy (*E.-L. A. Fallot, French physician, 1850–1911*). A congenital heart dis-

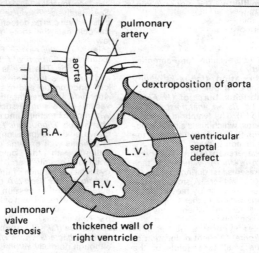

FALLOT'S TETRALOGY

ease with four characteristic defects: (*a*) pulmonary artery stenosis, (*b*) inter-ventricular defect of the septum, (*c*) over-riding of aorta, i.e. opening into both right and left ventricles, (*d*) hypertrophy of the right ventricle.

false. Not true. *F. pains.* Abdominal pains occurring in pregnancy which are not the real pains of labour. *F. pelvis.* The area between the brim of the true pelvis and the crest of the ilium. *F. joint.* Fibrous union of a fractured bone, which gives unnatural mobility. It may result from infection in an open fracture.

falx cerebri (*fal-ks ser'-e-bri*). The fold of dura mater which separates the two cerebral hemispheres.

familial (*fam-il'-e-al*). Affecting several members of one family.

Fanconi's syndrome (*G. Fanconi, Swiss paediatrician, 1892– *). Inherited disorder of metabolism in which reabsorption of phosphate, amino acids and sugar by the renal tubules is impaired. These substances then appear in the urine. The kidneys fail to produce acid urine, and resulting features are thirst, polyuria and rickets, leading to chronic renal failure.

fang. The root of a tooth.

fantasy (*fan'-tas-e*). An imaginative mental activity.

faradization (*M. Faraday, English physicist, 1791–1867*). Treatment by the application of an induced or faradic current of electricity. This is alternating, the negative and positive poles constantly reversing. The result is rapid and spasmodic contraction of the muscle to which it is applied.

farinaceous (*far-in-a'-shus*).

Foods having the nature of, or containing starch, e.g. wheat, oats, barley and rice.

farmer's lung. A disease occurring in those in contact with mouldy hay. It is thought to be due to a hypersensitivity, with widespread reaction in the lung tissue. It causes excessive breathlessness.

fascia (*fash'-e-ah*). A sheath of connective tissue, enclosing muscle.

fasciculation (*fas-ik-u-la'-shun*). Isolated fine muscle twitches which give a flickering appearance. It is seen in some cases of nerve impairment.

fasciculus (*fas-ik'-u-lus*). A small bundle of fibres.

fastigium (*fas-tij'-e-um*). The part of a fever when the temperature is at its height.

fat. Adipose. The white oily portion of animal tissue. *F. -soluble vitamins.* Vitamins A, D, E and K. *Brown f. See* Brown adipose tissue. *Wool f.* Lanolin (*q.v.*).

fatigue (*fat-eeg'*). A state of weariness which may range from mental disinclination for effort to profound exhaustion following great physical and mental effort. *Muscle f.* May occur during prolonged effort due to oxygen lack and accumulation of waste products.

fatty acids (*fat'-te as'-ids*). Substances which form fats with glycerol.

fatty degeneration (*fat'-te dejen-er-a'-shun*). A degenerative change in tissue cells due to the invasion of fat and consequent weakening of the organ.

fauces (*faw'-sez*). The opening from the mouth into the pharynx. *Pillars of the f.* The two folds of muscle covered with mucous membrane which pass from the soft palate on either side of the fauces. One fold passes into the tongue, the other into the pharynx, and between them is situated the tonsil.

favism (*fa'-vizm*). A condition in which certain individuals develop acute haemolysis as a result of sensitivity to certain kinds of bean, e.g. Italian lentil. They have a deficiency of glucose-6-phosphate dehydrogenase in their red blood cells.

favus (*fa'-vus*). A contagious skin disease, with formation of scabs, in appearance like a honeycomb. It usually affects the scalp and is due to a fungus infection.

fear. A feeling of acute apprehension or anxiety. It may give rise to any of the following symptoms; tachycardia, pallor, faintness, sweating, tightness of the chest, irregular breathing, giddiness, dilated pupils, frequency of micturition and diarrhoea. *Obsessional f.* A recurring irrational fear that is not amenable to ordinary reassurance. *States of f. See* Anxiety states.

febrile (*feb'-rile*). Characterized by or relating to fever. *F. convulsion.* Convulsion which occurs in childhood. It is associated with pyrexia.

fecundation (*fe-kun-da'-shun*). Fertilization.

feeblemindedness (*fee-bl-mind'-ed-ness*). Formerly a term for some degree of mental subnormality (*q.v.*).

Fehling's solution (*H. von Fehling, German chemist, 1812–85*). Solution which changes colour in the presence of reducing substances. Formerly used to detect glycosuria.

Felty's syndrome (*A. R. Felty, American physician,*

1895–). A variety of rheumatoid arthritis in which the spleen is enlarged and may require removal.

femoral (*fem'-or-al*). Pertaining to the femur. *F. artery.* That of the thigh from groin to knee. *F. canal.* The opening below Poupart's ligament through which the femoral artery, etc., passes from the abdomen to the thigh. *F. hernia. See* Hernia. *F. thrombosis. See* Phlegmasia.

femur (*fe'-mer*). The thighbone.

fenestra (*fen-es'-trah*). A window-like opening. *F. ovalis.* The oval window connecting the middle and the internal ear.

fenestration (*fen-es-tra'-shun*). An operation by which a window is made in the bony labyrinth of the ear to assist hearing when deafness is due to otosclerosis.

ferment (*fer'-ment*). A substance which can produce chemical changes in other substances, without itself undergoing change. *Syn.* Enzyme.

fermentation (*fer-men-ta'-shun*). (1) A process of breaking down by an enzyme or ferment as in the production of alcohol and bread. (2) A method of bacterial identification by the production of gas during culture in a carbohydrate medium.

ferrous (*fer'-rus*). Containing iron. *F. fumarate, F. gluconate, F. succinate* and *F. sulphate* are all iron compounds given orally. *F. succinate* and *F. sulphate* are the most widely used.

fertilization (*fer-til-i-za'-shun*). The impregnation of the female sex cell, the ovum, by a male sex cell, a spermatozoon.

fester (*fes'-ter*). Superficial inflammation with suppuration.

festination (*fes-te-na'-shun*). The involuntary acceleration of walking which occurs when the centre of gravity is displaced in paralysis agitans.

fetishism (*fet'-ish-izm*). A superstition in which an object is regarded with an irrational fear or a strong emotional attachment.

fetal (*fe'-tal*). Pertaining to the fetus (*q.v.*).

fetus (*fe'-tus*). The name given to the developing baby between the 8th and the 40th weeks of pregnancy.

fever. (1) A rise of body temperature above normal, accompanied by quickened pulse and respiration, dry skin, scanty highly-coloured urine, vomiting, and headache. (2) Pyrexia (*q.v.*).

fibre (*fi'-ber*). A thread-like structure.

fibreoptics (*fi-ber-op'-tiks*). By the means of very fine glass fibres light can be transmitted along flexible tubes. Use is made of this in endoscopic instruments such as the gastroscope. Using a fibreoptic cardiac catheter pulses of light can be picked up from which the oxygen saturation can be determined.

fibrillation (*fib-ril-a'-shun*). A quivering, vibratory movement of muscle fibres. *Auricular* or *atrial f.* Rapid contractions of the atrium causing irregular contraction of the ventricles in both rhythm and force. *Ventricular f.* Fine rapid twitchings of the ventricles as may occur during cardiac surgery. Rapidly fatal unless it can be controlled. *See* Defibrillation.

fibrin (*fi'-brin*). A protein formed from fibrinogen in blood plasma in the process of clotting. It is separated from the serum, and entangles the corpuscles. *F. ferment.* Thrombin. *See* Thrombokinase.

fibrinogen (*fi-brin'-o-jen*). A soluble albuminous substance present in the blood which is converted into fibrin by the action of *thrombin* (*q.v.*) when the blood clots.

fibrinolysin (*fi-brin-ol'-is-in*). A proteolytic enzyme that dissolves fibrin.

fibrinolysis (*fi-brin-ol'-is-is*). The dissolution of a clot after healing has taken place.

fibrinopenia (*fi-brin-o-pe'-ne-ah*). Due to a lack of plasma fibrinogen there is a tendency to bleed as the coagulation time is increased.

fibroadenoma (*fi-bro-ad-en-o'-mah*). A tumour of glandular and fibrous tissue.

fibroangioma (*fi-bro-an-je-o'-mah*). A new growth arising in both fibrous and vascular tissue.

fibroblast (*fi'-bro-blast*). Cells which form fibrous tissue.

fibrocartilage (*fi-bro-kart'-il-aj*). Cartilage with fibrous tissue in it.

fibrochondritis (*fi-bro-kon-dri'-tis*). Inflammation of fibrocartilage.

fibrocyst (*fi'-bro-sist*). Cystic degeneration in a fibroma.

fibrocystic disease of the pancreas. An inherited condition characterized by fatty stools and repeated lung infections. Treated by giving pancreatin to replace the pancreatic secretion which is missing. *Syn.* Mucoviscidosis.

fibroid (*fi'-broid*). Composed of fibrous and muscular tissue. A tumour common in the uterus. More correctly a fibromyoma.

fibroma (*fi-bro'-mah*). A benign tumour of fibrous tissue. *Cystic f.* Fibrocyst (*q.v.*).

fibromyoma (*fi-bro-mi-o'-mah*). A tumour consisting of fibrous and muscle tissue. Fre-

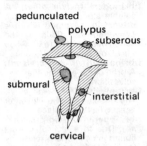

pedunculated

polypus

subserous

submural

interstitial

cervical

**FIBROMYOMA
OF UTERUS**

---

quently found in or on the uterus.

fibrosarcoma (*fi-bro-sar-ko'-mah*). A malignant tumour arising in fibrous tissue.

fibrosis (*fi-bro'-sis*). Fibrous tissue formation as occurs in scar tissue or as the result of inflammation. It is the cause of adhesions of the peritoneum or other serous membranes. *F. of lung.* This may precede bronchiectasis and emphysema.

fibrositis (*fi-bro-si'-tis*). A term loosely applied to pain and stiffness of sudden onset for which no other cause can be found although inflammation of fibrous tissue cannot be demonstrated. The condition is thought to arise from injury or strain to ligaments, causing muscle spasm.

fibula (*fib'-u-lah*). The slender bone from knee to ankle, on the outer side of the leg.

field of vision. That area that can be seen with the eye fixed. It can be plotted by a perimeter (*q.v.*).

fight response. The sympathetic nervous system activity involved in emotional excitement and exercise.

filament (*fil'-a-ment*). A small thread-like structure.

Filaria (*fil-air'-e-ah*). A genus of threadworms. Found mainly in the tropics and sub-tropics.

filariasis (*fil-ar-i'-as-is*). The condition of infection by *Filaria.* Elephantiasis (*q.v.*).

filiform (*fil'-e-form*). Hair-like. *F. papillae.* The fine hair-like processes that cover the anterior two-thirds of the tongue.

filix mas (*fi'-liks mas*). Male fern. A drug given to destroy tapeworms.

filtrate (*fil'-trate*). The fluid which passes through a filter.

fimbria (*fim'-bre-ah*). A fringe. *Fallopian f.* The fringed ends of the fallopian tubes in the centre of which is the abdominal ostium.

final common path. *See* Lower motor neurone.

finger (*fing'-er*). A digit. *Clubbed f.* A broadening and thickening of the ends of the fingers, common in chronic diseases of the heart and lungs.

first aid. Emergency treatment carried out before medical aid is available. *See* Appendix 1.

fission (*fish'-un*). A form of asexual reproduction by dividing into two equal parts as in bacteria. *Binary f.* The splitting in two of the nucleus and the protoplasm of a cell as in protozoa. *Nuclear f.* The splitting of the nucleus of an atom with the release of a great quantity of energy.

fissure (*fish'-ur*). A cleft. (1) *F. in ano.* A painful crack in the mucous membrane of the anus, generally caused by injury from hard faeces. (2) *F. of Rolando.* A definite fold in the cortex of each cerebral hemisphere dividing the sensory from the motor area.

fistula (*fis'-tu-lah*). An abnormal passage connecting the cavity of one organ with another or a cavity and the surface of the body. *F. in ano.* The result of an ischiorectal abscess where the channel is from the anus to the skin. *Biliary f.* A leakage of bile to the exterior, following operation on the gall-bladder or ducts. *Blind f.* One which is open at only one end. *Faecal f.* Following operations on the intestines in which sepsis is present, when the channel is from the intestine through the wound. *Vesicovaginal f.* An opening from the bladder to the vagina, either from error during operation, or from ulceration as may occur in carcinoma of the cervix. *Rectovaginal f.* Fistula from the rectum to the vagina that may result from severe perineal tear.

fits. Paroxysmal motor discharges leading to sudden convulsive movements. These may be: (*a*) *local*, as the carpopedal spasms of tetany; (*b*) *general*, as in epilepsy, eclampsia and hysteria. The term is sometimes applied to apoplexy (*q.v.*).

fixation (*fiks-a'-shun*). A term used to describe a failure to progress wholly or in part through the normal stages of psychological development to a fully developed personality. This is an unconscious process.

flaccid (*flak'-sid*). Soft, flabby. *F. paralysis.* See Paralysis.

flagellum (*flaj-el'-lum*). The whip-like protoplasmic filament by which some bacteria move. *Pl.* flagella.

flat-foot. *Pes planus.* A condition due to absence or sinking of the medial longitudinal arch of the foot, caused by weaken-

ing of the ligaments and tendons.

flatulence (*flat'-u-lens*). The presence of gas in the stomach which may be: (1) The result of air swallowing (*aerophagy*). Sometimes seen in nervous patients. (2) A sign of dyspepsia.

flatulent distension (*flat'-u-lent dis-ten'-shun*). This is due to gas in the intestines. It is a common complication after abdominal operations and is caused by intestinal stasis.

flatus (*fla'-tus*). Gas in the stomach or intestine.

Flaxedil (*flaks'-e-dil*). A proprietary muscle relaxant used in anaesthesia. Gallamine.

flea (*fle*). A blood-sucking insect parasite. *Human f. Pulex irritans* does not transmit disease. *Rat f. Xenopsylla cheopis* transmits plague.

flexibilitas cerea (*fleks-e-bil'-it-as se'-re-ah*). Waxy flexibility in which a patient retains the posture of the body or of a limb in which he or someone else has placed it. A symptom of some forms of schizophrenia.

flexion (*flek'-shun*). Bending. Moving a joint so the two or more bones forming it draw towards each other. *Dorsi-f.* Drawing the foot towards the lower limb. *Plantar f.* Bending the toes downwards.

Flexner's bacillus (S. Flexner, American bacteriologist, 1863–1946). A bacillus belonging to the *Shigella flexneri* group of pathogenic bacteria which cause bacillary dysentery.

flexor (*fleks'-or*). Any muscle causing flexion of a limb or part of the body.

flexure (*fleks'-ure*). A bend or angulation.

floaters (*flo'-ters*). Opacities in the vitreous of the eye that move about and appear as spots before the eye. Probably degenerative deposits. Muscae volitantes.

flocculent (*flok'-u-lent*). Woolly or flaky. Human milk forms a flocculent curd. Sodium citrate added to cows' milk humanizes the curd.

floppy infant (*flop'-e*). Infantile hypotonia in which there is absence of tone in the muscles, often due to impaired nerve supply.

flooding. Excessive loss of blood per vaginam. It may be associated with menstruation or miscarriage.

florid (*flor'-id*). A flushed facial appearance as seen in hypertension or after consuming alcohol.

flowmeter (*flo'-me-ter*). An instrument used to measure liquids or gas. *Oxygen f.* Measures oxygen in litres per minute. *Electro-magnetic f.* Used to measure blood flow.

fluctuation (*fluk-tu-a'-shun*). A wave-like motion felt on palpation of the abdomen. Varying from time to time.

fludrocortisone (*flu-dro-kor'-te-zone*). A synthetic steroid used to replace aldosterone.

fluid compartments (*flu'-id com-part'-ments*). The fluid-containing areas of the body. *See* Intracellular *and* Extracellular fluid.

fluid replacement (*flu'-id re-plase'-ment*). Term commonly used to describe the administration of intravenous fluids. *See* Appendix 8.

fluke (*flook*). A group of parasitic worms. Different varieties may affect the blood, the intestines, the liver or the lungs.

fluorescein (*flu-or-es'-in*). A dye used to detect corneal ulcer.

When it is dropped on the eye the ulcer stains green.

fluorescence (*flu-or-es'-ens*). The property of reflecting back light waves, usually of a lower frequency than that absorbed, so that invisible light (e.g. ultraviolet) may become visible.

fluorescent screen (*flu-or-es'-ent*). A specially prepared screen used in X-ray work which enables deep structures to be viewed and so more accurately examined.

fluoridation (*flu-or-id-a'-shun*). The adding of one part per million of fluorine to water in those areas where it is lacking.

fluorine (*flu'-or-een*). An element found in the water in some localities which if in excess causes a white mottled effect on the teeth but also helps to prevent dental decay. Where lacking it may be added to the water at the purification plant, making the fluoridation one part per million.

5-fluorocytosine (*flu-or-o-si'-to-seen*). An antifungal drug.

fluoroscope (*flu-or-o-scope*). A fluorescent screen used to view X-ray images.

flux (*fluks*). An excessive flow of any of the body secretions.

focus (*fo'-kus*). (1) The point of meeting of rays of light after passing through a lens (2) The local seat of a disease. *Pl.* foci.

focusing (*fo'-kus-ing*). The ability of the eye to alter its lens power so as to focus correctly at different distances.

Foelling's disease (*A. Foelling, contemporary Norwegian physician*). Phenylpyruvic oligophrenia. *See* Phenylketonuria.

foetal, foetus. *See* Fetal, Fetus.

foetor (*fe'-tor*). Unpleasant smell.

folic acid (*fo'-lik*). A constituent of the vitamin B complex which influences red blood cell formation. Used in the treatment of some forms of macrocytic anaemia and sprue. Given orally. *F. a. antagonists.* Antimetabolite drugs which inhibit the action of the folic acid enzyme. This is essential for nucleoprotein synthesis.

folie à deux (*fo'-le ah der'*). The sharing of delusions by two people living in close contact.

follicle (*fol'-likl*). A very small sac or gland. *F. of tonsil.* Invagination of the covering membrane forming a depression—in which infection often occurs (*follicular tonsillitis*). *Graafian f.* See Graafian follicle. *Hair f.* The sheath in which a hair grows. *F.-stimulating hormone (FSH).* A hormone produced by the anterior pituitary gland which controls the maturation of the graafian follicle in the ovary.

folliculitis (*fol-lik-u-li'-tis*). Inflammation of a group of follicles.

folliculosis (*fol-lik-u-lo'-sis*). Hypertrophy of follicles. *Conjunctival f.* A benign non-inflammatory overgrowth of follicles of the conjunctiva of the eyelids.

fomentation (*fo-men-ta'-shun*). A hot application. *Medical f.* Several thicknesses of flannel wrung out in boiling water, applied to relieve pain. *Surgical f.* A sterile, boiled foment of lint used to remove discharge and aid healing.

fomites (*fo'-mites*). Substances which have been in contact with a contagious disease and are capable of transmitting it, e.g. clothing, books and toys.

fontanelle (*fon-tan-el'*). A soft membranous space between the cranial bones of an infant. *Anterior f.* Between the parietal and frontal bones, which closes at about the age of 18 months. Rickets causes delay in this process. *Posterior f.* The junction of the occipital and parietal bones, at the sagittal suture, which closes at birth.

food-poisoning. A term commonly used to indicate an acute attack of gastro-enteritis after the consumption of unwholesome food. It may be due to chemical poisons such as antimony or arsenic or to poisonous fungi, but most frequently it is due to bacteria and their toxins, the commonest being: (1) Salmonella group, *Salmonella typhimurium* and *S. enteritidis*, infecting meat and fish preparations and duck eggs. (2) Staphylococci, often from infected milk or synthetic cream. The excreta of rats and mice, flies or lack of care by food handlers may be the cause of an outbreak, particularly if food is allowed to stand in a warm kitchen, when the organisms can multiply. Infected food and water may also transmit dysentery and typhoid fever. *See* Botulism.

foot. The termination of the lower limb. *Athlete's f.* Ringworm of the feet. *F. drop.* A preventable condition in most cases, due to inability to keep the foot at the correct angle owing to lack of support or exercises, or to paralysis of the flexors of the ankle. The foot must be fixed in position at a right-angle. *F. presentation.* The presentation of one or both legs instead of the head during labour. *Trench f.* A condition similar to frostbite occurring in soldiers, and due to prolonged standing in water of trenches.

foot and mouth disease. A bovine disease. Not the same as hand, foot and mouth disease (q.v.).

foramen (for-a'-men). An opening or hole, especially in a bone. *F. magnum.* The hole in the occipital bone through which the spinal cord passes. *F. ovale.* The hole between the left and right atrium in the fetus. *Obturator f.* The large hole in the os innominata.

forceps (for'-seps). Surgical instruments used for lifting or

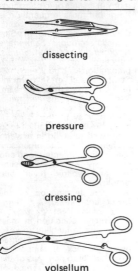

dissecting

pressure

dressing

volsellum

FORCEPS

compressing an object, e.g. *Artery f. (Spencer Wells f.)* These compress bleeding-points during an operation. *Cheatle's f.* are lifting forceps.

Midwifery f. are of various patterns, and are used in difficult labour to facilitate delivery. *Volsellum f.* have claw-like ends to grip the cervix of the uterus.

forensic (for-en'-sik). Applied to medicine, it is that concerned with the law and has bearing on legal problems.

foreskin (for'-skin). The prepuce (q.v.).

formaldehyde (for-mal'-de-hide). A gas used as a disinfectant, chiefly for rooms. A 40 per cent solution in water is known as *formalin* and is used as a spray, as a disinfectant.

formication (form-e-ka'-shun). A sensation as of insects creeping over the body.

formula (form'-u-lah). (1) A prescription. (2) A detailed statement of the ingredients of a chemical compound. (3) The presentation of the molecule of a chemical compound by chemical symbols.

formulary (form'-u-lar-e). A prescriber's handbook of drugs. *British National F.* One produced by the Joint Formulary Committee for easy reference for doctors and dispensers.

fornix (for'-niks). An arch: (1) Applied to an arched structure at the back and base of the brain. (2) The recesses at the top of the vagina in front (*anterior f.*), back (*posterior f.*), sides (*lateral f.*), of the cervix uteri. *Pl.* fornices.

Fortral (for'-tral). Pentazocine. A proprietary analgesic drug.

fossa (fos'-sah). A small depression or pit. Usually applied to those in bones. *Pituitary f.* In the sphenoid bone. *See* Sella turcica. *Pl.* fossae.

Fothergill's operation (W. E. Fothergill, English gynaecologist, 1865–1926). Amputation of the cervix, with anterior and posterior colporrhaphy for prolapse of the uterus.

fourchette (*foor-shet'*). The fold of membrane at the perineal end of the vulva.

fovea (*fo'-ve-ah*). A small depression or fossa. *F. centralis retinae.* The area of the retina which records the most distinct vision. *Syn.* Macula lutea.

Fowler's position (*G. R. Fowler, American surgeon, 1848–1906*). A position in which the trunk and thighs are raised, making the pelvis the lowest part of the body. Rarely used now.

fracture (*frak'-chur*). A broken bone. The signs and symptoms are: Pain, swelling, deformity, shortening of the limb, loss of power, abnormal mobility, and crepitus. The cause may be direct violence, as in a blow from a heavy object, or indirect, when falling on the hand causes fracture of the clavicle or severe muscle spasm such as that of the quadriceps muscle fracturing the patella. *Closed f. (simple).* A clean break with no communication with the skin. *Comminuted f.* The bone is broken in several places. *Compound f. (open).* There is a wound from the broken bone to the skin through which infection may enter. *Depressed f.* Of the cranium in which part of the bone is driven inwards. *Greenstick f.* In children, before complete ossification of bone, a partial break or bending may occur. *F. dislocation.* Occurs near a joint and is combined with dislocation of that joint. *Impacted f.* One end of the broken bone is driven into the other causing shortening. *Intracapsular f.* The break occurs within the joint capsule. *Pathological f.* Breaking occurring in diseased bones from slight injury. *Pott's f.* A fracture dislocation of the ankle involving the lower end of the fibula and

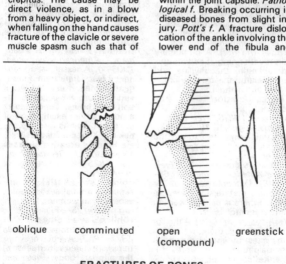

oblique   comminuted   open (compound)   greenstick

FRACTURES OF BONES

internal malleolus of the tibia. *Spontaneous f.* Occurs as a result of little or no violence, usually pathological. For first aid treatment, *see* Appendix 1.

fraenotomy (fren-ot´-o-me). The cutting of the fraenum linguae for tongue-tie.

fraenum (fre´-num). A fold of mucous membrane which checks or limits the movement of an organ. *F. linguae.* The fold under the tongue, which if too short causes difficulty in sucking and talking (tongue-tie) and is then partially severed.

fragilitas (fraj-il´-it-as). Brittleness. *F. ossium.* Abnormal fragility of bones, resulting in multiple fractures. It occurs in disorders of calcium metabolism.

framboesia (fram-be´-ze-ah). A tropical skin disease, known as 'yaws'. It is caused by a spirochaete susceptible to penicillin. It is not a venereal infection.

Franol (fra-nol). A proprietary drug containing ephedrine hydrochloride, theophylline and phenobarbitone, used for bronchitis and asthma.

free association. *See* Association.

Frei test (W. S. Frei, German dermatologist, 1885–1943). An intradermal test to aid the diagnosis of lymphogranuloma venereum.

Freiberg's disease (A. H. Freiberg, American surgeon, 1868–1940). Osteochondritis of the second metatarsal bone, in which there is pain on walking and standing.

fremitus (frem´-it-us). A thrill or vibration, e.g. that produced in the chest by speaking and felt on palpation.

Frenkel's exercises (H. S. Frenkel, German neurologist, 1860–1931). Exercises used in the treatment of tabes dorsalis to teach muscle and joint sense.

Freudian theory (S. Freud, Austrian psychiatrist, 1856–1939). Freud was the originator of psychoanalysis and psychoanalytical theory of the cause of neurosis.

Freyer's evacuator (Sir P. J. Freyer, English surgeon, 1851–1921). See Evacuator.

Freyer's operation. See Prostatectomy.

friable (fri´-ab-l). Crumbling.

friar's balsam (fri´-ars bal´-sam). Tincture of benzoin compound. See Balsam.

friction (frik´-shun). The act of rubbing. *F. murmur.* The grating sound heard in auscultation when two rough surfaces rub together, as in dry pleurisy.

Friedländer's bacillus (K. Friedländer, German pathologist, 1847–87). *Klebsiella pneumoniae,* cause of a rare form of pneumonia.

Friedman's test (M. H. Friedman, American physician, 1903–). A lesser used pregnancy test. Urine from a pregnant woman, if injected into a virgin rabbit, will cause ovulation in 18 hours. It necessitates a post-mortem examination of the rabbit. See Aschheim–Zondek and Xenopus toad tests.

Friedreich's ataxia or **disease** (N. Friedreich, German physician, 1825–82). A rare form of hereditary ataxia.

frigidity (frij-id´-it-e). An absence of normal sexual desire, especially in women.

frog plaster. See Plaster.

Fröhlich's syndrome (A. Fröhlich, Austrian neurologist, 1871–1953). A group of symptoms associated with disease of the pituitary body. These are: increased adiposity, atrophy of the genital organs, and development of feminine characteristics. *See* Dystrophic.

frontal (*fron'-tal*). Relating to the forehead. *F. sinus.* A pair of air sinuses situated above the nose in the frontal bone and communicating with the middle meatus of the nasal cavity.

frost-bite. Impairment of circulation chiefly affecting the fingers, the toes, the nose, and the ears, due to exposure to severe cold. The first stage is represented by chilblains. Advanced cases show thrombosis and dry gangrene (*q.v.*).

frozen shoulder. A stiff and painful shoulder. The cause is unknown.

fructose (*fruk'-toze*). Fruit sugar. A monosaccharide.

frusemide (*fru'-se-mide*). A diuretic with a rapid and powerful action. It may be administered orally or by injection.

FSH. *See* Follicle-stimulating hormone.

fuchsin (*fook'-zin*). A bright-red dye used in microscope work.

Fucidin (*fu-si-din*). A proprietary preparation of the antibiotic sodium fusidate which is highly effective against staphylococcal infection.

fugue (*fu'-g*). A period of altered awareness during which a person may wander for hours or days and perform purposive actions though his memory for the period may be lost. It may follow an epileptic fit or occur in hysteria or schizophrenia.

fulguration (*ful-gur-a'-shun*). Removal of papillomata of bladder by diathermy.

fuller's earth. Finely powdered aluminium silicate. A useful dusting powder which is very absorbent.

fulminating (*ful'-min-a-ting*). Sudden in onset and rapid in course.

fumigant (*fu'-mig-ant*). A substance which produces gas for fumigation.

fumigation (*fu-mig-a'-shun*). Disinfection by exposure to the fumes of a vaporized germicide.

functional disease. *See* Disease.

fundus (*fun'-dus*). The base of an organ or the part farthest removed from the opening. *F. of stomach.* That part above the cardiac orifice. *F. oculi.* The posterior part of the inside of the eye, as shown by the ophthalmoscope. *F. uteri.* The top of the uterus—that farthest from the cervix.

fungicide (*fun'-je-side*). A preparation that destroys fungal infection.

fungiform (*fun'-je-form*). Shaped like fungus or mushroom.

fungus (*fun'-gus*). A low form of vegetable life which includes mushrooms and moulds. Some varieties cause disease, such as actinomycosis, and ringworm.

funis (*fu'-nis*). The umbilical cord.

funnel chest (*fun'-el chest*). A developmental deformity in which there is a depression in the sternum and an inward curvature of the ribs and costal cartilages.

Furadantin (*fu'-rah-dan-tin*). A proprietary drug used in the treatment of urinary infections. Nitrofurantoin.

furor (*fu-ror'*). A state of intense excitement during which violent acts may be performed. This may occur following an epileptic fit.

furuncle (*fur-unk'-l*). A boil.

furunculosis (*fur-un-ku-lo'-sis*). A staphylococcal infection represented by many, or crops of, boils.

furunculus orientalis (*fur-*

un'-ku-lus or-e-en-ta'-lis). A protozoal infection mainly of the tropics, which causes a chronic ulceration. It is known by many place names, indicating districts in which it is common, e.g. *Delhi sore.*

fusidic acid (*fu'-si-dik as'-id*). An antibiotic which is effective against staphylococci that are drug resistant or penicillin sensitive.

fusiform (*fu'-se-form*). Shaped like a spindle.

Fusiformis (*fu-si-for'-mis*). A genus of anaerobic bacteria which may infect man and animals. Fusobacterium.

fusion (*fu'-shun*). (1) The union between two adjacent structures. (2) The co-ordination of separate images of the same object in the two eyes into one image.

G

Gadus morrhua (*ga'-dus-mor'-u-ah*). The codfish, from the liver of which oil is obtained.

Gaffky scale (*G. T. A. Gaffky, German bacteriologist, 1850–1918*). A method of sputum examination in which the tubercle bacilli present in a microscopic field are counted, e.g. G4 indicates two to three bacilli in each field.

gag. An instrument placed between the teeth, to keep the mouth open.

gait. Manner of walking. *Ataxic g.* The foot is raised high, descends suddenly, and the whole sole strikes the ground. *Cerebellar g.* A staggering walk indicative of cerebellar disease. *Spastic g.* Stiff, shuffling walk, the legs being kept together.

galactagogue (*gal-ak'-ta-gog*). An agent causing increased secretion of milk.

galactocele (*gal-ak'-to-seel*). A tumour containing milk, occurring in the breast.

galactorrhoea (*gal-ak-tor-re'-ah*). An excessive flow of milk.

galactosaemia (*gal-ak-to-se'-me-ah*). An inborn error of metabolism in which there is inability to convert galactose to glucose. This has proved to be one cause of retardation of mental development. If it is diagnosed early, a milk-free diet can be given with marked benefit.

galactose (*gal-ak'-toze*). Soluble sugar derived from lactose.

Galen, C. (*Greek physician in Rome, c. A.D. 130–200*). Galen's theories about the circulation of blood were accepted until William Harvey proved them to be incorrect nearly fifteen hundred years later.

galenical (*gal-en'-ik-al*). A preparation of a crude drug of animal or vegetable, rather than mineral or chemical origin.

gall (*gawl*). Bile, a digestive fluid secreted by the liver and stored in the gall-bladder. *G.-bladder.* The sac under the lower surface of the liver, which acts as a reservoir for bile. *G.-stone.* A concretion formed in the gallbladder. There are three varieties: (1) Cholesterol stone, usually a single large ovoid one of cholesterol. (2) Pigment stones, multiple small stones occurring in haemolytic diseases. (3) Mixed stones, multiple and faceted, they contain layers of cholesterol, calcium, and pigment and are associated with infection of the gall-bladder. *G.-stone colic. See* Biliary colic.

gallamine (*gal'-a-meen*). A synthetic muscle relaxant, chemically related to curare but less potent and shorter acting. Flaxedil is a proprietary brand.

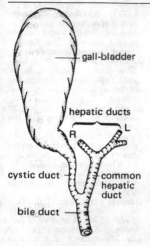

gall-bladder

hepatic ducts

R L

cystic duct

common hepatic duct

bile duct

GALL-BLADDER

Gallie's operation (*W. E. Gallie, Canadian surgeon, 1882–1959*). A living suture obtained from the fascia of a thigh muscle used to repair the abdominal wall after reduction of a hernia.

gallipot (*gal'-le-pot*). A small receptacle for lotions.

gallop rhythm (*gal'-op rithm*). Heart rhythm which may occur when there is ventricular overload. The sound is like that of horses' hooves galloping.

galvanism (*L. Galvani, Italian physician and physiologist, 1737–98*). Treatment by a continuous chemical battery. *See* Faradism.

galvanocauterization (*gal'-van-o-kaw-ter-i-za'-shun*). Burning by means of a wire heated by galvanic current.

galvanofaradization (*gal'-van-o-far-ad-i-za'-shun*). The

application of continuous and interrupted currents at the same time.

galvanometer (*gal-van-om'-e-ter*). An instrument for detecting or measuring the strength of a current of electricity.

gamete (*gam'-eet*). In reproduction, a sex cell which combines with another to form a zygote, from which a complete organism develops.

gametogenesis (*gam-et-o-jen'-e-sis*). The production of germ cells (*ova* or *sperm*) by the gonads.

gamgee tissue (*gam'-je*). Absorbent wool covered with gauze.

gamma (*gam'-mah*). The third letter in the Greek alphabet, γ.

gamma benzene hexachloride (*gam'-mah-ben'-zeen heks-a-klor'-ide*). A parasitic preparation used as a shampoo to treat head lice.

gamma camera (*gam'-mah kam'-er-ah*). A large stationary detector which views the whole of an organ at once. A method of scanning that shows the radioactivity pattern.

gamma encephalography (*gam'-mah en-kef-al-og'-raf-e*). A method of localizing a brain tumour by means of a radioactive isotope and scintillating machine.

gamma globulins (*gam'-mah glob'-u-lins*). Plasma proteins produced by the reticuloendothelial cells of the spleen, bone marrow and liver. They are concerned with antibody formation. *See* Globulin.

gamma rays (*gam'-mah*). The rays given off by radioactive substances, which are used to destroy tissues in the treatment of disease.

Gammexane (*gam-meks'-ane*). A powerful proprietary

insecticide used especially for destruction of the malarial mosquito.

ganglion (*gang'-le-on*). (1) A collection of nerve cells and fibres, forming an independent nerve centre, as is found in the sympathetic nervous system. (2) A cystic swelling on a tendon. *Pl.* ganglia.

ganglionectomy (*gang-le-on-ek'-to-me*). Excision of a ganglion.

ganglionic blocking agent. Drug used in the treatment of hypertension which blocks the transmission of impulses across the ganglia of the sympathetic nervous system.

gangrene (*gan'-green*). Death of tissue. Local death of bone is called *sequestrum*; of soft tissue, *slough. Dry g.* Due to failure of arterial blood supply, e.g. from injury or ligature of main artery, frostbite, or arterial disease. The affected part is painful, pale, and later becomes discoloured and black. There is a red line of demarcation between the living and dead tissues. *Moist g.* Caused by putrefactive changes. The part is swollen, blistered, and discoloured. There is little pain; the line of demarcation is not definite. General signs are: high fever, delirium and all signs of blood infection. This type may result from infective thrombosis or from pressure on veins as in strangulated hernia, etc. *Diabetic g.* A type likely to develop in diabetic patients, due to changes in blood vessels. *Gas g.* Infection of a wound with *Clostridium perfringens* (*welchii*). *See* Gas-gangrene. *Senile g.* Seen in the aged and due to impaired circulation.

Ganser state (*S. J. M. Ganser, German psychiatrist, 1853–*1931). Simulated madness. Giving approximate answers to questions, which show that the correct answers are known. Hysterical pseudodementia.

Gardiner-Brown test (*A. Gardiner-Brown, English otologist*). Tuning fork vibrations test of bone conduction in aural disease.

gargle (*gar'-gl*). A disinfectant solution for washing out the throat.

gargoylism (*gar'-goil-izm*). An inherited condition in which the coarse prominent features and large head are said to resemble a gargoyle. The vision is defective and there is mental subnormality.

Gärtner's bacillus (*A. G. Gärtner, German bacteriologist, 1848–1934*). A species of Salmonella, *S. enteritidis.*

gas. Molecules of a substance very loosely combined—a vapour. *Laughing g.* Nitrous oxide. *Marsh g.* Methane. *Sternutatory g.* One which causes sneezing. *Tear g.* Irritating to the eyes and causes excessive lacrimation.

gas-air analgesia (*an-al-je'-se-ah*). An authorized form of analgesia using nitrous oxide and air, by which the pains of labour are lessened without affecting uterine contractions.

gas-gangrene. The result of infection of a wound by anaerobic organisms, especially *Clostridium welchii*, normally found in the intestine of animals, and therefore likely to be present in cultivated soil, stable refuse, and road dirt. It has also occurred from the use of imperfectly sterilized catgut; accidental soiling of tissues if the gut has been opened during an operation, and from perforation of the rectum in fracture of the pelvis.

Gasser's ganglion (*J. L. Gasser, Austrian anatomist, 1723–65*). The ganglion of the sensory root of the fifth cranial nerve.

gasserectomy (*gas-er-ek'-to-me*). Excision of Gasser's ganglion.

gastralgia (*gas-tral'-je-ah*). Pain in the stomach of neuralgic type.

gastrectomy (*gas-trek'-to-me*). Excision of a part or whole of the stomach. *Partial g.* Commonly performed in the surgical treatment of peptic ulcer. *Billroth g.* Most of the lesser curvature and pyloric portion are removed and the duodenum joined to the refashioned stomach. This cuts down the production of secretin and of acid. *Polya g.* The first part of the duodenum and major portion of the stomach are removed and the stomach anastomosed to the jejunum. The blind portion

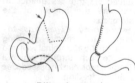

Billroth type I

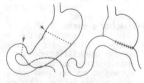

Polya type

GASTRECTOMY (PARTIAL)

of the duodenum supplies the bile, pancreatic and duodenal secretion.

gastric (*gas'-trik*). Pertaining to the stomach. *G. juice.* The clear fluid secreted by the glands of the stomach to assist digestion. It contains an enzyme called pepsin, which acts upon proteins in the presence of weak hydrochloric acid. *G. influenza.* A type of the infection in which vomiting, nausea, and lack of appetite are prominent signs. *G. ulcer.* Ulceration of the gastric mucosa associated with hyperacidity and often precipitated by stress.

gastrin (*gas'-trin*). A hormone secreted by the walls of the stomach, which excites continued secretion of digestive juice whilst the food is in the stomach.

gastritis (*gas-tri'-tis*). Inflammation of the stomach. *Acute g.* Severe irritation, of sudden onset, due to infected food or irritant poisons. *Chronic g.* Loss of appetite, nausea, flatulence and furred tongue, which may be due to repeated indiscretions of diet, alcohol or over-smoking. Hypochlorhydria is often present.

gastro-. A prefix relating to the stomach.

gastrocele (*gas'-tro-seel*). A hernia of the stomach.

gastrocnemius (*gas-trok-ne'-me-us*). The principal muscle of the calf in the leg.

gastrocolic reflex (*gas-tro-kol'-ik*). Following a meal increased peristalsis causes the colon to empty into the rectum. This gives rise to the desire to defaecate.

gastroduodenostomy (*gas-tro-du-o-den-os'-to-me*). A surgical anastomosis between the stomach and duodenum.

gastroenteritis (*gas-tro-en-ter-i'-tis*). Inflammation of the stomach and intestine. *Infantile g.* An acute condition of diarrhoea and vomiting producing severe dehydration. The cause may be (*a*) dietetic; (*b*) infective; (*c*) parenteral, when the condition is secondary to the infection elsewhere in the body, e.g. otitis media or bronchitis.

gastroenterology (*gas-tro-en-ter-ol'-o-je*). The study of diseases of the gastrointestinal tract.

gastroenteropathy (*gas-tro-en-ter-op'-ath-e*). Any disease condition affecting both the stomach and the intestine.

gastroenterostomy (*gas-tro-en-ter-os'-to-me*). A surgical anastomosis between the stomach and small intestine. Usually performed for pyloric obstruction.

gastrography (*gas'-trog-raf-e*). An X-ray examination using a fluorescent screen and a fluid radio-opaque dye that may be carried out early on a patient following or suffering from haematemesis.

gastroiliac reflex (*gas-tro-i'-*

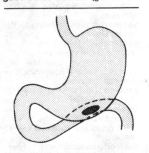

GASTROENTEROSTOMY

le-ak). Food entering the stomach sets up powerful peristalsis in the ileum and opening of the ileocaecal valve.

gastrojejunostomy (*gas-tro-je-ju-nos'-to-me*). A surgical anastomosis between the stomach and jejunum.

gastromalacia (*gas-tro-mal-a'-se-ah*). An abnormal softening of the walls of the stomach.

gastropathy (*gas-trop'-ath-e*). Any disease of the stomach.

gastroplasty (*gas-tro-plas'-te*). A reconstruction of the cardiac orifice of the stomach to rectify a hiatus hernia where fibrosis prevents replacement below the diaphragm.

gastroptosis (*gas-trop-to'-sis*). Downward displacement of the stomach owing to weakening of supporting ligaments or of its own musculature.

gastroscope (*gas'-tro-skope*). An instrument fitted with an electric bulb, which is introduced via the oesophagus to examine the interior of the stomach.

gastrostomy (*gas-tros'-to-me*). An artificial opening through the abdominal wall into the stomach, through which a feeding tube can be passed. *See* Artificial feeding.

gastrotorny (*gas-trot'-o-me*). Incision of the stomach.

gastrula (*gas'-tru-lah*). One stage in the development of the fertilized ovum.

Gaucher's disease (*P. C. E. Gaucher, French physician 1854–1918*). A rare familial disease in which fat is deposited in the reticulo-endothelial cells resulting in an enlarged spleen and anaemia. No cure is known.

gauze (*gaws*). A thin open-meshed material used for dressing wounds. It is sterilized by autoclave.

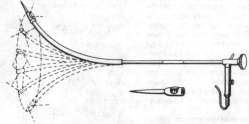

GASTROSCOPE

gavage (*gav´-arj*). Feeding by oesophageal tube.

Geiger counter (*H. Geiger, German physicist, 1882–1945*). An instrument for detecting radioactive substances. The apparatus is sensitive to the rays emitted.

gelatin (*jel´-at-in*). An albuminoid, obtained by boiling connective tissue or bones. It is used in *cooking* for the setting of jellies; in *pharmacy* for suppositories and capsules; and in *bacteriology* as a culture medium.

general paralysis of the insane (GPI). General paresis or dementia paralytica. A manifestation of tertiary syphilis, characterized by progressive mental and physical deterioration. The condition is uncommon now with the lessened incidence of tertiary syphilis and its early cure by penicillin.

generative (*jen´-er-a-tiv*). Referring to the reproduction of the species.

genes (*jeenz*). The hereditary factors present in the chromosomes in the germ cell which decide the physical and mental make-up of the offspring. *Dominant g.* Those that are capable

of transmitting their characteristics irrespective of the genes from the other parent. *Recessive g.* Those that can pass on the characteristics only if they are present with a similar recessive gene from the other parent, and then there is only a 1 in 4 chance. *See* Mendel's law.

genetic (*jen-et´-ik*). Concerned with origin or reproduction. *G. code.* Term given to the arrangement of genetic material stored in the DNA molecule of the chromosome. *G. counselling.* Service for prospective parents who can receive advice as to the likelihood of their children being born with congenital abnormalities.

genetics (*jen-et´-iks*). The study of heredity and natural development.

genital (*jen´-it-al*). Relating to the organs of generation.

genitalia (*jen-it-a´-le-ah*). The organs of reproduction.

genito-urinary (*jen-it-o-u´-rin-are-e*). Referring to both the reproductive organs and the urinary tract.

gentamicin (*gen-tah-mi´-sin*). Antibiotic commonly used in the treatment of infection with *Pseudomonas pyocyanea*.

gentian (*jen'-shun*). A vegetable extract, which is exceedingly bitter. It is prescribed as a tonic and stomachic. *G. violet.* An aniline dye, used in 1 per cent aqueous solution: (1) For small skin lesions. (2) Painting ulcers in stomatitis (*q.v.*). (3) By mouth as a treatment for threadworms.

genu (*jen'-u*). The knee. *G. valgum.* Knock-knee. *G. varum.* Bow-leg.

genupectoral position (*jen'-u-pek'-tor-al*). Knee-chest position. *See* Position.

genus (*je'-nus*). A classification of either animals or plants, each species having characteristics common to themselves, but differing from those of others.

Gerhardt's test (*C. F. Gerhardt, French chemist, 1816–56*). A method of testing urine for the presence of ketone bodies by using ferric chloride.

geriatrician (*jer-e-a-trish'-an*). A doctor who specializes in the diseases and care of the elderly.

geriatrics (*jer-e-at'-riks*). The study and treatment of the diseases of old age.

germ (*jerm*). A microbe.

German measles. *See* Rubella.

germicide (*jerm'-e-side*). An agent capable of destroying microbes and their spores.

gerontology (*jer-on-tol'-o-je*). The study of old age and the ageing processes.

Gessell's developmental charts (*A. Gessell, American psychologist, 1880– *). Charts which show the expected motor, social and psychological development of children.

gestation (*jes-ta'-shun*). Pregnancy. *Ectopic g.* Fetal development in some part other than the uterus—most usually the fallopian tube. At about the sixth week the tube is so dis-

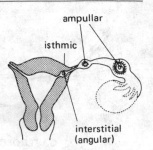

ECTOPIC GESTATION

tended that it ruptures and severe haemorrhage may occur, which is rapidly fatal if not promptly treated by operation.

Ghon's focus (*A. Ghon, Czechoslovakian pathologist, 1866–1936*). The primary lesion of pulmonary tuberculosis, as seen on an X-ray film, after it has healed by fibrosis and calcification.

giant-cell arteritis (*ji'-ant-sell ar-ter-i'-tis*). An inflammatory condition causing occlusion of arteries most often the carotid vessels and their branches. Alternative name temporal arteritis.

giardiasis (*A. Giard, French biologist, 1846–1908*). An infection with *Giardia lamblia* that causes a persistent mild diarrhoea. Intestinal malabsorption may also be caused especially in children. A tropical condition.

gibbosity (*gib-bos'-it-e*). A humped back.

gibbus (*gib'-bus*). The name applied to the prominence caused by collapse of the vertebral body and the acute angling of the spinous processes.

von Gierke's disease (*E. von*

Gierke, German pathologist, 1877–1945). See Glycogen storage disease.

gigantism (*ji-gant'-izm*). Abnormal growth of the body, due to over-activity of the anterior lobe of the pituitary gland.

Gilliam's operation (*D. T. Gilliam, American gynaecologist, 1844–1923*). For correction of retroversion of the uterus by shortening the round ligaments.

Gillies needle-holder (*Sir H. D. Gillies, British plastic surgeon, 1882–1960*). Combined scissors and fine suture needle-holder used in plastic surgery.

ginger (*jin'-jer*). The root of a tropical plant used in dyspepsia as a carminative.

gingiva (*jin-ji'-vah*). The gums or tissues surrounding the neck of a tooth.

gingivectomy (*jin-jiv-ek'-to-me*). An operation for pyorrhoea alveolaris (*q.v.*) in which the diseased gum is removed.

gingivitis (*jin-jiv-i'-tis*). Inflammation of the gums.

ginglymus (*jin'-glim-us*). A hinge joint.

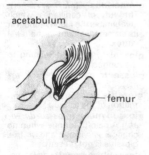

acetabulum

femur

GIRDLESTONE'S OPERATION

Girdlestone operation (*G. R. Girdlestone, English surgeon, 1881–1950*). G. pseudo-arthrosis of hip. A false joint made by excising the head and neck of femur and part of the acetabulum, and suturing a muscle mass between the bones' ends. A treatment for osteoarthritis.

gladiolus (*glad-e-o'-lus*). The blade-like portion of the sternum.

glanders (*glan'-ders*). A contagious disease of horses and asses, sometimes communicated to man through a crack in the skin.

glands. Special organs situated in many parts of the body. Their function is to secrete fluid prepared from the blood, either for use in the body, or for excretion as waste material. *Accessory g.* Detached glandular tissue near to one of similar structure. *Ductless g. Endocrine g.* One which produces an internal secretion but has no canal (duct) through which the secretion is carried away. An example is the thyroid gland. *Lymph g. See* Lymph nodes. *Mucous g.* One which secretes mucus. *Serous g.* One which secretes serum.

glandular fever (*gland'-u-lar*). Infective mononucleosis. A febrile condition of unknown cause, occurring chiefly in children and young adults. There is general enlargement and tenderness of lymph glands, especially those of the neck, axilla and groin, with leucocytosis. Rest during the fever but no specific treatment is known.

glans (*glanz*). An acorn-shaped body, such as the rounded end of the penis and the clitoris.

glare headache. A severe persistent headache occurring where there is strong sunlight and light-reflecting surfaces. Dark glasses are preventive.

glaucoma (*glaw-ko'-mah*). Raised intra-ocular pressure. *Primary g.* or *narrow angled g.* Glaucoma in which the aqueous fluid cannot drain. There is sudden onset with severe pain and blurred vision. *Chronic g.* Insidious in onset and causes progressive loss of vision by pressure on the optic nerve. *Secondary g.* Follows some pre-existing disease.

gleet. Chronic gonococcal urethritis marked by a transparent mucous discharge.

glenohumeral (*glen-o-hu'-mer-al*). Referring to the shoulder joint. The glenoid cavity of the scapula and the humerus.

glenoid (*glen'-oid*). Resembling a hollow. *G. cavity.* The socket of the shoulder-joint.

glia (*gli'-ah*). Neuroglia. The connective nerve tissue of the brain and spinal cord.

glioblastoma (*gli-o-blas-to'-mah*). A malignant glioma arising in the cerebral hemispheres.

glioma (*gli-o'-mah*). A new growth of neuroglia cells and fibres affecting the brain and spinal cord. The majority are malignant but seldom metastasize. *G. retinae. See* Retinoblastoma.

gliomyoma (*gli-o-mi-o'-mah*). A tumour of nerve and muscle tissue.

Glisson's capsule (*F. Glisson, British physician and anatomist, 1597–1677*). The connective tissue capsule of the liver which envelops the portal vein, hepatic artery and hepatic ducts.

globin (*glo'-bin*). A protein used in the formation of haemoglobin.

globulin (*glob'-u-lin*). A protein constituent of the blood (*serum-globulin*) and cerebro-spinal fluid. *Gamma g.* A blood fraction prepared from plasma containing antibodies which offers a temporary protection against measles, rubella, and sometimes poliomyelitis and other infections.

globulinuria (*glob-u-lin-u'-re-ah*). The presence of globulin in the urine.

globus (*glo'-bus*). A ball or globe. *G. hystericus.* A symptom of hysteria when a patient feels he cannot swallow because he has a lump in his throat.

glomerular filtration rate (*glo-mer'-u-lar*). The rate at which blood is filtered by the glomeruli of the kidneys. Normally this is 120 ml per minute.

glomerulonephritis (*glo-mer-u-lo-nef-ri'-tis*). Acute nephritis following a streptococcal infection in which there is inflammation of the glomeruli of the kidneys.

glomerulosclerosis (*glo-mer-u-lo-skler-o'-sis*). Degenerative changes in the glomerular capillaries of the renal tubule leading to renal failure.

glomerulus (*glo-mer'-u-lus*). The tuft of capillaries which invaginates the kidney tubule at its commencement in the renal cortex.

glossal (*glos'-sal*). Relating to the tongue.

glossectomy (*glos-sek'-to-me*). Excision of the tongue.

glossitis (*glos-si'-tis*). Inflammation of the tongue.

glossodynia (*glos-so-din'-e-ah*). A painful tongue when no change is visible and a true glossitis is not present.

glossopharyngeal (*glos-so-far-in-je'-al*). Pertaining to the tongue and pharynx. *G. nerve.* The ninth cranial nerve.

glossoplegia (*glos-so-ple'-je-ah*). Paralysis of the tongue.

glottis (*glot'-tis*). That part of the larynx which is associated with voice production.

glucagon (*glu'-ka-gon*). A polypeptide produced by the islets of Langerhans. It aids glycogen breakdown in the liver and raising of the blood sugar level.

glucocorticoids (*glu-ko-kor'-te-koids*). The adrenal steroids that are concerned with carbohydrate metabolism. They maintain the blood sugar level and aid in storing glycogen. They are anti-inflammatory.

glucogenesis (*glu-ko-jen'-e-sis*). The production of glucose. *Hepatic g.* The liberation of glucose from glycogen in the liver.

gluconeogenesis (*glu-ko-ne-o-jen'-e-sis*). The production of new glucose from the non-nitrogen portion of the amino acids after deamination.

glucose (*glu'-koze*). Dextrose or grape-sugar found in many fruits and honey. It is the absorbable sugar to which carbohydrates are reduced by digestion, and is therefore found in the blood in considerable quantity. It is present in the urine of patients with untreated diabetes mellitus. *G. tolerance test.* Test in which a glucose load is given and the concentration of glucose in the blood is estimated at intervals afterwards. Used mainly when diabetes mellitus (*q.v.*) is suspected.

glucose 6-phosphate dehydrogenase. A red-cell enzyme. Inherited deficiency causes a tendency to haemolytic anaemia. Most common in Negroes, Sephardic Jews, Mediterranean peoples and Orientals. *See* Favism.

glucuronic acid (*glu-ku-ron'-ik*). An enzyme in the liver that acts on the bilirubin from the

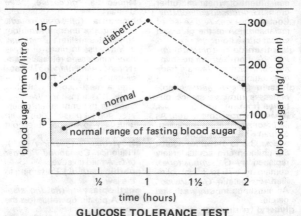

GLUCOSE TOLERANCE TEST

broken down red blood cells to form conjugated bilirubin.

glue ear (*gloo eer*). An accumulation of fluid in the middle ear.

glutamic acid (*glu-tam'-ik as-id*). One of the 22 amino acids formed by the digestion of dietary protein.

glutamic pyruvic transaminase (*glu-tam'-ik pi-ru'-vik trans-am'-in-ase*). Enzyme ·found in the liver and also in cardiac muscle. After a myocardial infarction there is a marked increase in the blood level of the enzyme.

glutamine. *See* Glutamic acid.

glutaraldehyde (*glu-tar-al'-de-hide*). Antiseptic solution used in the sterilization of equipment which cannot be heat-treated.

gluteal (*glu-te'-al*). Relating to the buttocks. *G. muscles.* Three in number which form the fleshy part of the buttocks.

gluten (*glu'-ten*). A nitrogenous constituent of wheat and other grains. *G.-induced enteropathy.* Coeliac disease. A disease of malabsorption of the gluten in wheat or rye flour.

glutethimide (*glu-teth'-im-ide*). A non-barbiturate hypnotic. Doriden is a trade preparation.

glycerin (*glis'-er-een*). A colourless syrupy substance obtained from fats and fixed oils. It has a hygroscopic action. As an emollient it is an ingredient of many skin preparations. *G. enema.* 3·5 to 14 ml for adults. For children and adults largely replaced by *G. suppositories,* containing 1·75 to 3·5 ml solidified with gelatin. *G. of thymol.* An antiseptic mouth wash and gargle.

glyceryl trinitrate (*glis'-er-il tri-ni'-trate*). Sublingual tablets

that relieve anginal pain by dilating the coronary arteries.

glycine. *See* Glutamic acid.

glycocholate of sodium (*gli'-ko-ko'-late*). One of the salts of bile.

glycogen (*gli'-ko-jen*). The form in which carbohydrate is stored in the liver and muscles. Animal starch. *G. storage disease.* Inherited disease in which there is a deficiency in the synthesis of glycogen. This accumulates in the liver causing enlargement.

glycogenesis (*gli-ko-jen'-e-sis*). The process of glycogen formation from the blood glucose.

glycogenolysis (*gli-ko-jen-ol'-is-is*). The breakdown of glycogen in the body so that it may be utilized.

glycoside (*gli'-ko-side*). A crystalline body in plants which when acted on by acids or ferments produces sugar. If the sugar is glucose it may be termed a *glucoside. See* Digitalis.

glycosuria (*gli-ko-su'-re-ah*). Sugar in the urine, a symptom of diabetes mellitus. *Emotional g.* May arise in times of stress due to increased release of adrenaline. *Alimentary g.* The appearance of sugar in the urine after a meal rich in carbohydrate. It is transitory. *Renal g.* Sugar in the urine in an otherwise normal person, due to an unusually low renal threshold (*q.v.*).

glycyrrhiza (*glis-ir-i'-zah*). Liquorice. *Compound Powder of G.* A mild laxative.

gnathic (*nath'-ik*). Pertaining to the jaw.

gnathoplasty (*na'-tho-plas-te*). A plastic operation on the jaw.

Goa powder (*go'-ah*). Derived

from a tropical tree, and the source of chrysarobin (q.v.).

goblet cells. Special secreting cells of goblet shape found in mucous membrane.

Goeckerman regimen (ger'-ker-man). A treatment for psoriasis which consists of warm baths, ultra-violet light and crude coal tar paste.

goitre (goi'-ter). Enlargement of the thyroid gland, causing a marked swelling in front of the neck, which sometimes results in pressure on the trachea. It may be endemic and give rise to no other symptoms, e.g. Derbyshire neck is of this type. *Colloid g.* An enlarged but soft thyroid gland with no signs of hyperthyroidism. *Exophthalmic g.* Hyperthyroidism with marked protrusion of eyeballs. *Lymphadenoid g.* An enlargement in which there is infiltration by lymphocytes and deposits of lymphoid tissue. *Primary toxic g.* Signs of excess of thyroxine in the blood, where the gland has not been previously enlarged. *Secondary toxic g.* In which the gland has been previously enlarged, and signs of hyperthyroidism suddenly develop. *Substernal g.* The enlargement of the gland behind the sternum and obvious swelling in the neck may not be apparent. *Syn.* Graves's disease; thyrotoxicosis. *See* Myxoedema.

goitrogens (goi'-tro-jens). Substances that block the synthesis of thyroxine and so cause goitre. The cause may be an inability to utilize iodine.

Golgi (C. Golgi, Italian histologist, 1844–1926). *G. bodies in cell.* Specialized structures seen near the nucleus of a cell during microscopic examination. *Organ of G.* The sensory end organs in muscle tendons that are sensitive to stretch.

gonad (gon'-ad). A sexual gland. The testicle or ovary.

gonadotrophic (gon-ad-o-tro'-fic). Having influence on the gonads. *G. hormones.* Those of the pituitary gland which control the ovaries and testes.

gonadotrophin (gon-ad-o-trof'-in). Any hormone that stimulates either the ovaries or testes.

gonioscopy (gon-e-os'-ko-pe). A method of examining the iris-corneal angle by means of a contact lens, light source and magnifying device.

gonococcus (gon-o-kok'-us). *Neisseria gonorrhoeae.* A diplococcus which causes gonorrhoea.

gonorrhoea (gon-or-re'-ah). A common venereal disease caused by the *Neisseria gonorrhoeae* infecting the genital tract, causing a discharge with pain and frequency of micturition. Spread by the blood stream may give rise to iritis or arthritis. Scar tissue formation may give rise to urethral stricture or infertility owing to occlusion of the uterine tubes. Most cases can be quickly treated by penicillin but reinfection is not uncommon.

gonorrhoeal (gon-or-re'-al). Relating to gonorrhoea. *G. arthritis.* Intractable infection of joints causing great pain and disability. *G. ophthalmia.* In the newly born (ophthalmia neonatorum) a notifiable disease and a cause of blindness. Good antenatal care should prevent infection and early intensive treatment with penicillin prevent blindness.

Goodpasture's syndrome (E. W. Goodpasture, American pathologist, 1886–1960). A rare haemorrhagic lung disorder associated with glomerulonephritis.

Gordh needle (*T. Gordh, contemporary Swedish anaesthetist*). An intravenous needle in which there is a rubber diaphragm through which repeated injections can be given.

gorget (*gor'-jet*). A grooved instrument used in lithotomy.

gouge (*gowj*). A strong grooved instrument, used for scooping out diseased bone, or other hard substances.

gout (*gowt*). A metabolic disease associated with an excess of uric acid in the blood. It is characterized by painful inflammation and swelling of the smaller joints, especially those of the big toe and thumb. Inflammation is accompanied by the deposit of urates around the joints. Colchium is the drug of choice in an acute attack and Probenecid may be used between attacks.

graafian follicles (*B. de Graaf, Dutch physician and anatomist, 1641–73*). Small vesicles

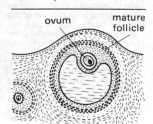

GRAAFIAN FOLLICLE

formed in the ovary, each containing an ovum. One follicle matures during each menstrual cycle.

Graefe's knife (*F. W. A. von Graefe, German ophthalmologist, 1828–70*). Scalpel used in ophthalmic surgery.

graft. Transplantation of healthy tissue from one part of the body to remedy a defect in a corresponding structure. *Autogenous g.* Graft taken from and given to the same individual. *Bone g.* Transplantation of bone. *Homogenous g.* A graft taken from one person and given to another individual of the same species. *Pedicle g.* Consists of the full thickness of the skin and subcutaneous tissue. *Pinch g.* Small pieces of skin of varying depth placed on a raw area. *Thiersch g.* Considerable pieces of partial thickness of skin used to cover large areas.

grain. (1) A minute hard particle. (2) A unit of weight in the Apothecaries' measure. *See* Appendix 7.

gram (*gramme*). The unit of weight of the metric system. In prescriptions the abbreviation G is recommended to avoid confusion with gr. *See* Appendix 7.

Gram's stain (*H. Gram, Danish physician, 1853–1938*). A special stain used in bacteriology, by the taking up of which some organisms are recognized. Indicated thus:

   Gram+ (*positive*);
   Gram− (*negative*).

grand mal (*grond mal'*). Major epilepsy. *See* Epilepsy.

granular (*gran'-u-lar*). Containing small particles. *G. cells. See* Leucocytes. *G. casts.* The degenerated cells from the lining of renal tubules excreted in the urine.

granulation (*gran-u-la'-shun*). The growth of new tissue by which wounds heal when the edges are not in apposition. It consists of new capillaries and fibroblasts which fill in the space and later form fibrous tissue. The resulting scar is liable to be hard and unsightly. A barrier of this tissue forms the walls of an abscess cavity, and the floor of an ulcer. By it inflammation is localized.

granule (*gran'-ule*). A small particle or grain.

granulocyte (*gran'-u-lo-site*). Polymorphonuclear white blood cells that may be either neutrophils, basophils, or eosinophils.

granulocytopenia (*gran-u-lo-si-to-pe'-ne-ah*). A marked reduction in the polymorphonuclear cells in the blood. The condition may precede agranulocytosis (*q.v.*).

granuloma (*gran-u-lo'-mah*). A tumour composed of granulation tissue.

granulosa cells (*gran-u-lo'-sah*). Cells present in the graafian follicle. *G. c. tumour.* A rare new growth of the ovary that produces excessive oestrogen.

grape-sugar. Dextrose.

gravel. Small calculi formed in the kidneys and bladder, and sometimes excreted with the urine.

Graves's disease (*R. J. Graves, Irish physician, 1796–1853*). Exophthalmic goitre. Hyperthyroidism (*q.v.*).

gravid (*grav'-id*). Pregnant.

gravity. Weight. *Specific g.* of any liquid is its weight compared with that of an equal volume of water, i.e. affected by the amount of solids dissolved in it.

greenstick fracture. *See* Fracture.

Grenz rays. A source of superficial X-rays that may be used to treat skin diseases.

Griffith's types (*F. Griffith, 20th century British bacteriologist*). A method of determining varieties of streptococci by agglutination tests. Applied mainly to haemolytic streptococci of Lancefield's Group A (*q.v.*).

gripe (*gripe*). Colic.

griseofulvin (*gri-se-o-ful'-vin*). An oral antifungal antibiotic that is used in the treatment of tinea.

group psychotherapy (*groop si-ko-ther'-ap-e*). A method of treatment whereby patients and staff, under the guidance of a psychotherapist, meet regularly to discuss the patients' problems. Insight is gained into the patients' way of meeting stress. The patient learns to understand and tries to change his behaviour as a result of the group process. He also contributes to the well-being of the other group members.

grouped breathing. Biot's respiration. *See* Biot.

guanethidine (*gwan-eth'-e-deen*). A hypotensive drug that acts by blocking the sympathetic nerve impulses to plain muscle without affecting the parasympathetic. Ismelin is a proprietary preparation.

guanine (*gwan'-een*). One of the purine bases found in the molecule of deoxyribonucleic acid.

guardianship. Under the Mental Health Act 1959, a method of compulsory care on an informal basis for mentally ill patients and for those suffering from psychopathic disorder, the mentally subnormal, or severely subnormal. The guardian may be a private person or a Local Health Authority.

gubernaculum (*gu-ber-nak'-u-lum*). A cord of fibromuscular tissue attached to the lower pole of the testis which has the power of retracting it.

Guillain–Barré syndrome (*G. Guillain, French neurologist, 1876–1961: A. Barré, French neurologist 1880–*). Condition in which there is advancing paralysis which frequently affects the respiratory muscles as well as the peripheral ones. Caused by a virus infection.

guillotine (*gil'-lo-teen*). A surgical instrument used for excising tonsils.

guinea worm. A tropical parasite which burrows into human tissues, particularly into the legs or feet.

gullet (*gul'-let*). The oesophagus.

gum-boil. An abscess at the root of a tooth.

gumma (*gum'-mah*). A soft, degenerating tumour characteristic of the tertiary stage of syphilis. It may occur in any organ or tissue.

gurgling. Caused by gas passing through liquid. *G. râle.* The sound heard on auscultation when the bronchi or lungs contain fluid.

gustatory (*gus'-ta-tor-e*). Relating to taste.

gut. The intestine.

gutta (*gut'-tah*). A drop.

gutta percha (*gut'-tah perk'-ah*). The dried juice of a tree utilized for surgical purposes, forming a thin sheet of waterproof tissue. It cannot be sterilized by heat.

gutter splint. A plaster of Paris or plastic splint moulded to a limb in gutter shape—not encasing it.

gynaecoid (*gi'-ne-koid*). Like the female. *G. pelvis.* One with a round brim and shallow cavity suited to childbearing.

gynaecologist (*gi-ne-kol'-o-jist*). One who specializes in the diseases of women.

gynaecology (*gi-ne-kol'-o-je*). The science treating of those diseases which are peculiar to women.

gynaecomastia (*gi-ne-ko-mas'-te-ah*). Excessive growth of the male breast.

gypsum (*jip'-sum*). Plaster of Paris (*calcium sulphate*).

gyrus (*ji'-rus*). A convolution as of the brain, cochlea, etc.

H

H. Symbol for hydrogen.

habit. Automatic response to specific situations acquired as a result of repetition and learning. *Drug h.* Drug addiction. *H. training.* A method used in psychiatric nursing whereby deteriorated patients can be rehabilitated and taught personal hygiene by constant repetition and encouragement.

haema-, haemo-, haemato- (*he'-mah, he'-mo, he'-mat-o*). Prefixes, denoting or relating to blood.

haemangioma (*he-man-je-o'-mah*). A new growth arising in a blood vessel.

haemarthrosis (*he-mar-thro'-sis*). An effusion of blood into a joint.

haematemesis (*he-mat-em'-e-sis*). Vomiting of blood. If it has been in the stomach for some time and become partially digested by gastric juice, it is of a dark colour and contains particles resembling coffee-grounds.

haematin (*he'-mat-in*). The iron-containing part of blood.

With globin it forms haemoglobin.

haematinic (*he-mat-tin'-ik*). An agent which increases the colouring matter in blood. *H. factors*. Those necessary for the proper formation of red blood cells. *See* Erythrocyte.

haematocele (*he'-mat-o-seel*). A swelling produced by effusion of blood; e.g. in the sheath surrounding a testicle or a broad ligament.

haematocolpos (*he-mat-o-kol'-pos*). Collection of blood in the vagina. *See* Cryptomenorrhoea.

haematology (*he-mat-tol'-o-je*). The science dealing with the nature, functions and diseases of blood.

haematoma (*he-mat-o'-mah*). A swelling containing blood.

haematometra (*he-mat-o-me'-trah*). Accumulation of blood in the uterus.

haematomyelia (*he-mat-o-mi-e'-le-ah*). An effusion of blood into the spinal cord.

haematomyelitis (*he-mat-o-mi-el-i'-tis*). An effusion of blood into the spinal canal with acute inflammation of the cord.

haematosalpinx (*he-mat-o-sal'-pinks*). Haemosalpinx. Accumulation of blood in the fallopian tubes.

haematoxylin (*he-mat-toks'-il-in*). Logwood. A stain used in bacteriology.

haematozoon (*he-mat-o-zo'-on*). Any animal parasite in the blood.

haematuria (*he-mat-tu'-re-ah*). Blood in the urine, due to injury or disease of any of the urinary organs. *See* Appendix 11.

haemochromatosis (*he-mo-kro-ma-to'-sis*). A condition in which there is high absorption and deposition of iron leading to a high serum level and pigmentation of the skin. *Syn.* Bronze diabetes.

haemoconcentration (*he-mo-kon-sen-tra'-shun*). A loss of circulating fluid from the blood with a high cell volume as is common in severe burns.

haemocytometer (*he-mo-si-tom'-e-ter*). An instrument for counting the blood corpuscles. It consists of a graduated pipette into which blood can be drawn and diluted, and a glass slide and cover disc ruled into squares of 0·05 mm. This allows for counting of blood cells under a microscope.

haemodialysis (*he-mo-di-al'-is-is*). The process of removing salts and urea from the blood by means of circulating the blood through a dialyser or artificial kidney, as in certain cases of renal failure.

haemoglobin (*he-mo-glo'-bin*). The complex protein molecule contained within the red blood cells which gives them their colour and by which oxygen is transported.

haemoglobinaemia (*he-mo-glo-bin-e'-me-ah*). The presence of haemoglobin in the blood plasma.

haemoglobinometer (*he-mo-glo-bin-om'-e-ter*). A simple instrument for estimating the haemoglobin level against a standard colour tube.

haemoglobinopathy (*he-mo-glo-bin-op'-ath-e*). Any one of a group of hereditary disorders in which there is an abnormality of the haemoglobin molecule. An example is sickle cell anaemia.

haemolysin (*he-mol'-is-in*). A substance which destroys red blood cells. It may be an enzyme, an antibody or a chemical compound.

haemolysis (*he-mol'-is-is*). Disintegration of red blood cells. In excess a characteristic of some diseases, causing severe anaemia and possibly jaundice.

haemolytic (*he-mo-lit'-ik*). Having the power to destroy red blood cells. *H. anaemia. See* Anaemia. *H. jaundice. See* Jaundice. *H. disease of the newborn.* A condition associated with the rhesus factor (*q.v.*). *H. uraemia. See* Uraemia.

haemopericardium (*he-mo-per-e-kar'-de-um*). Blood within the pericardium either due to a penetrating injury or following surgery.

haemophilia (*he-mo-fil'-e-ah*). A familial disease transmitted by females only, to their male offspring. Characterized by delayed, or entire absence of clotting power of the blood. Due to a lack of antihaemophilic globulin (AHG) or Factor VIII. Slight injuries may be fatal and any operation is dangerous. *Russell's viper venom* and *thrombin* will often arrest minor surface bleeding. Before operation or in an emergency an infusion of fresh frozen plasma or an injection of AHG concentrate can be given.

haemophiliac (*he-mo-fil'-e-ak*). A person afflicted with haemophilia.

Haemophilus influenzae (*he-mof-il-us in-flu-en'-ze*). A minute bacillus that may cause bronchitis and sinusitis.

haemophthalmia (*he-mof-thal'-me-ah*). Bleeding into the eye.

haemopneumothorax (*he-mo-nu-mo-thor'-aks*). Both blood and air are present in the pleural cavity as is likely following chest surgery or trauma of the chest wall.

haemopoiesis (*he-mo-poi-e'-sis*). Manufacture of red blood cells.

haemopoietic (*he-mo-poi-et'-ik*). Relating to red blood cell formation. *H. factors.* Those necessary for the development of red blood cells, e.g. vitamin B_{12} and folic acid.

haemopoietin (*he-mo-poi'-et-in*). Complex of intrinsic factor and vitamin B_{12} which stimulates haemopoiesis (*q.v.*).

haemoptysis (*he-mop'-tis-is*). Coughing up of blood. Being aerated, it is bright red and frothy if in any quantity, and if effort is used in expelling it. Blood from the lungs permeates sputum; from the upper passages a red streaked appearance is characteristic.

haemorrhage (*hem'-or-raj*). An escape of blood from its vessels. *Arterial h.* Bright red blood which escapes in rhythmic spurts, corresponding to the beats of the heart. *Venous h.* Dark red in colour and the blood flows evenly. *Capillary h.* Oozing of blood. Haemorrhage may also be: (*a*) *primary*—at the time of operation or injury; (*b*) *reactionary* or *recurrent*—occurring later when the blood pressure rises and a ligature slips or a vessel opens up; (*c*) *secondary*—as a rule about 10 days after injury, and always due to sepsis. Special types are: *Accidental h.* Bleeding from the uterus during pregnancy. It may be *revealed* or *concealed*. *Antepartum h.* That which occurs before labour starts. *See* Placenta praevia. *Cerebral h. See* Apoplexy. *Concealed h.* The blood collects in a cavity of the body. *Contrecoup h.* That which occurs at a distance from where the force was applied, e.g. a blow on the skull may cause the brain to strike the bony casing directly opposite the site of original force, causing bruising of the nerve tissues. *Extradural h.* Bleeding inside the head, but outside the dura. The result of injury to the skull causing signs of raised intracranial pressure. The cerebrospinal fluid is not blood-stained. It is treated by trephining, removal of clot, and ligature of bleeding vessel. *Inevitable h.* That which is unavoidable, as in placenta praevia. *Intradural h.* Bleeding beneath the dura mater. It may be due to injury and causes signs of compression. The cerebrospinal fluid will be blood-stained. *Post-partum h.* That which occurs after childbirth. *Revealed h.* Bleeding which is obvious. *Subarachnoid h.* Of the cerebral vessels between the pia and arachnoid mater.

haemorrhagic (*hem-or-raj'-ik*). Pertaining to or accompanied by haemorrhage. *H. purpura.* Purpura haemorrhagica (*q.v.*).

haemorrhoidectomy (*hem-or-oid-ek'-to-me*). The surgical removal of haemorrhoids.

haemorrhoids (*hem'-or-oids*). 'Piles' or locally dilated rectal veins. They may be either external or internal to the sphincter ani. Pain is caused on defaecation, and bleeding may occur. Acute attacks of inflammation intensify the symptoms. Treatment may be by surgical removal, or by injection of phenol in almond oil which causes fibrosis of the affected veins.

haemosalpinx (*he-mo-sal'-pinks*). Blood in the fallopian tube, usually caused by a tubal pregnancy. Haematosalpinx.

haemosiderosis (*he-mo-sid-er-o'-sis*). The deposition of iron in the tissues as brownish granules following excessive haemolysis of red blood cells.

haemostasis (*he-mo-sta'-sis*). The arrest of bleeding or the slowing up of blood flow in a vessel.

haemostatic (*he-mo-stat'-ik*). A drug or remedy for arresting haemorrhage.

haemothorax (*he-mo-thor'-aks*). Blood in the thoracic cavity, e.g. from injury to soft tissues as a result of fracture of rib.

Hageman factor (*ha'-gem-an*). The twelfth factor which facilitates the clotting of blood (called after the first patient found to be suffering from a deficiency of it).

hair. A delicate epidermal filament growing out of the skin. *H. follicle.* See Follicle.

halazone (*hal'-a-zone*). A chlorine antiseptic similar to chloramine. Used for the purification of drinking water.

Haldane apparatus (*J. S. Haldane, British physiologist, 1860–1936*). A piece of apparatus used in the analysis of respiratory gases.

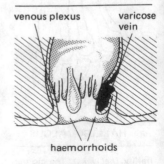

venous plexus   varicose vein

haemorrhoids

HAEMORRHOIDS

half-life. The term is applied to radioactive isotopes and denotes that period of time in which the element loses half activity by the process of disintegration.

halibut oil (*hal'-e-but*). Derived from the liver of halibut, and rich in vitamins A and D.

halitosis (*hal-e-to'-sis*). Foul-smelling breath.

hallucination (*hal-lu-sin-a'-shun*). A false perception in which the patient believes he see, smells, hears, tastes or feels an object or person when there is no basis in the external environment for the belief.

hallucinogens (*hal-lu-sin'-o-jens*). Drugs, e.g. LSD, that induce in a patient false sensory impressions or cause hallucinations (*q.v.*).

other toes. *H. varus.* In which the big toe is bent inwards, towards the other foot.

halogens (*hal'-o-jens*). The chemical elements chlorine, iodine, bromine and fluorine.

haloperidol (*hal-o-per'-id-ol*). A drug used in the treatment of hypomania and mania.

halothane (*hal'-o-thane*). A volatile anaesthetic liquid derived from ether.

hamamelis (*ham-a-me'-lis*). Witch-hazel, employed as an astringent, especially in haemorrhoids.

hammer toe. A deformity in which the first phalanx is bent upwards, with plantar flexion of the second and third phalanx.

hamstring muscles. The flexors of the knee joint that are situated at the back of the thigh.

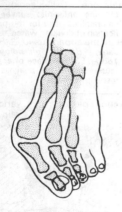

HALLUX VALGUS

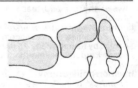

HAMMER TOE

hallux (*hal'-luks*). The big toe. *H. valgus.* A deformity in which the big toe is bent towards the

hand, foot and mouth disease. Disease caused by a coxsackievirus which results in vesicle formation on all three sites. Not the same as foot and mouth disease.

Hand – Schüller – Christian disease (*A. Hand, American paediatrician, 1868–1949: A. Schüller, Austrian neurologist, 1874– : H. A. Christian, American physician, 1876–1951*). A disease of the reticulo-endothelial system in which granulomas containing cholesterol are formed, chiefly in the skull.

handicapped (*hand'-e-kapt*). The term applied to a person with a mental or physical disability that interferes with normal living and earning capacity.

Hanot's disease (*V.-C. Hanot, French physician, 1844–96*). A form of cirrhosis of the liver in which the fibrosis is found mainly around the ductules of the biliary system.

haploid (*hap'-loid*). The condition in which the cell contains one set of chromosomes after division. In man they divide into twenty-three in each gamete (*q.v.*).

haptens (*hap'-tens*). Carbohydrates which become antigens when combined with body proteins.

hare-lip. A congenital fissure in the upper lip, often accompanied by cleft-palate. Treated by surgical repair when the child is very young.

harlequin rash (*har'-le-kwin*). A flushing of the skin in infants. Only one half of the body is affected. The mid line forms the demarcation point, which clearly separates it from the normal side.

Harris's operation (*S. Harris, Australian surgeon, 1880–1936*). See Prostatectomy.

Harrison's sulcus (*E. Harrison, British physician, 1789–1838*). A depression in the chest wall above the diaphragm noticed in difficult breathing, especially in children.

Hartmann's solution (*A. Hartmann, American physician, 1898– *). A valuable infusion fluid as it contains potassium and calcium chloride and lactic acid as well as sodium chloride. Used in the treatment of dehydration.

Harvey, W. (*English physician, 1578–1657*). In 1628 Harvey described his theory that blood circulates around the body. This was contained in his book *De Motu Cordis*.

Hashimoto's disease (*H. Hashimoto, Japanese surgeon, 1881–1934*). A lymphadenoid goitre caused by the formation of antibodies to thyroglobulin. It is an autoimmune condition giving rise to hypothyroidism.

hashish (*hash'-ish*). Indian hemp. See Cannabis indica.

Hassall's corpuscles (*A. H. Hassall, British chemist and physician, 1817–94*). Small striated bodies in the thymus gland which are the remains of tissue found in the early stages of development of this gland.

haustrations (*haws-tra'-shuns*). The pouches or sacculations of the colon.

haversian canals (*C. Havers, British physician and anatomist, 1650–1702*). Minute canals permeating bone, containing blood and lymph vessels to maintain its nutrition. See Bone.

hay fever. An acute catarrh affecting the nasal mucous membrane and the conjunctiva, and caused by hypersensitiveness to the pollen of grasses, etc. See Allergy.

Heaf test (*F. G. R. Heaf, British physician, 1894– *). A form of tuberculin testing. A drop of tuberculin solution on the skin is injected by a means of a number of very short needles mounted on a spring-loaded device.

healing. The process of return to normal function, after a period of disease or injury. *H. by first intention* signifies union of the edges of a clean incised wound without visible granulations, and leaving only a faint linear scar. *H. by second intention* is union of the edges of an open wound, by the formation of granulations which fill it in from the bottom and sides. These form fibrous tissue which contracts and causes an unsightly scar.

health. A state of physical, mental, and social well being.

heart. A hollow, muscular organ which pumps the blood throughout the body, situated behind the sternum slightly towards the left side of the thorax. *H. block.* A form of heart disease in which the passage of impulses down the bundle of His is interrupted. It may be partial, in which every second or third beat is missed, or complete, in which there is a very slow myogenic beat uninfluenced by the nervous system. *See* Stokes-Adams syndrome. *H. failure.* May be acute, as in coronary thrombosis or chronic. *H. murmur.* Abnormal sound heard in the heart, frequently caused by disease of the valves. Occurs when the blood flow through the heart exceeds a certain velocity. *H. sounds.* The sounds heard when listening to the heart beat. They are caused by the closure of the valves. *Chronic congestive h. failure.* Increasing congestion in the portal and pulmonary circulation and marked oedema.

heartburn. *See* Pyrosis.

heat exhaustion. Under very hot conditions there may be abdominal cramp, a rapid pulse, dizziness and dyspnoea caused by a lack of sodium chloride lost during excessive sweating.

heat spots. A skin eruption due to poorly developed sweat ducts. These become blocked and irritant retention cysts are formed.

heat stroke. A person exposed to great heat may fall unconscious, with a temperature of 40° to 42°C because the sweat secretion is suppressed and the body cannot lose heat.

hebephrenia (*he-be-fre'-ne-ah*). A form of schizophrenia characterized by thought disorder and emotional incongruity. Behaviour is often silly and childish. Delusions and hallucinations are common.

Heberden's nodes (*W. Heberden, British physician, 1710–1801*). Bony or cartilaginous outgrowths causing deformity of the terminal finger joints in osteo-arthritis.

hectic (*hek'-tik*). Habitual. *H. fever. See* Fever. *H. flush.* A malar flush seen in cases of phthisis.

hedonism (*he'-don-izm*). Excessive devotion to pleasure.

Hegar's dilators (*A. Hegar, German gynaecologist, 1830–1914*). A series of graduated dilators used to dilate the cervix uteri.

Hegar's sign. The marked softening of the cervix that takes place in early pregnancy.

heliotherapy (*he-le-o-ther'-ap-e*). Treatment of disease by exposure of the body to sunlight.

helium (*he'-le-um*). A gas used in conjunction with oxygen to facilitate respiration in obstructional types of dyspnoea (*q.v.*) and for decompressing deep-sea divers.

helix (*he'-liks*). A spiral twist. Used to describe the configuration of certain molecules, e.g. deoxyribonucleic acid (DNA).

Heller's operation (*E. Heller, German surgeon, 1877–1964*). For the relief of dysphagia in achalasia of the cardia, by dividing the muscle coat at the lower end of the oesophagus.

helminthiasis (*hel-min-thi'-*

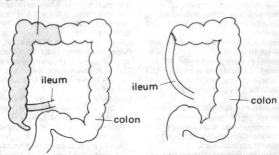

area removed

ileum

ileum

colon

colon

HEMICOLECTOMY AND TRANSVERSE ILEOCOLOSTOMY

as-is). The condition due to infestation with worms.

hemeralopia (*hem-er-al-o'-pe-ah*). Inability to see in a bright light. *See* Nyctalopia.

hemi- (*hem'-e*). Prefix meaning one half.

hemianopia (*hem-e-an-o'-pe-ah*). Partial blindness in which the patient can see only one-half of the normal field of vision.

hemiballismus (*hem-e-bal-is'-mus*). Involuntary chorea-like movements on one side of the body only.

hemicolectomy (*hem-e-ko-lek'-to-me*). The removal of the ascending and part of the transverse colon with an ileotransverse colostomy.

hemiglossectomy (*hem-e-glos-sek'-to-me*). Removal of approximately half the tongue.

hemiparesis (*hem-e-par-e'-sis*). A partial paralysis on one side of the body.

hemiplegia (*hem-e-ple'-je-ah*). Paralysis of one half of the body, usually due to cerebral

disease. The lesion is in the side of the brain opposite to the side paralysed, as the pyramidal fibres from each cerebral hemisphere cross in the medulla oblongata. If the right side is paralysed, speech is liable to be affected, as control of this is mainly in the left cerebrum. *Pontine h.* The cause is a lesion in the pons.

hemispheres (*hem'-is-feers*). The two halves of the cerebrum or cerebellum.

henbane (*hen'-bane*). *See* Hyoscyamus.

Henle's canals (*F. G. J. Henle, German anatomist, 1809–85*). Section of the kidney tubule in which there is a movement of sodium salts between it and the tissue fluid, and a certain adjustment of osmolarity.

Henoch's purpura (*E. H. Henoch, German paediatrician, 1820–1910*). *See* Purpura.

hepar (*he'-par*). The liver.

heparin (*hep'-ar-in*). An anticoagulant formed in the liver and circulated in the blood. Injected intravenously it prevents the conversion of prothrombin into thrombin, and is used in the treatment of thrombosis.

hepatalgia (*hep-at-al´-je-ah*). Pain in the liver.

hepatectomy (*hep-at-ek´-to-me*). Excision of a part or the whole of the liver.

hepatic (*he-pat´-ik*). Relating to the liver.

hepaticocholedochostomy (*hep´-at-ik-o-ko-le-dok-os´-to-me*). An anastomosis between the hepatic duct and the common bile duct.

hepaticojejunostomy (*hep-at´-ik-o-je-jun-os´-to-me*). The anastomosis of the hepatic duct to the jejunum usually following extensive excision for carcinoma of the pancreas.

hepaticostomy (*hep-at-ik-os´-to-me*). A surgical opening into the hepatic duct.

hepatitis (*hep-at-i´-tis*). Inflammation of the liver. *Amoebic h.* May arise during amoebic dysentery and lead to liver abscesses. *Infective h.* Caused by a virus (A or IH) spread by faecal contamination. Incubation 2 to 6 weeks. *Serum h.* Occurs 6 weeks to 6 months after parenteral inoculation of the virus (B or SH) usually in blood or its products. Can be fatal.

hepatization (*hep-at-i-za´-shun*). Changing of tissues into substance resembling liver. *Red h.* The red solid appearance of the consolidated lung in specific pneumonia, due to the invasion of the alveoli by red blood cells and fibrin. *Grey h.* The grey appearance later in the disease before resolution occurs, when white blood cells invade the area to destroy the infection.

hepatocele (*hep´-at-o-seel*). Hernia of the liver.

hepatocellular (*hep-at-o-sel´-u-lah*). Referring to the parenchymal cells of the liver.

hepatocirrhosis (*hep-at-o-sir-ro´-sis*). Cirrhosis of the liver.

hepatogenous (*hep-at-oj´-en-us*). Arising in the liver. Applied to jaundice where the disease arises in the parenchymal cells of the liver.

hepatojugular reflex (*hep-at-o-jug´-u-lar re´-fleks*). A test used to determine heart failure. Pressure over the liver causes distension of the neck veins, due to an increase in the venous return to the heart, and a rise in right atrial pressure.

hepato-lenticular (*hep-at-o-len-tik´-u-lar*). Applied to a degenerative condition of hepatic fibrosis with neurological symptoms of Parkinsonism which is secondary to excessive copper absorption.

hepatolithiasis (*hep-at-o-lith-i´-as-is*). Calculi formation in the liver.

hepatoma (*hep-at-o´-mah*). A primary malignant tumour arising in the liver cells.

hepatomegaly (*hep-at-o-meg´-al-e*). An enlargement of the liver.

hepatosplenomegaly (*hep´-at-o-splen-o-meg´-al-e*). Enlargement of the liver and spleen as may be found in kala-azar (*q.v.*).

hepatotoxic (*hep-at-o-toks´-ik*). Applied to drugs and substances that cause destruction of liver cells.

herd immunity (*herd im-mu´-nit-e*). Immunity which develops either naturally or as a result of artificial immunization in a whole population.

hereditary (*her-ed´-it-ar-e*).

Derived from ancestry. Inherited.

heredity (*her-ed'-it-e*). The characteristics both physical and mental derived from the parents and transmitted to the offspring. Recessive characteristics may miss one or two generations and reappear later.

Hering–Breuer reflex (*K. E. K. Hering, German physiologist, 1834–1918: J. Breuer, German physician, 1842–1925*). A reflex in which the depth of respiration is determined by the nervous impulses which affect the muscle spindles of the intercostal muscles and the diaphragm.

hermaphrodite (*her-maf'-ro-dite*). An individual whose gonads contain both testicular and ovarian tissue. These may be combined as an ovotestis or a testis on one side and an ovary on the other. The external genitalia may be indeterminate or of either sex. *Pseudo-h.* One whose gonads are histologically of one sex but the genitalia have the appearance of the opposite sex.

hernia (*her'-ne-ah*). Rupture. A protrusion of any part of the internal organs through the structures enclosing them. *Cerebral h.* A protrusion of brain through an opening in the skull. *Diaphragmatic h.* and *Hiatus h.* One part of the stomach through the oesophagal opening in the diaphragm. *Femoral h.* The loop of intestine protrudes through the femoral canal. More common in females. *Incisional* or *ventral h.* This occurs at the site of an old wound. *Inguinal h.* Protrusion of the intestine through the inguinal canal. This may be congenital or acquired, and is commonest in males. *Irredu-*

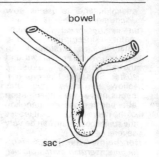

bowel

sac

HERNIA

cible h. One that cannot be replaced by manipulation. *Reducible h.* One that can be returned to its normal position by manipulative measures. *Strangulated h.* The neck of the sac containing the bowel is so constricted that the venous circulation is impeded, and gangrene will result if not treated promptly. Constipation is complete. *Umbilical h.* Protrusion of bowel through the umbilical ring. This may be congenital or acquired. *Vaginal h.* Rectocele or cystocele (*q.v.*).

hernioplasty (*her'-ne-o-plas-te*). A plastic repair of the abdominal wall performed after reducing the hernia. This may be by fascia, nylon or filigree wire.

herniorrhaphy (*her-ne-or'-raf-e*). Removal of the hernial sac and repair of the abdominal wall.

herniotomy (*her-ne-ot'-o-me*). An operation to remove the hernial sac.

heroin (*her'-o-in*). A diacetate of morphine used as an analgesic; it is a strong drug of addiction and its use is now discouraged.

herpes (*her'-peez*). An inflammatory skin eruption showing small vesicles. *H. simplex.* An eruption which appears around the mouth due to a virus. *H. zoster.* Shingles. The eruption follows the course of a cutaneous nerve; the inflammation affecting the sensory ganglion of the nerve root just as it leaves the spinal cord. Pain can be very severe.

Herxheimer reaction (*K. Herxheimer, German dermatologist, 1861–*). An inflammatory reaction in the tissues in cases of syphilis, which can occur on starting treatment.

Hess's test (*W. R. Hess, Swiss physiologist, 1881–*). A test used to diagnose purpura. An inflated blood pressure cuff causes an increase in capillary pressure and rupture of the walls, causing purpuric spots to develop.

hetero-. A prefix meaning other or different.

heterochromia (*het-er-o-kro'-me-ah*). A difference in colour in the two eyes. It may be congenital or secondary due to inflammation.

heterogenous (*het-er-oj'-en-us*). Composed of diverse constituents or derived from different sources.

heteroplasty (*het'-er-o-plas-te*). A plastic operation in which the graft is obtained from an animal not of the same species.

heterosexual (*het-er-o-seks'-u-al*). Attracted to and desiring to establish an emotional relationship with someone of the opposite sex.

heterotropia (*het-er-o-tro'-pe-ah*). A marked deviation of the eyes. Strabismus or squint.

heterozygous (*het-er-o-zi'-gus*). Possessing dissimilar alternative genes for a physical characteristic that are inherited one from each parent. One gene is dominant and the other is recessive.

hexachlorophane (*heks-a-klor'-o-fane*). An antiseptic often added to soap, soap solutions, or dusting powder and which greatly reduces the bacteria on the skin.

hexamethonium (*heks-a-metho'-ne-um*). A ganglionic blocking agent formerly used in the treatment of hypertension.

hexamine (*heks'-am-een*). A urinary antiseptic which releases formaldehyde in an acid urine.

Hg. Symbol for mercury (hydrargyrum).

hiatus (*hi-a'-tus*). A space or opening. *H. hernia.* Protrusion of the fundus of the stomach through the oesophageal opening in the diaphragm.

hiccup (*hik'-kup*). Hiccough. A spasmodic contraction of the diaphragm causing an abrupt inspiratory sound.

hidrosis (*hi-dro'-sis*). Excretion of sweat.

Higginson's syringe (*A. Higginson, British surgeon, 1808–*). An indiarubber syringe with a bulb in the centre which, when compressed, forces fluid forward through the nozzle. It can be used with suitable attachments for irrigation of any cavity of the body, e.g. antra, rectum or vagina.

high-temperature short-time. The process of pasteurization of milk by which it is heated to 71°C for 15 seconds. *See* Pasteurization.

higher centres. The cerebral cortex of the brain.

hilum (*hi'-lum*). A recess in an

organ, by which vessels enter and leave it.

hip. The upper part of the thigh at its junction with the pelvis. *H. replacement.* An operation in which the head of the femur and cup of the acetabulum are replaced by a metal prosthesis. *See* Arthroplasty.

hippocratic (*hip-po-krat'-ik*). Relating to Hippocrates, the Father of Medicine (*Greek physician, 460–377* BC). *H. oath.* The still accepted standard of medical ethics, attributed to Hippocrates. *H. facies. See* Facies.

hippuric acid (*hip-u'-rik as'-id*). A waste product of metabolism which is excreted in the urine.

hippuric acid test (*hip-u'-rik*). *See* Test.

Hirschsprung's disease (*H. Hirschsprung, Danish physician, 1831–1916*). *See* Megacolon.

hirsute (*hur'-sute*). Hairy.

hirudin (*hi-ru'-din*). The active principle in the secretion of the leech which prevents clotting of blood.

Hirudo (*hi-ru'-do*). The leech (*q.v.*).

histamine (*hist'-am-een*). An enzyme that causes local vasodilatation and increased permeability of the blood vessel walls. It is readily released from body tissues and is a factor in allergy response. Injected subcutaneously, it greatly increases gastric secretion of hydrochloric acid and is used to test for the same.

histidinaemia (*his-tid-in-e'-me-ah*). A congenital inability to metabolize histidine, causing mental retardation.

histidine (*his'-tid-een*). One of the 22 amino acids formed by the digestion of dietary protein.

histiocytes (*his'-te-o-sites*). The macrophage cells of connective tissue. Derived from the reticulo-endothelial cells they act as scavengers.

histiocytoma (*his-te-o-si-to'-mah*). A benign tumour of histiocytes causing a vascular nodule.

histiocytosis (*his-te-o-si'-to-sis*). A group of diseases of bone in which granulomas appear containing histiocytes and eosinophil cells. *See* Letterer–Siwe disease.

histocompatibility (*his-to-kom-pat-ib-il'-it-e*). The ability of cells to be accepted and to function in a new situation. Tissue typing reveals this and ensures a higher success rate in organ transplantation.

histology (*his-tol'-o-je*). The science dealing with the minute structure of tissues.

histolysis (*his-tol'-is-is*). Disintegration of tissues.

histoplasmosis (*his-to-plas-mo'-sis*). Inhalation of a yeast-like fungus causing a lung infection and rarely spreading throughout the reticulo-endothelial system.

hobnail liver. *See* Liver.

Hodgkin's disease (*T. Hodgkin, British physician, 1798–1866*). Lymphadenoma. A progressive malignant condition of the reticulo-endothelial cells. There is progressive enlargement of lymph nodes and lymph tissue all over the body. Treated by radiotherapy and cytotoxic drugs.

Hogben test. *See* Test.

Homans' sign (*J. Homans, American surgeon, 1877–1954*). Pain elicited in the calf when the foot is dorsiflexed. Indicative of venous thrombosis.

homatropine (*ho-mat'-ro-pin*). A mydriatic (*q.v.*) derived from *atropine*, and used in ophthalmic practice. Its effect is more transitory than that of atropine, and therefore it is used to dilate the pupil for examination of the disc, and not as treatment.

homeo- (*ho'-me-o*). A prefix meaning 'similar'.

homeopathy (*ho-me-op'-athe*). A system promulgated by C. F. S. Hahnemann (*German physician, 1755–1843*) and based upon the principle that 'like cures like'. Drugs are given which produce in the patient the signs of the disease to be cured, but they are usually prescribed in very small doses.

homeostasis (*ho-me-o-sta'-sis*). Automatic self-regulation of man to maintain the normal or standard state of the body under variations in the environment.

homeothermic (*ho-me-o-ther'-mik*). Warm-blooded animals, where the heat regulating mechanism maintains a constant body temperature in spite of the environment.

homicide (*hom'-e-side*). The killing of a human being, whether intentional (murder) or accidental (manslaughter).

homogenize (*ho-moj'-en-ize*). To reduce to the same consistency. A complete meal can be reduced in this way to a liquid or semi-solid state when there is difficulty in feeding.

homogeneous (*ho-mo-je'-ne-us*). Uniform in character. Similar in nature and characteristics.

homograft (*ho'-mo-graft*). A tissue or organ transplanted from one individual to another of the same species.

homolateral (*ho-mo-lat'-er-al*). On the same side.

homologous (*ho-mol'-o-gus*). Having a corresponding origin, structure and position. *H. chro-*

mosomes. Those that pair during meiosis and contain an identical arrangement of genes in the DNA pattern.

homologue (*ho'-mo-log*). A part or organ which has the same relative position or structure as another one.

homoplasty (*ho'-mo-plas-te*). Replacement by operation of a part or tissue of similar structure from another person of the same species.

homosexual (*hom-o-seks'-u-al*). Of the same sex.

homosexuality (*hom-o-seks-u-al'-it-e*). The attraction for and desire to establish an emotional relationship with a member of the same sex.

homozygous (*ho-mo-zi'-gus*). Possessing an identical pair of genes for a physical characteristic. *See* Heterozygous.

hookworm. *See* Ancylostoma.

hordeolum (*hor-de-o'-lum*). A stye. Inflammation of sebaceous glands of eyelashes.

hormone (*hor'-mone*). A chemical substance which is generated in one organ, and carried by the blood to another in which it excites activity.

hormonotherapy (*hor'-mon-o-ther'-ap-e*). Treatment by the use of hormones.

Horner's syndrome (*J. F. Horner, Swiss ophthalmologist, 1831–86*). A condition in which there is a lesion on the path of sympathetic nerve fibres.

horse serum (*hors'-se'-rum*). Serum (*q.v.*) containing antibodies which neutralize the toxins of diphtheria and tetanus. It is obtained from horses which have developed these antibodies.

horseshoe kidney. *See* Kidney.

Horton's syndrome (*B. T. Horton, American physician, 1895– *). Severe headache caused by the release of histamine.

host. The animal or tissue on which a parasite lives and multiplies. *Intermediate h.* One that shelters the parasite during a non-reproductive period.

host defences. The defence mechanisms of the body against pathogenic organisms.

hour-glass contraction. A contraction near the middle of a hollow organ, such as the stomach or uterus, producing an outline resembling that shape. Due to muscle spasm or scar tissue formation as the result of inflammation.

housemaid's knee. Prepatellar bursitis. Inflammation of the prepatellar bursa, which becomes distended with serous fluid. It is caused by constant kneeling on hard surfaces.

Houston's folds (*J. Houston, Irish surgeon, 1802–45*). Three oblique folds in the mucous membrane of the rectum.

human chorionic gonadotrophin, HCG (*kor-e-on'-ik gon-ad-o-tro'-fin*). A hormone produced by the placenta during pregnancy, the detection of which in the urine forms the basis of pregnancy tests.

human growth hormone. Hormone produced by the anterior pituitary gland which stimulates body growth.

humerus (*hu'-mer-us*). The bone of the upper arm.

humidity (*hu-mid'-it-e*). The amount of moisture in the air. *Relative h.* The humidity of the atmosphere compared with what it would be if the air were saturated.

humoral defences (*hu'-mor-al*). The defence mechanisms against invading organisms contained in the body fluids.

humour (*hu'-mor*). Any fluid of the body, such as lymph, aqueous humour, etc.

hunger pain. Pain associated with peptic ulcer which is relieved by taking food.

hunger stool. *See* Stool.

Huntington's chorea (*G. S. Huntington, American physician, 1851–1927*). A rare, degenerative inherited disorder of the brain in which there is progressive chorea and mental deterioration (dementia).

Hurler's syndrome (*G. Hurler, contemporary Austrian paediatrician*). An inherited disorder in which mental subnormality is caused by excess mucopolysaccharides being stored in the brain and reticuloendothelial system.

Hutchinson's teeth (*Sir J. Hutchinson, British surgeon, 1828–1913*). Typical notching of the borders of the incisor teeth occurring in congenital syphilis.

hyaline (*hi'-al-een*). Resembling glass. *H. cartilage. See* Cartilage. *H. casts. See* Casts. *H. cells.* Clear white blood cells. *H. degeneration.* A form which occurs in tumours due to deficiency of blood supply. It precedes cystic degeneration. *H. membrane disease. See* Respiratory distress syndrome.

hyalitis (*hi-al-i'-tis*). Inflammation of the hyaloid membrane or vitreous humour in the eyeball.

hyaloid membrane (*hi'-al-oid*). A delicate transparent membrane surrounding the vitreous humour of the eye.

hyaluronidase (*hi-al-u-ron'-e-daze*). An enzyme which facilitates the absorption of fluids in subcutaneous tissues. Hyalase is a proprietary preparation of the enzyme.

hybrid (*hi'-brid*). The offspring

of distinct but related members of a species.

hydatid (*hi-dat'-id*). A cystic swelling containing the embryo of *Echinococcus granulosus* (*q.v.*). It may be found in any organ of the body, e.g. in the liver. 'Daughter cysts' are produced from the original. Infection is from contaminated foods, e.g. salads.

hydatidiform mole (*hi-dat-id'-e-form*). *See* Mole.

hydraemia (*hi-dre'-me-ah*). A high fluid content in the blood rendering it more dilute.

hydragogue (*hi'-drah-gog*). A purgative causing copious liquid evacuations, e.g. magnesium sulphate, jalap.

hydramnios (*hi-dram'-ne-os*). An excessive amount of amniotic fluid.

hydrargyrism (*hi-drar'-je-rizm*). Chronic mercurial poisoning.

hydrarthrosis (*hi-drar-thro'-sis*). A collection of fluid in a joint.

hydrate (*hi'-drate*). A compound of an element with water.

hydro- (*hi'-dro*). A prefix referring to either water or hydrogen.

hydroa (*hi-dro'-ah*). A hypersensitivity of the skin to light, resulting in the formation of a vesicular eruption on the exposed parts with intense irritation.

hydrocarbon (*hi-dro-kar'-bon*). A compound of hydrogen and carbon. Fats are of this type.

hydrocele (*hi'-dro-seel*). A swelling caused by accumulation of fluid, especially in the tunica vaginalis surrounding the testicle.

hydrocephalus (*hi-dro-kef'-al-us*). 'Water on the brain'. Enlargement of the skull due to an abnormal collection of cerebrospinal fluid around the brain or in the ventricles. It may be congenital or acquired from inflammation of the meninges during infancy. *See* Toxoplasmosis.

hydrochloric acid (*hi-dro-klor'-ik*). HCl. A colourless compound of hydrogen and chlorine. In 0·2 per cent solution it is present in gastric juice and aids digestion.

hydrochlorothiazide (*hi'-dro-klor-o-thi'-az-ide*). A valuable oral diuretic similar to but more potent than chlorothiazide. Proprietary preparations are Esidrex and Hydrosaluric.

hydrocortisone (*hi-dro-kor'-te-zone*). Cortisol. A hormone isolated from the secretion of the adrenal cortex. It affects carbohydrate and protein metabolism and is anti-inflammatory. Used for topical application in eye, ear and skin conditions. Also used as intra-articular injection for arthritis and intravenously in status asthmaticus and in acute adrenocortical insufficiency.

hydrocyanic acid (*hi-dro-si-an'-ik*). A highly poisonous acid from bitter almonds. Prussic acid.

hydroflumethiazide (*hi-dro-flu-meth-i'-az-ide*). An oral thiazide diuretic. Naclex is a proprietary preparation.

hydrogen (*hi'-dro-jen*). A combustible gas, present in nearly all organic compounds which, in combination with oxygen, forms water. *H. ion concentration.* The amount of hydrogen in a liquid, which is responsible for its acidity. Expressed as the hydrogen exponent pH. The concentration in the blood is of importance in acidosis. *H. peroxide* (H_2O_2). An antiseptic. When in contact with pus the oxygen is released and causes frothing. It has also a bleaching action.

hydrolysis (*hi-drol'-is-is*). The process of splitting up into smaller molecules by uniting with water.

hydrometer (*hi-drom'-e-ter*). An instrument for estimating the specific gravity of fluids, e.g. a urinometer.

hydrometra (*hi-dro-me'-trah*). A collection of watery fluid in the uterus.

hydronephrosis (*hi-dro-nef-ro'-sis*). A collection of urine in the pelvis of the kidney, resulting in atrophy of the kidney structure, due to the constant pressure of the fluid, until finally the whole organ becomes one large cyst. The condition may be: (1) Congenital, due to malformation of the kidney or ureter. (2) Acquired due to any obstruction of the ureter by tumour or stone, or to back pressure from stricture of the urethra or enlarged prostate gland.

hydropathy (*hi-drop'-ath-e*). The treatment of disease by the use of water internally and externally.

hydropericarditis (*hi-dro-per-e-kard-i'-tis*). Inflammation of the pericardium resulting in serous fluid in the pericardial sac.

hydroperitoneum (*hi-dro-per-e-ton-e'-um*). *See* Ascites.

hydrophobia (*hi-dro-fo'-be-ah*). An acute infectious disease contracted by man through a bite from an animal infected with *rabies*. Caused by a virus present in the saliva. The symptoms include violent spasms of the muscles of deglutition, which are greatly aggravated by the sight of water. There are mental delusions, fever and a profuse flow of saliva. There is a long incubation period, so

immediate inoculation, with *anti-rabies vaccine* provides complete protection.

hydropneumothorax (*hi-dro-nu-mo-thor'-aks*). The presence of fluid and air in the pleural space.

hydrops (*hi'-drops*). Dropsy. *H. abdominis*. Ascites. *H. foetalis*. Severe form of erythroblastosis foetalis (*q.v.*). *H. tubae*. Hydrosalpinx.

hydrorrachis (*hi-dror'-rak-is*). Effusion into the spinal canal.

hydrorrhoea gravidarum (*hi-dror-re'-ah grav-id-ar'-um*). An abnormal discharge of fluid during pregnancy due to excessive mucous secretion from the endometrium.

hydrosalpinx (*hi-dro-sal'-pinks*). Distension of the fallopian tube by fluid.

Hydrosaluric (*hi-dro-sal-ur'-ik*). A proprietary preparation of hydrochlorothiazide. An oral diuretic.

hydrostatic test (*hi-dro-stat'-ik*). Determining that live birth has taken place by floating the fetal lungs in water.

hydrotherapeutics (*hi-dro-ther-ap-u'-tiks*). The treatment of disease by water.

hydrothorax (*hi-dro-thor'-aks*). Fluid in the pleural cavity due to serous effusion as in cardiac, renal and other diseases.

hydroxyproline (*hi-droks-e-pro'-leen*). One of the 22 amino acids which is glucogenic.

5-hydroxtryptamine (*hi-droks-e-trip'-tam-een*). Serotonin substance which acts as a chemical transmitter. It also stimulates smooth muscle.

hygiene (*hi'-jeen*). The science of health. *Communal h*. Deals with the maintenance of the health of the community by provision of a pure water supply, efficient sanitation good housing, etc. *Industrial h.* Care of the health of workers in the industry. *Mental h.* Deals with the healthy development of the mental outlook and emotional reactions. *Mouth h.* The efficient care and cleanliness of the mouth and teeth, especially important in illness. *Personal h.* Deals with measures taken by the individual to preserve his own health.

hygroma (*hi-gro'-mah*). A swelling caused by fluid. *Subdural h.* A collection of clear fluid in the subdural space.

hygrometer (*hi-grom'-et-er*). An instrument for measuring the water vapour in the air.

hygroscopic (*hi-gro-skop'-ik*). Readily absorbing moisture. *Glycerin* is used in medical treatment because it has this power, e.g. in treating chapped hands. Also used as a suppository to relieve constipation.

hymen (*hi'-men*). A fold of mucous membrane partially closing the entrance to the vagina.

hymenectomy (*hi-men-ek'-to-me*). The surgical removal of the hymen.

hymenotomy (*hi-men-ot'-o-me*). A surgical incision of the hymen to render the orifice larger.

hyoid bone (*hi'-oid*). A U-shaped bone above the thyroid cartilage, to which the tongue is attached.

hyoscine (*hi'-os-sin*). Scopolamine. An alkaloid obtained from solanaceous plants. It is a powerful cerebral depressant and may be used in acute mania. It diminishes glandular secretions, so it is used with papaveretum preoperatively and is a recognized preventive to sea sickness.

hyoscyamus (*hi-o-si'-am-us*). Henbane. The dried leaves have an antispasmodic action which relieves the pain of excessive peristalsis or of cystitis.

hypaemia (*hi-pe'-me-ah*). Deficiency of blood in a part.

hypaesthesia (*hi-pes-the'-ze-ah*). Impairment of sensation.

hypamnios (*hi-pam'-ne-os*). Lessened fluid in the amniotic sac.

hyper-. Greek prefix meaning 'above'.

hyperacidity (*hi-per-as-id'-it-e*). Excessive acidity. *Gastric h.* Hyperchlorhydria (*q.v.*).

hyperaemia (*hi-per-e'-me-ah*). Excess of blood in any part.

hyperaesthesia (*hi-per-es-the'-ze-ah*). Excessively acute feeling in any part.

hyperalgesia (*hi-per-al-ge'-ze-ah*). Excessive sensibility to pain.

hyperasthenia (*hi-per-as-the'-ne-ah*). Extreme weakness.

hyperbaric (*hi-per-bar'-ik*). At greater pressure than normal. *H. oxygen.* See Appendix 3.

hyperbilirubinaemia (*hi-per-bil-e-ru-bin-e'-me-ah*). An excess of bilirubin in the blood.

hypercalcaemia (*hi-per-kal-se'-me-ah*). Rise in blood calcium.

hypercalcuria (*hi-per-kal-sur'-e-ah*). A high level of calcium in the urine leading to renal stone formation.

hypercapnia (*hi-per-kap'-ne-ah*). An increased amount of carbon dioxide in the blood causing over stimulation of the respiratory centre.

hypercarbia (*hi-per-kar'-be-ah*). An increase in the carbon dioxide content of blood.

hypercatabolism (*hi-per-kat-ab'-ol-izm*). An excessive rate of catabolism. The rapid breakdown of protein or tissue.

hyperchlorhydria (*hi-per-*

klor-hi'-dre-ah). Excess of hydrochloric acid in the gastric juice.

hyperchromic (hi-per-kro'-mik). Highly coloured or stained.

hyperdynamia (hi-per-di-nam'-e-ah). Excessive muscle activity. *H. uteri*. Excessive uterine contractions in labour.

hyperemesis (hi-per-em'-es-is). Excessive vomiting. *H. gravidarum*. A complication of pregnancy which may be serious.

hyperextension (hi-per-eks-ten'-shun). A form of over-extension used to correct orthopaedic deformities.

hyperflexion (hi-per-flek'-shun). Over-flexion of a limb.

hyperglycaemia (hi-per-gli-se'-me-ah). Excess of sugar in the blood (*normal* 2·5–4·7 mmol/litre (45–80 mg/100 ml) when fasting); a sign of diabetes mellitus.

hyperhidrosis (hi-per-hi-dro'-sis). Excessive perspiration.

hyperimmune gammaglobulin (hi-per-im-mu'-n). *See* Immunoglobulin.

hyperkalaemia (hi-per-kal-e'-me-ah). A higher than normal concentration of potassium in the blood.

hyperkeratosis (hi-per-ker-a-to'-sis). A hyperplasia or overgrowth of the horny layers of the skin.

hyperkinesis (hi-per-ki-ne'-sis). A condition in which there is excessive movement.

hyperlipaemia (hi-per-lip-e'-me-ah). An increase in the fat content of blood. There may also be a rise in blood cholesterol.

hypermetropia (hi-per-met-ro'-pe-ah). Hyperopia. Farsightedness. The light rays converge beyond the retina and a biconvex lens (*q.v.*) is required to correct it.

hypermnesia (hi-perm-ne'-ze-ah). Outstanding power of memory; may be found in infant prodigies or in some forms of mania.

hypermotility (hi-per-mo-til'-it-e). Increased movement. *Gastric h.* Increased muscle action of the stomach wall, associated with increased secretion of hydrochloric acid.

hypernatraemia (hi-per-nat-re'-me-ah). An increase in the sodium content of the blood. Seen in infants when an excess of milk powder has been used in the preparation of feeds, giving an incorrect proportion of powder to water.

hypernephroma (hi-per-nef-ro'-mah). A malignant tumour of the kidney.

hyperosmolarity (hi-per-os-mo-lar'-it-e). A greater osmotic pressure than normal, usually applied to that exerted by salts and plasma proteins in the blood.

hyperostosis (hi-per-os-to'-sis). Thickening of bone. A bony outgrowth.

hyperparathyroidism (hi-per-par-ah-thi'-roid-izm). Excessive activity of the parathyroid glands, causing drainage of calcium from the bones, with consequent fragility and liability to spontaneous fracture.

hyperphagia (hi-per-fa'-ge-ah). Over-eating.

hyperpiesis (hi-per-pi-e'-sis). Abnormally high blood-pressure. *See* Hypertension.

hyperpituitarism (hi-per-pit-u'-it-ar-izm). Over-activity of the pituitary body causing acromegaly or gigantism.

hyperplasia (hi-per-pla'-ze-ah). Excessive formation of tissue.

hyperpnoea (*hi-perp-ne'-ah*). Deep breathing with marked use of abdominal muscles. Present in diseases in which there is acidosis (*q.v.*).

hyperpyrexia (*hi-per-pi-reks'-e-ah*). Excessively high body temperature, i.e. over 41°C (106°F).

hypersecretion (*hi-per-se-kre'-shun*). Profuse secretion.

hypersensitive (*hi-per-sen'-sit-iv*). (1) Abnormally sensitive. (2) An allergic state. *See* Allergy.

hypersplenism (*hi-per-splen'-izm*). Over-activity of an enlarged spleen in the destruction of blood cells and platelets.

hypertension (*hi-per-ten'-shun*). A raised blood pressure. It is dependent on cardiac output and the resistance of the blood vessels. Systolic and diastolic readings are taken. Also termed hyperpiesis. *Essential h.* High blood pressure without demonstrable change in kidneys, blood vessels or heart. *Malignant h.* A form of hyperpiesis which develops at a comparatively early age, and in which the prognosis is poor. *Portal h.* A raised pressure in the portal system, most often due to hepatic cirrhosis.

hyperthermia (*hi-per-ther'-me-ah*). Applied to a treatment in which a high body temperature is induced.

hyperthyroidism (*hi-per-thi'-roid-izm*). The symptoms produced by excessive thyroid secretion. This affects: (1) The metabolic process which is speeded up. The appetite is large but weight is lost. The temperature tends to be above normal, and respirations are increased. (2) The nervous system. The patient is very excitable and restless. Sleeplessness is present. Stimulation of the sympathetic nerves causes diarrhoea and excessive sweating. Exophthalmos may be present. The pulse is rapid and auricular fibrillation is common.

hypertonic (*hi-per-ton'-ik*). (1) Excessive tone or tension as in a blood vessel or muscle. (2) Applied to solutions which are stronger than physiological saline. *H. saline.* May be used for treating infected wounds and as an enema to treat thread worms.

hypertrichiasis (*hi-per-trik-i'-as-is*). Excessive growth of hair on any part of the body.

hypertrophy (*hi-per'-tro-fe*). Excessive thickening of a part or organ by increase of its own tissues. *Compensatory h.* of cardiac muscle occurs in valvular disease of the heart to maintain the circulation by giving increased power.

hyperuricaemia (*hi-per-u-re-se'-me-ah*). A high level of uric acid in the blood as may be found in gout.

hyperventilation (*hi-per-ven-til-a'-shun*). Over-breathing often associated with emotional upset. This lowers the dissolved carbon dioxide in the blood plasma which tends to alkalinity.

hyphaemia (*hi-fe'-me-ah*). Haemorrhage into the anterior chamber of the eye.

hypnosis (*hip-no'-sis*). An artificially induced state resembling sleep, in which there is increased suggestibility which may be used to abolish symptoms in hysterical states. It may also be favoured as a means of anaesthesia in childbirth and tooth extraction.

hypnotic (*hip-not'-ik*). An agent which causes sleep.

hypnotism (*hip'-not-izm*). The practice of hypnosis.

hypo- (*hi'-po*). Greek prefix meaning 'below'.

hypoalbuminaemia (*hi-po-al-bu-min-e'-me-ah*). A lack of serum albumin in the blood plasma leading to oedema in the tissues.

hypocalcaemia (*hi-po-kal-se'-me-ah*). Deficiency of blood calcium.

hypochlorhydria (*hi-po-klor-hi'-dre-ah*). A less than normal amount of hydrochloric acid in the gastric juice.

hypochlorite (*hi-po-klor'-ite*). A chlorine compound that is an effective disinfectant of clean articles but not in the presence of blood.

hypochondria (*hi-po-kon'-dre-ah*). A morbid preoccupation or anxiety about one's health. The sufferer feels that first one part of his body and then another part is the seat of some serious disease.

hypochondriac (*hi-po-kon'-dre-ak*). One affected by hypochondria. *H. region.* The upper abdominal region situated on either side under the lower ribs and costal cartilages.

hypochondrium (*hi-po-kon'-dre-um*). The upper region of the abdomen on each side of the epigastrium.

hypochromic (*hi-po-kro'-mik*). Deficient in pigmentation or colouring.

hypodermic (*hi-po-der'-mik*). Beneath the skin; applied to subcutaneous injections.

hypofibrinogenaemia (*hi-po-fib-rin-o-jen-e'-me-ah*). A lack of fibrinogen in the blood. This may occur in severe trauma or haemorrhage or with over-activity of fibrinolysins.

hypogammaglobulinaemia (*hi-po-gam-mah-glob-u-lin-e'-me-ah*). A deficiency of gamma globulin in the blood rendering the person susceptible to infection.

hypogastrium (*hi-po-gas'-tre-um*). The lower middle area of the abdomen, immediately below the umbilical region.

hypoglossal (*hi-po-glos'-sal*). Under the tongue. *H. nerve.* The twelfth cranial nerve.

hypoglycaemia (*hi-po-gli-se'-me-ah*). The blood-sugar is less than normal. Usually arising in diabetic patients having insulin, due to too high a dose, delay in eating or a rapid combustion of carbohydrate. *See* Hyperglycaemia.

hypokalaemia (*hi-po-kal-e'-me-ah*). A low potassium level in the blood plasma. This is likely to be present in dehydration and with repeated use of diuretics.

hypomania (*hi-po-ma'-ne-ah*). A degree of elation, excitement and activity higher than normal but less severe than that present in mania.

hyponatraemia (*hi-po-nat-re'-me-ah*). A deficiency of sodium in the blood. This is accompanied by an excess of water over electrolytes.

hypo-osmolarity (*hi-po-os-mo-lar'-it-e*). In medicine the term for decreased osmotic pressure in the blood.

hypoparathyroidism (*hi-po-par-ah-thi'-roid-izm*). A lack of parathyroid secretion leading to a low blood calcium and tetany.

hypophysectomy (*hi-po-fis-sek'-to-me*). Excision of the pituitary gland.

hypophysis cerebri (*hi-pof'-is-is ser'-e-bri*). The pituitary gland.

hypopiesis (*hi-po-pi-e-sis*). Abnormally low blood pressure.

hypopituitarism (*hi-po-pit-*

u'-it-ar-izm). Deficiency of secretion from the anterior lobe of the pituitary gland, causing excessive deposit of fat and infantilism in children. *See* Fröhlich's syndrome. Dwarfism (Lorain type) may result. In adults asthenia, drowsiness, and increased sugar tolerance, adiposity and sometimes polyuria are present.

hypoplasia (*hi-po-pla'-ze-ah*). Imperfect development of a part or organ.

hypoproteinaemia (*hi-po-pro-tin-e'-me-ah*). A deficiency of serum proteins in the blood. The cause may be dietary or excessive loss.

hypopyon (*hi-po'-pe-on*). A collection of pus in the anterior chamber of the eye.

hyposecretion (*hi-po-se-kre'-shun*). Under secretion from any glandular structure or secreting cells.

hypospadias (*hi-po-spa'-de-as*). A malformation in which the canal of the urethra opens upon the under surface of the penis.

hypostasis (*hi-pos'-ta-sis*). (1) A sediment or deposit. (2) Congestion of blood in a part, due to slowing of the circulation.

hypostatic (*hi-po-stat'-ik*). Relating to hypostasis. *H. pneumonia. See* Pneumonia.

hyposthenia (*hi-pos-the'-ne-ah*). Weakness; decreased strength.

hypotension (*hi-po-ten'-shun*). A low blood pressure. *Controlled* or *induced h.* An artificially produced lowering of the blood pressure so that an operation field is rendered practically bloodless.

hypotensive (*hi-po-ten'-siv*). Producing a reduction in tension, especially a drug that lowers the blood pressure.

hypothalamus (*hi-po-thal'-am-us*). Part of the brain situated at its base and concerned with temperature control, hunger, thirst and emotional changes.

hypothermia (*hi-po-ther'-me-ah*). Cooling of the body to reduce the oxygen requirements of the tissues. *Mild h.* Reduction of the body temperature to 34°C (93°F) may be induced by surface cooling with cold air and may be used for head injuries. *Conventional h.* Reduction to 30°C (86°F) may be done by immersion in cold water and allows arrest of the circulation for 9 min, without cerebral damage. Short heart operations may be performed. *Profound h.* A reduction to 10° to 15°C (50° to 59°F) allows 1 h for open-heart surgery but the blood must still receive oxygen. This may be done by using a pump oxygenator (*heart–lung machine*) and heat exchanger or by using a heat exchanger and the patient's own lungs to oxygenate the blood. The latter appears to damage the blood less and give a smoother convalescence.

hypothesis (*hi-poth'-e-sis*). A theory which attempts to explain, e.g. the cause of a disease.

hypothrombinaemia (*hi-po-throm-bin-e'-me-ah*). A diminished amount of thrombin in the blood with a consequent tendency to bleed.

hypothyroidism (*hi-po-thi'-roid-izm*). Insufficiency of thyroid secretion. *See* Myxoedema.

hypotonia (*hi-po-to'-ne-ah*). (1) Deficient muscle tone. (2) Diminished tension in the eyeball.

hypotonic (*hi-po-ton'-ik*). Describes solutions which are more diluted than normally used. Less than isotonic. *See* Hypertonic.

hypoventilation (*hi-po-ven-til-a'-shun*). Diminished breathing or inadequate ventilation by mechanical means.

hypovolaemia (*hi-po-vol-e'-me-ah*). A reduction in the circulating blood volume due to external loss of body fluids or to loss from the blood into the tissues as in shock.

hypoxaemia (*hi-poks-e'-me-ah*). An insufficient oxygen content in the blood.

hypoxia (*hi-poks'-e-ah*). A diminished amount of oxygen in the tissues. *Anaemic h.* Due to deficiency of haemoglobulin in the blood. *Histotoxic h.* Due to failure of the cells to extract oxygen from the blood. Occurs in cyanide poisoning. *Hypoxic h.* Due to lung disease or shortage of oxygen in inspired air so that oxygen cannot enter blood. *Stagnant h.* Due to reduction in blood flow.

hysteralgia (*his-ter-al'-je-ah*). Neuralgic pain in the uterus.

hysterectomy (*his-ter-ek'-to-me*). Removal of the uterus. *Abdominal h.* Removal via an abdominal incision. *Pan-h.* An old term for removal of uterus and adnexa. *Subtotal h.* Removal of the body of the uterus only. *Total h.* Removal of the body and the cervix. *Vaginal h.* Removal per vaginam. *Wertheim's h.* The parametrium, upper vagina and lymph glands are excised in addition.

hysteria (*hi-te'-re-ah*). A psychoneurosis manifesting itself in various disorders of the mind and body. There are mental and physical symptoms, not of organic origin, produced and maintained by motives of which the patient is unconscious, but directed at some real or fancied gain to be derived from them. *Conversion h.* The hysteria takes the form of loss of function of some part of the body. This may be loss of memory, vision or hearing or loss of muscle power or feeling in a hand or leg. The so-called 'paralysis' or numbness does not correspond to the nerve distribution.

hysterical (*his-ter'-ik-l*). Relating to hysteria.

hysterocele (*his'-ter-o-seel*). A hernia containing part of the uterus.

hysteromyoma (*his-ter-o-mi-o'-mah*). A muscle tumour of the uterus.

hysteromyomectomy (*his-ter-o-mi-o-mek'-to-me*). Excision of a hysteromyoma.

hysteropathy (*his-ter-op'-ath-e*). Any uterine disease.

hysteropexy (*his'-ter-o-peks-e*). Fixation of the uterus to the abdominal wall, to remedy displacement. *See* Ventrofixation.

hysteroptosis (*his-ter-op-to'-sis*). Prolapse of the uterus.

hysterosalpingography (*his'-ter-o-sal-ping-gog'-raf-e*). An X-ray examination of the uterus and uterine tubes following the injection of a radio-opaque dye.

hysterosalpingostomy (*his'-ter-o-sal-ping-gos'-to-me*). Establishing an opening between the distal portion of the uterine tube and the uterus in an effort to overcome infertility when the medial portion is occluded or excised.

hysterotomy (*his-ter-ot'-o-me*). Incision of the uterus. *See* Caesarean section.

I

I. The symbol for iodine.

-iasis (*i'-as-is*). A suffix meaning 'condition of'.

iatrogenic (*i-at-ro-jen'-ik*). Brought about by surgical or medical treatment, e.g. unwanted effects of drugs.

ice. Water in a solid state, at or below freezing-point. *I. bag.* A rubber bag half-filled with pieces of ice and applied near or to a part. *I. compress.* Compress made of lint wrung out of ice-cold water. *I.-water enema.* A treatment used to reduce temperature in hyperpyrexia.

ichor (*i'-kor*). A thin colourless discharge from ulcers and raw wounds.

ichthyol (*ik'-the-ol*). A mineral preparation rich in the remains of fossilized fishes. Used for skin diseases, and as an application for erosion of the cervix.

ichthyosis (*ik-the-o'-sis*). A congenital abnormality of the skin in which there is dryness, roughness, and the horny layer is thickened and large scales appear. These patients are liable to eczema and industrial dermatitis.

icterus (*ik'-ter-us*). Jaundice. *I. gravis.* A fatal form of jaundice occurring in pregnancy. *I. gravis neonatorum.* Haemolytic disease of the newborn. *See* Rhesus factor.

id. The most primitive part of the personality, containing the instinctive drives, which lives in the unconscious.

idea (*i-de'-ah*). A mental image and the meaning attached to it. *Association of i.s.* Ideas that recall to the mind associated objects or occasions due to some similarity or contrast. *Flight of i.s.* A mode of speech in which the person passes rapidly from one idea to the next with only a slight association between them, being unable to

maintain a course of thought. *I.s of reference.* Thoughts based on some external circumstances that the patient thinks refers to himself when no such thing is intended. *I.s of unreality.* The patient feels as if everything has changed and that things look different and unreal or do not exist.

ideation (*i-de-a'-shun*). The formulation of ideas.

idée fixe (*e-da feeks*). A fixed idea, a delusion that impels towards some abnormal action.

identification (*i-den-te-fik-a'-shun*). A mental mechanism by which an individual adopts the attitudes and ideas of another, often admired, person. *Patient i.* The wearing of a label with the name and hospital number of the patient.

ideomotor (*i-de-o-mo'-tor*). The association of ideas and muscle action as in absent-minded acts.

ideophrenic (*i-de-o-fren'-ik*). Relating to mental disorder with perverted ideas.

idiopathic (*id-e-o-path'-ik*). Self-originated; applied to a condition the cause of which is not known.

idiosyncrasy (*id-e-o-sin'-kras-e*). A peculiarity of constitution or temperament. It may exist in relation to drugs, e.g. when small doses of iodine or quinine will cause symptoms of poisoning in some people; or foods, such as shell-fish or strawberries, give rise to urticaria in others.

idiot (*id'-e-ot*). An obsolete term for one who would now be designated severely subnormal.

ileal (*i'-le-al*). Referring to the ileum. *I. conduit.* A surgical procedure in which the ureters are transplanted into the ileum, a loop of which is then brought to the surface of the abdomen in order to allow the urine to drain into a bag.

ileectomy (*i-le-ek'-to-me*). Excision of the ileum.

ileitis (*i-le-i'-tis*). Inflammation of the ileum. *Regional i.* Crohn's disease. A chronic condition of the terminal portion of the ileum in which granulation and oedema may give rise to obstruction.

ileocaecal valve (*i-le-o-se'-kal*). *See* Valve.

ileocolitis (*i-le-o-kol-i' tis*). Inflammation of the ileum and colon.

ileocolostomy (*i-le-o-kol-os'-to-me*). Making a permanent opening between the ileum and some part of the colon.

ileoproctostomy (*i-le-o-prok-tos'-to-me*). Making an opening between the ileum and the rectum.

ileorectal (*i-le-o-rek'-tal*). Referring to the ileum and rectum. *I. anastomosis.* The joining of the two, usually following total colectomy.

ileosigmoidostomy (*i-le-o-sig-moid-os'-to-me*). The surgical formation of an opening between the ileum and the sigmoid flexure.

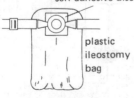

self-adhesive disc

plastic ileostomy bag

ILEOSTOMY APPLIANCE (SELF-ADHESIVE)

ileostomy (*i-le-os'-to-me*). An operation to make an opening into the ileum. *I. bags.* Disposable or rubber bags which can be adhesive or worn on a belt and add greatly to the comfort of the patient.

ileo-ureterostomy (*i'-le-o-u-re-ter-os'-to-me*). The transplantation of the ureters into a separated loop of ileum.

ileum (*i'-le-um*). The last part of the small intestine, terminating at the caecum.

ileus (*i'-le-us*). Obstruction of the bowel. *Paralytic i.* A condition resulting from local inflammation, the toxins of which affect the nerve supply to the bowel wall, and intestinal stasis results. One of the effects of peritonitis. Putrefaction takes place within the bowel, the poisons are absorbed, and the patient develops all the signs of toxaemia.

iliac (*il'-e-ak*). Pertaining to the ilium or flanks. *I. crest.* The crest of the hip-bone. *I. fossa.* The area of the abdomen over the concave surface of the iliac bone.

iliopsoas (*il-e-o-so'-as*). A name given to the flexor muscles of the hip, the iliacus and the psoas.

ilium (*il'-e-um*). The haunch-bone.

illumination (*il-lu-min-a'-shun*). The amount of light intensity falling on a surface. The unit of measurement that is used is the candela. *See* Appendix 6.

illusion (*il-lu'-zhun*). A mistaken perception due to a misinterpretation of a sensory stimulus; believing something to be what it is not.

image. (1) The mental recall of a former percept. (2) The optical picture transferred to the brain cells by the optic nerve.

imagery (*im'-aj-er-e*). Abstract thought about some object. The image may be recalled by a motor or sensory stimulus.

imago (*im-a'-go*). In psychology, an idea or fanciful image of the father or some other person based on fantasy or fear.

imbalance (*im-bal'-ans*). Lack of balance, e.g. between endocrine secretions, water and electrolytes or of muscles.

imbecile (*im'-be-seel*). A term no longer used. It denoted a severe degree of subnormality.

imipramine (*i-mip'-ram-een*). A drug, chemically related to chlorpromazine, that may be effective in relieving depression. Tofranil is a proprietary preparation.

immiscible (*im-mis'-sib-l*). Incapable of being mixed, e.g. oil and water.

immobilization (*im-mo-bil-i-za'-shun*). Making motionless. Used in the treatment of fractures and other conditions to promote healing. To immobilize a bone the joint above and below the break must be fixed.

immune (*im-mu'-n*). Protected against a disease, either by natural means or by inoculation. *I. body.* Antibody. *I. reaction.* That which causes a body to reject a transplanted organ.

immunity (*im-mu'-nit-e*). The resisting power of the body to the toxins of invading bacteria, shown by the presence in the blood of neutralizing antitoxins. *Natural i.* May be racial or familial, and is inborn. *Acquired i.* is produced by: (1) An attack of the disease. (2) Repeated small infections by organisms not in themselves able to produce signs of disease, but against which the body forms antibodies which accumulate in the blood. *Artificially acquired*

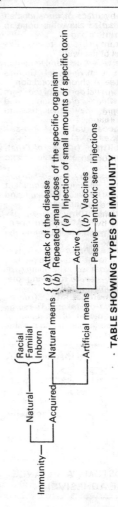

TABLE SHOWING TYPES OF IMMUNITY

i. is by: (1) Injections of small doses of toxins. (2) Injection of vaccines (*active i.*). (3) Introduction of antitoxic sera (*passive i.*).

immunization (*im-mu-ni-za'-shun*). The act of creating an active immunity.

immunoassay (*im-mu-no-ass'-a*). A quantitative estimate of the proteins contained in the blood serum.

immunocyte (*im'-mu-no-site*). A cell which is capable of producing antibodies.

immunoglobulins (*im-mu-no-glob'-u-lins*). Protein substances which are able to act as antibodies.

immunology (*im-mu-nol'-o-je*). The study of the body's reactions in overcoming invasion by bacteria or viruses.

immunosuppressive therapy (*im-mu'-no-sup-pres'-iv ther'-ap-e*). Use of drugs, e.g. actinomycin C, azothioprine and antilymphocyte serum (ALS) to prevent the rejection by the body of a transplanted organ.

impacted (*im-pak'-ted*). Driven into. *I. fracture. See* Fracture.

impalpable (*im-palp'-ab-l*). Incapable of being felt by manual examination. May apply to an organ or tumour.

imperforate (*im-per'-for-ate*). Without an opening. *I. anus.* A congenital defect in which this opening is closed. *I. hymen.* Complete closure of the vaginal opening by the hymen. *See* Cryptomenorrhoea.

impetigo (*im-pet-i'-go*). An acute contagious inflammation of the skin marked by pustules and scabs; of streptococcal or staphylococcal origin. *Bullous i.* A severe form, especially if occurring in the newly born, characterized by large blebs.

implantation (*im-plant-a'-shun*). The act of planting or setting in, e.g. of the fertilized ovum in the endometrium or of malignant cells into another structure.

implants (*im'-plants*). Pellets of synthetic hormones that may be introduced under the skin for slow absorption. They may be of deoxycortone acetate, oestradiol, progesterone or testosterone.

impotence (*im'-po-tens*). Absence of sexual power.

impregnate (*im'-preg-nate*). (1) To saturate or instil. (2) To render pregnant.

impulse (*im'-puls*). A natural or instinctive tendency to action without deliberation. *Cardiac i.* The beat of the apex of the heart as felt on the chest wall. *Morbid i.* An uncontrollable desire to act rashly. *Nerve i.* The force conveyed along nerve fibres.

inaccessibility (*in-ak-ses-ib-il'-it-e*). State of unresponsiveness characteristic of certain mental patients, e.g. schizophrenics.

inactivate (*in-ak'-tiv-ate*). To render inactive. To destroy the active principle bringing about change.

inanition (*in-an-ish'-un*). Wasting of the body from want of food.

inarticulate (*in-ar-tik'-u-late*). (1) Without joint. (2) Confused and jumbled, as applied to speech.

in articulo mortis (*ar-tik'-u-lo-mor'-tis*). In the act of dying.

inborn (*in'-born*). Inherited. *I. errors of metabolism.* An increasing number of known conditions in which there is an inherited deficiency or production of toxic substances.

incarcerated (*in-kar'-ser-a-ted*). Held fast. (1) Applied to a hernia which is immovable, and therefore only curable by operation. (2) A pregnant uterus held under the sacral brim.

incest (*in-sest'*). Sexual intercourse between blood relatives.

incipient (*in-sip'-e-ent*). Beginning to exist.

incision (*in-siz'-shun*). The act of cutting.

incisors (*in-si'-zors*). The cutting teeth. Four in the centre of each jaw.

inclusion bodies (*in-klu'-shun*). Any particles temporarily enclosed in the cytoplasm of a cell. For example in trachoma they are virus particles seen in the conjunctival epithelial cells.

incoherent (*in-ko-he'-rent*). Unable to be understood. Rambling speech that is disconnected.

incompatibility (*in-kom-pat-ib-il'-it-e*). The state of two or more substances being antagonistic, or destroying the efficiency of each other. Applied to mixtures of drugs, and to blood. *See* Blood grouping.

incompetence (*in-kom'-pe-tens*). Inefficiency. *Aortic i.* Failure of the aortic valves to regulate the flow of blood. *Mitral i. See* Mitral. *Valvular i.* Failure of a valve of the heart to work efficiently.

incontinence (*in kon'-tin-ens*). Inability to control natural functions or discharges. *I. of urine.* Enuresis (*q.v.*). *Paralytic i.* Loss of control of anal and urethral sphincters due to injury to nerve centres. *Stress i.* That which is due to defect in the urethral sphincters and is liable to occur when intra-abdominal pressure is increased as in coughing, lifting heavy weights, etc.

incoordination (*in-ko-or-din-a'-shun*). Inability to adjust har-

moniously the various muscle movements.

incrustation (*in-krus-ta'-shun*). The formation of a crust or scab on a wound.

incubation (*in-ku-ba'-shun*). Maintaining organisms in optimal conditions for their growth. *I. period.* The period between the date of infection and the appearance of symptoms.

incubator (*in'-ku-ba-tor*). (1) An apparatus in which prematurely born infants can be reared. (2) An apparatus used to develop bacteria at a uniform temperature suitable to their growth.

incus (*in'-kus*). The small anvil-shaped bone of the middle ear.

Indian hemp. *See* Cannabis indica.

indicanuria (*in-de-kan-u'-re-ah*). The presence of indican in the urine—a sign of protein putrefaction in the intestine. It may be present in chronic constipation or in intestinal obstruction.

indigenous (*in-dij'-en-us*). Occurring naturally in a certain locality.

indigestion (*(in-de-jes'-chun*). *See* Dyspepsia.

indigo carmine (*in'-de-go kar'-meen*). A harmless water-soluble blue dye used in the estimation of circulating blood volume.

indole (*in'-dol*). A product of protein decomposition in the bowel. Eliminated as indican in the urine.

indolent ulcer (*in'-do-lent ul'-ser*). One which heals slowly.

induced current (*in-duse'-d kur'-rent*). An electric current which, running through a primary coil of *thick* copper wire, induces through the air a current in a *thinner* wire which is wound round a bobbin and encircles the primary coil. The closer in proximity the stronger the current; this also makes the faradic current.

induction (*in-duk'-shun*). Causing to occur. In obstetrics, production of labour before term. *I. coil. See* Induced current. *Stage of i.* In anaesthetic administration, the initial or first stage.

induration (*in-du-ra'-shun*). The process of becoming hardened.

industrial (*in-dus'-tre-al*). Referring to industry. *I. diseases.* Those that are caused by the nature of the work. *Prescribed i. diseases.* Those for which sickness benefit is payable including those that are notifiable under the Factories Act.

inertia (*in-er'-she-ah*). Sluggishness; inability to move except when stimulated by an external force. *Uterine i.* Lack of muscle contraction during the first and second stage of labour.

in extremis (*in eks-tre'-mis*). At the point of death.

infant (*in'-fant*). Educationally a child under 7 years of age.

infant feeding. Breast milk is the ideal food for the baby and if breast feeding is established satisfactorily for the first few months it can aid physical and emotional development. Where it is not possible cow's milk or a dried milk preparation can be used. A baby requires 150 ml (110 calories or 420 J) per 1 kg of body weight in 24 hours.

infant mortality (*in'-fant mortal'-it-e*). Deaths of children under 1 year of age. *I.m. rate.* Deaths of children during the first year of life per 1000 live births.

infanticide (*in-fan'-te-side*). The killing of an infant by its mother during the first year of life.

infantile paralysis (*in'-fan-tile par-al'-is-is*). Poliomyelitis (*q.v.*).

infantilism (*in-fan'-til-izm*). Delayed maturity. *Coeliac i.* Failure to grow in coeliac disease (*q.v.*). *Pancreatic i.* Associated with fibrocystic disease of the pancreas (*q.v.*). *Pituitary i.* The perfectly formed dwarfs associated with hyposecretion of the growth hormone. *Renal i.* Also known as *renal rickets*: associated with disease of the kidney and upset in the calcium balance in the blood. There is dwarfism with signs of rickets (*q.v.*).

infarct (*in'-farkt*). The wedge-shaped area of necrosis in an organ produced by the blocking of a blood vessel, usually due to emboli. *White i.* The area is suddenly deprived of blood and is pale in colour. *Red i.* Red blood cells infiltrate into the area.

infarction (*in-fark'-shun*). The formation of an infarct. *Pulmonary i.* A small embolism in the lungs.

infection (*in-fek'-shun*). Invasion of the body by organisms causing disease. *Cross i.* Hazard occurring in hospitals when infection is transmitted from one patient to another owing either to their close proximity or to carelessness by the staff. *Droplet i.* Organisms are spread in minute particles of moisture exhaled, especially in coughing or sneezing. *Mass i.* Invasion of the blood stream by large numbers of organisms. *Pyogenic i.* Caused by pus-producing organisms. *Secondary i.* A superimposed second infection, when one is already present. *Water-borne i.* Organisms are

COMMON INFECTIOUS DISEASES

Disease	Incubation period (days)	Period of infectivity
Chickenpox (varicella)	10–20	2–3 days before until 10 days after onset of rash
Diphtheria	2–7	Until culture of 3 consecutive nose swabs proves negative
Enteric fevers		
Typhoid	6–21	Until at least one month after onset of disease and after 6 consecutive negative stools
Paratyphoid		
Measles (morbilli)	6–12	4 days before until 4 days after onset of rash
Mumps (parotitis)	12–28	48 hours before onset until resolution of symptoms
Pertussis (whooping cough)	7–14	7 days before until 3 weeks after onset of cough
Rubella (German measles)	14–21	During incubation period until 2 days after resolution of symptoms
Smallpox (variola)	2–3 to prodromal illness; 2–3 to rash	From early in incubation period until all scabs have disappeared

spread by the water supply, e.g. typhoid fever.

infectious diseases (*see* Table on p. 182)

infective (*in-fek'-tiv*). Of the nature of an infection. *I. exhaustive psychosis.* A psychosis developing during the course of another disease as in a severe infection, metabolic or glandular condition. It may subside as the disease is controlled but it may require psychiatric treatment. *I. mononucleosis.* Glandular fever (*q.v.*).

inferior. Lower, e.g. *i. vena cava,* the lower large vein.

inferiority (*in-fer-e-or'-it-e*). Of lesser rank, stature, position or ability. *Physical i.* Possession of some physical disability about which the person is sensitive, e.g. a club foot or squint. *I. complex.* See Complex.

infertility (*in-fer-til'-it-e*). Inability of a woman to conceive or of a man to produce viable sperm.

infestation (*in-fes-ta'-shun*). Invasion by animal parasites; applied to the presence of lice on the body or clothing, or in a house.

infiltration (*in-fil-tra'-shun*). The entrance and diffusion of some abnormal substance, either fluid or solid. *I. anaesthesia.* Injection of procaine or allied substances into the tissue for local effect.

inflammation (*in-flam-ma'-shun*). A series of changes in tissues indicating their reaction to injury, whether mechanical, chemical or bacterial, so long as the injury does not cause death of the affected part. The cardinal signs are: heat, swelling, pain and redness. *Acute i.* The onset is sudden, the symptoms marked and progressive. *Catarrhal i.* Attacks mucous surfaces

and stimulates exudation. *Caseous i.* A chronic form found in tuberculosis, in which the degenerative changes cause a cheesy material to form. *Chronic i.* Of slow development. Granulation tissue forms and tends to localize the infection. *Diffuse i.* An extensive type, as in nephritis and cellulitis. *Suppurative i.* In which the formation of pus results. *Traumatic i.* That which follows an injury and is non-bacterial.

influenza (*in-flu-en'-zah*). An acute infectious disease caused by either Virus A, giving rise to serious epidemics, or Virus B causing minor outbreaks. There is inflammation of the upper respiratory tract causing fever, headache, pain in the back, and limbs, anorexia and sometimes nausea and vomiting. The fever subsides in 2 to 3 days, leaving a feeling of lassitude and some mental depression. Secondary infection may lead to pneumonia and empyema.

infra- (*in'-frah*). A prefix meaning below or under.

infra-red rays. Invisible rays beyond the red end of the spectrum of long wavelength. *See* Ultra-violet rays.

infundibulum (*in-fun-dib'-u-lum*). A funnel-shaped passage or part.

infusion (*in-fu'-zhun*). (1) The process of extracting the soluble principles of substances (especially drugs) by soaking in water. (2) Treatment by the introduction of fluid into the body. *Saline i.* Subcutaneous or intravenous injection of salt and water. Dextrose may be added.

ingestion (*in-jest'-shun*). The introduction of food and drugs by the mouth.

inguinal (*in'-gwin-al*). Relating to the groin. *I. canal.* The channel through the abdominal wall, above Poupart's ligament through which the spermatic cord and vessels pass to the testis in the male, and which contains the round ligament of the uterus in the female. *I. hernia. See* Hernia.

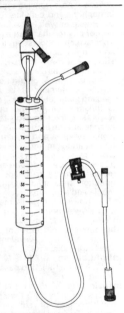

INTRAVENOUS DRIP SET (PAEDIATRIC)

inhalation (*in-hal-a'-shun*). The breathing of air, vapour or volatile drugs into the lungs. *Steam i.* By: (1) Maw's inhaler. (2) A jug, with a towel arranged funnel-wise to direct the steam into the respiratory passages. (3) A steam kettle and tent. Atomizers may be used to inhale drugs, e.g. penicillin and ephedrine. *I. anaesthesia.* By general anaesthetics, as ether, chloroform etc. *Oxygen i. See* Oxygen. *Carbon dioxide i. See* Carbon dioxide.

inherent (*in-heer'-ent*). Describing a characteristic that is innate or natural and essentially a part of the person.

inhibition (*in-hib-ish'-un*). Checking or restraining. Inhibitory nerves restrain muscle action, in contrast to accelerator nerves which stimulate it. Emotionally a person may be inhibited because he has certain ideas or feelings—often unconscious—which prevent him from acting as he would wish.

injection (*in-jek'-shun*). The act of introducing a liquid into the body by means of a syringe or other instrument. *Hypodermic i.* Below the skin. *Intramuscular i.* That made into the muscles. *Intrathecal i.* Into the theca of the spinal cord. *Intravenous i.* Into the veins. *Sclerosing i.* Of drugs, as quinine and urethane, to obliterate a blood vessel, as in treatment of varicose veins. *Subcutaneous (hypodermic) i.* Below the skin. Injections of fluid, stimulants etc. can be given into the rectum.

innate (*in'-ate*). Present in the individual at birth.

innervation (*in-ner-va'-shun*). Nerve supply to a part.

innocent (*in'-no-sent*). As applied to new growth, a harmless or non-malignant one.

innocuous (*in-nok'-u-ous*). Harmless.

innominate (*in-nom'-in-ate*). Unnamed. *I. artery.* A branch of the aorta now termed the brachiocephalic. *I. bone.* The united ilium, ischium and pubis.

inoculation (*in-ok-u-la'-shun*). Introduction through the skin of: (1) Infection by the bites of insects. (2) A vaccine to stimulate the production of antibodies against a disease.

inorganic (*in-or-gan'-ik*). Of neither animal nor vegetable origin.

inositol (*in-o'-se-tol*). A form of muscle or plant carbohydrate that has the same formula as simple sugar but not its other properties. It has been used in the treatment of dermatoses and also, combined with vitamin E, in cases of muscular dystrophy.

inotropic (*in-o-tro'-pik*). Affecting the force or energy of muscular contractions. The term may be applied to drugs acting on the heart muscle.

inquest (*in'-kwest*). In medicine a legal inquiry held by a coroner into the cause of sudden or unexpected death.

insanity (*in-san'-it-e*). An obsolete term for a state of severe mental disorder. Legally the person is not responsible for his actions and it is largely in this connection the term is retained. For examples, *see* Psychosis, Mania, Schizophrenia *and* Paranoia.

insecticides (*in-sek'-te-sides*). A large group of chemical compounds that kill insect pests. Some are very toxic and can cause irritability of the nervous system and gastrointestinal upsets in man and may accumulate in the body fat.

insemination (*in-sem-in-a'-shun*). (1) Fertilization of an ovum. (2) Introduction of the semen into the vagina. *Artificial i.* By means other than sexual intercourse. *AID.* The semen used is from a donor. *AIH.* The husband's semen is used.

insensible (*in-sen'-sib-l*). Not appreciated by the senses. *I. sweat.* That of which one is not aware.

insertion. The attachment of a muscle to the bone which it moves. *I. of tendon.* Insertion of a healthy tendon into a paralysed one at the periosteum of the joint so that normal function may result. *I. of nerve.* The operation which attaches a cut nerve by insertion of it into the sheath of another.

insidious (*in-sid'-e-us*). Approaching by stealth. A term applied to any disease which develops imperceptibly.

insight (*in'-site*). Mental awareness. The capacity of an individual to estimate a situation or his own behaviour or the connection between his present attitudes and past experiences. In psychiatry, a recognition by the patient that he is ill. Insight in this connection may be complete, partial or absent and may alter during the course of the illness.

in situ (*in sit'-u*). Latin term for in the original position.

insolation (*in-sol-a'-shun*). Exposure to sun's rays.

insomnia (*in-som'-ne-ah*). Inability to sleep.

inspiration (*in-spir-a'-shun*). Drawing in the breath.

inspissated (*in-spis'-a-ted*). Thickened, through evaporation or absorption. *I. serum.* A culture medium for bacteria. *I. sputum.* Occurs in pertussis and is difficult to cough up.

instillation (*in-stil-la'-shun*). Pouring a liquid into a cavity drop by drop, e.g. into the eye.

instincts. Inborn tendencies to act in a certain way without the influence of reason or previous education.

insufficiency (*in-suf-fish'-en-se*). Inadequacy. A term used to describe the failure of function in organs, as the heart, circulation, stomach, liver, muscles etc.

insufflation (*in'-suf-fla'-shun*). The act of blowing air or powder into a cavity.

insulate (*in'-su-late*). To surround an electrified body with a non-conducting substance, so that electricity cannot escape.

insulin (*in'-su-lin*). The endocrine secretion of the pancreas, which regulates sugar metabolism, and ensures complete fat combustion. It is extensively used in *diabetes mellitus*, controlling the blood sugar and preventing acidosis: thus enabling a less restricted diet to be taken. *Globin i., Isophane i., Protamine zinc i.* and *I. zinc suspension* are preparations in which the action is delayed and thus less frequent doses are necessary. A buffer dose of ordinary insulin may be given to tide over the period before it comes into effect. *I. coma.* See Coma. *I. test.* One carried out to determine if all the fibres have been severed in a vagotomy operation. *See* Diabetes mellitus *and* Aceto-acetic acid.

insulinase (*in'-su-lin-aze*). An enzyme that destroys the action of insulin and when present makes the control of diabetes difficult.

insulinoma (*in-su-lin-o'-mah*). A benign adenoma of the islet cells of the pancreas causing hypoglycaemia.

integument (*in-teg'-u-ment*). The skin.

intellect (*in'-tel-ekt*). The reasoning power, in contrast to the emotions or the will.

intelligence (*in-tel'-e-jens*). General mental ability. *I. tests.* Devised to measure the level of intelligence. *I. quotient* (IQ). The ratio of the mental age (*q.v.*) to chronological age expressed as a percentage.

intensive care unit (*in-ten'-siv kair' u'-nit*). A specialized unit in which the staff are especially trained and the equipment designed to care for critically ill patients.

intention tremor (*in-ten'-shun trem'-or*). *See* Tremor.

inter-. A prefix signifying 'between'.

intercellular (*in-ter-sel'-ul-ah*). Between the cells of a structure. May be applied to the connective tissue or fluid bathing the cells.

intercostal (*in-ter-kos'-tal*). Between the ribs. *I. muscles.* Those of the chest wall.

intercourse (*in-ter-kors'*). The sexual act of coitus.

intercurrent (*in-ter-kur'-ent*). Running between. *I. infection.* One which occurs during the course of another disease in the same person.

interferon (*in-ter-feer'-on*). A protein produced by cells which has an inhibitory effect on the multiplication of invading viruses.

interlobar (*in-ter-lo'-bar*). Between lobes. *I. empyema.* Pus collects between the lobes. It may be difficult to diagnose and the abscess may point and rupture into an air passage—the pus being coughed up.

interlobular (*in-ter-lob'-u-lar*). Between lobules. *I. veins.* Branches of the portal vein in the liver.

intermenstrual (*in-ter-men'-stru-al*). Between the menstrual periods, when the uterus is shedding its lining.

intermittent (*in-ter-mit'-tent*). Occurring at intervals. *I. claudication.* See Claudication. *I. fever.* See Fever. *I. positive airway pressure* (IPAP). A method of assisted ventilation, in which oxygen or air is used under pressure to inflate the lungs, when the patient is unable to breathe spontaneously.

interphase (*in'-ter-fase*). The period between two cell divisions during which the chromosomes are not easily visible.

intersex (*in'-ter-seks*). A congenital abnormality in which anatomical features of both sexes are evident.

interstitial (*in-ter-stish'-al*). Between the special tissues, i.e. in the connective tissues. *I. fluid.* The fluid in which body cells are bathed. It acts as an intermediary between the cells and the blood. See Extracellular fluid. *I. keratitis.* See Keratitis. *I. nephritis.* Chronic nephritis associated with fibrosis and hypertension.

intertrigo (*in-ter-tri'-go*). An irritating, eczematous skin eruption, from chafing where two moist surfaces are in close apposition causing interference with evaporation.

intervertebral (*in-ter-vert'-e-bral*). Between the vertebrae. *I. disc.* The pad of fibro-cartilage between the bodies of the vertebrae. Protrusion of the contents of the disc may give rise to sciatica by pressing on the nerve roots.

intestine (*in-tes'-tin*). That part of the alimentary canal which extends from the stomach to the anus. *Small i.* The first 6 m (20 ft), from the pylorus to the caecum, consisting of the duodenum, jejunum and ileum.

Large i. 2 m (6 ft) in length, consisting of the caecum, ascending, transverse and descending colon and rectum. The canal completes the process of digestion and eliminates waste matter.

intestinal (*in-tes'-tin-al*). Referring to the intestine.

intima (*in'-tim-ah*). The innermost coat of an artery or vein.

intolerance (*in-tol'-er-ans*). Lack of power to withstand. Applied to the effect of some drugs on individuals, e.g. *iodine* and *quinine.* See Idiosyncrasy.

intoxication (*in-toks-ik-a'-shun*). (1) Poisoning by drugs or harmful substances. (2) A state of drunkenness by taking too much alcohol.

intra- (*in'-trah*). A prefix signifying 'within'.

intra-abdominal (*in-trah-ab-dom'-in-al*). Within the abdomen.

intra-articular (*in-trah-ar-tik'-u-lar*). Within a joint capsule. *I-a. injections.* Those that may be injected in this way such as hydrocortisone.

intra-atrial (*in-trah-a'-tre-al*). Within the atrium. *I-a. thrombosis.* A blood clot formed in the atrium of the heart.

intracapsular (*in-trah-kap'-su-lar*). Within the capsule of a joint. *I. fracture.* See Fracture.

intracellular (*in-trah-sel'-u-lar*). Within a cell. *I. fluid.* the water and its dissolved salts found within the cells. *I. organisms.* Those which invade cells, e.g. the gonococcus.

intracerebral (*in-trah-ser'-e-bral*). Within the brain substance. *I. haemorrhage.* Arising in the cerebrum most often from the middle cerebral artery or from an aneurysm.

intracranial (*in-trah-kra'-ne-al*). Within the skull. *I. abscess.*

One arising within the brain or meninges. *I. aneurysm.* Arising in one of the cerebral vessels. It may be congenital or acquired. *I. pressure.* The pressure within the cranium measured by lumbar puncture.

intradermal (*in-trah-der'-mal*). Between the layers of the skin as in tests carried out for antibody formation.

intradural (*in-trah-du'-ral*). Within the dura mater. *I. haemorrhage. See* Haemorrhage.

intragastric (*in-trah-gas'-trik*). Within the stomach. *I. tube feeding.* Artificial feeding usually by nasogastric tube.

intrahepatic (*in-trah-hep-at'-ik*). Within the liver. Referring to a condition of the liver cells or connective tissue.

intralobular (*in-trah-lob'-u-lar*). Within the lobule. *I. veins.* Collect blood from within the lobules of the liver.

intramedullary (*in-trah-med-ul'-lar-e*). Within the bone marrow. *I. nail.* One for fixation of a fracture.

intramuscular (*in-trah-mus'-ku-lar*). Within muscle tissue.

intranasal (*in-trah-na'-zal*). Within the nose. *I. oxygen. See* Appendix 3.

intra-ocular (*in-trah-ok'-u-lar*). Within the eyeball.

intra-osseous (*in-trah-os'-se-us*). Into a bone.

intraperitoneal (*in-trah-per-it-o-ne'-al*). Within the peritoneal cavity.

intrathecal (*in-trah-the'-kal*). Within the meninges of the spinal cord, usually in the subarachnoid space.

intratracheal (*in-trah-trak'-e-al*). Within the trachea. *I. anaesthesia.* The anaesthetic inhaled through a tube passed into the trachea via the nose or mouth.

intrauterine (*in-trah-u'-ter-ine*). Within the uterus. *I. device. See* IUD. *I. douche.* Irrigation of the uterine cavity; for which a special nozzle is used, having a groove in it, so that the fluid can return and is not forced into the fallopian tubes. *I. life.* Fetal development in the uterus.

intravenous (*in-trah-ve'-nus*). Within a vein.

intraventricular (*in-trah-ven-trik'-u-lah*). Within a ventricle. It may apply to a cerebral or cardiac ventricle.

intrinsic factor (*in-trin'-sik*). An enzyme formed in gastric glands in the presence of HCl which is necessary for the absorption of the extrinsic factor (vitamin B_{12}).

introitus (*in-tro'-it-us*). An opening or entrance.

introjection (*in-tro-jek'-shun*). A mental process by which an individual takes into himself personal characteristics of another person, usually those of someone much loved or admired.

introspection (*in-tro-spek'-shun*). A subjective study of the mind and its processes, in which an individual studies his own reactions.

introversion (*in-tro-ver'-shun*). The looking inwards.

introvert (*in'-tro-vert*). A cool, thoughtful, reflective person who tends to be self-sufficient and is a poor mixer in society. *See* Extrovert.

intubation (*in-tu-ba'-shun*). The introduction of a tube into the air passages to allow air to enter the lungs. Used for administration of an anaesthetic, e.g. by Magill's catheter.

intumescence (*in-tu-mes'-ens*). A swelling or increase in bulk, like nasal mucous membrane in catarrh.

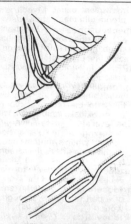

INTUSSUSCEPTION

intussusception (*in-tus-sus-sep'-shun*). A condition in which one part of the intestine becomes pushed or invaginated into another part beyond. It occurs mostly among children at the ileocaecal junction, and causes intestinal obstruction, with pain, vomiting, and small blood-stained evacuations. Prompt surgical treatment is necessary.

intussusceptum (*in-tus-sus-sep'-tum*). The invaginated part of the intestine in intussusception.

intussuscipiens (*in-tus-sus-sip'-e-ens*). The outer part of the intestine which encloses the intussusceptum.

inunction (*in-unk'-shun*). The act of rubbing an oily or fatty preparation into the skin.

inulin (*in'-u-lin*). A substance used to estimate the efficiency of renal function. It is filtered, but not re-absorbed or secreted, and its clearance rate therefore equals that of glomerular filtration.

invagination (*in-vaj-in-a'-shun*). Pushing of a part inwards, thus forming a pouch. The original condition of intussusception.

invasion (*in-va'-shun*). The onset of a disease.

inverse (*in'-vers*). Reverse of the normal. *I. temperature. See* Temperature. *I. respiration. See* Respiration. *I. uterus.* The organ is turned inside out. This occasionally occurs following labour.

invertase (*in-vert'-aze*). A ferment of intestinal juice acting on cane sugar.

in vitro (*in ve'-tro*). In a glass. As in a test tube. Refers to observations made outside the body. *See* In vivo.

in vivo (*in ve'-vo*). Within the living body. *See* In vitro.

involucrum (*in-vol-u'-krum*). New bone which forms a sheath around necrosed bone, as in chronic osteomyelitis.

involuntary (*in-vol'-un-tar-e*). Independent of the will.

involution (*in-vol-u'-shun*). (1) Turning inward; describes the contraction of the uterus after labour. (2) Sometimes applied to the slowing down process of aging.

involutional (*in-vol-u'-shun-al*). Relating to the changes of retrogression which occur during later life. *I. melancholia.* Depression occurring for the first time in later life and characterized by agitation and delusions of a hypochondriacal nature.

iodide (*i'-o-dide*). A compound of iodine.

iodine (*i'-o-deen*). A non-metallic element with a distinctive odour, obtained from sea-weed. *Tincture of i.* A $2\frac{1}{2}$ per cent spirit solution used as a skin antiseptic. *Lugol's i.* Aqueous solution used orally in the pre- and postoperative treatment of thyrotoxicosis. *Radioactive i.*(^{131}I). Used in the treatment and diagnosis of thyroid conditions.

iodism (*i'-o-dizm*). Poisoning from the prolonged use of iodine or iodides.

iodoform (*i-o'-do-form*). A yellow, crystalline, antiseptic powder containing iodine.

iodopsin (*i-o-dop'-sin*). A cone pigment in the retina of the eye. It is composed of a protein fraction and retinene (*q.v.*).

iodoxyl (*i-o-doks'-il*). A radio-opaque dye used in pyelography.

ion (*i'-on*). One of the components into which an electrolyte (*q.v.*) is broken up by electrolysis. *Hydrogen i. concentration.* The estimation of free hydrogen particles in the blood which govern its reaction. *I. exchange resin.* A special resin which has the ability to absorb certain ions.

ionization (*i-on-i-za'-shun*). When an electric current is passed through an electrolyte solution the molecules break up into electrically charged particles or ions. By this method, although it is not often used, substances can be introduced through the skin, e.g. copper sulphate to treat tinea pedis.

iopanoic acid (*i-o-pan'-o-ik a'-sid*). A radio-opaque dye used in X-ray examination of the gall-bladder and ducts. Telepaque is a proprietary preparation.

iophendylate (*i-o-fen'-de-late*). A radio-opaque dye that may be used in examination of the spinal canal. Myodil is a proprietary preparation.

ipecacuanha (*ip-e-kak-u-an'-ah*). The dried root of a Brazilian shrub, given in small doses as a stimulant expectorant.

IPP. Intermittent positive pressure.

iproniazid (*ip-ro-ni'-az-id*). An antidepressant drug that belongs to the group of mono-amine oxidase inhibitors.

ipsilateral (*ip-se-lat'-er-al*). Occurring on the same side. Applied when symptoms occur on the same side as the cerebral lesion.

iridectomy (*ir-di-ek'-to-me*). Excision of a part of the iris.

iridocele (*ir-id'-o-seel*). Hernia of a part of the iris, through a wound.

iridocyclitis (*ir-id-o-si-kli'-tis*). Inflammation of the iris and ciliary body.

iridodialysis (*ir-id-o-di-al'-is-is*). The separation of the outer border of the iris from its ciliary attachment, often a result of trauma.

iridoplegia (*ir-id-o-ple'-je-ah*). Paralysis of the iris.

iridoptosis (*ir-id-op-to'-sis*). Prolapse of iris.

iridotomy (*ir-id-ot'-o-me*). Incising the iris to make an artificial pupil.

iris (*i'-ris*). The coloured part of the eye made of two layers of muscle, the contraction of which alters the size of the pupil.

irritable bowel syndrome (*ir'-it-abl bow'-el sin'-drome*). A condition in which the patient complains of disordered bowel function but no organic disease can be discovered, despite thorough investigation.

irritable hip (*ir'-it-abl hip*). Transient synovitis of the hip in children of 5–10 years which causes a limp and pain.

iritis (*i-ri'-tis*). Inflammation of the iris causing pain, photophobia, contraction of pupil and discoloration of the iris.

iron (*ir-on*). A metallic element given in tonic mixtures and for the treatment of anaemia. It causes black discoloration of the stools. *I. lung.* See Respirator. *Radioactive i.* Used to estimate blood volume.

iron dextran (*ir-on deks-tran*). A solution for intravenous and intramuscular injection. Trade name is Imferon.

iron sorbitol (*ir-on sor'-be-tol*). A solution of iron for intramuscular injection. Jectofer is the trade preparation.

irradiation (*ir-ra-de-a'-shun*). Exposure to the action of rays, e.g. ultra-violet rays in the treatment of rickets.

irreducible (*ir-re-du'-sib-l*). Incapable of being replaced in a normal position. *I. hernia.* See Hernia.

irrigation (*ir-re-ga'-shun*). Washing out a cavity or wound, usually with a hot lotion.

irritant (*ir'-rit-ant*). An agent causing stimulation or excitation.

irritation (*ir-rit-a'-shun*). (1) A condition of undue nervous excitement, through abnormal sensitiveness. (2) Itching of the skin. *Cerebral i.* A stage of excitement present in many brain conditions, and typical of the recovery stage of concussion.

ischaemia (*is-ke'-me-ah*). Lack of blood to a part. *Cardiac i.* Heart muscle is deprived of blood as in coronary thrombosis. See Volkmann's ischaemic contracture.

ischiorectal abscess (*is-ke-o-rek'-tal*). A collection of pus in the ischiorectal connective tissue. A *fistula in ano* may result.

ischium (*is'-ke-um*). The lower posterior bone of the pelvic girdle.

Ishihara colour charts (*S. Ishihara, Japanese ophthalmologist, 1879–*). Consist of a pattern of dots of the primary colours on a similar background. The patterns can be seen by a normal sighted person, but one who is colour blind will only be able to identify some of them.

islets of Langerhans (*P. Langerhans, German pathologist, 1847–88*). The groups of cells in the pancreas that produce insulin.

isocarboxazid (*i-so-kar-boks'-az-id*). A drug used to relieve depression. Marplan is a proprietary preparation.

iso-immunization (*i-so-im-mu-ni-za'-shun*). Development of antibodies against an antigen derived from an individual of the same species.

isolation (*i-so-la'-shun*). The separation of a person with an infectious disease from those non-infected. *I. period.* The length of time during which a patient with an infectious fever is considered capable of infecting others by contact.

isolator (*i-so-la'-tor*). A term applied to a specially constructed chamber or unit in which a patient can be nursed or undergo treatment.

isoleucine (*i-so-lu'-seen*). One of the eight amino acids which are essential for health in the adult.

isometric (*i-so-met'-rik*). Having equal proportions. *I. exercises.* Those carried out without producing movement; used to maintain muscle tone following a fracture.

isoniazid (*i-so-ni'-az-id*). A

drug given orally in combination with streptomycin or sodium *para*-aminosalicylate which is effective in treating tuberculosis.

isoprenaline (*i-so-pren'-a-leen*). An oral synthetic drug which has an action like adrenaline and can be used to treat asthma.

isotonic (*i-so-ton'-ik*). Having uniform tension. *I. solution* is of the same osmotic pressure as the fluid with which it is compared. Normal saline is isotonic with blood plasma.

isotopes (*i'-so-topes*). Atoms of the same element but having different mass numbers. There are eleven isotopes of iodine. *Radioactive i.* Unstable isotopes which emit electrons (beta rays). Many also emit gamma rays. They may be used in the diagnosis and treatment of disease.

itch. (1) Scabies. (2) A skin eruption with irritation. *Baker's i.* Eczema of the hands due to the proteins of flour. *Barber's i.* Sycosis (*q.v.*). *Dhobie i.* A form of ringworm prevalent in the tropics. *Washer-woman's i.* Eczema of the hands due to the use of soda. *I. mite. Sarcoptes scabiei.*

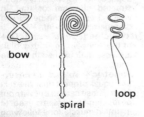

bow

spiral

loop

INTRAUTERINE DEVICES

-itis. A suffix denoting 'inflammation'.

IUD. Intrauterine device. Contraceptive device introduced into the uterine cavity.

J

Jacksonian epilepsy (*J. H. Jackson, British neurologist, 1835–1911*). *See* Epilepsy.

Jacquemier's sign (*T. Y. Jacquemier, French obstetrician, 1806–79*). Blueness of the lining of the vagina seen in the early weeks of pregnancy.

jactitation (*jak-tit-a'-shun*). The extreme restlessness of a patient.

jail fever. An old name for typhus fever because of its prevalence in prisons.

jargon (*jar'-gon*). The terminology used and generally understood only by those who have knowledge of that speciality, i.e. medical jargon, legal jargon.

jaundice (*jawn'-dis*). Syn. Icterus. A yellow discoloration of the skin and conjunctivae, due to the presence of bile pigment in the blood. It may be: (1) *Haemolytic j.* Due to excessive destruction of red blood cells, causing increase of bilirubin in the blood. The liver is not involved. *Acholuric j.* is of this type. It is characterized by increased fragility of red blood cells. Splenectomy effects a cure in most cases. (2) *Hepatocellular j.* In this the liver cells are damaged either by infection or drugs, most commonly the virus of *infective hepatitis.* Toxic agents may be chloroform, phosphorus, arsenic or gold. (3) *Obstructive j.* Bile is prevented from reaching the duodenum owing to obstruction by gallstone, growth or stricture of the common bile duct. (4) *Physiological j.* Jaundice occurring within the first few days of life, caused by the breakdown of red blood cells present in the newborn.

jejunectomy (*je-ju-nek'to-me*). Excision of a piece of the jejunum.

jejuno-ileostomy (*je-ju'-no il-e-os'-to-me*). The operation of making an anastomosis between the jejunum and the ileum.

jejunostomy (*je-ju-nos'-to-me*). Incision of the jejunum to make an opening through which food can be administered, in cases of cancer of the duodenum, etc.

jejunotomy (*je-ju-not'-o-me*). An incision into the jejunum.

jejunum (*je-ju'-num*). The portion of the small intestine (about 2·4 m (8 ft) in length), from the duodenum to the ileum.

Jenner's vaccination (*E. Jenner, British physician, 1749–1823*). Arm-to-arm vaccination with fluid from the lesions of cowpox, from which modern methods of smallpox vaccination were developed.

jigger (*jig'-er*). A type of flea found in the tropics which burrows into the soles of the feet and causes severe irritation.

Johne's bacillus (*H. A. Johne, German pathologist, 1839–1910*). *Mycobacterium johnei.*

Johne's disease (*H. A. Johne, German pathologist, 1839–1910*). A chronic enteritis of bovines, not pathogenic for man.

joint. An articulation. The point of junction of two or more bones. *J. receptors.* Specialized nerve tissues located in joint capsules which relay information to the brain so that the

position of the limbs in space is consciously recognized.

Joule (*J. P. Joule, British physicist 1818–89*). The unit of energy which is employed in the Système International d'Unités (SI units). *See* Appendix 6.

judgement (*juj'-ment*). The ability of an individual to estimate a situation, to arrive at reasonable conclusions, and to decide on a course of action.

jugular (*jug'-u-lar*). Relating to the neck. *J. veins.* Two large veins in the neck, which convey most of the blood from the head.

juvenile (*joo'-ven-ile*) Relating to young people.

juxtaglomerular (*juks-tah-glom-er'-u-lar*). Specialized cells found in the kidney which appear to play an important part in the control of aldosterone release.

juxtaposition (*juks-tah-po-sish'-un*). Close at hand. Adjacent.

K

Kahn test (*B. L. Kahn, American bacteriologist, 1887–   *). An agglutination test for syphilis.

kala-azar (*kah-lah-ah'-zar*). A tropical disease caused by the Leishman–Donovan parasite, and marked by enlargement of the spleen and anaemia. Leishmaniasis.

kanamycin (*kan-a-mi'-sin*). An antibiotic drug for severe infections with Gram-negative organisms where penicillin is ineffective. Kannasyn is a proprietary preparation.

kaolin (*ka'-o-lin*). China clay used as a dusting powder and for poulitces. *Refined k.* Aluminium silicate. Given orally to treat diarrhoea.

Kaposi's spots (*M. K. Kaposi, Austrian dermatologist, 1837–1902*). A serious complication of eczema occurring on exposure to herpes simplex virus infection. More commonly known as Kaposi's varicelliform eruption.

karyotype (*kar'-e-o-tipe*). The pattern which is seen when human chromosomes are photographed during metaphase. The pictures are then enlarged and paired according to the length of their short arm.

katabolism (*kat-ab'-ol-izm*). The breaking-down process in tissue structure. Catabolism. *See* Metabolism.

kataphoresis (*kat-a-for-e'-sis*). Ionization (*q.v.*).

katonium (*kat-one-e'-um*). A diuretic in which positively charged ions are used to produce an acidosis to which the kidneys respond by an increased output of acid urine.

Kayser–Fleischer ring (*B. Kayser, German ophthalmologist, 1869–1954: B. Fleischer, German ophthalmologist, 1874– *). Brownish pigmented ring seen in the cornea of patients with Wilson's disease.

Keller's operation (*W. L. Keller, American surgeon, 1874–1959*). A bone operation for correcting hallux valgus.

keloid (*ke'-loid*). A hard, whitish tumour of the skin. A type occurs in a healed wound due to overgrowth of fibrous tissue, causing the scar to be raised above the skin level. With X-ray treatment it disappears.

Kennedy's syndrome (*F. Kennedy, American neurologist, 1884–1952*). A frontal lobe tumour which involves one of the optic nerves.

keratectasia (*ker-a-tekt-a'-se-ah*). Protrusion of the cornea.

keratectomy (*ker-a-tek'-to-me*). Excision of the cornea.

keratin (*ker'-a-tin*). An albuminous substance which forms the base of all horny tissues.

keratinize (*ker'-a-tin-ise*). To become horny.

keratitis (*ker-a-ti'-tis*). Inflammation of the cornea. *Interstitial k.* A syphilitic manifestation, seen chiefly in the congenital type.

keratoconjunctivitis (*ker-a-to-kon-junk-tiv-i'-tis*). Inflammation of both the cornea and the conjunctiva of the eye.

keratoconus (*ker-a-to-ko'-nus*). A bilateral degenerative ocular condition in which the cornea becomes thin and protruded into a cone-shape.

kerato-iritis (*ker-a-to-i-ri'-tis*). Inflammation of cornea and iris.

keratoma (*ker-a-to'-mah*). An overgrowth of horny tissue.

keratomalacia (*ker-a-to-mal-a'-se-ah*). Ulceration and softening of the cornea. Due to deficiency of vitamin A. *See* Appendix 10.

keratome (*ker'-a-tome*). A knife with trowel-shaped blade, for incising the cornea.

keratometer (*ker-a-tom'-e-ter*). Ophthalmometer. An instrument by which the amount of corneal astigmatism can be measured accurately.

keratoplasty (*ker'-a-to-plas-te*). Plastic operation on the cornea including that of transplantation.

keratoscope (*ker'-a-to-skope*). A battery and disc of concentric circles for examining the eye to detect keratoconus.

keratosis (*ker-a-to'-sis*). A skin disease marked by excessive growth of the epidermis or horny tissue.

keratotomy (*ker-a-tot'-o-me*). Incision of the cornea.

kerion (*ke'-re-on*). A complication of ringworm of the scalp, with formation of pustules.

kernicterus (*kern-ik'-ter-us*). A complication of haemolytic jaundice of the newly born in which there is pigmentation of, and damage to, the brain cells.

Kernig's sign (*V. M. Kernig, Russian physician, 1840–1917*). A sign of meningitis. When the thigh is supported at right angles to the trunk, the patient is unable to straighten his leg at the knee-joint.

ketogenic diet (*ke-to-jen'-ik*). A high fat diet given to produce ketosis. Now seldom used.

ketones (*ke'-tone*). Compounds containing the carboxyl group (COOH). Products of incomplete fat metabolism in the body. *See* Aceto-acetic acid.

ketonuria (*ke-ton-ur'-e-ah*). The presence of ketones in urine.

ketosis (*ke-to'-sis*). The condition in which ketones are formed in excess in the body. *See* Acidosis.

17-ketosteroids (*ke-to-ster'-oids*). Steroids excreted in the urine and formed from the adrenal corticosteroids, testosterone, and to a lesser extent from oestrogens.

kidney (*kid'-ne*). One of two glandular, urine-secreting organs situated in the lumbar region. *Artificial k.* The apparatus used to remove retained waste products from the blood when kidney function is impaired. *K. failure.* The condition in which renal function is severely impaired and the organs are unable to maintain the

fluid and electrolyte balance of the body. *Granular k.* The small fibrosed kidney of chronic nephritis. *Horseshoe k.* The congenital fusion of the two kidneys into a horseshoe shape. *Large white k.* Present in subacute, hydraemic or parenchymatous nephritis. *Polycystic k.* A congenital bilateral condition of multiple cysts replacing kidney tissue. *K. transplant.* The surgical implantation of a kidney taken from a live donor or from one who has recently died. Used in the treatment of renal failure.

Killian's operation (*G. Killian, German otolaryngologist, 1860–1921*). Opening the frontal sinus to curette it and the ethmoid cells.

kilogram (*kil'-o-gram*). One thousand grams. *See* Appendix 6.

Kimmelstiel–Wilson's disease (*P. Kimmelstiel, German pathologist, now in the USA, 1900– : C. Wilson, British physician, 1906–)*. Nephrotic syn-

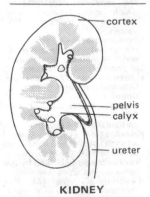

KIDNEY

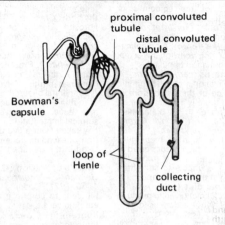

proximal convoluted tubule

distal convoluted tubule

Bowman's capsule

loop of Henle

collecting duct

NEPHRON OF KIDNEY

drome associated with diabetes mellitus.

kinaesthesis (*kin-es-the'-sis*). The combined sensations by which position, weight and muscular position are perceived.

kinanaesthesia (*kin-an-es-the'-se-ah*). Impaired sensation. An inability to recognize position or objects not seen.

kinase (*ki'-naze*). Activator. *See* Enterokinase *and* Thrombokinase.

kinematics (*kin-e-mat'-iks*). The science of movement, in particular that of the body.

kineplastic stump (*kin-e-plas'-tik*). An amputation stump so made that the patient can control the artificial limb by the remaining muscles.

Kirschner's wire (*M. Kirschner, German surgeon, 1879–1942*). A thin wire that

may be passed through a bone to exert skeletal traction.

kiss of life. The expired air method of artificial respiration, by either mouth-to-nose or mouth-to-mouth breathing. *See* Appendix 2.

Klebsiella (*kleb-se-el'-ah*). A genus of bacteria. They are short rods, Gram-negative, non-spore-forming, and encapsulated. They may cause infection of the lung, intestines and urinary tract.

Klebs–Löffler bacillus (*T. A. E. Klebs, German bacteriologist, 1834–1913: F. A. J. Löffler, German bacteriologist, 1852–1915*). The *Corynebacterium diphtheriae*, the cause of diphtheria.

kleptomania (*klep-to-ma'-ne-ah*). An irresistible urge to steal when there is often no need and no particular desire for the objects.

Klinefelter's syndrome (*H. F. Klinefelter, American physician, 1912– *). Due to a chromosome abnormality in which each cell has XXY sex chromosomes making a total of 47 (normal 46). Affected men have female breast development, small testes and are infertile.

Klippel–Feil syndrome (*M. Klippel, French neurologist, 1858–1942: A. Feil, French physician 1884– *). A congenital abnormality in which the neck is very short due to absence or fusion of several vertebrae in the cervical region.

Klumpke's paralysis (*A. Déjerine-Klumpke, French neurologist, 1859–1927*). Affects the hand and arm and is due usually to a birth injury to the brachial plexus.

kneading (*ne'-ding*). A method used in massage. Pétrissage.

knee. The joint between the femur and the tibia. *K. jerk.* An upward jerk of the leg, obtained by striking the patellar tendon when the knee is passively flexed. *Housemaid's k. See* Bursitis. *Knock k. Genu valgum.* A condition in which the knees turn inwards towards each other.

Koch's bacillus (*R. Koch, German bacteriologist, 1843–1910*). The *Mycobacterium tuberculosis,* the causative organism of tuberculosis.

Köhler's disease (*A. Köhler, German physician and roentgenologist, 1874–1947*). A type of osteochondritis.

koilonychia (*koil-on-ik'-e-ah*). Spoon-shaped nails as present in iron deficiency anaemia.

Koplik's spots (*H. Koplik, American paediatrician, 1858–1927*). Small white spots in an area of hyperaemia, sometimes occurring on the cheeks inside the mouth as an early sign of measles. They appear on the second day of onset, before the general rash, and are diagnostic.

Korotkoff's method (*N. S. Korotkoff, Russian physician, 1874– *). The method of finding the systolic and diastolic blood pressure by listening to the sounds produced in an artery while the pressure in a previously inflated cuff is gradually reduced.

Korsakoff's syndrome or psychosis (*S. S. Korsakoff, Russian neurologist, 1854–1900*). A chronic condition in which there is impaired memory, particularly for recent events and the patient is disorientated for time and place. It may be present in psychosis of infective, toxic, or metabolic origin or in chronic alcoholism.

Krabbe's leucodystrophy (*K. H. Krabbe, Danish neurologist, 1885–1961*). Mental subnormality due to degenerative disease of the white matter of the brain.

kraurosis vulvae (*kror-o'-sis vul'-ve*). A degenerative condition of the vagina treated by giving oestrin preparations.

Krebs' cycle (*Sir H. Krebs, German biochemist in England, 1900– *). A series of reactions during which the aerobic oxidation of pyruvic acid takes place. This is part of carbohydrate metabolism. *K. urea c.* The way in which urea is formed in the liver.

Kretschmer's types (*E. Kretschmer, German physician, 1888–1964*). The method of classifying potential psychopathic personalities in relation to their body shape, e.g. short and fat: tendency to manic depression; tall and thin: a tendency to schizophrenia.

Krukenberg tumour (*G. P. H. Krukenberg, German gynaecologist, 1871–1946*). A large secondary growth in an ovary. The primary one is usually in the stomach and is small.

Kuntscher nail (*G. Kuntscher, German orthopaedic surgeon, 1902–*). An intramedullary nail

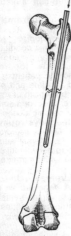

KUNTSCHER INTRAMEDULLARY NAIL

for treating fracture of long bones, especially the shaft of femur.

Kupffer's cells (*K. W. von Kupffer, German anatomist, 1829–1902*). Reticuloendothelial cells of the liver concerned in the organization of bile.

Kupperman test (*kup'-perman*). Test for pregnancy by injecting urine into immature female rats. Results are available in 2 hours.

kwashiorkor (*kwosh-e-or'-kor*). A condition of protein malnutrition occurring in children in under-privileged populations. Fatty infiltration of the liver arises and may cause cirrhosis.

kymograph (*ki'-mo-graf*). An apparatus consisting of a rotating drum upon which graphic records can be traced of physiological or psychological processes.

kyphoscoliosis (*ki-fo-skol-e-o'-sis*). A curvature of the spine in which there is backward and sideways displacement.

kyphosis (*ki-fo'-sis*). Posterior curvature of the spine; humpback.

L

labial (*la'-be-al*). Pertaining to the lips or labia.

labile (*la'-bile*). Unstable. Applies to those drugs and preparations that are subject to change or readily altered by heat.

lability of mood (*la-bil'-e-te*). The tendency to sudden changes of mood of short duration.

labioglossopharyngeal paralysis (*la'-be-o-glos-o-fa-rin'-je'-al*). Bulbar paralysis. *See* Paralysis.

labium (*la'-be-um*). A lip. *Pl.* labia, *L. majus pudendi.* The large fold of flesh surrounding the vulva. *L. minus pudendi.* The lesser fold within.

labour. Parturition or child-birth, which takes place in three stages. (1) Dilatation of the cervix uteri. (2) Passage of child through the birth canal. (3) Expulsion of placenta. *Induced l.* Brought on by artificial means before term, as in cases of contracted pelvis or if overdue. *Obstructed l.* Due to a mechanical hindrance. *Precipitate l.* Labour in which the baby is delivered extremely rapidly. *Premature l.* That which occurs before term. *Spurious l.* Pains which sometimes precede true labour pains.

labyrinth (*lab'-ir-inth*). The structures forming the internal ear, i.e. the cochlea and semicircular canals. *Bony l.* The bony canals of the internal ear. *Membranous l.* The membrane inside the bony canals.

labyrinthectomy (*lab-ir-inth-ek'-to-me*). Destruction of the membranous labyrinth of the inner ear. A possible treatment for Ménière's disease if medical treatment has failed.

labyrinthitis (*lab-ir-inth-i'-tis*). Inflammation of the labyrinth.

lac (*lak*). Milk.

laceration (*las-er-a'-shun*). A wound with torn and ragged edges—not clean cut.

lacrimal apparatus (*lak'-rim-al*). The structures secreting the tears and draining the fluid from the conjunctival sac.

lacrimation (*lak-rim-a'-shun*). An excessive secretion of tears.

lacrimators (*lak'-rim-a-tors*). Substances which cause excessive secretion of tears, e.g. tear gas.

lactagogue (*lak'-ta-gog*). See Galactagogue.

lactalbumin (*lakt-al'-bu-min*). An albumin of milk.

lactase (*lak'-taze*). The enzyme of succus entericus which splits lactose to glucose and galactose.

lactate (*lak'-tate*). A salt of lactic acid. *L. dehydrogenase.* An enzyme which is found in the liver.

lactation (*lak-ta'-shun*). (1) The period during which the infant is nourished from the breast. (2) The process of milk secretion, carried on by the mammary glands.

lacteals (*lak'-te-als*). The lymphatics of the intestine which absorb split fats.

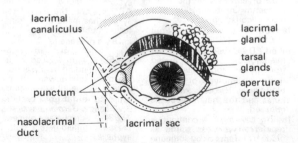

LACRIMAL APPARATUS

lactic acid (*lak'-tik*). An acid formed by the fermentation of lactose or milk sugar. It is produced naturally in the vagina before the menopause. May be used in vaginal pessaries for its antiseptic action.

lactiferous (*lak-tif'-er-us*). Conveying or secreting milk.

lactifuge (*lak'-te-fuj*). A drug or agent which retards the secretion of milk.

lactobacillus (*lak-to-bas-il'-us*). A member of a genus of micro-organisms, many of which produce fermentation.

lactoflavin (*lak'-to-flav-in*). Riboflavine (*q.v.*).

lactogenic (*lak-to-jen'-ik*). Stimulating the production of milk. *See* Luteotrophin.

lactometer (*lak-tom'-e-ter*). An instrument for measuring the specific gravity of milk.

lactose (*lak'-toze*). Milk sugar.

lactosuria (*lak-to-su'-re-ah*). Lactose in the urine.

lacuna (*lak-u'-nah*). A small cavity or depression in any part of the body. *Pl.* lacunae.

Laënnec's cirrhosis (*R. T. H. Laënnec, French physician, 1781–1826*). The commonest type of cirrhosis of the liver, frequently attributable to high alcohol consumption.

laevulose (*lev'-u-loze*). Fruit sugar.

laked. Describes blood when haemoglubin has separated from the red blood cells.

laking. Haemolysis of the red blood cells. The cells swell and burst and the haemoglobin is released.

lalling (*lal'-ing*). A continuous repetitive, wordless sound as made by infants or by someone who is severely subnormal.

lambdoidal suture (*lamb-doid'-al*). The junction of the occipital bone with the parietals.

lamellae (*la-mel'-le*). (1) Very thin superimposed layers of bone. (2) Minute medicated discs used in applying drugs to the eye, where they dissolve. *Sing.* lamella.

lamina (*lam'-in-ah*). A bony plate or layer. *L. cribrosa*. The portion of sclera where the fibres of the optic nerve pass through it at the optic disc.

laminectomy (*lam-in-ek'-to-me*). Excision of the posterior arch of a vertebra, sometimes performed to relieve pressure on the spinal cord or nerves.

Lancefield's groups (*R. C. Lancefield, American bacteriologist, 1895– *). Divisions of haemolytic streptococci. Twelve groups are recognized, most human infections being due to Group A. Other groups are mainly responsible for animal infections.

lancinating (*lan'-sin-a-ting*). Sharp, cutting; it describes some pains.

Landsteiner classification (*K. Landsteiner, Austrian biologist in the USA, 1868–1943*). A system of blood groups, the ABO system. The use of this system has made blood transfusion much safer.

Landry's disease (*J. B. G. Landry, French physician 1826–1865*). A term applied to an acute ascending paralysis from the lower limbs upwards. It may arise in polyneuritis or myelitis.

Lange colloidal gold test (*C. F. A. Lange, German physician, 1883– *). A test made on cerebrospinal fluid to detect syphillis.

Langerhans, islets of (*P. Langerhans, German pathologist, 1847–88*). The groups of cells in the pancreas which produce insulin.

Langhans' cell (*T. Langhans, Swiss pathologist, 1839– *). The deep cellular tissues of the chorionic villi (*q.v.*).

lanolin (*lan'-o-lin*). A fat obtained from sheep's wool, and used as a basis for ointments. *See* Adeps.

lanugo (*lan-u'-go*). A fine layer of hair seen on the body of newly born infants.

laparoscopy (*lap-ar-os'-ko-pe*). Viewing the abdominal cavity by passing a telescopic instrument through the abdominal wall.

laparotomy (*lap-ar-ot'-o-me*). Incising the abdominal wall for exploratory purposes.

lard. The fat of the pig; used as a basis for ointments.

lardaceous (*lar-da'-she-us*). The same as amyloid.

large intestine. The part of the alimentary tract which extends from the ileocaecal valve to the anus. *See* Intestine.

laryngeal (*la-rin'-je-al*). Pertaining to the larynx.

laryngectomy (*lar-in-jek'-to-me*). Excision of the larynx.

laryngismus stridulus (*lar-in-jiz'-mus strid'-u-lus*). A crowing sound on inspiration following a period of apnoea due to spasmodic closure of the glottis. It occurs in rickets when the calcium content of the blood is low. Treatment is as for rickets.

laryngitis (*lar-in-ji'-tis*). Inflammation of the larynx causing hoarseness or loss of voice due to acute infection or improper use (*chronic l.*). *L. stridulosa.* Spasm of the larynx, dyspnoea and stridulant inspiration at night. Occurs in nervous children with enlarged tonsils. *Tuberculous l.* A variety

that responds well to antituberculous drugs.

laryngologist (*lar-in-gol'-o-jist*). A specialist in diseases of the larynx.

laryngoparalysis (*lar-in'-go-par-al'-is-is*). Paralysis of the larynx.

laryngopharynx (*lar-in'-go-far'-inks*). The lower part of the pharynx.

laryngoscope (*lar-in'-go-skope*). An endoscopic instrument for examining the larynx

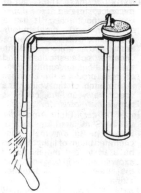

LARYNGOSCOPE

or for aiding the insertion of endotracheal tubes or the bronchoscope.

laryngospasm (*lar-in'-go-spazm*). A reflex prolonged contraction of the laryngeal muscles that is liable to occur on insertion or withdrawal of an intratracheal tube.

laryngostenosis (*lar-in-go-sten-o'-sis*). Contraction or stricture of the larynx.

laryngostomy (*lar-in-gos'-to-*

me). Incision of the larynx to provide an artificial air-passage.

laryngotracheal (*lar-in-go-trak'-e-al*). Referring to both the larynx and trachea.

laryngotracheitis (*lar-in-go-trak-e-i'-tis*). Inflammation of both the larynx and trachea.

laryngotracheobronchitis (*lar-in-go-trak-e-o-brong-ki'-tis*). An acute viral infection of the respiratory tract which occurs in young children.

larynx (*lar'-inks*). The organ of the voice, situated at the upper end of the trachea. It has a muscular and cartilaginous frame, lined with mucous membrane. Across it are spread the vocal cords of elastic tissue, and the vibrations and contractions of these produce the changes in the pitch of the voice. The space between the cords is termed the *glottis*.

laser (*la'-zer*). Light Amplification by Stimulated Emission of Radiation. An extremely concentrated beam of light that can be used to cut metals. Used experimentally in surgery and in the treatment of detached retina.

Lasix (*la'-sik*). A proprietary preparation of frusemide.

Lassa fever (*las-sah*). A disease caused by a virus, usually found in West Africa. The illness is severe and is likely to be fatal, particularly if contracted by Europeans. First reported from Lassa in northern Nigeria.

Lassar's paste (*G. Lassar, German dermatologist, 1849–1907*). A soothing paste used in skin diseases, containing salicylic acid, powdered zinc, starch and petroleum jelly.

latent (*la'-tent*). Temporarily concealed; not manifest. *L. heat.* That which brings about

a change in state, i.e. from water into steam. When condensation occurs this heat is released.

lateral (*lat'-er-al*). Relating to the side. *L. ventricles.* The ventricles in the brain in which the cerebrospinal fluid is formed.

lateroversion (*lat-er-o-ver'-shun*). Turning to one side, such as may occur of the uterus.

laudanum (*lod'-an-um*). Tincture of opium; a preparation used as a narcotic.

laughing gas. Nitrous oxide (*q.v.*).

lavage (*lav-arj'*). Washing out a cavity. *Colonic l.* Washing out the colon. Some litres of fluid are used. *Gastric l.* Of the stomach. *Rectal l.* Of the rectum.

Lawrence's line ration diet (*R. D. Lawrence, British physician, 1892–1968*). A diabetic diet in which one line ration consisted of carbohydrates 10 g, protein 7·5 g and fat 9 g. Now superseded by the 5 g interchangeable portions diet. *See* Appendix 10.

laxative (*laks'-at-iv*). A mild aperient (*q.v.*).

lead (*led*). A metal, the salts of which are applied externally as an astringent lotion to inflamed surfaces and bruises. *L. poisoning.* A disease which usually occurs in children as the result of excessive lead in the atmosphere, or from chewing toys and other objects covered with paint containing lead. The symptoms and signs include malaise, colic, peripheral neuropathy and encephalitis. There is often pallor and a blue line around the gums.

lecithin (*les'-ith-in*). A nitrogenous and fatty substance found in nerve tissues, blood, and bile and also in eggs.

leech (*le'-tch*). *Hirudo medicinalis.* An aquatic worm which sucks blood and is sometimes used as a counter-irritant.

leg. The lower limb, from knee to ankle. *Barbados l.* Elephantiasis. *Bow l.* Genu valgum. *White l.* Phlegmasia alba dolens (*q.v.*). *Scissor l.* Cross legged, as occurs in Little's disease.

legumin (*leg'-u-min*). A protein of peas, beans, and all pulses.

Leishman–Donovan bodies (*Sir W. B. Leishman, English pathologist, 1865–1926; C. Donovan, Irish physician, 1863–1951*). The intracellular forms of *Leishmania donovani*, the parasite producing kala-azar. These bodies occur in the spleen and liver of patients.

Leishmania (*leesh-ma'-ne-ah*). Parasitic protozoa having flagellae which infect the blood of man and are the cause of leishmaniasis.

leishmaniasis (*leesh-man-i'-a-sis*). Kala-azar (*q.v.*).

Lembert's suture (*A. Lembert, French surgeon, 1802–51*). For wounds of the intestine. So arranged that the edges are turned inwards and the peritoneal surfaces are in contact.

lenitive (*len'-it-iv*). A soothing agent.

lens (*lens*). (1) The transparent, cystalline body situated behind the pupil of the eye. It serves as a refractive medium for rays of light. (2) Pieces of glass shaped to focus or scatter rays of light. They can be of varied shapes in order to improve sight. *Contact l.* A thin sheet of glass or plastic moulded to fit directly over the cornea. Worn instead of spectacles.

lentigo (*len-ti'-go*). A freckle.

leontiasis (*le-on-ti'-as-is*). A disease of the face in which osseous deformity produces a lion-like appearance. It occurs

sometimes in leprosy, elephantiasis, etc.

lepidosis (*lep-id-o'-sis*). Any scaly eruption of the skin.

leprosy (*lep'-ro-se*). A chronic infectious disease affecting the skin and nerves, owing to the *Mycobacterium leprae*. There are three recognized forms: (1) Tuberculoid, in which the tissue defence is good. (2) Lepromatous, in which the tissue defence is poor or absent. (3) Dimorphous, in which there is partial tissue defence. Signs and symptoms include anaesthesia, especially of hands and feet; skin lesions (various types anywhere on the body); and the thickening of certain nerves. The last sometimes culminates in paralysis of certain muscles of the hands, feet, or face (i.e. primary deformity). Fingers and toes do *not* die and drop off, but can be 'lost' due to the fact that there is lack of sensation and therefore ulceration and sepsis ensues and the small bones of the extremities become affected (i.e. secondary deformity). Modern physiotherapeutic and operative surgical techniques can prevent much of this deformity. Sulphone preparations are used successfully in treatment.

leptazol (*lep'-ta-zol*). A respiratory stimulant used in poisoning cases where there is respiratory depression.

leptomeningitis (*lep-to-men-in-ji'-tis*). Inflammation of the pia mater and arachnoid membranes.

Leptospira (*lep-to-spi'-rah*). A class of spirochaete. *L. icterohaemorrhagiae.* The cause of Weil's disease (*q.v.*).

leptospirosis (*lep-to-spi-ro'-sis*). Weil's disease (*q.v.*).

Leriche syndrome (*R. Leriche, French surgeon, 1879-1955*). A condition in which atherosclerosis of peripheral arteries is accompanied by obstruction of the lower end of the aorta.

neutrophil

eosinophil

basophil

polymorphonuclear

lymphocyte

monocyte

LEUCOCYTES

lesbianism (*les'-be-an-izm*). Sexual attraction of one woman to another.

lesion (*le'-zhun*). An injury, wound, or morbid structural change in an organ. The word is used as a general term for some local disease condition.

let-down reflex. The sensation felt by a mother in anticipation of feeding her baby. It occurs as the breasts fill with milk.

lethargy (*leth'-ar-je*). A condition of drowsiness or stupor which cannot be overcome by the will.

Letterer–Siwe disease (*E. Letterer, German physician, 1895– : S. A. Siwe, German physician, 1897– *). A disease occurring in young children in which histiocytic granules appear during the first year of life. The spleen and liver become enlarged as do the lymph glands. The disease runs a rapid and fatal course.

leucine (*lu'-sin*). An essential amino acid of the protein molecule; it may be excreted in the urine from excessive endogenous breakdown of protein, as in acute atrophy of the liver.

leucocyte (*lu'-ko-site*). A white blood corpuscle. There are three types: (a) *granular* (polymorphonuclear cells) formed in bone marrow, consisting of neutrophils, eosinophils and basophils; (b) lymphocytes (formed in the lymph glands), and (c) monocytes. *L. count* (normal):

	per mm³
Neutrophils	5000
Lymphocytes	2000
Monocytes	350
Eosinophils	100
Basophils	50
Total	7500

leucocytolysis (*lu-ko-si-tol'-is-is*). Destruction of white blood cells.

leucocytosis (*lu-ko-si-to'-sis*). Increased number of leucocytes in the blood.

leucoderma (*lu-ko-der'-mah*). A congenital absence of pigment in patches or bands, producing abnormal whiteness of the skin.

leucodystrophy (*lu-ko-dis'-tro-fe*). A degenerative disorder of the brain which starts during the first few months of life and leads to mental, visual and motor deterioration.

leucoma (*lu-ko'-mah*). A white spot on the cornea, following an injury to the eye.

leuconychia (*lu-ko-nik'-e-ah*). White patches on the nails due to air underneath.

leucopenia (*lu-ko-pe'-ne-ah*). A decreased number of white cells, usually granulocytes, in the blood. It may be present in tuberculosis, enteric fever, influenza or undulant fever.

leucoplakia (*lu-ko-pla'-ke-ah*). A chronic inflammation, characterized by a white thickened surface. *L. buccalis.* A condition that affects the mucous membrane of the mouth. *L. vulvae.* The mucous membrane and skin of the labia become thickened and scattered white patches appear. It is a precancerous condition and the treatment is vulvectomy.

leucopoiesis (*lu-ko-poi-e'-sis*). The formation of white blood cells.

leucorrhoea (*lu-kor-re'-ah*). A thick whitish discharge from the vagina, which occurs when there is congestion in the pelvic organs. Blennorrhagia.

leucotomy (*lu-kot'-o-me*). Severing of white fibres. *Prefrontal l.* An operation in which the fronto-thalamic connection fibres passing into the frontal lobes of the brain are severed.

It may considerably relieve symptoms of worry, tension, and fear but there may also be changes in personality, such as lack of initiative and perseverence. The process is irreversible.

leukaemia (*lu-ke'-me-ah*). A blood disease of unknown cause, in which there is great increase in the number of white cells. There are two chief forms. (1) *Lymphatic* (or *lymphocytic*) *l.* in which there is enlargement of the lymphatic glands and spleen. (2) *Myeloid l.* Associated with disease of the bone marrow and enlargement of the spleen. Both forms may be *acute*, lasting only a few weeks or months, or *chronic* lasting a number of years with long periods of remission following treatment.

levallorphan (*lev-al-or'-fan*). A respiratory stimulant that antagonizes the action of morphine. Lorfan is a proprietary preparation.

levator (*lev-a'-tor*). A muscle which raises a part. *L. palpebrae.* Raises the eye lid.

levorphanol (*lev-or'-fan-ol*). An analgesic somewhat resembling morphine in its action and addiction potentialities. In tablet or injection form, it is subject to the Misuse of Drugs Act. Dromoran is a proprietary preparation.

libido (*lib-e'-do*). (1) The vital force or impulse which brings about purposeful action. (2) Sexual drive. In Freudian psychoanalysis the motive force of all human beings.

lice. *See* Louse.

lichen (*li'-ken*). A group of inflammatory affections of the skin, in which the lesions consist of papular eruptions. *L. planus.* Raised flat patches of dull, reddish-purple colour, with smooth or scaly surface. The skin is stained when they disappear.

lichenification (*li'-ken-if-e-ka'-shun*). The stage of an eruption when it resembles lichen.

lichenoid (*li'-ken-oid*). A rash that resembles lichen.

lid lag. A sign of thyrotoxicosis. A rim of sclera is apparent over the cornea when the patient's gaze is lowered.

lie. A position or direction. *L. of fetus.* The position of the fetus in the uterus.

Lieberkühn's glands (*J. N. Lieberkühn, German anatomist, 1711–56*). Tubular glands of the small intestine.

lien (*li'-en*). The spleen.

lienculus (*li-en'-ku-lus*). An accessory spleen.

lienitis (*li-en-i'-tis*). Inflammation of the spleen (splenitis).

lienorenal (*li-en-o-re'-nal*). Relating to the spleen and kidney. *L. anastomosis.* The joining of the splenic vein to the left renal vein. A method of reducing the blood supply to the liver in portal hypertension.

lienunculus (*li-en-un'-ku-lus*). A detached portion of spleen.

ligament (*lig'-a-ment*). A band of fibrous tissue connecting bones forming a joint. *Annular l.* The ring-like band which fixes the head of the radius to the ulna. *Cruciate l.* Crossed ligaments within the knee joint. *Poupart's l.* Between the pubic bone and anterior iliac crest. *Round l.* For example one of the two anterior ligaments of the uterus, passing through the inguinal canal and ending in the labia majora.

ligation (*lig-a'-shun*). The application of a ligature.

ligature (*lig'-at-chur*). A thread of silk, catgut or other material used for tying vessels.

light. Electromagnetic waves which by stimulating the retina of the eye give the sensation of light. *L. baths.* Ultra-violet rays are administered by an electric arc, made by two poles (*tungsten* or *carbon rods*) or the mercury vapour lamp. These have a tonic effect and kill bacteria near the surface. Vitamin D is produced by their action on ergosterol of subcutaneous tissues. *Wood l.* That from which visible rays have been eliminated. Used in the diagnosis of skin diseases.

light coagulation. A method of treating retinal detachment by directing a beam of strong light from a carbon arc through the pupil to the affected area.

lightening. The relief experienced in the late stages of pregnancy when the uterus sinks into the pelvis and ceases to press on the diaphragm.

lightning pains. Intense, sharp, and cutting pains in the legs characteristic of locomotor ataxia.

lignocaine (*lig'-no-kane*). A local anaesthetic for infiltration or surface application. Xylocaine is a proprietary preparation.

limbus (*lim'-bus*). Applied to the eye, the border where the cornea joins the sclera.

lime. (1) A citrus fruit resembling a small lemon. (2) Calcium oxide, the salts of which help to form bone (CaO). *Chlorinated l.* Bleaching powder. *L. water.* Calcium hydrate solution. Given to counteract acidity.

lincomycin (*lin-ko-mi'-sin*). An antibiotic derived from the *Streptomyces* genus.

linctus (*link'-tus*). A thick syrup given to soothe and allay coughing. It should not be diluted. *Opiate l. of squill* contains opium. *Codeine l.* and *methadone l.* are similar.

linea (*lin'-e-ah*). A line. *L. alba.* The tendinous area in the centre of the abdominal wall into which the transversalis and part of the oblique muscles are inserted. *L. albicantes.* White streaks that appear on the abdomen when it is distended by pregnancy or a tumour. *L. aspera.* The rough ridge on the back of the femur into which muscles are inserted. *L. nigra.* The pigmented line which often appears in pregnancy on the abdomen between the umbilicus and pubis.

lingual (*ling'-gwal*). Pertaining to the tongue.

lingula (*ling'-u-la*). A tongue-like projection of lung tissue from the left upper lobe.

liniment (*lin'-e-ment*). A liquid to be applied externally by rubbing. *Camphor l.* is of camphor and olive oil.

linseed. Seeds of the common flax, which contain an oil with a demulcent action. *L. meal* is crushed linseed used for poultices.

lint. A loosely woven cotton fabric, one side of which is fluffy, and the other smooth.

liothyronine (*li-o-thi'-ro-neen*). A preparation of thyroid hormone used in the treatment of hypothyroidism where rapid results are desired.

liothyroxine (*li-o-thi-roks'-een*). A preparation of thyroid extract for the treatment of cretinism and myxoedema.

lipaemia (*li-pe'-me-ah*). The presence of excess fat in the blood. Sometimes a feature of diabetes.

lipase (*lip'-aze*). The fat-splitting ferment of pancreatic juice. Also called steapsin.

lipids (*lip'-ids*). The fat particles found in blood serum.

Lipiodol (*lip-i'-o-dol*). A proprietary compound of iodine and oil, which being opaque to X-rays may be introduced to outline cavities; e.g. spinal canal, bronchial tubes, etc.

lipodystrophy (*lip-o-dis'-tro-fe*). A disorder of fat metabolism. *Progressive l.* Chiefly affects females in which there is progressive loss of fat over the upper half of the body.

lipoid (*lip'-oid*). Resembling fat or oil. *L. nephrosis.* A condition of the kidney in which fat is deposited.

lipoidoses (*lip-oid-o'-ses*). A group of diseases in which there is an error in lipoid metabolism. Xanthomata (*q.v.*) are common.

lipolysis (*lip-ol'-is-is*). The breakdown of fats by the action of bile salts and enzymes to a fine emulsion and fatty acids.

lipoma (*lip-o'-mah*). A tumour composed of fatty tissue, arising in any part of the body, and developing in connective tissue. *Diffuse l.* A tumour of fat in an irregular mass without a capsule.

lipoproteins (*lip-o-pro'-teens*). The total fat concentration in the serum.

lipotrophic substances (*lip-o-tro'-fik*). Dietary factors which have the power to remove fat and so help to prevent fatty infiltration of the liver, e.g. choline and methionine.

lipuria (*lip-u'-re-ah*). The presence of fat in urine.

liquefaction (*lik-we-fak'-shun*). Reduction to liquid form.

liquor (*lik'-er*; Latin *li'-kwor*). A watery fluid. Drugs are administered in this form. *L. amnii.* The fluid in which the fetus floats. *L. arsenicalis.* A solution of arsenic to be taken by mouth.

L. epispasticus. Blistering fluid.
L. sanguinis. The plasma, or fluid part of blood.

Lister, J. (*British surgeon, 1827–1912*). In 1867 Lord Lister described the antiseptic technique which prepared the way for modern surgery.

lithagogue (*lith'-a-gog*). A drug which helps to expel calculi.

lithiasis (*lith-i'-as-is*). Formation of calculi. *Conjunctival l.* Small white chalky areas on the under surface of the eyelids.

lithium carbonate (*lith'-e-um kar'-bon-ate*). A drug used in the treatment of manic-depressive illness.

litho- (*lith'-o*). A prefix signifying 'a stone'.

lithonephrotomy (*lith-o-nef-rot'-o-me*). Incision of the kidney to remove a stone. Nephrolithotomy.

lithopaedion (*lith-o-pe'-de-on*). A dead fetus that has been retained and become calcified.

lithosis (*lith-o'-sis*). Disease resulting from inhalation of particles of silica, etc., into the lungs. Pneumoconiosis.

lithotome (*lith'-o-tome*). A knife used in lithotomy.

lithotomy (*lith-ot'-o-me*). Incision of the bladder for the removal of calculi. *L. position.* See Position.

lithotripsy (*lith'-o-trip-se*). Lithotrity. The crushing of calculi in the bladder.

lithotrite (*lith'-o-trite*). An instrument used for lithotripsy.

lithuresis (*lith-u-re'-sis*). Passage of small calculi or gravel in the urine.

litmus (*lit'-mus*). A blue pigment obtained from lichen and used for testing the reaction of fluids. *Blue l.* is turned red by an acid. *Red l.* is turned blue by an alkali.

litre (*le'-ter*). The unit of capacity in the metric system. One thousand millilitres. *See* Appendix 6.

Little's disease (*W. J. Little, British surgeon, 1810–94*). Spastic diplegia. A congenital muscle rigidity of the lower limbs, causing 'scissor leg' deformity. The cause may be haemorrhage into, or bruising of the brain before or during birth.

liver (*liv'-er*). The large gland situated in the right upper area of the abdominal cavity. Its chief functions are: (1) The secretion of bile. (2) The maintenance of the composition of the blood. (3) The regulation of metabolic processes. *Cirrhotic l.* Fibrotic changes which occur in the liver as the result of chronic inflammation. *Hobnail l.* The appearance of the cirrhotic liver. *Nutmeg l.* A mottled condition, typical of the effect of congestive heart failure.

livid (*liv'-id*). A bluish-grey complexion, produced by congestion of blood.

LMP. Last menstrual period.

LOA. Left occipitoanterior. The position of the fetus in the uterus.

lobar (*lo'-bar*). Relating to a lobe.

lobe. A section of an organ, separated from neighbouring parts by fissures.

lobectomy (*lo-bek'-to-me*). Removal of the lobe, e.g. of the lung. Performed in lung abscess or unilateral bronchiectasis.

lobotomy (*lob-ot'-o-me*). An operation in which the nerve fibres in the prefrontal area of the brain are severed to effect a change of behaviour. *Syn.* Leucotomy.

lobular (*lob'-u-lar*). Relating to a lobule.

lobule (*lob'-ule*). A small lobe.

localize (*lo'-kal-ize*). To limit the spread, e.g. of disease or infection, to a certain area.

lochia (*lo'-ke-ah*). The discharge of blood and tissue debris from the uterus following childbirth. *L. alba.* The later pale discharge. *L. rubra.* The earlier discharge first containing bright blood and later dark blood. *L. serosa.* A thin clear discharge.

lochiometra (*lo-ke-o-me'-trah*). A collection of lochia in the uterus.

locked twins. The condition of twins with their bodies so placed that neither can be born naturally.

lock-jaw. Tetanus.

locomotor ataxia (*lo-ko-mo'-tor a-taks'-e-ah*). Tabes dorsalis. *See* Ataxia.

loculated (*lok'-u-la-ted*). Divided into small locules or cavities.

loculus (*lok'-u-lus*). A small cystic cavity, one of a number.

logarithmic growth (*log-ar-ith'-mik*). The growth phase of bacteria in which the organisms double their numbers at regular intervals.

loiasis (*lo-i'-as-is*). Infestation of the conjunctiva and eyelids with a parasite worm, the *Loa loa.* A tropical condition.

loin. The area at the back, between the thorax and the pelvis.

Lomotil (*lo'-mo-til*). A proprietary mixture of diphenoxylate and atropine, used to reduce motility of the intestine.

long-acting thyroid stimulator (LATS). A substance found in the plasma of some patients with thyrotoxicosis. Thought to be formed as the result of an autoimmune reaction.

long-sight (*long-site*). Hypermetropia (*q.v.*).

loop (1) A complete bend. (2)

A platinum wire in a handle used for transferring bacteriological material. It is always flamed to red heat before and after use.

LOP. Left occipitoposterior. The position of the fetus in the uterus.

lordosis (*lor-do'-sis*). A form of spinal curvature in which there is an abnormal forward curve of the lumbar spine.

lotion (*lo'-shun*). A medicinal solution, used for bathing wounds, etc. *Calamine l.* A soothing mixture containing calamine and zinc oxide. *Evaporating l.* A dilute alcoholic solution applied to bruises. *Lead l.* A weak solution of lead acetate used for sprains and bruises where the skin is unbroken. *Red l.* Zinc oxide in solution. A stimulating lotion for sluggish tissues.

loupe (*loop*). A magnifying lens which may be used in eye examination.

louse (*lows*). A parasite which infests mammals. *Head l. Pediculus capitis. Body* or *clothes l. Pediculus corporis. Pubic* or *crab l.* Infests the hair on the body. Diseases known to be transmitted by the louse are typhus fever, relapsing fever and trench fever.

low birth weight (*low berth wate*). The term used for infants whose birth weight was less than 2·5 kg.

lozenge (*loz'-enj*). A medicated tablet, with sugar basis.

LSD. *See* Lysergide.

lubb-dupp. Describes the sounds heard through the stethoscope when listening to the normal heart. *Lubb* when the atrioventricular valves shut, and *dupp* when the semilunar valves meet each other.

lucid (*lu'-sid*). Clear, particularly

of the mind. *L. interval.* May occur in cerebral injury between two periods of unconsciousness or as a sane interval in a mental disorder.

Ludwig's angina (*W. F. von Ludwig, German surgeon, 1790–1865*). *See* Angina.

Lugol's solution (*J. G. A. Lugol, French physician, 1786–1851*). A preparation of iodine and potassium iodide. It is best given in milk and is largely used in the treatment of toxic goitre.

lumbago (*lum-ba'-go*). A painful rheumatic affection of the muscles and fibrous tissues of the loin, usually the result of exposure to the cold.

lumbar (*lum'-bar*). Pertaining to the loins. *L. puncture.* A trocar and cannula are inserted into the spinal canal, and cerebrospinal fluid is withdrawn. The manometer attached to the cannula gives a reading of the intraspinal pressure. Normally this is 120 mm.

lumbosacral (*lum-bo-sa'-kral*). Relating to both the lumbar vertebrae and the sacrum.

Lumbricus (*lum'-brik-us*). (1) A genus of worms, including the earthworm. (2) *Ascaris* spp. which are parasitic in the intestine of man.

lumen (*lu'-men*). The space inside a tube.

lunacy (*lu'-nas-e*). A term formerly applied to insanity (*q.v.*).

lunar caustic. Nitrate of silver.

lung. One of a pair of conical organs of the respiratory system, consisting of an arrangement of air tubes terminating in air vesicles (*alveoli*) and filling almost the whole of the thorax. The right lung has three lobes and the left lung two. They are connected with the air by means of the bronchi and trachea.

lunula (*lu'-nu-lah*). The white semicircle, near the root of each nail.

lupus (*lu'-pus*). A skin disease, having many manifestations. *L. erythematosus.* An urticaria which finally produces a round plaque-like area of hyperkeratosis. It is thought to be due to an autoimmune reaction to sunlight, infection or other unknown cause. *L. vulgaris.* A tuberculous disease of the skin treated with isoniazid.

luteinizing hormone (*lu'-te-in-i-zing hor'-mone*). One of three hormones produced by the anterior pituitary gland which control the activity of gonads.

luteotrophin (*lu-te-o-tro'-fin*). An anterior pituitary hormone. The name now given to prolactin as it is known to influence both the secretion of milk and the corpus luteum.

luxation (*luks-a'-shun*). Dislocation.

lying. Making an untruthful statement. *Pathological l.* A disorder of conduct which may occur as a symptom in behaviour disorders of children or in certain mental disorders such as addiction or psychopathic personality.

lying-in. The puerperium.

lymph (*limf*). The fluid from the blood which has transuded through capillary walls to supply nutriment to tissue cells. It is collected by lymph vessels which ultimately return it to the blood. *L. nodes* or *glands.* Structures placed along the course of lymph vessels, through which the lymph passes and is filtered of foreign substances, e.g. bacteria. These nodes also make lymphocytes. *Plastic l.* Exuded in inflammation, which tends to cause adhesion between structures and so limit spread of infection, e.g. in peritonitis. *Vaccine I.* Used for vaccination against smallpox.

lymphadenectomy (*limf-ad-en-ek'-to-me*). Excision of a lymph gland or nodes.

lymphadenitis (*limf-ad-en-i'-tis*). Inflammation of a lymph gland.

lymphadenoma (*limf-ad-en-o'-mah*). A malignant disease of lymphoid tissue. Hodgkin's disease (*q.v.*).

lymphadenopathy (*limf-aden-op'-ath-e*). Any disease condition of the lymph nodes.

lymphangiectasis (*limf-an-je-ek'-tas-is*). Dilated lymph vessels due to some obstruction of the lymph current.

lymphangiogram (*limf-an'-je-o-gram*). An X-ray of lymph vessels made possible by the insertion of a dye.

lymphangioma (*limf-an-je-o'-mah*). A swelling composed of dilated lymph vessels.

lymphangioplasty (*limf-an'-je-o-plas-te*). Any plastic operation which aims at making an artificial lymph drainage.

lymphangitis (*limf-an-ji'-tis*). Inflammation of lymph vessels, manifested by red lines on the skin over them. It occurs in cases of severe infection through the skin, usually by streptococci.

lymphatic (*limf-at'-ik*). Referring to the lymph. *L. leukaemia.* See Leukaemia. *L. system.* The system of vessels and glands through which the lymph is returned to the circulation. The vessels end in the thoracic duct (*q.v.*).

lymphoblasts (*limf'-o-blasts*). Early developmental cells that mature into lymphocytes.

lymphocytes (*limf'-o-sites*). White blood cells formed in the lymphoid tissue. Their function is the production of immune bodies to overcome and protect against infection.

lymphocythaemia (*limf-o-si-the'-me-ah*). Excessive numbers of lymphocytes in the blood.

lymphocytosis (*limf-o-si-to'-sis*). Lymphocythaemia (*q.v.*).

lymphoedema (*limf-e-de'-mah*). A condition in which the intercellular spaces contain an abnormal amount of lymph due to obstruction of lymph drainage.

lymphogranuloma venereum (*limf-o-gran-u-lo'-mah ven-e'-re-um*). A sexually-transmitted disease due to a virus, primarily a tropical condition.

lymphoid (*limf'-oid*). Relating to the lymph.

lymphoma (*limf-o'-mah*). A tumour of lymphoid tissue.

lymphorrhagia (*limf-o-raj'-e-ah*). The escape of lymph from a ruptured lymphatic vessel.

lymphosarcoma (*limf-o-sar-ko'-mah*). Sarcoma arising in a lymph gland.

lyophilized skin (*li'-o-fil-ized*). Skin from cadavers may be treated by lyophilization, reconstituted and used for temporary skin replacement in severe burns.

lyophilization (*li-o-fil-i-za'-shun*). A method of preserving biological substances in a stable state by freeze drying. It may be used for plasma, sera, bacteria and tissues.

lysergide (*li-ser'-jide*). Lysergic acid diethylamide. LSD. A psychotomimetic drug that may cause visual hallucination and increased auditory acuity but may prove very disrupting to the personality and affect mental ability.

lysin (*li'-sin*). A specific antibody that can destroy cells or tissues. *See* Bacteriolysin.

lysine (*li'-seen*). One of the 22 amino acids formed by the digestion of dietary protein. It is essential for normal health.

lysis (*li'-sis*). (1) The gradual decline of a disease, especially of a fever. The temperature falls gradually as in typhoid. (*See* Crisis.) (2) The action of a lysin.

lysozyme (*li'-so-zime*). An enzyme present in tears, nasal mucus, and saliva that can kill most organisms coming into contact with it.

lytic mixture (*lit'-ik*). One used to assist in inducing and maintaining hypothermia (*q.v.*). It consists of chlorpromazine, pethidine and promethazine. It acts as a sedative and prevents shivering.

M

m. Abbreviation of: *misce*, mix; *metre*, a unit of length.

maceration (*mas-er-a'-shun*). Softening of a solid by soaking it in liquid.

McArdle's disease (*B. Mc-Ardle, contemporary British biochemist*). Myopathy resulting from the absence in voluntary muscle of the enzyme phosphorylase.

McBurney's point (*C. McBurney, American surgeon, 1845–1913*). The spot midway between the *anterior iliac spine* and the *umbilicus* where pain is felt on pressure if the appendix is inflamed.

Mackenrodt's ligaments (*A. K. Mackenrodt, German gynaecologist, 1859–1925*). The transverse or cardinal ligaments that support the uterus in the pelvic cavity.

McNaghten's Rules on Insanity at Law. The rules which define the factors on which a defence to a charge of murder on grounds of insanity may be established. These were evolved after Sir Robert Peel's Secretary was killed by McNaghten in 1843. He was suffering from delusions and the judge ordered that he be found not guilty.

macrocephalus (*mak-ro-kef'-al-us*). Possessing an abnormally large head.

macrocheilia ((*mak-ro-ki'-le-ah*). Excessive development of the lips caused by dilated lymphatic spaces.

macrocyte (*mak'-ro-site*). An abnormally large red corpuscle found in the blood in some forms of anaemia.

macrocythaemia (*mak-ro-si-the'-me-ah*). Abnormally large red cells in the blood.

Macrodex (*mak'-ro-deks*). A proprietary intravenous dextran solution useful as a plasma substitute in treating shock.

macroglossia (*mak-ro-glos-se-ah*). Abnormal enlargement of the tongue.

macromastia (*mak-ro-mas'-te-ah*). Abnormal increase in the size of the breast.

macrophage (*mak'-ro-fage*). A large reticulo-endothelial cell which has the power to ingest cell debris and bacteria.

macrophthalmos (*mak-rof-thal'-mos*). A congenital condition of bilateral large eyes.

macroscopic (*mak-ro-skop'-ik*). Discernible with the naked eye.

macrostomia (*mak-ros'-to-me-ah*). An abnormal development of the mouth in which the mandibular and maxillary processes do not fuse.

macula (*mak'-u-lah*) or **ma-**

cule. A spot or discoloured area of the skin, not raised above the surface. *M. lutea.* The central area of the retina, where vision is clearest.

maculopapular eruption (*mak'-u-lo-pap'-u-lar*). A rash of red raised spots or papules, as in measles.

Madura foot (*mad-u'-rah*). See Mycetoma.

Magendie's foramen (*F. Magendie, French physiologist, 1783–1855*). Aperture in the roof of the fourth ventricle of the brain through which cerebrospinal fluid passes into the subarachnoid space.

magnesium (*mag-ne'-ze-um*). A bluish-white metal. *M. sulphate* is a saline purgative. *M. trisilicate* an antacid powder taken after food for dyspepsia and peptic ulceration. *M. carbonate* and *M. hydroxide* are neutralizing antacids used in hyperacidity.

magnet operation (*mag'-net*). See Operation.

main en griffe (*man-on-greef*). A claw-like deformity of the hand.

mal. Disease. *M. de mer.* Seasickness. *Grand m., petit m.* Forms of epilepsy.

malabsorption (*mal-ab-sorp'-shun*). Inability to absorb. May be the cause of deficiency disease due to the lack of an essential factor.

malacia (*mal-a'-se-ah*). Softening of tissues. *Osteo-m.* Softening of bone tissue. *Kerato-m.* Softening of the cornea.

malachite green (*mal'-ah-kite*). A substance used as part of the diluting fluid for white cells of the blood when they are being counted.

maladie de Roger (*H. L. Roger, French physician, 1811–91*). A small ventricular septal defect which causes no symptoms unless bacterial endocarditis (*q.v.*) supervenes.

maladjustment (*mal-ad-just'-ment*). Failure to adjust to society.

malaise (*mal-aze'*). A feeling of general discomfort and illness.

malar (*ma'-lar*). Relating to the cheek or cheekbone. *M. flush.* See Hectic.

malaria (*mal-air'-e-ah*). A febrile disease caused by a parasite introduced into the blood by mosquitoes of the genus *Anopheles.* The attacks are periodic every 48 to 72 hours according to the type of plasmodium (*q.v.*). A typical malarial paroxysm consists of three stages. (1) The shivering fit. (2) High fever. (3) The sweating stage.

malarial therapy (*mal-air'-e-al ther'-ap-e*). A hyperpyrexia is induced by infecting a patient with malaria. Sometimes used in the treatment of neurosyphilis.

malaxation (*mal-aks-a'-shun*). A kneading movement in massage.

male fern. *Filix mas.* A drug given by mouth, to expel tapeworms.

malformation (*mal-form-a'-shun*). Deformity. A structural defect.

Malgaigne's bulgings (*J. F. Malgaigne, French surgeon, 1806–65*). Bulging of the lower abdominal muscles when there is a lack of tone in them. Thought to predipose to inguinal hernia.

malignant (*mal-ig'-nant*). A term applied to any disease of a virulent and fatal nature. *M. growth* or *tumour.* Cancer. *M. pustule.* Anthrax. *M. endocarditis.* See Endocarditis. *M. hypertension.* See Hypertension. *M. exophthalmos.* A condition seen in thyrotoxicosis where there is raised intraocular pressure causing pain and the threat of damage to the optic nerve.

malingering (*mal-ing'-ger-ing*). The shamming of illness.

malleolus (*mal-le-o'-lus*). The projection on the tibia (*internal m.*) and on the fibula (*external m.*) at the ankle-joint.

malleus (*mal'-le-us*). The hammer-shaped bone in the middle ear.

malnutrition (*mal-nu-trish'-un*). The condition in which nutrition is defective in quantity or quality.

mallet finger (*mal'-let*). A deformity whereby there is flexion of the distal phalanx of one finger.

malocclusion (*mal-o-klu'-shun*). An abnormality of dental development which causes overlapping of the bite.

malpighian body (*M. Malpighi, Italian anatomist, physician and physiologist, 1628–94*). The glomerulus and Bowman's capsule of the kidney.

malposition (*mal-po-zi'-shun*). An abnormal position of any part.

malpractice (*mal-prak'-tis*). Failure to maintain accepted ethical standards.

malpresentation (*mal-pres-en-ta'-shun*). Any abnormal position of the fetus at birth, which renders delivery difficult or impossible.

malrotation of gut (*mal-ro-ta'-shun*). A condition in which there is an abnormal attachment of the intestine to the mesentery. It is liable to cause a volvulus to occur.

malt (*mawlt*). Grain which has been soaked, made to germinate, and dried. It is used as a nutrient in wasting diseases. *M.*

extract. Aids the digestion of starches. *M. sugar.* Maltose.

Malta fever. *See* Undulant fever.

maltase (*mawl'-taze*). A sugar splitting enzyme which converts maltose to dextrose. Present in pancreatic and intestinal juice.

maltose (*mawl'-toze*). The sugar formed by the action of digestive enzymes on starch.

malunion (*mal-u'-ne-on*). Faulty repair of a fracture.

mamilla (*mam-il'-lah*). The nipple.

mammae (*mam'-me*). The breasts or milk-secreting glands.

mammaplasty (*mam'-mah-plas-te*). A plastic operation to reduce the size of abnormally large pendulous breasts.

mammary (*mam'-mar-e*). Relating to the breasts.

mammography (*mam-og'-raf-e*). X-ray examination of the breast to try and detect early cancer.

mammothermography (*mam-o-therm-og'-raf-e*). An examination of the breast that depends on the more active cells producing heat that can be shown on a thermograph, and may indicate a precancerous stage.

Manchester operation. *See* Fothergill's operation.

mandible (*man'-dib-l*). The lower jaw-bone.

manganese (*man'-gan-ees*). A grey-white metal, from the salts of which the permanganates are formed.

mania (*ma'-ne-ah*). Elevation of the mood accompanied by acceleration of thought and action. *M. à potu.* Transient alcoholic excitement.

manic-depressive psychosis (*man'-ik de-pres'-iv si-ko'-sis*).

A mental illness characterized by mania or endogenous depression (*q.v.*). The attacks may alternate between mania and depression or the patient may just have recurrent attacks of mania or depression.

manipulation (*man-ip-u-la'-shun*). Using the hands in a skilful manner, such as in reducing a fracture or hernia or changing the position of the fetus.

mannerisms (*man'-er-izms*). Small actions performed without thought that are characteristic of the individual. They assume psychiatric significance when they become exaggerated or excessive and are associated with emotional stress.

mannitol (*man'-e-tol*). A synthetic carbohydrate given intravenously to reduce intracranial pressure by its diuretic action.

manometer (*man-om'-e-ter*). An instrument for measuring the volume or tension of liquids or gases. *See* Sphygmomanometer.

manometry (*man-om'-et-re*). The science of pressure measurement of liquids and gases.

Mantoux test (*C. Mantoux, French physician, 1877–1947*). An intradermal injection of old tuberculin to determine susceptibility to tuberculosis. If positive a weal develops in 24 to 48 hours.

manubrium (*man-u'-bre-um*). The upper part of the sternum to which the clavicle is attached.

MAOI. *See* Monoamine oxidase.

maple syrup urine disease (*ma'-pul si'-rup*). An inborn error of metabolism in which there is an accumulation in the blood of valine, leucine and isoleucine. The urine smells like maple syrup and there[...] subnormality, spast[...] convulsions.

marasmus (*mar-as'-mus*). Gradual wasting of the tissues, owing to insufficient or unassimilated food, occurring especially in infants. It is not always possible to discover the cause.

marble bone disease (*mar'-bul bone*). A condition in which there is increased density of bone which is visible on X-ray. *See* Albers–Schönberg's disease.

Marburg virus (*mar'-berg*). A virus found in Africa which may be transmitted to man from monkeys. The resulting illness is severe and likely to be fatal particularly if contracted by Europeans. An outbreak occurred among laboratory workers in Marburg, Germany, in 1967.

Marfan's syndrome (*B.-J. A. Marfan, French paediatrician, 1858–1942*). A hereditary disorder in which there are very long digits, a high arched palate, hypertonus and cardiac lesions, the most common of which is atrial septal defect.

marihuana (*mar-e-hwar'-nah*). *Cannabis indica*, Indian hemp or hashish. *See* Cannabis.

Marmite (*mar'-mite*). A proprietary extract from yeast containing vitamin B in large quantities.

Marplan (*mah'-plan*). A proprietary preparation of isocarboxazid. An antidepressive drug.

marrow (*mar'-ro*). (1) The substance contained in the middle of long bones and in the cancellous tissue of all types. *Red m.* Found in all cancellous tissue. Blood cells are made in it. *Yellow m.* The fatty substance contained in the centre of long bones. *M. puncture.* Investigatory procedure in which marrow cells are aspirated from the sternum or iliac crest. (2) *Spinal m.* The spinal cord.

masochism (*mas'-o-kizm*). Punishing oneself. This may be a conscious or unconscious process.

massage (*mas-sarj'*). A scientific method of rubbing, kneading, and manipulating the body to stimulate circulation, improve metabolism and break down adhesions. *External cardiac m.* Applying rhythmic pressure to the lower sternum to cause expulsion of blood from the ventricles and restart circulation in cases of sudden heart failure.

masseter (*mas'-se-ter*). The muscle of the cheek chiefly concerned in mastication.

masseur (*mas-sur'*). A man who performs massage. *Feminine:* Masseuse.

mastalgia (*mas-tal'-je-ah*). Pain in the breast.

mastatrophia (*mast-a-tro'-fe-ah*). Atrophy of the breast.

mast cells. Connective tissue cells found in many body tissues including the heart, liver and lungs.

mastectomy (*mast-ek'-to-me*). Amputation of the breast. *Radical m.* Removal of the breast, axillary lymph glands and pectoralis muscle (modified Halsted's operation).

mastication (*mas-tik-a'-shun*). The act of chewing food.

mastitis (*mas-ti'-tis*). Inflammation of the breast.

mastodynia (*mas-to-din'-e-ah*). Pain in the breasts which frequently occurs during the premenstrual phase.

mastoid (*mas'-toid*). Nipple-shaped. *M. process.* The prominence on the temporal bone which projects downwards behind the ear and into which the sternocleidomastoid muscle is inserted. *M. antrum.* The cavity in this part of the temporal bone which communicates with the middle ear, and contains air. *M. cells.* Hollow spaces in the mastoid bone. *M. operation.* For drainage of these cells when infection spreads from the middle ear.

mastoidectomy (*mas-toid-ek'-to-me*). Removal of diseased bone and drainage of purulent mastoiditis.

mastoiditis (*mas-toid-i'-tis*). Inflammation of the mastoid antrum and cells.

mastoidotomy (*mas-toid-ot'-o-me*). Surgical opening of the mastoid antrum.

masturbation (*mas-ter-ba'-shun*). Production of sexual excitement by friction of the genitals.

materia medica (*mat-e'-re-ah med'-ik-ah*). The science of the source and preparation of drugs used in medicine.

matrix (*ma'-triks*). (1) That tissue in which cells are embedded. (2) The uterus or womb.

matter. Substance. *Grey m.* A collection of nerve cells or non-medullated nerve fibres. *White m.* Medullated nerve fibres massed together, as in the brain.

mattress suture (*su'-chur*). *See* Suture.

maturation (*mat-u-ra'-shun*). Ripening or developing.

maxilla (*maks-il'-lah*). The upper or lower jawbone.

maxillary (*maks-il'-lar-e*). Pertaining to either jawbone.

MCHC. Mean corpuscular haemoglobin concentration.

MCV. Mean corpuscular volume.

measles (*meez'-ls*). Morbilli. An acute infectious disease of childhood caused by a virus spread by droplets. Onset is catarrhal before the rash appears at the 4th day. Koplik's spots (*q.v.*) are diagnostic earlier. Secondary infection may give rise to the serious complications of otitis media or bronchopneumonia. The severity of the attack may be lessened by giving gammaglobulin between the 5th and 9th days following contact. *German m.* See Rubella.

meatus (*me-a'-tus*). An opening or passage. *Auditory m.* The opening leading into the auditory canal. *Urethral m.* Where the urethra opens to the exterior.

mecamylamine (*mek-am-il'-am-een*). A ganglion-blocking drug which given by mouth causes a marked fall in blood pressure, used in treating arterial hypertension. Inversine is a proprietary preparation.

mechanism of labour (*mek'-an-izm*). The sum of the forces which extrude the fetus through the genital passages, and the opposing resisting forces which restrain it and affect its position.

Meckel's diverticulum (*J. F. Meckel, German anatomist and surgeon, 1781–1833*). The remains of a passage which, in the embryo, connected the yolk sac and intestine, evident as an enclosed sac or tube in the region of the ileum.

meconium (*me-ko'-ne-um*). The first intestinal discharges of a newly born child. Dark green in colour and consisting of epithelial cells, mucus and bile. *M. ileus.* Intestinal obstruction due to blockage of the bowel by a plug of meconium.

median (*me'-de-an*). In the middle.

mediastinum (*me-de-as-ti'-num*). The space in the middle of the thorax, between the two pleurae.

medical (*med'-e-kal*). Pertaining to medicine. *M. jurisprudence.* Medical science as applied to aid the law, e.g. in case of death by poisoning, violence, etc.

medical social worker. A trained hospital worker who looks after the patients' social welfare. Known formerly as Almoner.

medicated (*med'-e-ka-ted*). Impregnated with a medicinal substance.

medication (*med-e-ka'-shun*). Administration of remedies.

medicine (*med'-e-sin*). (1) A drug or preparation given for the cure of disease. (2) The science of healing by use of internal remedies. *Forensic m.* Medical jurisprudence (*q.v.*). *Industrial m.* That concerned with the prevention and treatment of diseases due to manufacturing processes. *Preventive m.* Medical measures taken to prevent disease, e.g. spread of infection. *Proprietary m.* A drug commercially produced and patented as suitable for use in treatment of diseases. *Psychosomatic m.* The study of the relationship of physical and mental illness. *Social m.* The study of the influences of environment and economic conditions on physical and mental illnesses.

medico-chirurgical (*med'-e-ko-ki-rur'-je-kal*). Applying to both medicine and surgery.

medico-social (*med-e-ko-so'-shal*). Applying to both medicine and the social factors involved.

Mediterranean anaemia. See Thalassaemia.

Mediterranean fever. Undulant fever (*q.v.*).

medium (*me'-de-um*). A bacteriological preparation on which bacteria are grown.

Medresco (*me-dres'-ko*). The standard hearing aid obtainable in the United Kingdom under the National Health Act 1948.

medulla (*med-ul'-lah*). Marrow. *M. oblongata.* That portion of the spinal cord which is contained inside the cranium. In it are the nerve centres which govern respiration and the action of the heart, etc.

medullary (*med-ul'-lar-e*). Pertaining to marrow. *M. cavity.* The hollow in the centre of long bones.

medullated (*med'-ul-la-ted*). Having a covering or sheath. *M. nerve fibre.* That with a fatty sheath, a myelin sheath.

medulloblastoma (*med-ul'-lo-blast-o'-mah*). A rapidly growing tumour of neuro-epithelial origin mostly arising in the roof of the fourth ventricle in children.

megacolon (*meg-a-ko'-lon*). Extreme dilatation of the large intestine. Hirschsprung's disease.

megaduodenum (*meg-a-du-o-de'-num*). A gross enlargement of the duodenum.

megalo- (*meg'-al-o*). A prefix meaning 'great'.

megaloblast (*meg'-al-o-blast*). A large cell from which the finished red blood cell is derived.

megalocephalic (*meg-al-o-kef-al'-ic*). Large headed.

megalokaryocyte (*meg-al-o-kar'-e-o-site*). A large cell of the bone marrow, responsible for blood platelet formation.

megalomania (*meg-al-o-ma'-ne-ah*). Delusion of grandeur or self-importance.

mega-ureters (*meg'-ah-u-re'-ters*). A condition in which there is more than one ureter leading

from the kidney. Caused by a developmental abnormality.

megrim (*me'-grim*). Migraine (*q.v.*).

meibomian cyst (*H. Meibom, German anatomist, 1638–1700*). A small swelling containing the secretion of the glands. A chalazion.

meibomian glands (*H. Meibom, German anatomist, 1638–1700*). Small sebaceous glands situated beneath the conjunctiva of the eyelid.

meibomianitis (*mi-bo-me-an-i'-tis*). A bilateral chronic inflammation of the meibomian glands.

Meigs' syndrome (*J. V. Meigs, American surgeon, 1892– *). A fibroma or benign solid tumour of the ovary causing ascites and pleural effusion.

meiosis (*mi-o'-sis*). A stage of reduction cell division when the chromosomes are halved in number ready for union at fertilization.

Meissner's plexus (*G. Meissner, German anatomist and physiologist, 1829–1905*). The submucous plexus. *See* Plexus.

mel. Honey. Oxymel or purified honey is an ingredient of cough mixtures.

melaena (*mel-e'-nah*). The discharge of black faeces due to blood which has undergone change in the alimentary tract. A symptom of gastric or duodenal ulcer.

melancholia (*mel-an-ko'-le-ah*). A state of extreme depression.

melanin (*mel'-an-in*). Dark pigment found in hair, choroid coat of the eye and the skin.

melanism (*mel'-an-izm*). A condition marked by abnormal deposit of dark pigment in any organ.

melanocyte (*mel'-an-o-site*).

Cell responsible for the formation of the skin pigment melanin. *M.-stimulating hormone (MSH).* Hormone produced in the pituitary which stimulates the formation of melanin.

melanoderma (*mel-an-o-der'-mah*). A patchy pigmentation of the skin, usually of face or neck, which may be caused by light sensitization or provoked by oil of bergamot used in the perfumery and cosmetics industry.

melanoma (*mel-an-o'-mah*). Brown pigmentation. *Simple m.* A birth mark. *Malignant m.* A tumour arising in any pigment-containing tissues especially the skin and the eye.

melanosis (*mel-an-o'-sis*). *See* Melanism.

melanotic sarcoma (*mel-an-ot'-ik*). *See* Sarcoma.

melanuria (*mel-an-u'-re-ah*). Black pigment in the urine. Present in melanotic sarcoma.

melasma (*mel-az'-mah*). Dark discoloration of the skin, e.g. in Addison's disease.

membrane (*mem'-brane*). A thin elastic tissue covering the surface of certain organs and lining the cavities of the body. *Basement m.* The delicate layer of cells beneath the surface cells of mucous membrane. *Mucous m.* Contains secreting cells and lines all cavities connected directly or indirectly with the skin. *Serous m.* Lubricating membrane lining the abdominal cavity and thorax and covering most of organs within.

menaphthone (*men-af'-thone*). A synthetic preparation of vitamin K.

menarche (*men-ar'-ke*). The first appearance of menstruation.

Mendel's law (*G. J. Mendel, Austrian monk, 1822–84*). A theory that the offspring do not inherit the characteristics of the parents in equal proportion, but that some are *dominant* while others are *recessive*.

mendelian characteristics (*G. J. Mendel, Austrian monk, 1822–84*). Characteristics which are dominant and transmitted from parents to children in full measure.

Mendelson's syndrome (*C. L. Mendelson, contemporary American obstetrician*). A condition in which there is severe oedema and spasm of the bronchioles due to the inhalation of acid gastric contents. *Syn.* Acid aspiration syndrome.

Ménière's disease or **syndrome** (*P. Ménière, French physician, 1799–1862*). Attacks of vertigo and tinnitus with progressive nerve deafness. The cause is unknown.

meningeal (*men-in-je'-al*). Relating to the meninges.

meninges (*men-in'-jees*). The membranes covering the brain and spinal cord. There are three: the dura mater (outer), arachnoid (middle) and pia mater (inner).

meningioma (*men-in-je-o'-mah*). A tumour developing from the arachnoid and pia mater.

meningism (*men'-in-jizm*). Signs of cerebral irritation similar to meningitis, but no inflammation is present.

meningitis (*men-in-ji'-tis*). Inflammation of the meninges. *Meningococcal m.* or *Cerebrospinal fever.* An epidemic form with a rapid onset but quickly responds to treatment by sulphadiazine tablets or intravenous sulphadimidine if the patient is unconscious. *Tuberculous m.* Inflammation of tuberculous origin. If diagnosed early, can now be treated successfully with streptomycin, isoniazid and sodium aminosalicylate.

meningocele (*men-in'-go-seel*). A protrusion of the meninges through the skull or spinal column, appearing as a cyst filled with cerebrospinal fluid. *See* Spina bifida.

The normal cessation of menstruation, usually occurring between the 45th and 50th year of life. *Artificial m.* An induced cessation by operation or treatment with radium.

menorrhagia (*men-or-raj'-e-ah*). Menorrhoea, an excessive flow of the menses.

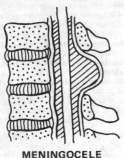

MENINGOCELE

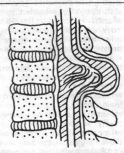

MENINGOMYELOCELE

meningococcus (*men-in-go-kok'-kus*). *Neisseria meningitidis*. A diplococcus, the micro-organism of cerebrospinal fever.

meningo-encephalitis (*men-in-go-en-kef-al-i'-tis*). Inflammation of the brain and meninges.

meningomyelocele (*men-in-go-mi'-el-o-seel*). A protrusion of the spinal cord and meninges through a defect in the vertebral column. *Syn.* Myelomeningocele. *See* Spina bifida.

meniscectomy (*men-is-ek'-to-me*). Removal of a semilunar cartilage.

meniscus (*men-is'-kus*). (1) The convex or concave surface of a liquid as observed in its container. (2) A semilunar cartilage.

menopause (*men'-o-paws*).

menses (*men'-sez*). The discharge from the uterus during menstruation.

menstrual (*men'-stru-al*). Relating to the menses. *M. cycle.* The monthly cycle commencing with the first day of menstruation, when the endometrium is shed, through a process of repair and hypertrophy till the next period. It is governed by the anterior pituitary gland and the ovarian hormones, oestrogens, and progesterone.

menstruation (*men-stru-a'-shun*). A monthly discharge of blood and endometrium from the uterus, starting at the age of puberty and lasting until the menopause. *Vicarious m.* Discharge of blood at the time of menstruation from some other organ than the uterus, e.g. epistaxis is not uncommon.

mental (*men'-tal*). Pertaining to the mind. *M. age.* The measurement of the intelligence level of an individual in terms of the average chronological age of children showing the same mental standard, as measured by a scale of mental tests. *M. disorder.* A term defined by the Mental Health Act 1959 to cover all forms of mental illness and disability and includes mental illness, severe subnormality and psychopathic disorder. *M. mechanisms.* A method of resolving a situation by reverting to an earlier pattern of behaviour when the individual feels unable to reach a more realistic solution. *M. subnormality.* A condition of arrested or incomplete development of the mind existing before the age of 18 years, whether congenital or arising from disease or injury. As children they are unable to profit by the normal school education, and as adults to maintain themselves in anything but the simplest manner.

Mental Health Review Tribunal. A board to whom persons detained under compulsory admission orders or taken into guardianship have the right of appeal at stated intervals.

mental welfare officer. He is appointed by the Local Health Authority and has many duties regarding the care of mentally disordered children and adults, including their compulsory admission to hospital or into guardianship (*q.v.*).

mentha (*men'-thah*). Mint. *Aq. menth. pip.* Peppermint water.

menthol (*men'-thol*). Mint camphor. A crystalline substance derived from oil of peppermint and used in neuralgia and rhinitis, as a local anodyne and antiseptic.

mepacrine (*mep'-a-krin*). A synthetic drug once widely used as an antimalarial agent.

mephitic (*mef-it'-ik*). Offensive or foul. Applied to gangrene with a noxious odour.

mepyramine maleate (*mep-e'-ram-een*). An antihistamine drug used in the treatment of allergic reactions. Anthisan is a proprietary preparation.

mercaptopurine (*mer-kap'-to-pu-reen*). A drug which prevents nucleic acid synthesis and may be used in treating acute leukaemia in children.

mercurialism (*mer-ku'-re-al-izm*). Chronic poisoning due to absorption of mercury.

mercurochrome (*mer-ku'-ro-krome*). An antiseptic preparation of mercury with a dye. Less toxic than other forms, so is used for mucous surfaces, especially of the genitourinary tract.

mercury (*mer'-ku-re*). Quicksilver. A heavy liquid metal, the salts of which are used occasionally as antiseptics and disinfectants. *Yellow oxide of m.* An eye ointment. *M. ointments* are used for some skin diseases. *M. vapour lamp.* Made of quartz glass which permits the ultraviolet rays to pass through. Air is exhausted from the tube and replaced by mercury vapour, through which passes a strong electric current resulting in a powerful ultra-violet light.

mersalyl (*mer'-sal-il*). A mercurial diuretic which prevents reabsorption of water in the renal tubules, so reducing oedema in heart failure and renal insufficiency.

mesarteritis (*mes-ar-ter-i'-*

tis). Inflammation of the middle coat of an artery.

mesencephalon (*mes-en-kef'-al-on*). The middle brain.

mesenchyme (*mes'-en-kime*). Mesoderm (*q.v.*).

mesenteric (*mes-en-ter'-ik*). Pertaining to the mesentery.

mesentery (*mes'-en-ter-e*). A fold of the peritoneum which connects the intestine to the posterior abdominal wall.

mesmerism (*F. A. Mesmer, Austrian physician, 1734–1815*). Hypnotism.

mesocolon (*mes-o-ko'-lon*). A fold of the peritoneum which connects the colon with the posterior abdominal wall.

mesoderm (*mes'-o-derm*). The middle of the three primary layers of cells in the embryo from which the connective tissues develop.

mesometrium (*mes-o-me'-tre-um*). The broad ligaments connecting the uterus with the sides of the pelvis.

mesosalpinx (*mes-o-sal'-pinks*). That part of the broad ligament around the fallopian tubes.

mesothelioma (*me-so-the-le-o'-mah*). A rapidly growing tumour of the pleura, which may be seen in patients with asbestosis.

mesovarium (*mes-o-var'-e-um*). A fold of peritoneum connecting the ovary to the broad ligament.

messenger RNA (*mes'-en-jer*). The ribonucleic acid which acts as a template for the linking of amino acids during the formation of protein in the cells.

metabolic (*met-ah-bol'-ik*). Referring to metabolism.

metabolism (*met-ab'-ol-izm*). The process of life, by which tissue cells are destroyed by combustion (*catabolism*); and

renewed from chemical substances carried in the blood and derived from digested foods (*anabolism*). *Basal m. See* Basal metabolic rate.

metabolite (*met-ab'-o-lite*). Any product of or substance taking part in metabolism. *Essential m.* A substance that is necessary for normal metabolism.

metacarpals (*met-ah-kar'-pals*). The five bones of the hand which join the fingers to the wrist. *See* Metacarpus.

metacarpophalangeal (*met-ah-kar-po-fal-an'-je-al*). Usually referring to the joint between the metacarpal bones and the phalanges.

metacarpus (*met-ah-kar'-pus*). The five bones of the hand uniting the carpus with the phalanges of the fingers.

metamorphosis (*met-ah-mor-fo'-sis*). A structural change or transformation.

metaphase (*met'-ah-fase*). The second stage of mitosis or cell division.

metaphysis (*met-af'-is-is*). The junction of the epiphysis with the diaphysis in a long bone.

metastasis (*me-tas'-tas-is*). The transfer of a disease from one part of the body to another, through the blood vessels or lymph channels, e.g. (1) Secondary deposits may occur from a primary malignant growth. (2) Septic infection may arise in other organs from some original focus.

metatarsalgia (*met-ah-tar-sal'-je-ah*). Neuralgia in the fore part of the foot.

metatarsals (*met-ah-tar'-sals*). The five bones of the foot. *See* Metatarsus.

metatarsus (*met-ah-tar'-sus*). The five bones of the foot uniting the tarsus with the phalanges of the toes.

meteorism (*me'-te-or-izm*). Distension of the intestines with gas. Tympanites (*q.v.*).

methadone (*meth'-a-done*). A powerful analgesic with no sedative action. Amidone.

methaemoglobin (*meth-hem-o-glo'-bin*). An alteration in haemoglobin caused by the action of a drug on the red blood corpuscles. Most commonly phenacetin and other aniline derivatives.

methaemoglobinaemia (*meth-hem'-o-glo-bin-e'-me-ah*). Cyanosis and inability of the red blood cells to transport oxygen due to the presence of methaemoglobin.

methandienone (*meth-an-di'-en-one*). An anabolic steroid used to build up body tissues. Dianabol is a proprietary preparation.

methane (*me'-thane*). Marsh gas.

methicillin (*meth-e-sil'-in*). A form of penicillin that is resistant to staphylococcal penicillinase. Celbenin is a proprietary preparation.

methionine (*meth-i'-o-neen*). An essential amino acid containing sulphur; it is necessary for fat metabolism.

methohexitone (*meth-o-heks'-e-tone*). A barbiturate anaesthetic agent. Given intravenously it has a quick recovery time. Brietal is a proprietary preparation.

methotrexate (*meth-o-treks'-ate*). A cytotoxic drug that antagonizes folic acid and prevents cell formation. It may be used to treat acute leukaemia in childhood.

methylamphetamine (*meth-il-am-fet'-am-een*). A synthetic drug which stimulates the central nervous system and raises the blood pressure. Useful in the treatment of morphine and barbiturate poisoning.

methylated spirit. A preparation of methyl-alcohol, to which pyridine is now added. Also called *industrial alcohol* and *surgical spirit.*

methyldopa (*meth-il-do'-pah*). A hypotensive drug whose action is increased if used with thiazide diuretics. Used to treat hypertension. Aldomet is a proprietary preparation.

methylene blue (*meth'-il-een*). An aniline dye. Chiefly used to test renal function. If injected intravenously, it can be seen entering the bladder from the ureter within five minutes.

methylpentynol (*meth-il-pen'-tin-ol*). A sedative and tranquilizing drug which allays apprehension and may be used before operation or other procedures that might cause the patient discomfort. It is a Schedule 4 poison. Oblivon is a proprietary preparation of it.

methylphenidate (*meth-il-fen'-e-date*). An antidepressant drug that stimulates the central nervous system. Ritalin is a proprietary preparation.

methyl salicylate (*meth'-il sal-is'-e-late*). A compound used externally for rheumatic pains, lumbago, etc. Oil of wintergreen contains it.

metra (*me'-trah*). The uterus.

metralgia (*me-tral'-je-ah*). Pain in the uterus.

metre (*me'-ter*). The unit of length in the metric system. *See* Appendix 6.

metric system (*met'-rik sis'-tem*). The system of weights and measures in which the units are multiplied and divided by powers of ten. Method of measurement in the Système International d'Unités (SI units) (*q.v.*). See Appendix 6.

metritis (*me-tri'-tis*). Inflammation of the uterus.

metrocolpocele (*me-tro-kol'-po-seel*). The protrusion of the uterus into the vagina, the wall of the latter being pushed forward also.

metrodynia (*me-tro-din'-e-ah*). Pain in the uterus.

metronidazole (*me-tro-nid'-az-ole*). A drug that is effective in overcoming *Trichomonas* infection of the genital tract of both sexes when taken as oral tablets. Flagyl is a proprietary preparation.

metropathia haemorrhagica (*me'-tro-path'-e-ah*). A condition of excessive menstruation due to increased vascularity of the endometrium associated with follicular cysts of the ovary.

metroptosis (*me-trop-to'-sis*). Prolapse of the uterus.

metrorrhagia (*me-tror-raj'-e-ah*). Irregular bleeding from the uterus not associated with menstruation.

metrostaxis (*me-tro-staks'-is*). Persistent slight haemorrhage from the uterus.

Michel's suture clips (*G. Michel, French surgeon, 1875–1937*). Small metal clips for suturing wounds.

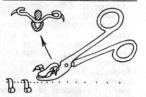

MICHEL'S CLIP (REMOVAL)

micro- (*mi'-kro*). A prefix meaning 'small'.

microbe (*mi'-krobe*). A minute living organism, especially those causing disease. See Bacteria, Rickettsia, Virus.

microbiology (*mi-kro-bi-ol'-o-je*). The study of micro-organisms and their effect on living cells.

microcephalic (*mi-kro-kef-al'-ik*). Having an abnormally small head.

Micrococcus (*mi-kro-kok'-kus*). A genus of bacteria, each individual of which has a spherical shape.

microcurie (*mi-kro-ku'-re*). 1/1000 000 of a curie. A measurement of radioactivity.

microcythaemia (*mi-kro-si-the'-me-ah*). Abnormally small red cells in the blood.

microcytic (*mi-kro-sit'-ik*). Relating to small cells. As found in iron deficiency anaemia.

micrognathia (*mi-kro-nath'-e-ah*). Failure of development of the lower jaw causing a receding chin.

microgram (*mi'-kro-gram*). A unit of weight. See Appendix 6.

micron (*mi'-kron*). 1/1000th of a millimetre. A measurement used for bacteria, and represented by the Greek letter μ. Not an approved measurement under the SI system.

micro-organism (*mi-kro-or'-gan-izm*). A microbe.

microphage (*mi'-kro-fage*). A minute phagocyte.

microphthalmos (*mi-krof-thal'-mos*). An eye that is smaller than normal, its function may or may not be impaired.

microscope (*mi'-kro-skope*). An instrument which enlarges objects that are normally invisible to the human eye.

microscopic (*mi-kro-skop'-ik*).

Visible only by means of the microscope.

Microsporum (*mi-kro-spor'-um*). A fungus; the cause of some skin diseases, especially ringworm.

micturating cystogram (*mik'-tu-ra-ting sist'-o-gram*). X-ray investigation of the bladder. Micturition is observed after the instillation of a radio-opaque dye through a catheter.

micturition (*mik-tu-rish'-un*). The act of passing urine.

midbrain (*mid'-brane*). The portion which connects the cerebrum with the pons and cerebellum. The mesencephalon.

midriff (*mid'-rif*). The diaphragm.

midwifery (*mid-wif'-er-e*). Obstetrics.

migraine (*me'-grane*). A condition in which dilatation of the cranial arteries causes episodes of severe headache, often with nausea, vomiting and visual disturbance.

milestones (*mile'-stones*). The 'norms' against which the motor, social and psychological development of a child is measured.

miliaria (*mil-e-a'-re-ah*). Prickly heat, an acute itching eruption common among white people in tropical and sub-tropical areas.

miliary (*mil'-e-ar-e*). Resembling millet seed. *M. tuberculosis*. See Tuberculosis.

milk. The secretion of mammary glands.

Composition of Milk (%)

	Cows' milk	Human milk
Protein	3·5	2·0
Fats	3·5	3·5
Carbohydrates	4·0	6·0
Mineral salts	0·7	0·2
Water	88·0	88·0

Designations of m. (1) *Tuber-*

culin tested from herds certified free from tuberculosis. (2) *Pasteurized m.* One of several recognized methods of heat treating the milk may be used. (3) *Sterilized m.* Milk that has been heated to 100°C (212°F). *M. teeth.* The first set of teeth.

milk sugar. Lactose, a disaccharide.

Miller–Abbott tube (*T. G. Miller, American physician, 1886– ; W. O. Abbott, American physician, 1902–43*). A double-channel intestinal tube for treating obstruction—especially that due to *paralytic ileus* of the small intestine. It has an inflatable balloon at its distal end.

milliampere (*mil-le-am'-pair*). 1/1000th of an ampere, the measurement of intensity of the electrical current.

millicurie (*mil-le-ku'-re*). The unit of radio-activity, i.e. the amount of radon which equals that of 1 mg of radium. *M. hour.* The action of one millicurie for one hour.

milliequivalent (*mil-e-e-quiv'-al-ent*). The amount of a substance that balances or is equivalent in combining power to 1 mg of hydrogen. A method of assessing the body's acid–base balance or needs during electrolyte upset.

milligram (*mil'-le-gram*). mg. 1/1000th of a gram. *See* Appendix 6.

millilitre (*mil'-le-le-ter*). ml. 1/1000th of a litre. *See* Appendix 6.

millimetre (*mil'-le-me-ter*). mm. 1/1000th of a metre. *See* Appendix 6.

Milroy's disease (*W. F. Milroy, American physician, 1855–1942*). A disease in which there is a congenital obstruction of the lymph channels in the legs.

Milton. A proprietary antiseptic consisting of a standardized 1 per cent solution of electrolytic sodium hypochlorite. It is used especially for the sterilization of babies' feeding bottles.

mineralocorticoids (*min-er-al-o-kor´-te-koids*). The steroids from the adrenal cortex that maintain the salt and water balance in the body.

miners' elbow. Swelling of the bursa over the olecranon process; due to pressure on the elbow whilst lying on the side.

miosis (*mi-o´-sis*). *Also* meiosis. Constriction of the pupil of the eye as to a bright light.

miotic (*mi-ot´-ik*). A drug which causes contraction of the pupil. Myotic.

miscarriage. Abortion (*q.v.*). The expulsion of the fetus before the 28th week of pregnancy, i.e. before it is legally viable.

mitochondria (*mi-to-kon´-dre-ah*). Bodies which occur in the cytoplasm of cells and are concerned with energy production and oxidation. *Sing.* mitochondrion.

mitosis (*mi-to´sis*). The usual method of multiplication of cells by a specific process of division.

mitral (*mi´-tral*). Shaped like a mitre. *M. incompetence.* A term applied to a defective mitral valve allowing a back flow or regurgitation when the valve is closed. *M. stenosis.* The formation of fibrous tissue causing a narrowing of the valve, usually due to rheumatic heart disease and endocarditis. *M. valve.* The bicuspid valve between the left atrium and left ventricle of the heart. *M. valvotomy.* An operation for overcoming stenosis by dividing the fibrous tissue to free the cusps.

mittelschmerz (*mit´-tel-shmer-tz*). Pain occurring in the period between the menses, accompanying ovulation.

ml. Abbreviation for millilitre. *See* Appendix 6.

MNS blood system. Minor blood group in which the antigens are described as M, N and S. In the English population 28 per cent have M; 22 per cent have N; and 50 per cent have S antigens.

modiolus (*mo-de-o´-lus*). The central pillar of the cochlea, around which the bony labyrinth winds.

Mogadon (*mog´-ad-on*) A proprietary preparation of nitrazepam. A hypnotic drug used to induce sleep. It is favoured for its safety and lack of side effects.

molar teeth (*mo´-lar*). The grinders, twelve in number, three on either side of each jaw.

molarity (*mo-lar´-it-e*) The term used to describe the concentration of a fluid. *See* Appendix 6.

mole. (1) A pigmented naevus or dark-coloured growth on the skin. They are of various sizes, and sometimes covered with hair. (2) A uterine tumour. *Carneous m.* The result of a missed abortion (*q.v.*). Organized blood clot surrounds a shrivelled fetus in the uterus. *Hydatidiform m.* (*vesicular m.*) A condition in pregnancy in which the chorionic villi of the placenta degenerate into clusters of cysts like hydatids (*q.v.*). Malignant growth is very likely to follow if any remnants are left in the uterus. *See* Chorion epithelioma. (3) The term used in the metric system to describe the molecular weight of a substance in grams. *See* Appendix 6.

molecule (*mol´-e-ku-l*). The chemical combination of two or more atoms which form a specific chemical substance, e.g. H_2O (water).

mollities ossium (*mol-lish'-e-eez os'-se-um*). Osteomalacia (*q.v.*).

molluscum (*mol-lus'-kum*). A class of skin diseases. *M. contagiosum.* A benign tumour arising in the epidermis caused by a virus, transmitted by direct contact or fomites. It is a round white elevation with a central dimple.

monarticular (*mon-ar-tik'-u-lah*). Referring to one joint only.

Mönckeberg's sclerosis (*J. G. Mönckeberg, German pathologist, 1877–1925*). Extensive degeneration, with atrophy and calcareous deposits in the middle muscle coat of arteries, especially the small ones.

Mongolian blue spots. Pigmentation of the skin found in the newborn of negroid and oriental origin. There is a bluish discoloration of the back which resembles a large bruise.

mongolism (*mon'-gol-izm*). Down's syndrome. A type of congenital mental subnormality. Associated with an extra chromosome. There is retarded mental and physical growth with characteristic facial appearance (resembling the mongolian races) and often congenital cardiac lesions are present.

Monilia (*mon-il'-e-ah*). Former name for the genus of fungi now known as *Candida* (*q.v.*).

monitoring (*mon'-it-or-ing*). Recording. *Patient m.* Electrodes or transducers are attached to the patient so information such as temperature, pulse, respiration, and blood pressure can be seen on a screen or automatically recorded.

Monitron (*mon'-it-ron*). An apparatus by which temperature, pulse, respiration, and systolic and diastolic blood pressures can be automatically recorded.

mono- (*mon'-o*). A prefix meaning 'single'.

monoamine oxidase (*mon-o-am' een oks'-e-daze*). An enzyme that breaks down noradrenaline and serotonin in the body. *M. o. inhibitors* (MAOI). Drugs that prevent the breakdown of serotonin and lead to an increase in mental and physical activity. Foods containing tyramine, such as cheese, Marmite, Bovril and broad beans, should be avoided as severe headache and hypertension occur.

monocular (*mon-ok'-u-lar*). Pertaining to, or affecting one eye only.

monocyte (*mon'-o-site*). A white blood cell having one nucleus, derived from the reticular cells, and having a phagocytic action.

mononucleosis (*mon-o-nu-kle-o'-sis*). *Infective m.* An infectious disease probably due to a virus, in which there is an increase of monocytes. Glandular fever.

monophasia (*mon-o-fa'-ze-ah*). Aphasia in which speech is limited to one word or phrase.

monoplegia (*mon-o-ple'-je-ah*). Paralysis of one limb or of a single muscle or group of muscles.

monorchid (*mon-or'-kid*). An individual with only one testicle.

monosaccharide (*mon-o-sak'-ar-ide*). A simple sugar. The end result of carbohydrate digestion. Examples are glucose, fructose and galactose.

monosomy (*mon-o-so'-me*). A congenital defect in the number of human chromosomes. There is one less than the normal 46.

Monro's foramen (*A. Monro,*

British anatomist and surgeon, 1733–1817). The communication between the lateral ventricles and third ventricles of the brain.

mons (*monz*). A prominence or mound. *M. pubis* or *m. veneris*. The eminence, consisting of a pad of fat, which lies over the os pubis in the female.

monster (*mon'-ster*). A maldevelopment of the fetus which results in a grossly abnormal individual.

Montgomery's glands or **tubercles** (*W. F. Montgomery, Irish obstetrician, 1797–1859*). Sebaceous glands around the nipple, which grow larger during pregnancy.

mood. Emotional reaction. A small swing between a serious or an elated mood is natural but in certain psychiatric conditions there is severe depression in some cases and wild excitement in others, or alternations between both.

moon face. One of the features occurring in Cushing's syndrome (*q.v.*) and as the result of prolonged treatment with steroid drugs.

Mooren's ulcer (*A. Mooren, German ophthalmologist, 1829–99*). A rare superficial ulcer of the cornea in elderly persons.

morbid (*mor'-bid*). Diseased, or relating to an abnormal or disordered condition.

morbidity (*mor-bid'-it-e*). The susceptibility of a population to a certain disease. Usually shown statistically as the number of cases which occur per thousand of population.

morbilliform (*mor-bil'-e-form*). A rash resembling that of measles.

Morgagni, hydatids of (*G. B. Morgagni, Italian anatomist and pathologist, 1682–1771*). Translucent cysts which develop at the fibrinated end of the fallopian tube in the female and in the epididymis in the male.

moribund (*mor'-ib-und*). In a dying condition.

Morison's pouch (*J. B. Morison, British surgeon, 1853–1939*). See Pouch.

morning sickness. Nausea and vomiting which occurs in pregnancy during the 4th to 16th week.

moron (*mor'-on*). A former term for persons suffering from severe subnormality of the mind.

morphine (*mor'-feen*). The principal alkaloid obtained from opium, and given hypodermically as a narcotic and analgesic.

morphology (*mor-fol'-o-je*). The study of the structure of organisms.

Moro reflex (*E. Moro, German paediatrician, 1874–1951*). The reaction to loud noise or sudden movement which should be present in the newborn. Startle reflex (*q.v.*). There is extension of the trunk and abduction of the arms and fingers and also, to a lesser degree, the legs. This is followed by a return to normal posture. The baby may cry at the same time.

mortality rate (*mor-tal'-it-e*). Death-rate. The ratio of the number of deaths to the total population.

mortification (*mor-tif-ik-a'-shun*). Gangrene or death of tissue.

morula (*mor'-u-lah*). An early stage of development of the ovum when it is a solid mass of cells.

mosaic (*mo-za'-ik*). An individual who has cells of varying genetic composition.

motile (*mo'-tile*). Capable of movement. With bacteria this may be inherent in the cell or by means of flagellae.

motion sickness (*mo'-shun sik'-ness*). Sickness occurring as the result of travel by land, sea or air. Appears to be caused by excessive stimulation of the vestibular apparatus.

motions. The evacuations of the bowels.

motivate (*mo'-te-vate*). To provide an incentive or purpose for a course of action.

motivation (*mo-te-va'-shun*). The reason or reasons, conscious or unconscious behind a particular attitude or behaviour.

motive (*mo'-tiv*). The incentives that determine a course of action or its direction.

motor end plate (*mo'-tor end plate*). The nuclei and cytoplasm of muscle fibres at the termination of motor nerves.

motor nerves. Those which convey an impulse from a nerve centre to a muscle or gland to promote activity.

motor neurone disease. A disease in which there is degeneration of the anterior cells in the spinal cord, the motor nuclei of cranial nerves and the corticospinal tracts. The cause is unknown.

mould (*mo-ld*). A species of fungus.

moulding (*mo'-ld-ing*). The compression of the infant's head as it is forced through the maternal passages during labour.

mountain sickness. Dyspnoea, headache, rapid pulse and vomiting, which occur on sudden change to the rarefied air of high altitudes.

movements (**fetal**). *See* Quickening.

moving beam radiotherapy. Method of radiotherapy in which the dose to the target tissue is increased whilst that to the skin is reduced.

mucilage (*mu'-sil-aj*). A solution of gum and water.

mucin (*mu'-sin*). The chief constituent of mucus.

mucocele (*mu'-ko-seel*). A mucous tumour. *M. of gall-bladder* occurs if a stone obstructs the cystic duct.

mucocutaneous (*mu-ko-ku-ta'-ne-us*). Pertaining to mucous membrane and skin.

mucoid (*mu'-koid*). Resembling mucus.

mucolysis (*mu-kol'-is-is*). The act of dissolving mucus.

mucolytics (*mu-ko-lit'-iks*). Drugs that have a mucus softening effect and so reduce the viscosity of the bronchial secretion.

mucopurulent (*mu-ko-pu'-ru-lent*). Containing mucus and pus.

mucosa (*mu-ko'-sah*). Mucous membrane.

mucous (*mu'-kus*). Pertaining to or secreting mucus. *M. membrane. See* Membrane.

mucoviscidosis (*mu-ko-vis-kid-o'-sis*). Fibrocystic disease of the pancreas. *See* Fibrocystic.

mucus (*mu'-kus*). The viscid secretion of mucous membranes.

müllerian ducts (*J. P. Müller, German physiologist, 1801–58*). A pair of ducts in the female fetus that develop into the uterine tube, uterus and vagina.

multigravida (*mul-te-grav'-id-ah*). Multipara (*q.v.*).

multilocular (*mul-te-lok'-u-lah*). Having many locules. *M. cyst. See* Cyst.

multinuclear (*mul-te-nu'-kle-ah*). A cell possessing many nuclei.

multipara (*mul-tip'-ar-ah*). A woman who has had more than one pregnancy. Multigravida.

mumps. Epidemic parotitis. A contagious disease common amongst children, and characterized by inflammation and swelling of the parotid glands. The symptoms are fever, and a painful swelling in front of the ears, making mastication difficult. *See* Infectious diseases.

muriatic acid (*mu-re-at'-ik*). Hydrochloric acid (*q.v.*).

murmur (*mer'-mer*). A blowing sound, heard on auscultation. *Aortic m.* Indicates disease of the aortic valve. *Diastolic m.* One heard after the second heart sound. *Friction m.* Present when two inflamed surfaces of serous membrane rub on each other. *Mitral m.* A sign of incompetence of the mitral valve. *Systolic m.* Heard during systole.

Murphy's sign (*J. B. Murphy, American surgeon, 1857–1916*). The sign which denotes inflammation of the gall-bladder. Continuous pressure over the organ will cause the patient to 'catch' his breath at the zenith of inspiration.

Musca domestica (*mus'-kah do-mes'-tik-ah*). The house fly.

muscae volitantes (*mus'-ke vol-e-tan'-tes*). Floating bodies in the vitreous humour which are visible to the patient.

muscarine (*mus'-kar-in*). A poisonous alkaloid found in certain fungi, and causing muscle paralysis.

muscle (*mus'-l*). Strong tissue composed of fibres which have the power of contraction, and thus produce movements of the body. *Cardiac m.* Partially striped interlocking cells but not under the control of the will. *Striped* or *striated m.* Voluntary muscle; transverse bands across the fibres give the characteristic appearance. It is under the control of the will. *Smooth* or *non-striated m.* Involuntary muscle of spindle-shaped cells contracts independently of the will, e.g. that of the intestinal wall.

muscular dystrophies (*mus-ku-lah dis'-tro-fes*). A number of inherited diseases in which there is progressive muscle wasting which leads to death in the second or third decade of life. *See* Duchenne muscular dystrophy.

musculocutaneous nerves (*mus'-ku-lo-ku-ta'-ne-us*). Those which supply the muscles and the skin.

musculoskeletal (*mus-ku-lo-skel'-e-tal*). Referring to both the osseus and muscular systems.

mustine hydrochloride (*mus'-teen hi-dro-klor'-ide*). Nitrogen mustard. A cytotoxic drug which may be given intravenously for malignant disease of lymph glands and reticuloendothelial cells, e.g. Hodgkin's disease.

mutation (*mu-ta'-shun*). A chemical change in the genes of a cell causing it to show a new characteristic. Some produce evolutional changes, others disease.

mute (*mewt*). Without the power of speech.

myalgia (*mi-al'-je-ah*). Pain in the muscles.

myasthenia (*mi-as-the'-ne-ah*). Muscle weakness. *M. gravis.* An extreme form of muscle weakness which is progressive. A rapid onset of fatigue, thought due to the too rapid destruction of acetylcholine at the neuromuscular junction. Commonly affected muscles are

231 MYO

those of vision, speaking, chewing and swallowing. Neostigmine injections are useful. Thymectomy has been curative in some cases.

mycetoma (*mi-se-to'-mah*). Madura foot. A fungus infection of the foot causing ulcers; a tropical disease.

Mycobacterium (*mi-ko-bak-te'-re-um*). Rod-shaped, acid-fast bacterium. *M. leprae*. The causative organism of leprosy. *M. tuberculosis*. The cause of tuberculosis.

mycosis (*mi-ko'-sis*). Any disease which is caused by a fungus. *See* Actinomycosis.

mydriasis (*mid-ri'-as-is*). Abnormal dilatation of the pupil of the eye.

mydriatics (*mid-re-at'-iks*). Drugs which cause mydriasis.

myectomy (*mi-ek'-to-me*). Excision of a portion of muscle.

myelin (*mi'-el-in*). The fatty covering of medullated nerve fibres.

myelitis (*mi-el-i'-tis*). Inflammation (1) of the marrow of the spinal cord; if affecting the grey matter it is called *poliomyelitis*. (2) of bone marrow. *See* Osteomyelitis.

myeloblast (*mi'-el-o-blast*). A primitive cell in the bone marrow from which develop the granular leucocytes.

myelocele (*mi'-el-o-seel*). Myelomeningocele. A hernia-like protrusion of the meninges containing a portion of the spinal cord. *See* Spina bifida.

myelocytes (*mi'-el-o-sites*). Cells of the bone marrow, derived from myeloblasts.

myelocytic leukaemia (*mi-el-o-sit'-ik lu-ke'-me-ah*). *See* Leukaemia.

myelogram (*mi'-el-o-gram*). Radiograph of the spinal cord.

myelography (*mi-el-og'-raf-e*). Radiographic examination of the spinal cord following the insertion of a radio-opaque substance into the subarachnoid space by means of lumbar puncture.

myeloid (*mi'-el-oid*). Resembling bone marrow or referring to the spinal cord. *M. leukaemia*. A malignant disease in which there is excessive production of leucocytes in the bone marrow.

myeloma (*mi-el-o'-mah*). A tumour in the medullary cavity of bone.

myelomatosis (*mi-el-o-mat-o'-sis*). Multiple myeloma.

myelomeningocele (*mi-el-o-men-in'-go-seel*). Meningomyelocele (*q.v.*).

myocarditis (*mi-o-kar-di'-tis*). Inflammation of the myocardium.

myocardium (*mi-o-kar'-de-um*). The muscle tissue of the heart.

myocele (*mi'-o-seel*) Protrusion of muscle through a rupture of its sheath.

myoclonus (*mi-o-klo'-nus*). Spasmodic contraction of muscle.

myofibrosis (*mi-o-fi-bro'-sis*). Fibrous tissue changes in a muscle. This may follow trauma where insufficient exercise impairs reabsorption of fibrin.

myogenic (*mi-o-jen'-ik*). Originating in muscle tissue. *M. contraction* of cardiac muscle is independent of nerve stimulus.

myoglobin (*mi-o-glo'-bin*). *See* Myohaemoglobin.

myohaemoglobin (*mi-o-he-mo-glo'-bin*). The haemoglobin present in muscle, having a lower molecular weight than blood haemoglobin. It colours muscle and transports oxygen.

myohaemoglobinuria (*mi-o-he-mo-glo-bin-u'-re-ah*). The presence of myohaemoglobin in the urine. It occurs in crush syndrome.

myoma (*mi-o'-mah*). A tumour of muscle tissue. *See* Fibromyoma.

myomectomy (*mi-o-mek'-to-me*). Removal of a myoma—usually referring to a uterine tumour.

myometritis (*mi-o-me-tri'-tis*). Inflammation of the myometrium.

myometrium (*mi-o-me'-tre-um*). The uterine muscle.

myoneural (*mi-o-nu'-ral*). Relating to both muscle and nerve. *M. junction.* Where nerve endings terminate in a muscle.

myopathy (*mi-op'-ath-e*). Muscular dystrophy. One of a group of hereditary degenerative diseases of muscle groups in which there is wasting and weakness.

myopia (*mi-o'-pe-ah*). Nearsightedness. The light rays focus in front of the retina and need a biconcave lens (*q.v.*) to focus them correctly.

myoplasty (*mi'-o-plas-te*). Any operation in which muscle is detached and utilized, as may be done to correct deformity.

myosarcoma (*mi-o-sar-ko'-mah*). A sarcomatous tumour in muscle.

myosin (*mi'-o-sin*). Muscle protein.

myositis (*mi-o-si'-tis*). Inflammation of a muscle. *M. ossificans.* A condition in which bone cells deposited in muscle continue to grow and cause hard lumps. It may occur after fractures, if passive movements are used. Active exercises only should be carried out.

myotics (*mi-ot'-iks*). Drugs which cause miosis and contract the pupil. Miotics.

myotonia (*mi-o-to'-ne-ah*). Lack of muscle tone. *M. congenita.* An hereditary disease in which the muscle action has a prolonged contraction phase and slow relaxation.

myotomy (*mi-ot'-o-me*). The division or dissection of a muscle.

myringa (*mir-ing-ah*). The ear drum or tympanic membrane.

myringitis (*mir-in-ji'-tis*). Inflammation of the tympanic membrane.

myringoplasty (*mir-ing'-o-plas-te*). A repair of perforation of the ear drum. This may be by a skin graft taken from the anterior meatal wall.

myringotome (*mir-ing'-o-tome*). An instrument for puncturing the tympanic membrane in myringotomy.

myringotomy (*mir-in-got'-o-me*). Incision of the tympanic membrane to drain pus from the middle ear.

myxoedema (*miks-e-de'-mah*). Hypothyroidism. A disease caused by atrophy of the thyroid gland. Marked by oedematous swelling of face, limbs, and hands; dry and rough skin; loss of hair; slow pulse; subnormal temperature; slowed metabolism; and mental dullness. It is treated with preparations of thyroid gland. *Congenital m.* Cretinism (*q.v.*).

myxoma (*miks-o'- mah*). A benign tumour arising from mucous membrane.

myxosarcoma (*miks-o-sar-ko'-mah*). A sarcoma containing mucoid tissue.

myxovirus (*miks'-o-vi-rus*). The group name of a number of related viruses including the causal viruses of influenza, para-influenza, mumps and Newcastle disease (of fowls).

N

N. Chemical symbol for nitrogen.

Naboth's follicle (*M. Naboth, German anatomist, 1675–1721*). Cystic swelling of a cervical gland as its duct has become blocked by regenerating squamous epithelium.

NaCl. Chemical symbol for sodium chloride (common salt).

NAD. Abbreviation meaning 'nothing abnormal diagnosed'.

naevus (*ne'-vus*). A birthmark; a circumscribed area of pigmentation of the skin due to dilated blood vessels. A haemangioma. *N. flammeus.* A flat bluish-red area usually on the neck or face; popularly known as 'port-wine stain'. *N. pilosus.* A hairy naevus. *Spider n.* A small red area surrounded by dilated capillaries. *Strawberry n.* A raised tumour-like structure of connective tissue containing spaces filled with blood.

nail. The keratinized portion of epidermis covering the dorsal extremity of the fingers and toes. *N. bed.* The area covered by a nail. *Hang n.* A strip of epidermis hanging at one side of a nail. *Ingrowing n.* Where the flesh overlaps the nail. *Spoon n.* A nail with depression in the centre and raised edges. Sometimes present in iron deficiency anaemia.

nalidixic acid (*nal-e-diks'-ik a'-sid*). Chemotherapeutic agent used in the treatment of urinary infections.

nalorphine (*nal-or'-feen*). An antidote for morphine, pethidine and methadone overdosage. It antagonizes respiratory depression. Lethidrone is a proprietary preparation of it.

nandrolone (*nan'-dro-lone*). An anabolic steroid that promotes protein metabolism and skeletal growth and has a masculinizing effect. Durabolin is a proprietary preparation.

nape. The back of the neck.

napkin rash. An erythematous rash which may occur in infants in the napkin area. Often caused by the passage of frequent loose stools containing fatty acids which cause breakdown of urea in the urine, producing ammonia which burns the skin. Treatment is by cleanliness of the skin, boracic acid dusting powder and exposure to the air. Alterations in the diet may be indicated.

narcissism (*nar-sis'-izm*). From the Greek legend. The stage of infant development when the child is mainly interested in himself and his own bodily needs.

narco- (*nar'-ko-*). A prefix denoting 'stupor'.

narcoanalysis (*nar-ko-an-al'-is-is*). A form of psychotherapy in which an injection of a barbiturate drug produces a drowsy, relaxed state during which a patient will talk more freely, and in this way much repressed material may be brought to consciousness. This may cause emotional stress. The interview may be terminated by giving more of the drug to produce a deep sleep.

narcolepsy (*nar'-ko-lep-se*). A condition in which there is an uncontrollable desire for sleep.

narcosis (*nar-ko'-sis*). A state of unconsciousness produced by a narcotic drug. *Basal n.* A state of unconsciousness produced prior to surgical anaesthesia. The drugs that may be used are avertin, paraldehyde or a barbiturate (not so commonly used now). *Continuous n.* A less frequently used form of treatment in which the patient is kept asleep for 2 or 3 weeks at a time. It may be used in cases of extreme excitement or agitation. The patient needs to be kept quiet and under constant observation but be rousable to eat and drink, and where he does not move himself, he must be regularly turned by the nurses.

narcosynthesis (*nar-ko-sin'-thes-is*). The inducement of an hypnotic state by means of drugs. An aid to psychotherapy.

narcotic (*nar-kot'-ik*). A drug that produces narcosis or unnatural sleep.

nares (*nar'-eez*). *Sing.* naris. The nostrils. *Posterior n.* The opening of the nares into the nasopharynx.

nasal (*na'-zal*). Pertaining to the nose.

nascent (*nas'-ent*). (1) At the time of birth. (2) Incipient.

nasogastric (*na-zo-gas'-trik*). Referring to the nose and stomach. *N. tube.* One passed into the stomach via the nose.

nasolacrimal (*na-zo-lak'-re-mal*). Concerning both nose and lacrimal apparatus. *N. duct.* The duct draining the tears from the inner aspect of the eye to the inferior meatus of the nose.

nasopharynx (*na-zo-far'-inks*). The upper part of the pharynx; that above the soft palate.

nasosinusitis (*na-zo-si-nu-si'-tis*). Inflammation of the nose and adjacent sinuses.

nates (*na'-teez*). The buttocks.

natural childbirth. A delivery which utilizes the minimum of medical attention.

nausea (*naw'-se-ah*). A sensation of sickness with inclination to vomit.

navel (*na'-vel*). The umbilicus.

navicular (*nav-ik'-u-lah*). One

of the tarsal bones of the foot. A former name for the scaphoid of the wrist.

nebula (*neb'-u-lah*). A slight opacity or cloudiness of the cornea.

nebulizer (*neb'-u-li-zer*). An apparatus for reducing a liquid to a fine spray.

neck (*nek*). (1) The narrow part of an organ or bone. *Anatomical n.* The constriction of the humerus just below the articulating surface. *Surgical n.* The narrowed part of the humerus between the shaft and the tuberosities. (2) The part of the body which connects the head and the trunk. *Derbyshire n.* Simple goitre. *Wry n.* Torticollis (*q.v.*).

necro- (*nek'-ro*). A prefix meaning 'dead'.

necrobiosis (*nek-ro-bi-o'-sis*). Localized death of a part as a result of degeneration.

necropsy (*nek-rop'-se*). Examination of a dead body. A post mortem.

necrosis (*nek-ro'-sis*). Death of a portion of tissue.

necrotomy (*ne-krot'-o-me*). An operation to remove a sequestrum.

needling (*need'-ling*). (1) Discission; the operation for cataract of lacerating and splitting up the lens so that it may be absorbed. (2) Capsulotomy. Tearing a hole in the remaining lens capsule after an extracapsular cataract extraction.

negative pole (*neg'-at-iv pole*). The pole or cathode that attracts the positive current and repels the negative current.

negativism (*neg'-a-tiv-izm*). A symptom of mental illness in which the patient does the opposite of what is required of him and so presents an uncooperative attitude. Common in schizophrenia.

Neisseria (*ni-ser'-e-ah*). Paired Gram-negative cocci. *N. gonorrhoeae*. The causative organism of gonorrhoea. *N. meningitidis*. The cause of meningococcal meningitis.

Nematoda (*nem-at-o'-dah*). A family of worms, including the *Ascaris* or roundworm and the *Oxyuris* or threadworm.

neo- (*ne'-o*). A prefix meaning 'new'.

neoarthrosis (*ne-o-ar-thro'-sis*). A false joint.

neocortex (*ne-o-kor'-teks*). The cerebral cortex excluding the hippocampal formation and piriform area.

neoglycogenesis (*ne-o-gli-ko-jen'-es-is*). The formation of liver glycogen from noncarbohydrate sources. Glyconeogenesis.

neologism (*ne-ol'-o-jizm*). The formation of new words, either a completely new one or a contraction of two separate words. This is done particularly by schizophrenic patients.

neomycin (*ne-o-mi'-cin*). An antibiotic drug of wide range that may be used to sterilize the gut or as an ointment against skin infections.

neonatal (*ne-o-na'-tal*). Referring to the first month of life. *N. mortality*. Death rate during this period as compared with the remaining 11 months of the first year. *N. ophthalmia*. *See* Ophthalmia.

neonate (*ne'-o-nate*) Term applied to a baby under one month old.

neoplasm (*ne'-o-plazm*). A morbid new growth. It may benign or malignant.

neostigmine (*ne-o-stig'-meen*) A synthetic preparation of physostigmine used in the treatment of myasthenia gravis and as an antidote to curare.

nephralgia (*nef-ral'-je-ah*). Pain in the kidney of neuralgic type. It may be due to tuberculosis or stone.

nephralgic crises (*nef-ral'-jik kri'-ses*). Spasms of pain in the lumbar region in tabes dorsalis.

nephrectomy (*nef-rek'-to-me*). Excision of a kidney.

nephritis (*nef-ri'-tis*). Inflammation of the kidneys (Bright's disease). *Acute glomerulo-n.* or *Ellis type I.* Thought to be due to hypersensitivity to toxins from the haemolytic streptococcus; there is oliguria and haematuria. *Subacute n., Ellis type II* or *hydraemic n.* Characterized by excessive albuminuria and massive oedema. Cause may be unknown or it may follow acute glomerulonephritis. *Chronic n.* or *azotaemic n.* The kidneys are fibrosed and contracted. It is associated with hypertension and gradually increasing uraemia. Treatment aims at general rest, warmth and low protein diet to rest the kidneys in the acute stage. Restriction of salt and water, and a high protein diet to replace loss in the subacute case. *Acute tubular n.* May be caused by damage to tubular cells by drugs, crush syndrome or incompatible blood transfusion. Treatment is by giving glucose and restricting protein or by using renal dialysis. *Embolic n.* Small emboli in the kidney cause haematuria.

nephro- (*nef'-ro*). Pertaining to the kidney.

nephroblastoma (*nef-ro-blas-to'-mah*). *See* Wilms' tumour.

nephrocalcinosis (*nef-ro-kal-sin-o'-sis*). A condition in which there is deposition of calcium in the renal tubules resulting in calculi formation and renal insufficiency.

nephrocapsulectomy (*nef-ro-kap-su-lek'-to-me*). Operation for removal of the capsule of the kidney.

nephrocele (*nef'-ro-seel.* Hernia of the kidney.

nephrogenic diabetes insipidus (*nef-ro-jen'-ik di-a-be'-teez in-sip'-id-dus*). An X-linked congenital disorder in which the renal tubules fail to respond to antidiuretic hormone, resulting in polydipsia and polyuria.

nephrolith (*nef'-ro-lith*). Stone in the kidney; renal calculus.

nephrolithotomy (*nef-ro-lith-ot'-o-me*). Removal of a renal calculus.

nephroma (*nef-ro'-mah*). Tumour of the kidney.

nephron (*nef'-ron*). A uriniferous tubule, consisting of Bowman's capsule the first and second convoluted tubule with the connecting loop of Henle, which opens into a collecting tubule. It is the essential structure for extraction of waste materials from the blood in the form of urine.

nephropathy (*nef-rop'-ath-e*). Any disease condition of the kidney substance.

nephropexy (*nef-ro-pek'-se*). The fixation of a floating (mobile) kidney, usually by sutures to neighbouring muscle.

nephroptosis (*nef-rop-to'-sis*). Downward displacement, or undue mobility, of kidney found on palpation.

nephropyeloplasty (*nef-ro-pi'-el-o-plast-te*). A plastic operation on the pelvis of the kidney.

nephropyosis (*nef-ro-pi-o'-sis*). Suppuration in the kidney.

nephrosclerosis (*nef-ro-skler-o'-sis*). Constriction of the ar-

terioles of the kidney. Seen in benign and malignant hypertension and in arteriosclerosis in old age.

nephrosis (*nef-ro'-sis*). Any disease of the kidney. Especially that which is characterized by oedema, albuminuria and a low plasma albumin. Caused by non-inflammatory degenerative lesions of the tubules.

nephrostomy (*nef-ros-to'-me*). Drainage of a kidney by passing a catheter at operation through the kidney substance.

nephrotic syndrome (*nef-rot'-ik*). A clinical syndrome in which there are albuminuria, low plasma protein, and gross oedema. Due to increased capillary permeability in the glomeruli. It may occur as a result of acute glomerulonephritis; in subacute nephritis, diabetes mellitus amyloid disease, systemic lupus erythematosus and renal vein thrombosis.

nephrotomy (*nef-rot'-o-me*). Incision of the kidney.

nephro-ureterectomy (*nef-ro-u-re-ter-ek'-to-me*). Removal of the kidney and the ureter.

nerve (*nerv*). A bundle of nerve fibres enclosed in a sheath called the epineurium. Its function is to transmit impulses between any part of the body and a nerve centre. *Sensory n.* (*afferent*) conveys sensations from an area to a nerve centre. *Motor n.* (*efferent*) conveys impulses causing activity from a nerve centre to a muscle or gland. *N. block.* A method of producing regional anaesthesia by injecting procaine into the nerves supplying the area to be operated on. *N. fibre.* The prolongation of the nerve cell, which conveys the impulse to or from the part which controls. *Vaso-*

motor n. Either dilator or constrictor to blood vessels to control the muscle wall. *See* Dorsal root.

nervous. Pertaining to, or composed of, nerves.

nervousness. Excitability of the nervous system, characterized by a state of mental and physical unrest.

nettle-rash. An irritating rash. Urticaria.

neural (*nu'-ral*). Pertaining to the nerves. *N. arch.* The bony arch on each vertebra which encloses the spinal cord.

neuralgia (*nu-ral'-je-ah*). Sharp stabbing pain, along the course of a nerve owing to neuritis or functional disturbance.

neurapraxia (*nu-rap-raks'-e-ah*). An injury to a nerve resulting in temporary loss of function and paralysis.

neurasthenia (*nu-ras-the'-ne-ah*). An outdated term for a state of general debility, both physical and mental.

neurectasis (*nu-rek'-tas-is*). The surgical operation of stretching a nerve.

neurectomy (*nu-rek'-to-me*). Excision of part of a nerve.

neurilemma (*nu-ril-em'-mah*). The membranous sheath surrounding a nerve-fibre.

neurinoma (*nu-rin-o'-mah*). An innocent tumour arising in the neurilemma of a nerve fibre. *Acoustic n.* This arises in the eighth cranial nerve.

neuritis (*nu-ri'-tis*). Inflammation of a nerve with pain, tenderness, and loss of function. *Multiple n.* That involving several nerves. Polyneuritis. *Nutritional n.* That which may be caused by alcoholism or lack of vitamin B complex. *Peripheral n.* That involving the terminations of nerves. *Sciatic n.* Scia-

tica (*q.v.*). *Optic n.* Of the optic nerve. Papilloedema. *Tabetic n.* A type occurring in tabes dorsalis. *Traumatic n.* That which results from an injury.

neuroblast (*nu'-ro-blast*). An embryonic nerve cell.

neuroblastoma (*nu-ro-blas-to'-mah*). A malignant tumour of immature nerve cells, most often arising in the very young.

neurodermatitis (*nu-ro-der-mat-i'-tis*). A localized prurigo of somatic and psychogenic origin. It irritates and rubbing causes thickening and pigmentation.

neuro-epithelioma (*nu-ro-ep-e-the-le-o'-mah*). A tumour of undifferentiated cells of nervous origin usually, but not always, occurring in the brain.

neurofibroma (*nu-ro-fi-bro'-mah*). An innocent tumour of nerve and fibrous tissue.

neurofibromatosis (*nu-ro-fi-bro-mat-o'-is*). Von Recklinghausen's disease. A generalized hereditary disease in which there are numerous tumours of the skin and nervous system.

neurogenic (*nu-ro-jen'-ik*). Derived from or caused by nerve stimulation. *N. shock. See* Shock.

neuroglia (*nu-rog'-le-ah*). The special form of connective tissue supporting nerve tissues.

neurohypophysis (*nu-ro-hi-pof'-is-is*). Posterior pituitary gland.

neurologist (*nu-rol'-o-jist*). One who is an expert in knowledge of diseases of nerves.

neurology (*nu-rol'-o-je*). The scientific study of the nervous system.

neuroma (*nu-ro'-mah*). A tumour of nerve tissue.

neuromuscular (*nu-ro-mus'-ku-lah*). Refers to the fine nerve endings which stimulate the contraction of muscle fibres. *N. junction*. The small gap between the end of the motor nerve and the motor endplate of the muscle fibre supplied. This gap is bridged by the release of acetylcholine whenever a nerve impulse arrives.

neuromyelitis optica (*nu-ro-mi-el-i'-tis op-tik-ah*). A disease in which there ia a bilateral optic neuritis and paraplegia. It may be a form of multiple sclerosis.

neurone (*nu'-ron*). A complete nerve cell, with its processes, including those which bring *afferent* impulses to it and those which convey *efferent* impulses from it. *Lower motor n.* The anterior horn cell and its neurone which conveys impulses to the appropriate muscles. Also known as the final common path. *Upper motor n.* That in which the cell is in the cerebral cortex and the fibres conduct impulses to associated cells in the spinal cord.

neuropathic (*nu-ro-path'-ik*). Relating to nervous disorder.

neuropathy (*nu-rop'-ath-e*). A disease process of nerve degeneration and loss of function. *Diabetic n.* That associated with diabetes. *Ischaemic n.* That caused by a lack of blood supply.

neuroplasty (*nu'-ro-plas-te*). Operation for transplantation of nerves.

neurorrhaphy (*nu-ror'-raf-e*). The operation of suturing a divided nerve.

neurosis (*nu-ro'-sis*). A mental disorder, which does not affect the whole personality, characterized by exaggerated anxiety and tension. *Anxiety n.* There is persistent anxiety and the accompanying symptoms of fear, rapid pulse, sweating, trembling, loss of appetite and insomnia. *Obsessive–compulsive n.* This is characterized by compulsions and rumination (*q.v.*). See Hysteria *and* Phobia.

neurosurgery (*nu-ro-sur'-jer-e*). That branch of surgery dealing with the brain, spinal cord and nerves.

neurosyphilis (*nu-ro-sif'-il-is*). A manifestation of third stage syphilis in which the nervous system is involved. The three commonest forms are: (1) Meningovascular syphilis affecting the blood vessels to the meninges. (2) Tabes dorsalis, *see* Ataxia. (3) General paralysis of the insane.

neurotic (*nu-rot'-ik*). A loosely applied adjective denoting association with neurosis.

neurotmesis (*nu-rot-me'-sis*). A severing of a nerve sheath and its fibres which may be partial or complete. The usual cause is a penetrating wound.

neurotomy (*nu-rot'-o-me*). The division of a nerve.

neurotoxic (*nu-ro-toks'-ik*). Poisonous or destructive to nervous tissue.

neurotripsy (*nu-ro-trip'-se*). Bruising or crushing a nerve.

neurotropic (*nu-ro-tro'-pik*). Having an affinity for nerve tissue. *N. viruses*. Those that particularly attack the nervous system.

neutral (*nu'-tral*). Neither acid nor alkaline.

neutropenia (*nu-tro-pe'-ne-ah*). A lack of neutrophils in the blood.

neutrophils (*nu'-tro-fils*). White blood cells which stain with neutral dyes.

new growth. Abnormal growth of tissue in type or location. *Malignant n. g.* Cancer (*q.v.*).

Newton (*Sir I. Newton, British scientist, 1642–1727*). The unit

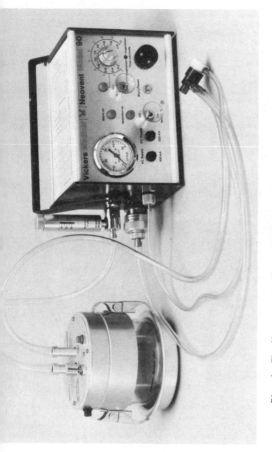

Plate I. The Neovent, a ventilator specifically designed to assist respiration in very young babies. (*By courtesy of Vickers Medical*)

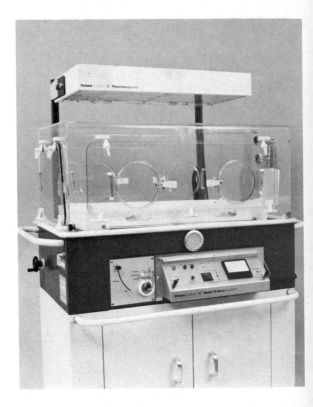

Plate II. An infant incubator provides continuous monitoring of the temperature of sick or premature babies and automatically alters the environmental temperature. The temperature of the baby is therefore maintained within finely controlled limits. (*By courtesy of Vickers Medical*)

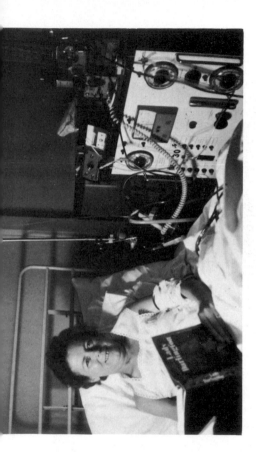

Plate III. A haemodialysis unit. Patients with renal failure are treated regularly on dialysis machines which perform the function normally undertaken by the kidney. The patients are taught to manage their own dialysis in hospital until they are capable of undertaking this in their own homes. (*By courtesy of Dr R. Gabriel, St Mary's Hospital, London*)

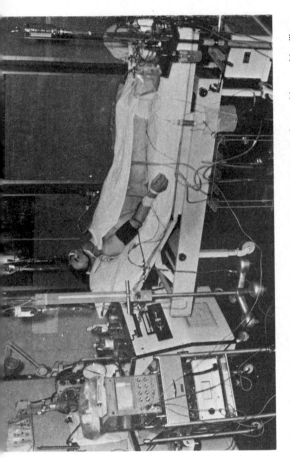

Plate IV. An intensive care unit. Patients who are critically ill as the result of an accident, sudden illness or major surgery are nursed in intensive care units where highly skilled staff and specialized equipment are available.

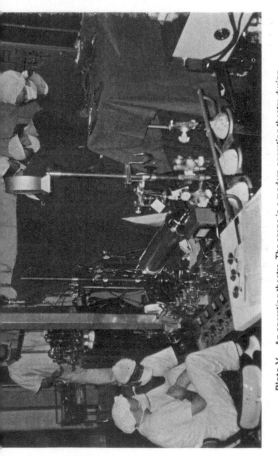

Plate V. An operating theatre. The scene in a modern operating theatre during a major operation.

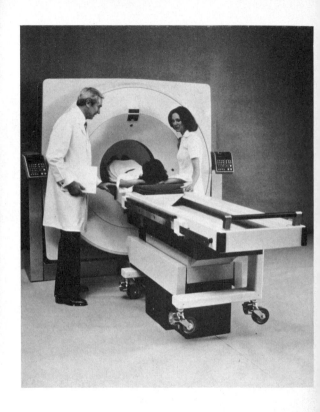

Plate VI. A whole-body scanner. This piece of modern equipment assists doctors to detect and diagnose disease at an early stage. The scanner takes X-ray photographs through sections of the body and produces its results with the aid of a computer. The scanner is able to penetrate tissues which previously could not be photographed. (*By courtesy of E.M.I. Medical Ltd*)

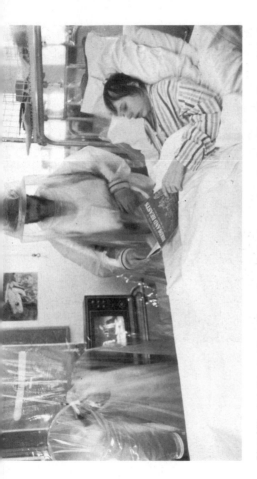

Plate VII. An isolator tent is used for nursing patients who are extremely vulnerable to infection or who have a very contagious disease. Direct contact with other people is prevented and all care is carried out by nurses wearing the suits which are incorporated into the sides of the tent. (*By courtesy of Dr R. L. Fowles, Royal Marsden Hospital*)

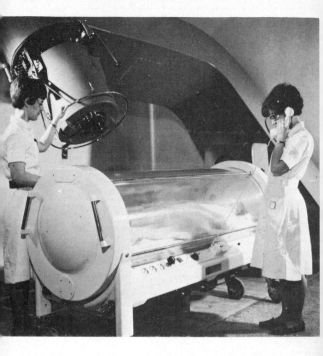

Plate VIII. A hyperbaric oxygen chamber. This chamber is used to administer oxygen under increased pressure. It has been successful in the treatment of patients with carbon monoxide poisoning, frostbite and gas gangrene. It is also used for patients undergoing radiotherapy, since the increased oxygen supply to the tumour renders it more susceptible to radiation. (*By courtesy of Vickers Medical*)

of force used in the Système International d'Unités. *See* Appendix 6.

niacin (*ni'-as-in*). Nicotinic acid (*q.v.*).

nicotine (*nik'-o-tin*). A poisonous alkaloid in tobacco.

nicotinic acid (*nik-o-tin'-ik as-id*). A factor found in vitamin B complex. *See* Appendix 10.

nictitation (*nik-tit-a'-shun*). The act of winking.

nidus (*ni'-dus*). A nest. A place in which an organism finds conditions suitable for its growth and development.

Niemann–Pick disease (*A. Niemann, German paediatrician, 1880–1921: F. Pick, German physician, 1868–1935*). Rare inherited disease in which there is lipoid storage abnormality and widespread deposition of lecithin in the tissues. Mental retardation is usual.

night-blindness (*nite blindnes*). Nyctalopia. Difficulty in seeing in the dark. This may be a congenital defect or a vitamin A deficiency.

night-sweat (*nite swet*). Profuse perspiration during sleep, especially typical of tuberculosis.

night-terrors (*nite ter'-ors*). Dreams causing acute fear.

nihilism (*ni'-hil-izm*). In psychiatry a term used to describe feelings of not existing and hopelessness, that all is lost or destroyed.

nikethamide (*nik-eth'-am-ide*). A cardiac and respiratory stimulant. Coramine is a proprietary preparation.

nipple (*nip'-pl*). The small conical projection in the centre of the breast. *Depressed n.* This should be drawn out during pregnancy, so that later the infant can suck. *Retracted n.* A sign of cancer of the breast.

Nissl granules (*F. Nissl, German neuropathologist, 1860–1919*). RNA-containing units found in the cytoplasm of cells. Probably associated with protein synthesis.

nit (*nit*). The egg of the head louse attached to the hair near the scalp.

nitrofurantoin (*ni-tro-fu-ran-to'-in*). A urinary antiseptic which is bacteriocidal and is effective against a wide range of organisms. Furadantin is a proprietary preparation of it.

nitrofurazone (*ni-tro-fu'-raz-one*). A local application used as an antibacterial agent for skin conditions. Furacin is a proprietary preparation.

nitrogen (*ni'-tro-jen*). A gaseous element of which air is largely composed, and the essential constituent of all protein foods.

nitrogen mustard hydrochloride (*ni'-tro-jen mus'-tard*). A cytotoxic drug. *See* Mustine hydrochloride.

nitroglycerin (*ni-tro-glis'-er-een*). Trinitrin. Glyceryl trinitrate. A drug which causes dilatation of the coronary arteries. In angina pectoris a tablet should be dissolved sublingually before exertion.

nitrous oxide (*ni'-trus oks'-ide*). N_2O. Laughing gas. A general anaesthetic ensuring a brief spell of unconsciousness, and used largely for dental operations. With oxygen it is extensively used as a light anaesthetic, but does not give sufficient muscle relaxation for abdominal operations unless combined with other drugs.

noci-association (*no'-se as-so-se-a'-shun*). The discharge of nervous energy which occurs unconsciously in trauma, as in surgical shock. *See* Anoci-association.

nocturia (*nok-tu'-re-ah*). The production of large quantities of urine at night.

nocturnal (*nok-tur'-nal*). Referring to the night. *N. enuresis.* Bed wetting. Incontinence of urine during sleep.

node. A swelling or protuberance. *Atrioventricular* (*auriculoventricular*) *n.* The specialized tissue between the right atrium and ventricle, at the point where the coronary vein enters the atrium, from which is initiated the impulse of contraction down the bundle of His. *Sinoatrial* (*sino-auricular*) *n.* The pacemaker of the heart. The specialized neuromuscular tissue at the junction of the superior vena cava and the right atrium, which, stimulated by the right vagus nerve, controls the rhythm of contraction in the heart. *N. of Ranvier.* A constriction occurring at intervals in a nerve fibre to enable the neurilemma with its blood supply to reach and nourish the axon of the nerve.

nodule (*nod'-ule*). A small swelling or protuberance.

noma (*no'-mah*). Cancrum oris (*q.v.*).

nomenclature (*no-men'-klature*). The terminology of a science; a classified system of names.

non compos mentis (*non kom'-pos men'-tis*). A person whose mental state is such that he is unable to manage his own affairs.

non-specific urethritis (*non-spes-if'-ik u-re-thri'-tis*). Venereal disease caused by a variety of organisms. Frequently seen in young men. *See* Urethritis.

noradrenaline (*nor-ad-ren'-al-een*). A hormone present in extracts of the suprarenal medulla. It causes vasoconstriction and raises both the systolic and diastolic blood pressure but does not stimulate general metabolism.

norethandrolone (*nor-eth-an'-dro-lone*). An anabolic steroid that aids in the utilization of protein. May be used to treat severe wasting and in osteoporosis.

norethisterone (*nor-eth-is'-ter-one*). An anabolic steroid. *See above.* Primolut N is a proprietary preparation.

normal (*nor'-mal*). Conforming to a standard; regular or usual. *N. flora.* Bacteria which normally live on body tissues and have a beneficial effect. *N. saline.* Isotonic (*q.v.*) solution of sodium chloride. *Syn.* Physiological (*q.v.*) solution.

normoblast (*nor'-mo-blast*). A nucleated red blood cell in bone marrow. *See* Erythrocyte.

normochromic (*nor-mo-kro'-mik*). When the haemoglobin level in the red blood corpuscle is within normal limits.

normoglycaemia (*nor-mo-glise'-me-ah*). When the blood sugar level is within the normal range.

normotension (*nor-mo-ten'-shun*). Normal tone, tension or pressure. Usually used in relation to blood pressure.

normovolaemic shock (*nor-mo-vol-e'-mik*). A state of shock in which the blood volume is normal. Coronary thrombosis is an example.

nose. The organ of smell and of respiration.

nosology (*nos-ol'-o-je*). The scientific classification of diseases.

nostalgia (*nos-tal'-je-ah*). Home-sickness.

nostril (*nos'-tril*). One of the anterior orifices of the nose.

notifiable (*no-te-fi'-ab-l*). A term applied to such diseases as must be reported to the Medical Officer of Health. These include measles, scarlet fever, typhus and typhoid fever, cholera, smallpox, diphtheria and tuberculosis.

novobiocin (*nov-o-bi'-o-sin*). A wide-range oral antibiotic that is effective against *Proteus* organisms.

noxious (*nok'-she-us*). Harmful. The term may be applied to drugs or other substances liable to cause injury.

nucha (*nu'-kah*). The nape of the neck.

nuclear (*nu'-kle-ar*). Pertaining to a nucleus. *N. pacemaker.* An artificial heart pacemaker which derives its energy from nuclear power. It requires changing much less frequently than a battery-powered pacemaker.

nucleic acids (*nu'-kle-ik as-ids*). Purine and pyrimidine compounds found in deoxyribonucleic acid and ribonucleic acid.

nucleolus (*nu-kle'-o-lus*). Small dense body in the cell nucleus which contains ribonucleic acid. Its function is still obscure, but it disappears during mitosis (*q.v.*).

nucleoproteins (*nu'-kle-o-pro'-teens*). Constituents of cell nuclei from which purines are derived.

nucleotide (*nu'-kle-o-tide*). Compound formed from pentose sugar, phosphoric acid and a nitrogen-containing base.

nucleus (*nu'-kle-us*). (1) The essential part of a cell, governing nutrition and reproduction, its division being essential for the formation of new cells. (2) A group of nerve cells in the central nervous system. *Caudate n., lenticular n.* are part of the basal ganglia (*q.v.*). *N. pulposus.* The jelly-like centre of an intervertebral (*q.v.*) disc, which may prolapse and cause pressure upon one of the spinal nerve roots; most commonly the sciatic.

nullipara (*nul-ip'-ar-ah*). A woman who has never given birth to a child.

nutation (*nu-ta'-shun*). Uncontrollable nodding of the head.

nutmeg liver. *See* Liver.

nutrition (*nu-trish'-un*). The process by which food is assimilated into the body in order to nourish it.

nutritional disease (*nu-trish'-un-al*). One that is due to the continued absence of a necessary food factor.

nux vomica (*nuks vom'-ik-ah*). The seed of an East Indian tree, from which strychnine (*q.v.*) is derived. In small doses it is a tonic.

nyctalgia (*nik-tal'-je-ah*). Pain occurring during the night.

nyctalopia (*nik-tal-o'-pe-ah*). Night blindness. Defective vision in a dim light especially due to deficiency of vitamin A. *See* Appendix 10.

nycturia (*nik-tu'-re-ah*). Incontinence of urine at night or excessive production of urine.

nymphae (*nim'-fe*). The labia minora. *See* Labia.

nymphomania (*nim-fo-ma'-ne-ah*). Excessive sexual desire in a woman.

nystagmus (*nis-tag'-mus*). An involuntary, rapid movement of the eyeball. It may be hereditary, result from disease of the semi-circular canals or of the central nervous system. It can occur from visual defect or be associated with other muscle spasms. *Miner's n.* An occupational form.

nystatin (*ni'-stat-in*). An antibiotic drug particularly useful in treating thrush and moniliasis of the vagina.

O

O. Chemical symbol for oxygen.

obesity (*o-be'-sit-e*). Corpulence; excessive development of fat throughout the body.

objective signs (*ob-jek-tiv sines*). Those which the observer notes, as distinct from symptoms of which the patient complains (*subjective*).

oblique muscles (*o-bleek' mus'-ls*). (1) A set of muscles which assist in movement of the eye. (2) Muscles found in the wall of the abdomen.

obsession (*ob-ses'-shun*). An idea which persistently recurs to an individual although he resists it and regards it as being senseless. A compulsive thought. *See* Compulsion.

obsessive neurosis. *See* Neurosis.

obstetrician (*ob-stet-rish'-un*). One who is trained and specializes in obstetrics.

obstetrics (*ob-stet'-riks*). The branch of medicine dealing with pregnancy and labour.

obturator (*ob'-tur-a-tor*). That which closes an opening. *O. foramen.* The large hole in the os innominatum closed by fascia and muscle.

obtusion (*ob-tu'-shun*). Weakening or blunting of normal sensations, a condition produced by certain diseases.

occipital (*ok-sip'-it-al*). Relating to the occiput.

occipito-anterior (*ok-sip'-it-o an-te'-re-or*). When the back of the head is to the front of the pelvis as the child's head comes through the birth canal. *Occipito-posterior* is the reverse position.

occiput (*ok'-sip-ut*). The back of the head.

occlusion (*ok-klu'-shun*). Closure, applied particularly to alignment of the teeth in the jaws, or the lumen of a blood vessel.

occlusive therapy (*ok-klu-siv ther'-ap-e*). A form of treatment used for children with strabismus (squint). They are encouraged to use the affected eye by having the healthy one covered. (2) A method of treatment used in certain skin conditions.

occult blood. A term applied to blood excreted in the stools in such small quantity as to require chemical tests to detect.

occupational disease (*ok-ku-pa'-shun-al dis-eez'*). One due to the nature of one's work. Industrial disease.

occupational therapy (*ok-ku-pa'-shun-al ther'-ap-e*). *See* Therapy.

ocular (*ok'-u-lar*). Relating to the eye.

oculogyric (*ok-u-lo-ji'-rik*). Causing movements of the eyeballs.

oculentum (*ok-u-len'-tum*). An eye ointment.

oculomotor (*ok-u-lo-mo'-tor*). Relating to movements of the eye. *O. nerves.* The third pair of cranial nerves which control the eye muscles.

Oddi, sphincter of (*R. Oddi 19th century Italian physician*). The muscular sphincter situated at the junction of the common bile duct and the pancreatic duct.

odontalgia (*o-don-tal'-je-ah*). Toothache.

odontoid (*o-don'-toid*). Resembling a tooth. *O. process*. A projection from the axis vertebra upon which the head rotates.

odontolith (*o-don'-to-lith*). Tartar, the calcareous matter deposited upon teeth.

odontology (*o-don-tol'-o-je*). The science of treating teeth. Dentistry.

odontoma (*o-don-to'-mah*). A tumour of tooth structures.

odontoprisis (*o-don-to-pri'-sis*). Grinding of the teeth.

-odynia (*o-din'-e-ah*). Suffix meaning 'pain'.

oedema (*e-de'-mah*). Dropsy. An effusion of fluid into the tissues. If the finger is pressed upon an affected part, the surface pits and regains slowly its original contour. *Cardiac o*. That due to heart failure. *Famine o*. Due to diet deficiency. *Lymphatic o*. That due to blockage of the lymph vessels. *Pulmonary o*. Effusion of fluid into the alveoli and tissues between them. A serious cause of cyanosis. *See* Pulmonary. *Renal o*. That occurring in nephritis. *Venous o*. Fluid due to obstruction in veins.

Oedipus complex (*e'-dip-us*). From Greek mythology. The exaggerated affection of a son for his mother, with hostility towards the father. It is a normal stage in the early development of the child, but may become fixed or a complex if the child cannot solve the conflict during the early years or during adolescence.

oesophageal (*e-sof-aj-e'-al*). Pertaining to the oesophagus. *O. atresia*. A congenital abnormality in which the oesophagus is not continuous between the pharynx and the stomach. May be associated with a fistula into the trachea.

oesophagectasis (*e-sof-aj-ekt'-as-is*). Dilatation of the oesophagus.

oesophagitis (*e-sof-aj-i'-tis*). Inflammation of the oesophagus. *Reflux o*. That caused by regurgitation of acid stomach contents through the cardiac sphincter.

oesophagojejunostomy (*e-sof'-ag-o-je-ju-nos'-to-me*). An anastomosis of the jejunum with the oesophagus following a total gastrectomy.

oesophagoscope (*e-sof'-ag-o-skope*). An instrument for viewing the inside of the oesophagus.

oesophagoscopy (*e-sof-ag-os'-ko-pe*). An examination carried out with an oesophagoscope.

oesophagotomy (*e-sof-ag-ot'-o-me*). Incision of the oesophagus.

oesophagus (*e-sof'-ag-us*). The canal which extends from the pharynx to the stomach. It is about 23 cm (9 in) long.

oestradiol (*e-stra'-de-ol*). The chief naturally occurring oestrogen in the ovary and can be chemically prepared and is marketed in different forms, *e.g. o. benzoate or ethinyl o*.

oestrin (*e'-strin*). A general term to describe the endocrine secretion of the graafian follicle. *See* Oestrogens.

oestrogens (*e'-stro-jens*). Hormones that have the same action as oestradiol, and though largely produced in the ovary, can also be extracted from the placenta, adrenal cortex, and the testis.

ohm (*G. S. Ohm, German physicist, 1787–1854*). The unit of electrical resistance.

Oidium albicans (*o-id'-e-um al'-be-kans*). The former term for *Candida albicans* which causes thrush or moniliasis.

ointment (*oint'-ment*). An external application with a base of lard, lanolin or petroleum jelly in which the remedy is incorporated.

olecranon (*o-lek'-ran-on*). The curved process of the ulna which forms the point of the elbow.

oleum (*o'-le-um*). Oil. *O. morrhuae.* Cod-liver oil. *O. ricini.* Castor oil.

olfactory (*ol-fak'-tor-e*). Relating to the sense of smell. *O. nerves.* The first pair of cranial nerves; those of smell.

oligaemia (*ol-ig-e'-me-ah*). Deficient quantity of blood.

oligocythaemia (*ol-ig-o-si-the'-me-ah*). Blood cell deficiency.

oligohydramnios (*ol-ig-o-hi-dram'-ne-os*). Deficiency in the amount of amniotic fluid.

oligomenorrhoea (*ol-ig-o-men-or-e'-ah*). A diminished flow at the menstrual period. Scanty menstruation.

oligophrenia (*ol-ig-o-fre'-ne-ah*). Mental subnormality. The condition may be congenital or due to disease or injury. *Phenylpyruvic o.* An hereditary abnormality associated with an excessive excretion of phenylpyruvic acid (*q.v.*).

oligospermia (*ol-ig-o-sper'-me-ah*). A diminished output of sperm. Production may be stimulated by testosterone.

oliguria (*ol-ig-u'-re-ah*). Deficient secretion of urine.

olivary (*ol'-iv-ar-e*). Like an olive in shape. *O. body.* A mass of grey matter situated behind the anterior pyramid of the medulla oblongata.

olive oil. A vegetable oil used as a food and intestinal lubricant. *O. o. enema.* Given to soften faeces after rectal or perineal operations, or for obstinate constipation.

omentopexy (*o-men'-to-peks-e*). Fixation of the omentum. *Cardio-o.* The omentum may be attached to the heart to establish a collateral circulation when there is coronary occlusion.

omentum (*o-men'-tum*). A fold of peritoneum. *Greater o.* Reflected from the greater curvature of the stomach and lying in front of the intestines. *Lesser o.* Reflected from the lesser curvature and attaching the stomach to the under surface of the liver.

omphalitis (*om-fal-i'-tis*). Inflammation of the umbilicus.

omphalocele (*om'-fal-o-seel*). Umbilical hernia.

omphaloproptosis (*om-fal-o-prop-to'-sis*). Excessive protrusion of the umbilicus.

omphalus (*om'-phal-us*). The umbilicus.

Onchocerca volvulus (*on-ko-ser'-kah vol'-vu-lus*). A filarial worm that may give rise to skin and subcutaneous lesions and attack the eye.

onchocerciasis (*on-ko-ser-ki'-as-is*). A filariasis caused by *Onchocerca volvulus.*

oncogenic (*on-ko-jen'-ik*). Giving rise to tumour formation.

oncology (*on-kol'-o-je*). The scientific study of tumours.

oncometer (*on-kom'-e-ter*). An instrument for measuring the size of the spleen, kidneys and other organs. *See* Plethysmography.

onychia (*on-ik'-e-ah*). Inflammation of the matrix of a nail, with suppuration, which may cause the nail to fall off.

onychogryphosis (*on-ik-o-gri-fo'-sis*). Enlargement of the nails, with excessive curvature, most commonly affecting the big toes.

onychomycosis (*on-ik-o-mi-ko'-sis*). Infection of the nails by fungi. Ringworm of the nails.

onychosis (*on-ik-o'-sis*). Deformity of the nails or of a nail.

oöcyte (*o'-o-site*). The immature egg cell or ovum in the ovary.

oögenesis (*o-o-jen'-e-sis*). The development and production of the ovum.

oöphoralgia (*o-off-or-al'-je-ah*). Pain in the ovary.

oöphorectomy (*o-off-or-ek'-to-me*). Excision of an ovary.

oöphoritis (*o-off-or-i'-tis*). Inflammation of an ovary.

oöphoron (*o-off'-or-on*). The ovary (*q.v.*).

oöphorosalpingectomy (*o-off'-or-o-sal-pin-jek-to-me*). Removal of the ovary and its associated fallopian tube.

opacity (*o-pas'-it-e*). Cloudiness, lack of transparency.

open fracture. *See* Fracture.

operant conditioning (*op'-er-ant con-dish'-un-ing*). A form of behaviour therapy in which a reward is given when the subject performs the action required of him. The reward serves to encourage repetition of the action.

operation (*op-er-a'-shun*). A surgical procedure in which instruments or hands are used by the operator. *Avascular o.* One in which there is little or no bleeding achieved by applying an Esmarch's bandage from the extremity upwards on an elevated limb or by the use of drugs causing hypotension. *Magnet o.* The removal of a foreign body from the eye by means of a magnet. *Palliative o.* Relieves symptoms, but does not cure, e.g. gastroenterostomy in carcinoma of the pylorus.

ophthalmia (*off-thal'-me-ah*). Inflammation of the eye, involving especially the conjunctiva. *Gonorrhoeal o.* or *o. neonatorum.* A serious infection caused by *Neisseria gonorrhoea. Granular o.* An acute and purulent form when there is a gritty feeling on moving the eyelids. *Phlyctenular o. See* Conjunctivitis. *Purulent o.* When the discharge is pus. *See* Trachoma.

ophthalmic (*off-thal'-mik*). Relating to the eye.

ophthalmitis (*off-thal-mi'-tis*). Inflammation of the eyeball. *Sympathetic o.* A serious complication in the sound eye following a perforating wound in the opposite eye.

ophthalmologist (*off-thal-mol'-o-jist*). A specialist in diseases of the eye.

ophthalmology (*off-thal-mol'-o-je*). The study of the eye and its diseases.

ophthalmometer (*off-thal-mom'-e-ter*). An instrument for accurately measuring corneal astigmatism.

ophthalmometry (*off-thal-mom'-e-tre*). The use of the ophthalmometer.

ophthalmoplegia (*off-thal-mo-ple'-je-ah*). Paralysis of the muscles of the eye.

ophthalmoscope (*off-thal'-mo-skope*). An instrument fitted with a battery, light and lenses by which the retina of the eye can be illuminated and examined.

ophthalmoscopy (*off-thal-mos'-ko-pe*). The examination of the eye by the aid of an ophthalmoscope.

ophthalmotomy (*off-thal-mot'-o-me*). Incision into the eye.

ophthalmotonometer (*off-thal'-mo-ton-om'-e-ter*). An instrument for measuring the intraocular tension of the eye.

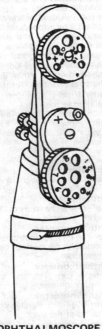

OPHTHALMOSCOPE

duces deep sleep, slows the pulse and respiration, contracts the pupils and checks all secretions of the body except sweat. *Alkaloids of o.* Morphine, codeine, papaverine, etc. *Tincture of o.* Laudanum.

opponens (*op-po'-nens*). Opposing. Adductor muscles of the fingers and toes. *O. pollicis.* Adducts the thumb so that it and the little finger can be brought together.

opsin (*op-sin*). A protein which combines with vitamin A aldehyde to form rhodopsin (visual purple) in the eye.

opsonic index (*op-son'-ik*). A measurement of the bactericidal power of phagocytes.

opsonins (*op'-son-ins*). Substances present in the blood which render bacteria more eas-

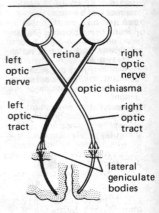

left retina right
optic optic
nerve nerve
optic chiasma
left right
optic optic
tract tract

lateral
geniculate
bodies

visual centres in
occipital lobes
of brain

OPTIC CHIASMA

opiate (*o'-pe-ate*). Any medicine containing opium.

opisthotonos (*op-is-thot'-on-os*). A muscle spasm causing the back to be arched and the head retracted, with great rigidity of the muscles of the neck and back. This condition may be present in acute cases of meningitis, tetanus, and strychnine poisoning.

opium (*o'-pe-um*). A drug derived from dried poppy-juice and used as a narcotic. It pro-

ily destroyed by the phagocytes. Each kind of bacteria has its specific opsonin.

optic (*op'-tik*). Relating to vision. *O. atrophy.* Degeneration of the optic nerve. *O. chiasma.* The crossing of the fibres of the optic nerves at the base of the brain. *O. disc.* Where the optic nerve enters the eyeball.

optical density (*op'-tik-al den'-si-te*). The refractive power of the transparent tissues through which light rays pass, changing the direction of the ray.

optician (*op-tish'-an*). One who makes and fits spectacles.

optimum (*op'-te-mum*). Most favourable.

optometry (*op-tom'-et-re*). The measuring of visual acuity and the fitting of glasses to correct visual defects.

oral (*or'-al*). Relating to the mouth. *O. eroticism.* Oral gratification which the infant gains from sucking and exploring objects with his mouth. It is still in evidence in later life in the pleasure derived from eating, gum-chewing, smoking and kissing.

Orbenin (*or-ben'-in*). A proprietary preparation of cloxacillin (*q.v.*).

orbicular (*or-bik'-u-lar*). Circular.

orbit (*or'-bit*). The bony cavity containing the eyeball.

orchidectomy (*or-kid-ek'-to-me*). Excision of a testicle.

orchidopexy (*or'-kid-o-pek-se*). An operation to free an undescended testicle and place it in the scrotum.

orchiepididymitis (*or-ke-ep-e-did-e-mi'-tis*). Inflammation of testicle and epididymis.

orchis (*or'-kis*). The testicle.

orchitis (*or-ki'-tis*). Inflammation of a testicle.

orf (*orf*). A virus infection transmitted from sheep to man. It may give rise to a boil-like lesion on the hands of meat handlers.

organ. A part of the body designed to perform a particular function. *End o.* The termination of nerve fibres. *O. of Corti.* The sensitive nerve terminals in the internal ear.

organic (*or-gan'-ik*). Pertaining to the organs. *O. disease* is of an organ and accompanied by structural changes.

organism (*or'-gan-izm*). An individual living being, animal or vegetable.

orgasm (*org'-azm*). The climax in sexual intercourse.

oriental sore (*or-e-en'-tal*). *See* Furunculus.

orientation (*or-e-en-ta'-shun*). A sense of direction. The ability of a person to estimate his position in regard to time, place and persons. Imparting relevant information at the onset of a course or conference so that its content and objects may be understood.

orifice (*or'-e-fis*). Any opening in the body.

ornithosis (*or-nith-o'-sis*). A newer term for psittacosis (*q.v.*) as it has been found the virus may be transmitted by a wider group of birds.

orogenital syndrome (*or-o-jen'-it-al sin'-drome*). A syndrome characterized by stomatitis, glossitis, cheilitis and an eczematous eruption around the genitalia. Caused by riboflavine deficiency.

oropharynx (*or-o-far'-inks*). The lower portion of the pharynx behind the mouth and above the oesophagus and larynx.

ortho (*or'-tho*). A prefix meaning 'straight'.

orthodontics (*or-tho-don'-tiks*). Dentistry which deals with the prevention and correction of irregularities of the teeth.

orthopaedic (*or-tho-pe'-dik*). Relating to the correction of deformities of bone.

orthopnoea (*or-thop-ne'-ah*). Difficulty in breathing unless in an upright position, i.e. sitting up in bed.

orthoptic (*or-thop'-tik*). Relating to correction of oblique vision (squint).

orthostatic (*or-tho-stat'-ik*). Standing erect. *O. albuminuria. See* Albuminuria.

Ortolani's sign (*M. Ortolani, contemporary Italian orthopaedic surgeon*). A test performed soon after birth to detect possible congenital dislocation of the hip. A 'click' is felt on reversing the movements of abduction and rotation of the hip while the child is lying with knees flexed.

os. (1) A bone: *O. calcis.* The heel-bone or calcaneum. (2) A mouth or opening. *External o.* The opening of the cervix into the vagina. *Internal o.* The junction of the cervical canal and body of the uterus.

oscheocele (*os'-ke-o-seel*). Scrotal hernia or swelling.

oscillation (*os-sil-a'-shun*). A swinging or tremulous motion.

oscilloscope (*os'-sil-o-skope*). An instrument that indicates when an electrical current is passed through it.

Osler's nodes (*Sir W. Osler, Canadian physician, 1849–1919*). Small painful swellings which occur in or beneath the skin, especially of the extremities in subacute bacterial endocarditis, caused by minute emboli. They usually disappear in 1–3 days.

osmolality (*oz-mo-lal'-it-e*). The osmotic concentration of a fluid obtained by estimating the depression of freezing point of the water caused by the constituents contained therein.

osmole (*oz-mole*). Unit for measuring the ability of dissolved substances to cause osmosis and osmotic pressure. It is equal to the molecular weight of the constituents in grams divided by the number of ions into which the molecule dissociated.

osmoreceptors (*oz-mo-re-sep'-tors*). Specialized nerve cells located in the internal carotid arteries which monitor the osmotic pressure of the blood and the extracellular fluid. Impulses from these receptors are relayed to the hypothalamus.

osmosis (*oz-mo'-sis*). The diffusion of fluids through a semipermeable membrane.

osmotic pressure (*oz-mo'-tic pre'-shur*). Pressure exerted by large molecules in the blood, e.g. albumen and globulin proteins, which draws fluid into the bloodstream from the surrounding tissues.

osseous (*os'-se-us*). Bony.

ossicle (*os'-sik-l*). A small bone. *Auditory o.* Those of the middle ear: the malleus, incus, and stapes.

ossification (*os-sif-ik-a'-shun*). The formation of bone.

ostalgia (*os-tal'-je-ah*). Pain in a bone.

osteitis (*os-te-i'-tis*). Inflammation of bone. *O. deformans. See* Paget's disease. *O. fibrosa cystica* or *parathyroid o.* Defects of ossification, with fibrous tissue production, leading to weakening and deformity. It affects children chiefly, and is associated with parathyroid tumour, removal of which checks it. *See* von Recklinghausen's disease.

osteo-arthritis (*os-te-o-ar-thri'-tis*). A form of arthritis in which there is destruction of articular cartilage and bony outgrowths at the edges of joints. A painful disease of the elderly, occurring in the larger joints where most weight is carried.

osteo-arthrotomy (*os-te-o-ar-throt'-o-me*). Excision of the jointed end of a bone.

osteoblasts (*os'-te-o-blasts*). Bone-forming cells that aid in growth and repair and the deposition of calcium.

osteochondritis (*os-te-o-kondri'-tis*). A non-inflammatory disease of the epiphysis causing pain and deformity. When occurring in the hip it is termed *Perthes' disease*; in the tarsal scaphoid bone—*Köhler's disease*; in the tibial tubercle—*Schlatter's disease*.

osteochondroma (*os-te-o-kon-dro'-mah*). A new growth arising from both bone and cartilage.

osteoclasis (*os-te-o-kla'-sis*). The manual fracture of bones to correct a deformity such as bow-legs.

osteoclasts (*os'-te-o-klasts*). (1) Large bone cells that absorb and remove bone tissue and callus. (2) Instruments designed for surgical fracture of bone.

osteocyte (*os'-te-o-site*). A bone cell.

osteo-ectomy (*os-te-o-ek'-to-me*). Excision of bone.

osteogenesis (*os-te-o-jen'-e-sis*). The formation of bone. *O. imperfecta cystica*. X-ray examination shows cystic spaces in the bone. Due to over-secretion of the parathyroids causing decalcification of the bones and a high blood calcium.

osteogenic (*os-te-o-jen'-ik*). Originating in or derived from bone. *O. sarcoma*. A malignant growth of bone.

osteoma (*os-te-o'-mah*). An innocent new growth arising in a bone-forming cell or osteoblast.

osteomalacia (*os-te-o-mal-a'-se-ah*). A disease characterized by painful softening of bones. Due to vitamin D deficiency.

osteomyelitis (*os-te-o-mi-el-i'-tis*). Inflammation of the bone and marrow. *Acute o.* Commonly occurs in children due to a blood-borne staphylococcal infection. The vascular edge of the epiphyseal cartilage is first attacked. *Chronic o.* Can result from an acute attack or from an open fracture.

osteopath (*os'-te-o-path*). One who practises bone manipulation and treats bone conditions. Often medically unqualified.

osteopathic back (*os-te-o-path'-ik*). A term used to describe acute pain and muscle spasm following displacement of one of the small facet type joints of the spine.

osteopathy (*os-te-op'-ath-e*). Any bone disease. Also commonly used for the treatment of disease by manipulation of bones.

osteoperiostitis (*os'-te-o-per-e-os-ti'-tis*). Inflammation of bone and periosteum.

osteophony (*os-te-off'-on-e*). Conduction of sound by bone.

osteophyte (*os'-te-o-fite*). A small outgrowth of bone.

osteoplasty (*os'-te-o-plas-te*). Plastic operations on bone.

osteoporosis (*os-te-o-por-o'-sis*). Rarefaction of bone. The bones are lacking in mineral salts due to deficiency of bony matrix. This may be due to protein or hormone insufficiency.

osteosarcoma (os-te-o-sar-ko'-mah). A sarcoma in bone.

osteotome (os'-te-o-tome). A surgical instrument for cutting bone.

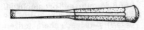

OSTEOTOME

osteotomy (os-te-ot'-o-me). The cutting of bone, usually performed to correct deformity. *O. of hip.* A method of treating osteo-arthritis by cutting the bone and altering the line of weight-bearing.

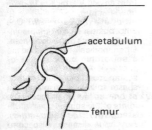

OSTEOTOMY OF HIP

ostium (os'-te-um). A mouth. *Abdominal o.* The opening at the end of the fallopian tube into the peritoneal cavity.

otalgia (o-tal'-je-ah). Ear-ache.

otic (o'-tik) Relating to the ear.

otitis (o-ti'-tis). Inflammation of the ear. *O. media.* Middle-ear disease.

otolaryngology (o-to-lar-in-gol'-o-je). The scientific study of the ear and the larynx and the diseases concerned with them.

otoliths (o'-to-liths). Ear stones. Calcareous concretions of the inner ear, at the base of semicircular canals.

otologist (o-tol'-o-jist). A specialist in diseases of the ear.

otomycosis (o-to-mi-ko'-sis). A fungal infection of the auditory canal.

otophone (o'-to-fone). Ear trumpet.

otorrhoea (o-tor-re'-ah). Discharge from the ear, especially of pus.

otosclerosis (o-to-skler-o'-sis). A thickening and ossification of the tissues and ligaments that convey the sound waves to the internal ear. The stapes becoming fixed in the oval window.

otoscope (o'-to-skope). Auriscope. An instrument for examining the ear.

otoscopy (o-tos'-ko-pe). An examination of the tympanic membrane and auditory canal by means of an otoscope.

ounce (ounse). An Imperial measurement of weight and of volume. *See* Appendix 7.

oval window (o'-val win'-do). The membrane through which vibrations are transmitted from the stapes bone in the middle ear to the cochlea in the inner ear. *See* Ear.

ovarian (o-vair'-e-an). Relating to an ovary. *O. cyst.* A tumour of the ovary containing fluid.

ovariectomy (o-vair-e-ek'-to-me). Excision of an ovary. Oöphorectomy.

ovariotomy (o-vair-e-ot'-o-me). Usually taken to mean removal of an ovary, but literally, incision of an ovary.

ovaritis (o-var-i'-tis). Oöphoritis (*q.v.*).

ovary (o'-var-e). One of a pair

of glandular organs in the female pelvis, associated with the uterus. Its function is the production of ova.

over-compensation (*o-ver-kom-pen-sa'-shun*). A mental mechanism by which a person tries to assert himself by aggressive behaviour or by talking or acting 'big' to compensate for a feeling of inadequacy.

overdosage (*o-ver-do'-saj*). Denotes the toxic effects resulting from too high a blood level of a drug. This may be from too large or repeated doses or from the cumulative effect.

overhydration (*o-ver-hi-dra'-shun*). The administration of too much intravenous fluid.

oviducts (*o'-ve-dukts*). The fallopian tubes (*q.v.*).

ovotestis (*o-vo-tes'-tis*). A gonad containing both ovarian and testicular tissue.

ovulation (*ov-u-la'-shun*) The process of rupture of the mature graafian follicle when the ovum is shed from the ovary.

ovum (*o'-vum*). An egg. The reproductive cell of the female. *Pl.* ova.

oxalate (*oks'-al-ate*). A salt of oxalic acid in which blood is stored prior to biochemical determination being made.

oxalic acid (*oks-al'-ik as'-id*). Salts of lemon. A corrosive poison that can be precipitated by lime water, milk, or a suspension of chalk.

oxaluria (*oks-al-u'-re-ah*). Oxalates in urine.

Oxford inflator. A simple hand pump with facemask for applying emergency artificial respiration.

oxidization (*oks-e-di-za'-shun*). Oxidation. The process of oxidizing by which combustion occurs and breaking up of matter takes place; e.g. oxida-

tion of carbohydrates gives carbon dioxide and water.

$$C_6H_{12}O_6 + 6O_2 = 6CO_2 + 6H_2O.$$

oximeter (*oks-im'-e-ter*). A photoelectric cell used to determine the oxygen saturation of blood. *Ear o.* One attached to the ear by which the oxygen content of blood flowing through the ear can be measured.

oxycyanide of mercury (*oks-e-si'-an-ide of mer-ku'-re*). A mercurial antiseptic that may be used for urethral or bladder irrigation.

oxygen (*oks'-e-jen*). A colourless, odourless gas constituting one-fifth of the atmosphere. It is stored in cylinders at high pressure or as liquid oxygen and released for inhalation in cases of dyspnoea. For methods of administration, *see* Appendix 3.

oxygenation (*oks-e-jen-a'-shun*). Saturation with oxygen; a process which occurs in the lungs to the haemoglobin of blood.

oxygenator (*oks'-e-jen-a-tor*). A machine through which the blood is passed to oxygenate it. *Pump o.* Machines substitute for both the heart and the lungs. Either of the above may be used in cardiac surgery.

oxyhaemoglobin (*oks-e-he-mo-glo'-bin*). Haemoglobin oxygenated, as in arterial blood.

oxyntic cells (*oks-in'-tik*). Those which secrete acid, e.g. HCl in the stomach is made by these cells of the gastric glands.

oxytetracycline (*oks-e-tet-rah-si'-kleen*). An antibiotic drug produced from a mould. Terramycin is a proprietary preparation of it.

oxytocic (*oks-e-to'-sik*). Any drug which stimulates uterine contractions and may be used to hasten delivery.

oxytocin (*oks-e-to'-sin*). That part of pituitrin which contracts the uterus. Pitocin is a proprietary form.

oxyuriasis (*oks-e-u-ri'-a-sis*). Infestation by thread worms.

Oxyuris (*oks'-e-u'-ris*). A genus of nematode worms found in the intestines. Family Ascaridae.

ozaena (*o-ze'-nah*). Atrophic rhinitis. A condition of the nose in which there is loss and shrinkage of the ciliated mucous membrane and of the turbinate bones.

ozone (*o'-zone*). An intensified form of oxygen containing three O atoms to the molecule, O_3, and often discharged by electrical machines such as X-ray apparatus. In medicine it is employed as an antiseptic and oxidizing agent.

P

pacchionian bodies (*A. Pacchioni, Italian anatomist, 1665–1726*). Arachnoid granulations by which the cerebrospinal fluid drains into the venous channels in the dura mater.

pace-maker. The sino-atrial node. *See* Node. *Artificial p.* An instrument that takes over the function of the sino-atrial node by sending small electrical impulses to the heart. An electrode may be sewn on to the epicardium and attached either to an *external p.* or to one that is implanted in the rectus abdominis muscle. Alternatively an electrode may be passed through a vein (in the elbow or neck) into the apex of the right ventricle and attached either to an *external p.* or to one that is

implanted under the skin in the axilla.

pachy- (*pak'-e*). A prefix meaning 'thick'.

pachydermatous (*pak-e-der'-mat-us*). Thick-skinned.

pachydermia (*pak-e-der'-me-ah*). A thick skin. *P. laryngis.* A chronic hypertrophy of the vocal cords.

pachymeningitis (*pak-e-menin-ji'-tis*). Inflammation with thickening of the dura mater of the brain.

pachysomia (*pak-e-so'-me-ah*). Much thickening of soft parts as in acromegaly.

Pacini's corpuscles (*F. Pacini, Italian anatomist, 1812–83*). Specialized end-organs, situated in the subcutaneous tissue of the extremities and near joints, that respond to firm pressure.

pack. Ribbon or folded gauze for placing in a cavity. *Abdominal p.* One used in the theatre to protect or seal off a part. *Cold p.* A little used method of reducing temperature. *Hot p.* Applied to a limb or part to relieve pain or reduce muscle spasm as in poliomyelitis.

packed cell volume (*pakt sel vol'-ume*). The percentage of blood which is made up of red cells. The normal range is 40–47 per cent.

paediatrician (*pe-de-at-rish'-an*). A specialist in the diseases of children.

paediatrics (*pe-de-at'-riks*). The branch of medicine dealing with diseases of children.

Paget's disease (*Sir J. Paget, British surgeon, 1814–99*). (1) Of bone in which over-activity of the osteoblasts and osteoclasts leads to dense bone formation with areas of rarefaction. Osteitis deformans. (2) Carcinoma of the nipple.

painter's colic. See Colic.

palate (*pal'-ate*). The roof of the mouth. *Hard p.* in front, is of bone. *Soft p.* continues from it, and is of muscle which forms the pillars of the fauces and the uvula. *Artificial p.* A plate made to close a cleft palate. *Cleft p.* A congenital deformity where there is lack of fusion of the two bones forming the palate.

palatine (*pal'-at-ine*). Two bones forming most of the hard palate. *P. processes.* The horizontal portions of the superior maxillae forming the anterior portion of the hard palate.

palatoplegia (*pal-at-o-ple'-je-ah*). Paralysis of the soft palate.

palliative (*pal'-le-at-iv*). An agent which relieves, but does not cure disease.

pallidectomy (*pal-le-dek'-to-me*). An operation performed to decrease the activity of the globus pallidum, the medial part of the lentiform nucleus in the base of the cerebrum. It has brought about a marked improvement in severely agitated cases of paralysis agitans.

pallor (*pal'-or*). Lack of colour.

palmar (*pal'-mar*). Relating to the palm of the hand. *P. crease.* Crease occurring on the palm of the hand which may vary from normal in certain inherited diseases. *P. fascia.* The arrangement of tendons in the palm of the hand. *Deep* and *superficial p. arches.* The chief arterial blood supply to the hand formed by anastomosis of ulnar and radial arteries.

palpation (*pal-pa'-shun*). Examination of the organs by touch or pressure of the hand over the part.

palpebra (*pal'-pe-brah*). The eyelid.

palpebral (*pal'-pe-bral*). Referring to the eyelids. *P. ligaments.* Stretch from the junction of the upper and lower lid to the orbital bones, both medially and laterally.

palpitation (*pal-pit-a'-shun*). Rapid and forceful contraction of the heart of which the patient is conscious.

palsy (*pawl'-ze*). Paralysis. *Bell's p.* Paralysis of the facial muscles on one side, supplied by the seventh cranial nerve. *Creeping p.* Progressive muscular atrophy. *Crutch p.* Due to pressure of the crutch on the radial nerve and a cause of 'dropped wrist'. *Erb's p.* Paralysis of one arm due to a birth injury to the brachial plexus. *Shaking p.* Paralysis agitans.

panacea (*pan-a-se'-ah*). A cure-all.

panarthritis (*pan-ar-thri'-tis*). Inflammation of all the structures of a joint.

pancarditis (*pan-kar-di'-tis*). Inflammation of all the structures of the heart—as may occur in rheumatic infection.

Pancoast's tumour (*H. K. Pancoast, American radiologist, 1875–1939*). Pain, wasting and weakness of the arm which occur as secondary features of carcinoma of the bronchus due to neurological involvement. The tumour is at the apex of the lung.

pancreas (*pan'-kre-as*). An elongated, racemose gland about 15 cm (6 in) long, lying behind the stomach, with its head in the curve of the duodenum, and its tail in contact with the spleen. It secretes a digestive fluid (*pancreatic juice*) containing ferments, which act on all classes of foods. The fluid enters the duodenum by the pancreatic duct which joins the common bile duct. The pancreas also secretes the hor-

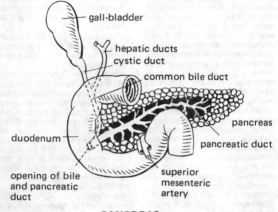

- gall-bladder
- hepatic ducts
- cystic duct
- common bile duct
- pancreas
- duodenum
- pancreatic duct
- opening of bile and pancreatic duct
- superior mesenteric artery

PANCREAS

mones insulin and glucagon (q.v.).

pancreatectomy (pan-kre-at-ek'-to-me). Excision of the head and the body of the pancreas for carcinoma.

pancreatico-duodenal (pan-kre-at'-ik-o du-o-de'-nal). Relating to the pancreas and duodenum. *P. artery.* That to the head of the pancreas and duodenum.

pancreatin (pan'-kre-at-in). An extract from the pancreas containing the digestive enzymes. Used to treat deficiency as in fibrocystic disease of the pancreas.

pancreatitis (pan-kre-at-i'-tis). Inflammation of the pancreas. *Acute p.* A severe condition in which the pancreatic enzymes can cause self digestion. *Subacute p.* May follow mumps or influenza infections. Usually a chronic form.

pancreozymin (pan-kre-o-zi'-min). A hormone secreted in the small intestine that stimulates the secretion of pancreatic enzymes.

pancytopenia (pan-si-to-pe'-ne-ah). A lack of all the blood cells due to failure of bone marrow formation.

pandemic (pan-dem'-ik). An epidemic spreading over a wide area.

panhysterectomy (pan-hister-ek'-to-me). *See* Hysterectomy.

panic-state. A feeling of overwhelming fear or terror. It may occur in anxiety states, war neurosis or acute schizophrenia.

panicula (pan-ik'-u-lah). A little swelling.

panleucopenia (pan-lu-ko-pe'-ne-ah). A lack of all the white blood cells.

panmyelopathy (pan-mi-el-

op'-ath-e). Disease affecting all the cells formed in the bone.

panniculis (*pan-ik'-u-lus*). A sheet of membranous tissue.

panniculitis (*pan-ik-ul-i'-tis*). A disease in which tender nodules appear in the subcutaneous fat accompanied by periods of fever.

pannus (*pan'-nus*). Increased vascularity of the cornea leading to granulation tissue formation and impaired vision.

panophthalmia (*pan-off-thal'-me-ah*). Panophthalmitis. Inflammation of all the tissues of the eyeball.

panophthalmitis (*pan-off-thal-mi'-tis*). Inflammation of the eye involving all three coats, the retina, choroid and sclera.

panosteitis (*pan-os-te-i'-tis*). Inflammation of all the structures of a bone.

panotitis (*pan-o-ti'-tis*). Inflammation of the internal, as well as of the middle ear.

pansystolic murmur (*pan-sis-tol'-ik mer'-mer*). A heart murmur heard throughout the time when the heart is in systole. *See* Murmur.

pantothenic acid (*pan-to-then'-ik as'-id*). One of the vitamins in the B complex.

pantropic (*pan-trop'-ik*). An adjective applied to organisms that attack a wide range of structures.

Papanicolaou test (*G. N. Papanicolaou, Greek physician, anatomist and cytologist, 1883–1962*). *See* Test.

papaveretum (*pap-av-er-e'-tum*). A preparation of the alkaloids of opium. Omnopon is a proprietary preparation.

papaverine (*pa-pav'-er-een*). An alkaloid of opium.

papilla (*pap-il'-lah*). A small nipple-like eminence. *Pl.* papillae. *Circumvallate p.* At the back of the tongue arranged in a V-shape, and containing taste buds. *Filiform p.* Fine, slender filaments on the main part of the tongue which give it its velvety appearance. *Fungiform p.* Mushroom-shaped papillae of the tongue. *Optic p.* The optic disc where the optic nerve leaves the eye-ball. *Tactile p.* The projections on the true skin containing touch corpuscles.

papillary (*pap'-il-lar-e*). Composed of or pertaining to papillae.

papilliferous cyst (*pap-il-lif'-er-us*). *See* Cyst.

papillitis (*pap-il-li'-tis*). Inflammation of the optic disc. It may also be termed optic neuritis.

papilloedema (*pap-il-e-de'-mah*). Oedematous swelling of the optic disc indicating increase of intracranial pressure.

papilloma (*pap-il-lo'-mah*). An innocent growth of epithelial tissue, e.g. a wart.

papillomatosis (*pap-il-lo-mat-o'-sis*). The occurrence of multiple papilloma.

papovavirus (*pap-o'-vah-vi-rus*). A family of viruses which cause, amongst other things, human warts.

papular (*pap'-u-lah*). Referring to papules.

papule (*pap'-ule*). A pimple, or small solid elevation of the skin.

papulopustular (*pap-u-lo-pus'-tu-lar*). Showing both papules and pustules.

papulosquamous (*pap-u-lo-skwa'-mus*). Eruptions of the skin involving the epidermis including such conditions as psoriasis and lichen planus.

para-aminobenzoic acid (*par-ah-am-in-o-ben-zo'-ik*). Filters the ultra-violet rays of the sun and in a cream protects against sunburn.

para-aminosalicylic acid (*par-ah-am-in-o-sal-is-il'-ik*). In the form of a calcium or sodium salt this is an antituberculous drug used with streptomycin and/or isoniazid. PAS.

paracentesis (*par-ah-sen-te'-sis*). Puncture of the wall of a cavity in order to draw off fluid as is performed in cases of dropsy and severe effusions. *P. abdominis.* Puncture of the abdomen to remove fluid. *P. thoracis.* Of the thoracic cavity. *P. tympani.* Removal of fluid from the middle ear by puncture of the drum.

paracetamol (*par-ah-set'-a-mol*). An analgesic and antipyretic. Panadol is a proprietary preparation.

parachlorometacresol (*par-ah-klor-o-met-ah-kre'-sol*). Chlorocresol (*q.v.*). A coal tar antiseptic preparation.

parachlorometaxylenol (*par'-ah-klor-o-met-ah-zi'-le-nol*). Chloroxylenol (*q.v.*). A group of antiseptics of which Dettol and Roxenol are examples.

paracusis (*par-ah-ku'-sis*). A perverted sense of hearing. *P. willisiana.* Hearing better in a noise, as in a railway train.

paradoxical breathing (*par-ah-doks'-ik-al*). This occurs when the two lungs are not working in unison as may occur in pneumothorax.

paraesthesia (*par-es-the'-ze-ah*). Disorder of sensation, e.g. a feeling of tingling or as of 'pins and needles'.

paraffin (*par'-af-in*). Any saturated hydrocarbon obtained from coal-tar. *P. molle.* Petroleum jelly. *P. wax.* A hard paraffin that can be used for wax treatment for chronic inflammation of joints. *Liquid p.* An intestinal lubricant, extensively used as a fine emulsion. Also applied to wounds to prevent the injury of new granulations when dressings are removed, e.g. flavine emulsion.

paraform (*par'-ah-form*). Paraformaldehyde. A preparation of formaldehyde used as an antiseptic and also for fumigating rooms.

paraldehyde (*par-al'-de-hide*). A drug with a most pungent taste. It is hypnotic and anaesthetic.

paralysis (*par-al'-is-is*). Loss of sensation and the power of movement of any part, as the

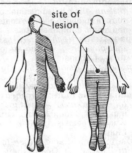

hemiplegia   paraplegia

PARALYSIS

result of interference with the nerve supply. *P. agitans* ('shaking palsy') is a disease occurring in people of middle age, slow in development and characterized by rigidity of the muscles of the face, producing a mask-like expression, typical tremors of the limbs, great muscle weakness and a peculiar gait. Also known as Parkinson's disease *Bulbar p.* (*labioglossopharyngeal p.*). Due to changes in the motor centres of the medulla oblongata. It affects the muscle of the mouth, tongue, and pharynx. *Diphtheritic p.* A complication of diphtheria, the soft palate being first affected. *Facial p. (Bell's palsy).* Affects the muscles of the face and is due to injury to or inflammation of the facial nerve. *Flaccid p.* Loss of tone and absence of reflexes in the paralysed muscles. *Infantile p.* A former term for acute anterior poliomyelitis (*see* Poliomyelitis). *Spastic p.* Characterized by rigidity of affected muscles.

paralytic (*par-ah-lit'-ik*). Affected by or relating to paralysis. *P. ileus.* Absence of peristalsis in a portion of the intestine associated with peritonitis.

paramedian incision (*par-ah-me'-de-an*). One to the side of the median line.

paramedical (*par-ah-med'-e-kal*). Having some association with the science or practice of medicine. The paramedical services include occupational, speech and physical therapy, and medical social work.

parametric (*par-ah-me'-trik*). Concerning the tissue surrounding the uterus.

parametritis (*par ah-me-tri'-tis*). Inflammation of the parametrium; pelvic cellulitis.

parametrium (*par-ah-me'-tre-um*). The connective tissue around the uterus.

paramnesia (*par-am-ne'-ze-ah*). A defect of memory in which there is a false recollection. The patient may fill in the forgotten period with imaginary events which he describes in great detail.

paramyotonia congenita (*par-ah-mi-o-to'-ne-ah con-jen'-it-ah*). Congenital muscle weakness and lack of muscle tone, only when the patient is exposed to cold.

paranoia (*par-ah-noi'-ah*). A mental disorder characterized by delusions of grandeur or persecution which may be fully systematized in logical form, with the personality remaining fairly well preserved.

paranoid (*par'-ah-noid*). Resembling paranoia. A condition that can occur in many forms of mental disease. Delusions of persecution are a marked feature. *P. schizophrenia.* See Schizophrenia.

paraparesis (*par-ah-par-e'-sis*). An incomplete paralysis, especially of the lower limbs.

paraphimosis (*par-ah-fi-mo'-sis*). Retraction of the prepuce behind the glans penis, with inability to replace it.

paraphrenia (*par-ah-fre'-ne-ah*). Schizophrenia occurring for the first time in later life and not accompanied by deterioration of the personality.

paraplegia (*par-ah-ple'-je-ah*). Paralysis of the lower extremities and lower trunk. All parts below the point of lesion in the spinal cord are affected. It may be of sudden onset from injury to the cord or develop slowly as the result of disease as in *locomotor ataxia, transverse myelitis,* etc.

parasite (*par'-ah-site*). Any animal or vegetable organism living upon or within another, from which it derives its nourishment.

parasiticide (*par-ah-sit'-is-ide*). A drug which kills parasites.

parasympathetic system (*par-ah-sim-path-et'-ik*). Part of the autonomic nervous system (*q.v.*).

parasympatholytic (*par-ah-sim-path-o-lit'-ik*). A drug that neutralizes the effect of the parasympathetic nerves.

parathormone (*par-ah-thor'-mone*). The endocrine secretion of the parathyroid glands.

parathyroid glands (*par-ah-thi'-roid*). Four small endocrine glands—two associated with each lobe of the thyroid gland, and sometimes embedded in it. The secretion from these has some control over calcium metabolism, and lack of it is a cause of tetany (*q.v.*).

parathyroidectomy (*par-ah-thi-roid-ek'-to-me*). Removal of parathyroid glands.

paratyphoid fever (*par-ah-ti'-foid*). An infection resembling typhoid, but usually of a milder nature and caused by a different bacillus. There are three forms, A, B and C, each due to a specific organism. In preventive inoculation, TAB vaccine, prepared from typhoid and paratyphoid A and B bacilli, may be given, or a vaccine to which paratyphoid C has been added.

paravertebral (*par-ah-ver'-te-bral*). Near or at the side of the vertebrae.

parencephalous (*par-en-kef'-al-us*). Having a congenital malformation of the brain.

parenchyma (*par-en-ki'-mah*). The essential active cells of an organ as distinguished from vascular and connective tissue.

parenteral (*par-en'-ter-al*). Apart from the alimentary canal. Applied to the introduction into the body of drugs or fluids by routes other than the mouth or rectum, e.g. intravenously or subcutaneously.

paresis (*par-e'-sis*). Partial paralysis.

parietal (*par-i'-et-al*). Relating to the walls of any cavity; e.g. *p. pleura*, the pleura attached to the chest wall. *P. bones.* The two bones forming part of the roof and sides of the skull. *P. cells.* Alternative name for the oxyntic cells in the gastric mucosa that secrete hydrochloric acid.

parietes (*par-i'-et-ez*). The walls of any cavity.

Paris technique. A method of treating carcinoma of the cervix of the uterus by irradiation with radium in large doses.

Parkinson's disease (*J. Parkinson, British physician, 1755–1824*). Paralysis agitans. *See* Paralysis.

paronychia (*par-on-ik'-e-ah*). An abscess near the finger-nail; a whitlow or felon. *P. tendinosa.* The spread of infection that involves the tendon sheath.

parosmia (*par-os'-me-ah*). A disordered sense of smell.

parotid (*par-ot'-id*). Situated near the ear. *P. glands.* Two salivary glands, one in front of each ear.

parotitis (*par-o-ti'-tis*). Inflammation of the parotid gland. Caused usually by ascending infection via its duct, e.g. when hygiene of the mouth is neglected or when the natural secretions are lessened, especially in severe illness or following operation. *Epidemic p.* Mumps (*q.v.*).

parous (*par'-us*). Having borne one or more children.

paroxysm (*par'-oks-izm*). A sudden attack or recurrence of a symptom of a disease.

paroxysmal (*par-oks-iz'-mal*). Occurring in paroxysms. *P. cardiac dyspnoea.* Cardiac asthma. Recurrent attacks of dyspnoea associated with pulmonary oedema and left-sided heart failure. *P. tachycardia.* Recurrent attacks of rapid heart beats that may occur without heart disease.

parrot disease. See Psittacosis.

parthenogenesis (par-then-o-jen'-es-is). Asexual reproduction by means of an egg without fertilization by the male.

parturient (par-tu'-re-ent). Giving birth; relating to child-birth.

parturition (par-tu-rish'-un). The act of giving birth to a child.

Parvobacteriaceae (par'-vo-bak-ter-e-a'-se-e). A group of bacteria which includes the causative organisms of whooping cough, brucellosis and plague.

pascal (B. Pascal, French scientist, 1623–68). Unit of pressure in the Système International d'Unités (SI units). Also known as Newton/metre². See Appendix 6.

Paschen bodies (E. Paschen, German pathologist, 1860–1936). Small granules demonstrable in the fluid of the vesicles of smallpox.

passive. Not active. P. immunity. See Immunity. P. movements. In massage, manipulations without the help of the patient.

passivity feelings (pas-iv'-e-te). Psychiatric term for a delusional feeling that a person is under some outside control.

Pasteurella (pas-tur-el'-lah). A genus of short rod-shaped bacilli. P. pestis. The causative organism of plague transmitted by rat fleas to man.

Pasteur, L. (French chemist and bacteriologist, 1822–95). Founded the science of microbiology and developed the technique of vaccination. P. treatment. Preventing hydrophobia (q.v.) by injecting a very weak form of the virus of rabies and gradually producing immunity.

pasteurization (pas-tur-i-za'-shun). The process of checking fermentation in milk and other fluids, by heating them to a temperature between 63° and 68°C (145° to 150°F) for 30 min and then rapidly cooling. This kills all pathogenic bacteria and has safeguarded the nation's milk supply. Variations of the above time and temperatures may be used.

patella (pat-el'-lah). The small, circular, sesamoid bone forming the knee-cap.

patellar (pat-el'-lar). Belonging to the patella (q.v.). P. bursae. Bursae around the patella.

patellectomy (pat-el-ek'-to-me). Excision of the patella.

patent (pa'-tent). Open. P. ductus arteriosus. When the ductus arteriosus (q.v.) fails to close at birth, so that some blood passes from the aorta into the pulmonary artery instead of into the systemic circulation.

patho- (path'-o). A prefix denoting 'disease'.

pathogenic (path-o-jen'-ik). Causing disease. P. bacteria. Disease-causing organisms.

pathogenicity (path-o-jen-is'-it-e). The ability of an organism to cause disease.

pathognomonic (path-og-no-mon'-ik). Specifically characteristic of a disease. Sign or symptom by which a pathological condition can be identified.

pathological (path-o-loj'-ik-al). Pertaining to the study of disease.

pathology (path-ol'-o-je). The branch of medicine treating of disease, and the changes in structure and function which it causes.

pathophobia (path-o-fo'-be-ah). Exaggerated dread of disease.

Paul–Bragg respirator (R. W.

Paul, contemporary British engineer; Sir W. H. Bragg, British physicist 1862–). An apparatus fitted around the chest by which artificial respiration may be carried out.

Paul–Bunnell test (*J. R. Paul, American physician, 1893– ; W. W. Bunnell, American physician, 1902–).* An agglutination test which, if positive, confirms the diagnosis of glandular fever.

Paul's tube (*F. T. Paul, British surgeon, 1851–1941).* A bent glass tube, used chiefly for colonic drainage.

Pavlov's method (*I. P. Pavlov. Russian physiologist, 1849–1936).* A method for the study of the conditioned reflexes. Pavlov noticed his experimental dogs salivated in anticipation of food when they heard a bell ring.

peak flow meter. Meter designed to measure the maximum velocity of air flow during a forced expiration.

peau d'orange (*po-dor-ahnj').* The appearance of the overlying skin in advanced carcinoma of the breast. Blockage of the skin lymphatics causes dimpling of the hair follicle openings which resembles orange skin.

pecten (*pek'-ten).* The middle third of the anal canal.

pectin (*pek'-tin).* A setting agent used in cookery, formed from pectose, a carbohydrate found in fruit.

pectoral (*pek'-tor-al).* Relating to the chest. *P. muscles.* The pectoralis major and minor.

pectus (*pek'-tus).* The chest.

pedicle (*ped'-ik-l).* The stem or neck of a tumour. *P. graft.* A tissue graft that is partially detached and inserted in its new position while temporarily still obtaining its blood supply from the original source.

pediculosis (*ped-ik-u-lo'-sis).* The condition of being infested with lice.

Pediculus (*ped-ik'-u-lus).* The louse, a small parasite infesting the skin and hairy parts of the body. *See* Louse.

peduncle (*ped-un'-kl).* A narrow part of a structure acting as a support. *P. of cerebellum.* One of the collections of nerve-fibres connecting the cerebellum with the medulla oblongata.

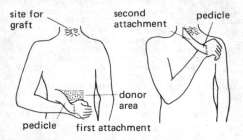

PEDICLE GRAFT

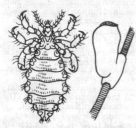

adult (x 10)   egg (nit)
                attached
                to hair

PEDICULUS

peeling. Desquamation (*q.v.*).

Pel–Ebstein's fever (*P. K. Pel, Dutch physician, 1852–1919: W. Ebstein, German physician, 1836–1912*). A recurrent pyrexia having a span of 15 to 21 days seen especially in cases of lymphadenoma.

pellagra (*pel-lag'-grah*). A deficiency disease due to lack of vitamin B (*nicotinic acid*). It is characterized by debility, spinal pains, digestive disorders and erythema with exfoliation of the skin. *See* Appendix 10.

pellicle (*pel'-lik-l*). (1) A scum on the surface of a liquid. (2) A thin skin or membrane.

pelvic (*pel'-vik*). Pertaining to the pelvis. *P. girdle.* The ossa innominata and sacrum. *P. peritonitis. See* Peritonitis.

pelvimeter (*pel-vim'-e-ter*). Calipers for measuring the diameter of the pelvis.

pelvimetry (*pel-vim'-et-re*). Measuring of the pelvis. *X-ray p.* Used to measure the internal pelvic diameters and late in pregnancy this can be assessed in relation to the fetal head. Cephalopelvimetry.

pelvirectal (*pel-ve-rek'-tal*). The term applied to the flexure where the pelvic colon joins the rectum at an acute angle.

pelvis (*pel'-vis*). A basin-shaped cavity. *Bony p.* The pelvic girdle formed of the innominate bones and the sacrum. *Contracted p.* Narrowing of the diameter of the pelvis. *See* Conjugate. It may be of the *true* conjugate or the *diagonal*. Effective antenatal care will recognize this condition, and caesarean section is often necessary to ensure live birth. The deformity may be the result of rickets. *False p.* The part formed by the concavity of the iliac bones above the ileopectineal line. *Renal p.* The dilatation of the ureter, which by enclosing the hilus surrounds the pyramids of the kidney substance. *True p.* The basin-like cavity below the false pelvis, its upper limit being the pelvic brim.

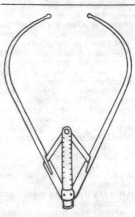

PELVIMETER

pemphigus (*pem'-fig-us*). An acute or chronic skin disease, characterized by an eruption of large blebs which leave pigmented areas on healing. Itching may be marked and the general health is usually impaired. It is of many varieties.

pempidine tartrate (*pem'-pe-deen*). A hypotensive drug which may be used to treat arterial hypertension. Perolysen and Tenormal are proprietary preparations.

pendulous (*pen'-du-lus*). Hanging down. *P. abdomen.* Due to weakness and laxity of abdominal muscles. In pregnancy it causes the uterus to fall forwards.

penicillamine (*pen-is-il'-am-een*). A chelating agent that is used in copper and lead poisoning to aid excretion of the metal.

penicillinase (*pen-is-il'-in-aze*). An enzyme that destroys penicillin. Many staphylococci produce this enzyme.

penicillins (*pen-is-il'-ins*). A group of antibiotics that are bacteriocidal for those organisms that are sensitive to the drug used. *Benzyl p.* A soluble form quickly absorbed giving high blood levels but rapidly excreted. *Procaine p.* A less soluble form, so there is slow release and absorption from intramuscular site. Effective for 24 hours. Other preparations are: ampicillin, cloxacillin, methicillin and phenoxymethylpenicillin (*q.v.*).

Penicillium notatum (*pen-is-il'-e-um no-tah'-tum*). A mould from which penicillin first derived.

penis (*pe'-nis*). The male organ of copulation.

pentagastrin (*pen-tah-gas-trin*). A synthetic hormone with a similar structure to gastrin

(*q.v.*). Replacing histamine in gastric secretion tests, as it has no side effects.

pentobarbitone (*pen-to-barb'-e-tone*). A basal narcotic of barbiturate group. Nembutal is a proprietary preparation of it.

pentose shunt (*pen'-tose*). Metabolic pathway by which glucose 6-phosphate is converted to pentose sugars which are necessary for the formation of DNA and RNA.

peppermint (*pep'-er-mint*). A carminative and flavouring agent.

pepsin (*pep'-sin*). An enzyme found in gastric juice. It partially digests proteins in an acid solution.

pepsinogen (*pep-sin'-o-jen*). The precursor of pepsin, activated by HCl.

peptic (*pep'-tik*). Applied to the gastric secretions and areas affected by them. *P. glands.* The gastric glands. *P ulcer.* One arising in the stomach or duodenum associated with hyperacidity.

peptone (*pep'-tone*). The result of the action of pepsin on protein.

peptonized foods (*pep'-ton-ized*). Foods partially digested by artificial methods.

peptonuria (*pep-ton-u'-re-ah*). Peptones in the urine.

percentile charts (*per-sen'-tile*). Charts which show the limits of normal height and weight in children against which physical development is measured.

percept or **perception** (*per'-sept, per-sep'-shun*). An awareness and understanding of an impression that has been presented to the senses. The mental process by which we perceive.

perchloride of mercury (*per-klor'-ide*). Corrosive sublimate.

percussion (*per-kush'-un*). A method of diagnosis by tapping with the fingers upon any part of the body. By the sounds produced, information can be gained as to the condition of organs below the skin.

perflation (*per-fla'-shun*). Ventilation by forcing air into a room.

perforation (*per-for-a'-shun*). A hole through the whole thickness of a wall of a cavity or organ. It may be caused by ulceration or trauma.

perfusion (*per-fu'-shun*). Pouring fluid over. *P. fluid.* One used to bathe a tissue usually to maintain its health, often by allowing a chemical exchange of necessary and waste products.

peri- (*per'-e*). Prefix meaning 'around'.

perianal (*per-e-a'-nal*). Surrounding or located around the anus. *P. abscess.* A small subcutaneous pocket of pus near the anal margin.

periarteritis (*per-e-ar-ter-i'-tis*). Inflammation of the outer coat of an artery.

periarthritis (*per-e-ar-thri'-tis*). Inflammation of the tissues surrounding a joint.

pericardiectomy (*per-e-kar-de-ek'-to-me*). Excision of a large part of the pericardium. Sometimes performed to check impaired cardiac action in constrictive pericarditis.

pericarditis (*per-e-kar-di'-tis*). Inflammation of the pericardium secondary to other disease such as rheumatic fever, tuberculosis or myocardial infarction. *Adhesive p.* Adhesions occur between the two layers of pericardium owing to a thick fibrinous exudate. *Constrictive p.* Progressive fibrosis causing constriction of heart movement.

Purulent p. Due to pyogenic infection. *Serous p.* Excessive serous exudate impairing heart function.

pericardium (*per-e-kar'-de-um*). The smooth membranous sac enveloping the heart, consisting of an outer fibrous and an inner serous coat. *Adherent p.* Fibrous tissue formation between the layers, the result of acute pericarditis.

pericardotomy (*per-e-kard-ot'-o-me*). An operation to open the pericardium, sometimes performed to break down adhesions following pericarditis.

perichondrium (*per-e-kon'-dre-um*). The membrane covering cartilaginous surfaces.

pericolpitis (*per-e-kol-pi'-tis*). Inflammation of the tissues around the vagina.

pericranium (*per-e-kra'-ne-um*). The periosteum of cranial bones.

pericystitis (*per-e-sis-ti'-tis*). Inflammation of the tissues surrounding the bladder.

perihepatitis (*per-e-hep-at-i'-tis*). Inflammation of the peritoneum covering the liver.

perilymph (*per'-e-limf*). Lymph separating bone and membrane in the bony labyrinth of the ear.

perimeter (*per-rim'-e-ter*). (1) The line marking the boundary of any area or geometrical figure; the circumference. (2) An instrument for measuring the field of vision.

perimetritis (*per-e-me-tri'-tis*). Inflammation of the perimetrium.

perimetrium (*per-e-me'-tre-um*). The peritoneal covering of the uterus.

perimetry (*per-im'-et-re*). The process of mapping the visual fields.

perinatal (*per-e-na'-tal*). Pertaining to the first week of life. Also incorporates pre- and postnatal periods.

perineal (*per-e-ne'-al*). Relating to the perineum.

perineorrhaphy (*per-e-ne-or'-raf-e*). Suture of the perineum to repair a laceration caused during childbirth.

perinephric (*per-e-nef'-rik*). Around the kidney.

perinephritis (*per-e-nef-ri'-tis*). Inflammation of the tissues enveloping the kidney.

perineum (*per-e-ne'-um*). The tissues between the anus and external genitals. *Lacerated p.* May result from childbirth but is often forestalled by performing an episiotomy (*q.v.*). Treatment is by perineorrhaphy.

periodic syndrome (*per-e-od'-ik sin'-drome*). Recurrent head, limb or abdominal pains in children for which no organic cause can be found. It often leads to migraine in adult life.

periodontitis (*per-e-o-don-ti'-tis*). Inflammation of the tissues surrounding a tooth.

periodontium (*per-e-o-don'-te-um*). The connective tissue between the teeth and their bony sockets.

periosteal (*per-e-os'-te-al*). Pertaining to or composed of periosteum. *P. elevator.* An instrument for separating the periosteum from bone.

periosteotome (*per-e-os'-te-o-tome*). An instrument for incising the periosteum and separating it from the bone.

periosteum (*per-e-os'-te-um*). The fibrous membrane covering the surface of bone. It consists of two layers, the inner or *osteogenetic*, which is closely adherent, and which forms new cells (by which the bone grows in girth) and in close contact with it the *fibrous* layer richly supplied with blood vessels.

periostitis (*per-e-os-ti'-tis*). Inflammation of the periosteum.

peripheral (*per-if'-er-al*). Relating to the periphery. *P. neuritis.* Inflammation of terminal nerves. *P. resistance.* The resistance in the walls of the arterioles, which is a major factor in the control of blood pressure. *See* Neuritis.

periphery (*per-if'-er-e*). The outer surface or circumference.

perisalpingitis (*per-e-sal-pin-ji'-tis*). Inflammation of the peritoneal covering of the fallopian tube.

perisplenitis (*per-e-splen-i'-tis*). Inflammation of the peritoneum over the spleen.

peristalsis (*per-e-stal'-sis*). A wave-like contraction, preceded by a wave of dilatation, which travels along the walls of a tubular organ, tending to press its contents onwards. It occurs in the muscle coat of the alimentary canal. *Reversed p.* The wave of contraction passes the reverse way towards the mouth. *Visible p.* The wave is visible on the surface of the abdomen. It can be seen in premature infants and in those who have pyloric stenosis.

peritomy (*per-it'-o-me*). Excision of a portion of the conjunctiva at the edge of the cornea, for the cure of pannus.

peritoneal (*per-it-o-ne'-al*). Referring to the peritoneum. *P. cavity.* The abdominal cavity lined by peritoneum. *P. dialysis.* A method of removing waste products from the blood by passing a cannula into the peritoneal cavity, running in a fluid, and after an interval, draining it off.

peritoneoscope (*per-it-o'-ne-o-skope*). An endoscopic instrument for viewing the peritoneal cavity through the abdominal wall.

peritoneoscopy (*per-it-o-ne-os'-ko-pe*). Visual examination of the peritoneum by means of a peritoneoscope.

peritoneum (*per-it-o-ne'-um*). The serous membrane lining the abdominal cavity and forming a covering for the abdominal organs. *Parietal p.* That which lines the abdominal cavity. *Visceral p.* The inner layer which closely covers the organs, and includes the mesenteries. *Pelvic p.* That which covers the pelvic organs.

peritonitis (*per-it-on-ī'-tis*). Inflammation of the peritoneum due to infection. This may occur from: (1) Perforation of a viscus, e.g. the stomach. (2) Infection of an organ, e.g. the appendix. (3) Intestinal obstruction, as in strangulated hernia. (4) Injury, as a stab wound. (5) Blood-borne infection, e.g. Streptococcus or pneumococcus. *Pelvic p.* That confined to the peritoneum or pelvic organs. *Septic p.* Due to a pyogenic organism. *Tuberculous p.* A chronic form due to the tubercle bacillus affecting chiefly mesenteric glands.

peritonsillar (*per-e-ton'-sil-lar*). Around the tonsil. *P. abscess. See* Quinsy.

perityphlitis (*per-e-tif-lī'-tis*).

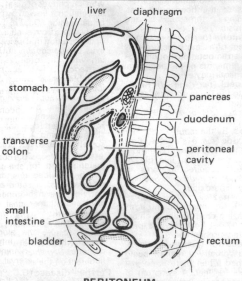

liver — diaphragm

stomach — pancreas

duodenum

transverse colon — peritoneal cavity

small intestine

bladder — rectum

PERITONEUM

Inflammation of peritoneum around the caecum and appendix.

perlèche (*pair-lesh'*). A superficial fissuring at the angles of the mouth often due to vitamin B deficiency.

permeability (*per-me-a-bil'-it-e*). The degree to which a fluid can pass from one structure through a wall or membrane to another.

pernicious (*per-nish'-us*). Highly destructive; fatal. *P. anaemia.* An anaemia due to lack of absorption of vitamin B_{12} for the formation of red blood cells. At one time a fatal condition.

perniosis (*per-ne-o'-sis*). Chilblains. A result of vascular spasm in the superficial arterioles of the hands and feet, causing thrombosis and necrosis.

peromelia (*per-o-me'-le-ah*). A defect of a limb which resembles an amputation though bud-like remnants of the peripheral segments may exist.

peroneal (*per-o-ne'-al*). Relating to the fibula. *P. muscles.* Of the leg.

peroral (*per-or'-al*). By the mouth.

per os. By the mouth.

peroxide (*per-oks'-ide*). A compound of any element with more than the normal quantity of oxygen required to form an oxide. *P. of hydrogen. See* Hydrogen peroxide.

perphenazine (*per-fen'-a-zeen*). An antiemetic and tranquillizing drug similar to chlorpromazine. Fentazin is a proprietary preparation.

persecution (*per-se-ku'-shun*). In psychiatry a fear of being harmed when there is no just cause for fear. A symptom of schizophrenia and paranoia.

perseveration (*per-sev-er-a'-shun*). The constant recurrence of an idea or the tendency to keep repeating the same words or actions.

persistant ductus arteriosus (*per-sist'-ant duk'-tus art-er-e-o'-sus*). Condition occurring when the ductus arteriosus (*q.v.*) does not close after birth. It causes a shunt from the aorta to the pulmonary artery. *See* Patent.

personality (*per-son-al'-it-e*). The sum total of heredity and inborn tendencies, with influences from environment and education, which goes to form the mental make-up of a person and influence his attitude to life. *Cycloid p.* An unstable person who has periods of great activity and elation followed by periods of depression. *Dual p.* The patient suffers from such a degree of dissociation that he leads two lives, one personality not knowing what the other is doing. *Hysterical p.* An emotionally unstable person whose behaviour is designed to attract attention. Such people are very open to suggestion, are self-centred and long for sympathy. *Schizoid p.* An introverted person who is shy and retiring. A poor mixer in society, given to day dreaming.

Perspex (*per'-speks*). A plastic material used for splinting. It can be moulded to individual requirements, is semitransparent, light, washable and is not affected by immersion in water.

perspiration (*per-spir-a'-shun*). The secretion of the sweat glands. *Insensible p.* Sweat which is not visible on the skin. *Sensible p.* Moisture apparent on the skin.

Perthes' disease (*G.C. Perthes, German surgeon, 1869–1927*). Osteochondritis.

pertussis (*per-tus'-sis*). Whooping cough.

perversion (*per-ver'-shun*). Morbid diversion from a normal course. *Sexual p.* Abnormality of expression of sexual instinct.

pes (*paze*). The foot, or any foot-like structure. *P. cavus.* A deformity of the foot occurring in various forms of paralysis, characterized by hollowness of the instep and retraction of the toes. *P. malleus valgus.* Hammer toe (*q.v.*). *P. planus.* Flat-foot (*q.v.*).

pessary (*pes'-sar-e*). (1) An instrument for supporting a displaced uterus, by insertion into the vagina. *Ring p.* Made of rubber or plastic material. *Hodge p.* Made of vulcanite or plastic. (2) A medicated suppository inserted into the vagina, for antiseptic purposes. *See* Vaginitis. (3) *Diaphragm p.* A contraceptive.

pesticides (*pes'-te-sides*). Chemical agents that destroy pests. They may give rise to poisoning.

pestilence (*pes'-til-ense*). Any deadly epidemic disease; a term commonly applied to plague.

pestis (*pes'-tis*). Plague (*q.v.*).

petechia (*pe-te'-ke-ah*). A small spot due to effusion of blood under the skin, e.g. the spots of purpura and typhus fever. *Pl.* petechiae.

pethidine (*peth'-e-deen*). A synthetic drug which relieves pain and has an antispasmodic action on plain muscle. In obstetrics it may be combined with hyoscine. Given by mouth or by hypodermic injection.

petit mal (*pet'-e-mal*). A form of epilepsy (*q.v.*).

Petri dishes (*R. J. Petri, German bacteriologist, 1852–1922*). Shallow glass dishes in which organisms are grown on a culture medium.

pétrissage (*pa-tris-sahj'*). A kneading action used in massage.

petroleum (*pet-ro'-le-um*). An oily liquid found in the earth of various parts of the world. In medicine, it is used as an antiseptic, a laxative, and for skin diseases.

petrositis (*pet-ro-si'-tis*). Inflammation of the petrous portion of the temporal bone usually spread from a middle ear infection.

petrous (*pet'-rus*). Stony. *P. bone.* Part of the temporal bone, containing the organ of hearing.

Peyer's glands or **patches** (*Johann Conrad Peyer, Swiss anatomist, 1653–1712*). Small lymph nodules situated in the

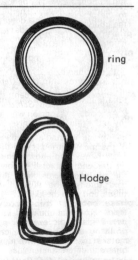

ring

Hodge

PESSARIES

mucous membrane of the lower part of the small intestine. In typhoid fever they become infected and ulcerated.

pH. A measure of the hydrogen ion concentration and so the acidity or alkalinity of a fluid. Expressed numerically 1 to 14; 7 is neutral, below this is acid and above alkaline.

phaeochromocytoma (*fe-o-kro-mo-si-to'-mah*). A tumour of the adrenal medulla which gives rise to paroxysmal hypertension.

phage (*faj*). Bacteriophage. A virus which lives on bacteria but is confined to particular strains. *P.-typing*. The identification of certain bacterial strains by determining the presence of strain-specific phages. Used in detecting the causative organisms of epidemics, especially food poisoning.

phagocytes (*fag'-o-sites*). Polymorphonuclear leucocytes and large lymphocytes which have the power of destroying harmful micro-organisms in the blood. *See* Leucocyte.

phagocytosis (*fag-o-si-to'-sis*). The action of phagocytes.

phalanges (*fal-an'-jez*). The bones of the fingers or toes. *Sing*. Phalanx.

phallitis (*fal-i'-tis*). Inflammation of the penis.

phallus (*fal'-lus*). The penis.

phantasy (*fan'-tas-e*). A mental activity in which imagination weaves thoughts and feelings which bear little relation to reality.

phantom limb (*fan'-tom*). Following amputation when the patient can still feel the limb.

phantom tumour or **cyst.** A tumour-like swelling of the abdomen caused by contraction of the muscles or by localized gas.

pharmaceutical (*far-mah-su'-tik-l*). Relating to drugs.

pharmacogenetics (*far-mah-ko-jen-et'-iks*). The study of genetically determined variations in drug metabolism and the response of the individual.

pharmacology (*far-mah-kol'-o-je*). The science of the nature and preparation of drugs.

pharmacopoeia (*far-mah-ko-pe'-ah*). An authoritative publication which gives the standard formulae and preparation of drugs as used in a given country. *British P.* That authorized for use in Great Britain.

pharmacy (*far'-mas-e*). The art of preparing, compounding, and dispensing medicines.

pharyngeal (*far-in'-je-al*). Relating to the pharynx.

pharyngectomy (*far-in-jek'-to-me*). Excision of a section of the pharynx.

pharyngitis (*far-in-ji'-tis*). Inflammation of the pharynx.

pharyngolaryngeal (*far-in-go-lar-in-je'-al*). Referring to both the pharynx and larynx.

pharyngotympanic tube (*far-in-go-tim-pan'-ik*). Eustachian tube leading from the pharynx to the middle ear.

pharynx (*far'-inks*). The muscular pouch lined with mucous membrane situated at the back of the mouth. It leads into the oesophagus, and also communicates with the nose through the posterior nares, with the ears through the eustachian tubes, and with the larynx.

phase contrast microscopy (*faze kon'-trast mi-kros'-ko-pe*). Microscopic examination of living unstained biological material by the use of two light beams at different intensities.

phenacetin (*fen-as'-e-tin*). An antipyretic, diaphoretic and analgesic drug. Often combined with aspirin and used to relieve minor pain.

phenelzine (*fen-el'-zeen*). A drug used in the treatment of depression. Nardil is a proprietary preparation.

Phenergan (*fen-er'-gan*). Proprietary preparation of promethazine. An antihistamine drug useful for alleviating skin irritation and for its sedative effect.

phenformin (*fen-for'-min*). An oral hypoglycaemic agent. A biguanide that aids the entry of glucose into the cells.

phenindione (*fen-in-di'-one*). A synthetic anticoagulant for oral administration given for the prevention and treatment of thrombosis, the dose depending on the prothrombin level in the blood. Dindevan is a proprietary preparation.

pheniodol (*fen-i'-o-dol*). A dye which is opaque to X-ray used for testing gall-bladder efficiency.

phenobarbitone (*fe-no-bar'-bit-one*). A barbiturate drug which depresses the cerebral cortex and is useful in small oral doses for mild sedation or in larger doses intramuscularly for violent states due to cerebral irritation.

phenol (*fe'-nol*). Carbolic acid. A disinfectant derived from coal tar.

phenothiazines (*fe-no-thi'-az-eens*). A group of drugs used in the treatment of severe psychiatric disorders. The first to be used was chlorpromazine (Largactil).

phenotype (*fen'-o-tipe*). The characteristics of an individual that are not due to his genetic makeup.

phenoxybenzamine (*fen-okse-benz'-am-een*). A vasodilator drug useful in treating peripheral conditions such as Raynaud's disease. Dibenyline is a proprietary preparation.

phenoxymethylpenicillin (*fen-oks-e-meth-il-pen-is-il'-in*). An acid resistant penicillin that can be administered orally. Penicillin V.

phenylalanine (*fen-il-al'-a-neen*). An essential amino acid that cannot be properly metabolized in persons suffering from phenylketonuria (*q.v.*).

phenylbutazone (*fen-il-bu'-taz-one*). An analgesic and antiseptic drug used in the treatment of gout and rheumatic disorders. Butazolidin is a proprietary preparation of it.

phenylketonuria (*fen-il-keton-u'-re-ah*). The presence in the urine of phenylpyruvic acid due to the incomplete breakdown of phenylalanine, an amino acid. It is a hereditary abnormality leading to severe mental deficiency which if detected early can be treated by a diet that is very low in protein.

phenylpyruvic acid (*fen-il-piru'-vik*). An abnormal constituent of the urine present in phenylketonuria (*q.v.*) which can be detected by the use of Phenistix. *See* Appendix 11.

phenytoin sodium (*fen'-e-to-in so'-de-um*). A drug with anticonvulsant properties particularly useful in controlling major epilepsy. Epanutin is a proprietary preparation of it.

phial (*fi'-al*). A small glass container or bottle for drugs.

phimosis (*fi-mo'-sis*). Constriction of the prepuce so that it cannot be drawn back over the glans penis. The usual treatment is circumcision.

phlebectomy (*fleb-ek'-to-me*). Excision of a portion of a vein.

phlebitis (*fleb-i'-tis*). Inflammation of a vein which tends to formation of a thrombus. The symptoms are: pain and swelling of the affected part, and redness along the course of the vein, which is felt later as a hard, tender cord.

phlebogram (*fleb'-o-gram*). An X-ray examination after dye insertion, to see the condition of deep veins prior to operation.

phlebolith (*fleb'-o-lith*). A calculus occasionally formed in a vein.

phlebothrombosis (*fleb-o-throm-bo'-sis*). Simple clotting of blood within a vein without local inflammation, so the clot does not become firmly attached and is likely to break away as an embolus.

Phlebotomus (*fleb-ot'-o-mus*). A genus of sandflies that transmits the protozoa *Leishmania* causing leishmaniasis.

phlebotomy (*fleb-ot'-o-me*). Venesection.

phlegm (*flem*). Mucus secreted by the lining of the air-passages and expectorated.

phlegmasia (*fleg-ma'-ze-ah*). Inflammation. *P. alba dolens* or '*white leg*' is due to lymphatic blockage and deep femoral thrombosis sometimes occurring after labour.

phlegmatic (*fleg-mat'-ik*). Dull and apathetic.

phlegmon (*fleg'-mon*). A brawny swelling resulting from inflammation of connective tissue. It may lead to suppuration or ulceration.

phlyctenules (*flik'-ten-ules*). Small vesicles on the conjunctiva. *See* Conjunctivitis.

phobia (*fo'-be-ah*). An irrational fear produced by a specific situation which the patient attempts to avoid.

phocomelia (*fo-ko-me'-le-ah*). A congenital deformity in which the long bones of the limbs are minimal or absent and the individual has 'seal' hands or feet or stump-like limbs of various lengths.

pholcodine (*fol'-ko-deen*). A linctus for the suppression of a non-productive or irritating cough.

phonation (*fo-na'-shun*). The art of uttering vocal sounds.

phonetic (*fo-net'-ik*). Representing sounds or pertaining to the voice.

phonic spasm (*fo'-nik spazm*). An affliction of singers and public speakers when they are unable to perform in public but can talk normally.

phonocardiogram (*fo-no-kar'-de-o-gram*). A record of the heart sounds made by a phonocardiograph.

phonocardiograph (*fo-no-kar'-de-o-graf*). An instrument that records heart sounds and murmurs.

phosgene (*fos'-jeen*). A lung-irritant gas.

phosphatase(s) (*fos'-fat-aze*). Enzymes involved in the metabolism of phosphate. *Alkaline p.* One formed by osteoblasts in the bone and by liver cells and excreted in the bile. A high blood level denotes obstructive jaundice or excessive bone activity. A moderate increase occurs in disease of the liver cells.

phosphates (*fos'-fates*). Salts of phosphoric acid, sometimes prescribed as tonics.

phosphaturia (*fos-fat-u'-re-ah*). Excess of phosphates in the urine.

phospholipids (*fos-fo-lip'-ids*). Esters of glycerol fats that are found in cells especially of the nervous system.

phosphorus (*fos'-for-us*). A non-metallic highly inflammable element. Not used in medicine except as phosphoric acid or its salts. It is poisonous, causing fatty degeneration of organs, especially the liver.

photalgia (fo-tal'-je-ah). Painful eyes from exposure to too much light.

photocoagulation (fo'-to-ko-ag-ul-a'-shun). The use of a powerful light source to induce inflammation of the retina and choroid to treat retinal detachment.

photophobia (fo-to-fo'-be-ah). Intolerance of light.

photosensitive (fo-to-sens'-e-tiv). Reacting to light rays.

phrenectomy (fren-ek'-to-me). The removal of a phrenic nerve. See Avulsion.

phrenemphraxis (fren-em-fraks'-is). The operation in which the phrenic nerve is crushed, not removed. The resulting paralysis is then likely to be only temporary. See Phrenectomy.

phrenic (fren'-ik). (1) Relating to the mind. (2) Pertaining to the diaphragm. P. avulsion. See Avulsion.

phrenicotomy (fren-e-kot'-o-me). Division of a phrenic nerve to paralyse one-half of the diaphragm. See Avulsion.

phthalylsulphathiazole (thal-il-sul-fah-thi'-a-zole). An insoluble sulphonamide, poorly absorbed in the intestine so used to kill intestinal bacteria prior to surgery.

Phthirus pubis (thi'-rus pu'-bis). The crab louse.

phthisis (thi'-sis). Advanced or chronic tuberculosis of the lungs, in which wasting is marked. Previously termed consumption, it is less often seen with the advance in the treatment of early cases.

physical (fiz'-ik-al). In medicine, relating to the body as opposed to the mental processes. P. signs. Those observed by inspection, percussion, etc.

physician (fiz-ish'-an). One who practises medicine as opposed to surgery.

physics (fiz'-iks). The study of the laws and phenomena of nature.

physiological (fiz-e-o-loj'-ik-al). Relating to physiology (q.v.). Normal, as opposed to pathological. P. jaundice. See Jaundice. P. solutions. Those of the same salt composition and same osmotic pressure as blood plasma.

physiology (fiz-e-ol'-o-je). The science of the functions of living bodies.

physiotherapy (fiz-e-o-ther'-ap-e). Treatment by natural forces, e.g. heat, light, electricity, massage, etc.

physique (fiz-eek'). The structure of the body.

physostigmine (fi-so-stig'-meen). Eserine. An alkaloid from the Calabar bean. It is an antidote to curare; it constricts the pupils and is used in the treatment of myasthenia gravis. Neostigmine is a similar synthetic drug.

phytomenadione (fi-to-men-ah-di'-one). An intravenous preparation of vitamin K, effective in treating haemorrhage occurring during anticoagulant therapy. Konakion is a proprietary preparation. Mephyton is an emulsion for oral administration.

pia mater (pi'-ah ma'-ter). The innermost membrane enveloping the brain and spinal cord consisting of a network of small blood vessels connected by areolar tissue. This dips down into all the folds of the nerve substance.

pica (pi'-kah). Unnatural craving for strange foods. It may occur in pregnancy, and sometimes in mental diseases.

Pick's disease (*A. Pick, Czechoslovakian physician, 1851–1924*). (1) Hepatic enlargement with ascites and pleural effusion, associated with constrictive pericarditis. (2) A form of presenile dementia with atrophy of the frontal lobes of the cerebrum.

Pickwickian syndrome (*pik-wik'-e-an*). Condition in which extreme obesity is associated with severe congestive cardiac failure. The victims are cyanosed and have polycythaemia and marked oedema. (After the fat boy 'Joe' in *Pickwick Papers*.)

picric acid (*pik'-rik*). A derivative of phenol. It is used chiefly as the reagent in Esbach's test for albuminuria. *See* Appendix 11.

pigeon breast (*pij'-un brest*). A deformity in which the sternum is unduly prominent. A result of rickets.

pigment (*pig'-ment*). Colouring matter. *Bile p.* Bilirubin and biliverdin. *Blood p.* Haematin. *Melanotic p.* Melanin (*q.v.*).

pigmentation (*pig-ment-a'-shun*). The deposition in the tissues of an abnormal amount of pigment.

piles. Haemorrhoids.

pill. A rounded mass of one or more drugs in powder form held together by glycerin and sometimes coated with sugar.

pilocarpine (*pi-lo-kar'-peen*). An alkaloid prepared from jaborandi leaves. It is used to constrict the pupils.

pilomotor nerves (*pi-lo-mo'-tor*). Those supplying plain muscle connected with hair follicles. Stimulation causes the hair to be erected, and also the condition of 'gooseflesh' of the skin.

pilonidal cyst (*pi-lo-ni'-dal*). A congenital infolding of hair-bearing skin over the coccyx. It may become infected and lead to sinus formation.

pilosebaceous (*pi-lo-se-ba'-shus*). Applied to sebaceous glands that open into the hair follicles.

pilosis (*pi-lo'-sis*). Abnormal growth of hair.

pilula (*pil'-u-lah*). Latin for pill.

pimple. A small papule or pustule.

pineal (*pin'-e-al*). Shaped like a pine cone. *P. body.* A small cone-shaped structure on the base of the brain and composed of glandular substance. It is supposed to have an endocrine secretion but this is not definitely established.

pine oil. A volatile oil from pine prescribed for inhalation in cases of laryngitis and bronchitis.

pinguecula (*pin-gwek'-u-lah*). Nodules of hyaline and yellow elastic tissue that occur on the cornea. A degenerative condition in which inflammation is common.

pink disease. Mercurial poisoning thought to be caused by teething powders. Erythroedema polyneuritis (*q.v.*).

pink eye. Infective conjunctivitis.

pinna (*pin'-nah*). The projecting part of the external ear; the auricle.

pinocytosis (*pi-no-si-to'-sis*). A process similar to phagocytosis by which molecules of protein enter or are absorbed by cells.

pint. Twenty fluid ounces. *See* Appendix 7.

pinta (*pin'-tah*). A non-venereal skin infection caused by the

Treponema carateum prevalent in the West Indies and Central America.

piperazine (*pi-per'-az-een*). An anthelmintic in tablet or elixir form given in the treatment of threadworms and roundworms.

pipette (*pip-et'*). A glass tube for conveying small quantities of liquid.

piriform fossae (*pir'-e-form foss-e*). Spaces between the larynx and pharyngeal walls that may be viewed with a laryngeal mirror.

pisiform (*pi'-se-form*). Pea-shaped; one of the carpal bones.

pitchblende (*pitch'-blend*). Uranium oxide, a black mineral from which radium is obtained.

pituitary gland (*pit-tu'-it-ar-e*). An endocrine gland suspended from the base of the brain and protected by the sella turcica in the sphenoid bone. It consists of two lobes. (1) *Anterior*, which has some influence in regulating growth and metabolism and influences the other endocrine glands. (2) *Posterior*, which secretes oxytocin and vasopressin (*q.v.*).

pityriasis (*pit-e-ri'-as-is*). A skin disease characterized by fine scaly desquamation. *P. rosea.* An inflammatory form, in which the affected areas are macular and ring-shaped.

placebo (*plas-e'-bo*). Any inactive substance resembling medicine given during controlled experiments or to satisfy a patient.

placenta (*plas-en'-tah*). The after-birth. A vascular structure inside the pregnant uterus supplying the fetus with nourishment through the connecting umbilical cord. The placenta develops about the third month of pregnancy, and is expelled after the birth of the child. *Battledore p.* In which the cord is attached to the margin and not the centre. *P. praevia.* One attached to the lower part of the uterine wall. As labour advances, it may be a cause of severe antepartum haemorrhage.

placidity (*plas-id'-e-te*). A calm state, the opposite of rage, in which it takes a strong stimulus to evoke a response.

plagiocephaly (*pla-je-o-kef'-al-e*). Asymmetry of the head resulting from the irregular closing of the sutures.

plague (*plaig*). An acute fever endemic in Asia and Africa. The causative organism is *Pasteurella pestis* transmitted by the bites of fleas that have derived the infection from diseased rats. *Bubonic p.* Characterized by buboes. *Pneumonic p.* The infection attacks chiefly the lung tissues. A very fatal form.

plantar (*plan'-tar*). Relating to the sole of the foot. *P. arch.* The arch made by anastomosis of the plantar arteries. *P. flexion.* Bending of the toes downward and so arching the foot. *P. reflex.* Contraction of the toes on stroking the sole of the foot.

plasma (*plaz'-mah*). The fluid part of blood. *Reconstituted p.* Dried plasma when again made liquid by addition of distilled water. *P. proteins.* Those present in the blood plasma: albumin, globulin and fibrinogen. *P. values.* The salt and chemical content of blood plasma. *See* Appendix 9.

plasmaphoresis (*plaz-mah-for-e'-sis*). A method of removing a portion of the plasma from circulation. Venesection is performed, the blood allowed to settle, then the cellular part returned to circulation.

plasmids (*plaz'-mids*). Extrachromosomal or free units of DNA found in bacteria.

plasminogen (*plas-min'-o-jen*). The inactive precursor of plasmin. Plasmin has the property of dissolving fibrin and so aids in the dispersal of blood clots.

Plasmodium (*plas-mo'-de-um*). The parasite which causes malaria. *P. falciparum*. The cause of malignant tertian malaria. *P. vivax* causes the benign tertian form.

plaster (*plah'-ster*). A substance for application to the surface of the body. It is prepared in various forms. *Adhesive p.* Used for (a) drawing together the edges of wounds; (b) holding in position small dressings; (c) for support, e.g. of a sprained ankle. *P. bandage. See* Plaster of Paris. *Bivalve p.* A plaster of Paris splint cut into two pieces. *See* Croft's splint. *Bohler's p.* Plaster for Pott's fracture. A leg splint of plaster of Paris, in which is embedded an iron stirrup extending below the foot, which enables the patient to walk without putting weight on the joint. *Corn p.* One impregnated with salicylic acid. *Frog p.* A plaster of Paris splint used to maintain the position after correction of the deformity due to congenital dislocation of the hip. *P. jacket.* One of plaster of Paris applied to support the spine. *P. of Paris.* Calcium sulphate or gypsum with which book muslin is impregnated and used to form a plaster cast to immobilize a part.

plastic (*plas'-tik*). Constructive. Tissue-forming. *P. surgery.* The grafting of tissue from a healthy area of the body, to restore an injured or deformed part. *P. lymph.* The exudate which in wounds and inflamed serous tissues is organized into fibrous tissue and promotes healing.

plasticity (*plas-tis'-e-te*). A stiffness as present in the limbs following a cerebral lesion.

platelets (*plate'-lets*). Thrombocytes. *See* Blood.

platinum (*plat'-in-um*). A metal. Used to encase radium (1 mm thick), as it prevents penetration of the *alpha* and *beta* rays which cause burning, but does not hold back the *gamma* rays.

pleocytosis (*ple-o-si-to'-sis*). An increase in cells, usually lymphocytes in the cerebrospinal fluid.

pleomorphism (*ple-o-morf'-izm*). Occurring in more than one form. Several distinct types of the same species.

pleoptics (*ple-op'-tiks*). A method of improving vision in a poorly functioning eye by stimulating the use of the fovea.

plethora (*pleth'-or-ah*). Fulness. Excess of blood in the vessels, characterized by florid complexion, full pulse, and tendency for the nose to bleed.

plethysmography (*pleth-is-mog'-raf-e*). The study of the circulation in the extremity by enclosing the limb in an oncometer and noting by means of an amplifier the changes in volume.

pleura (*plu'-rah*). The serous membrane lining the thorax and enveloping each lung. *Parietal p.* The layer which lines the chest wall. *Visceral p.* The inner layer which is in close contact with the lung.

pleurisy (*plu'-ris-e*). Inflammation of the pleura. *Diaphragmatic p.* When that part covering the diaphragm is affected most. *Dry p.* (*fibrinous*). In which the membrane is inflamed and roughened, but no fluid is formed. This causes a

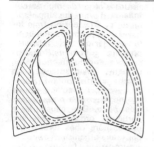

PLEURAL EFFUSION

purposeless cough and a sharp, stabbing pain on inspiration. *P. with effusion* (*wet pleurisy*). Characterized by inflammation and exudation of serous fluid into the pleural cavity. Pain is less, but cardiac and respiratory function may be impeded to such an extent that the fluid has to be aspirated. This may result from infection or irritation of the pleura. *Purulent p.* or *empyema*. When pus is formed in the pleural cavity. An operation for drainage is necessary.

pleurocele (*plu'-ro-seel*). Hernia of the lung or pleural tissue.
pleurodesis (*plu-ro-de'-sis*). Occluding the pleural space by the insertion of silver nitrate to cause adhesions in cases of chronic or recurrent pneumothorax.
pleurodynia (*plu-ro-din'-e-ah*). Pain in the intercostal muscles, probably rheumatic in origin.
pleurolysis (*plu-rol'-is-is*). Pneumolysis (*q.v.*).
plexor (*pleks'-or*). An instrument resembling a hammer, used in percussion.
plexus (*pleks'-us*). A network of veins or nerves. *Auerbach's p.*

The nerve ganglion situated between the longitudinal and circular muscle fibres of the intestine. They are motor nerves. *Brachial p.* The network of nerves of the neck and axilla. *Choroid p.* A capillary network situated in the ventricles of the brain which forms the cerebrospinal fluid. *Meissner's p.* The sensory nerve ganglion situated in the submucous layer of the intestinal wall. *Solar* or *coeliac p.* The network of nerves and ganglia at the back of the stomach, which supply the abdominal viscera. *Haemorrhoidal* or *rectal p.* The network of veins which surrounds the rectum and forms a direct communication between the systemic and portal circulations.
plicate (*pli'-kate*). Folded or plaited.
plumbism (*plum'-bizm*). Lead poisoning.
plumbum (*plum'-bum*). Lead.
Plummer–Vinson syndrome (*H. S. Plummer, American physician, 1874–1936: P. P. Vinson, American physician, 1890– *). Difficulty in swallowing associated with glossitis and iron deficiency anaemia.
pneumatocele (*nu-mat'-o-seel*). (1) A swelling, containing a collection of gas. (2) Hernia of the lung.
pneumaturia (*nu-mat-tu'-re-ah*). Flatus is passed with the urine owing to a vesicolic fistula and air from the bowel entering the bladder.
pneumocephalus (*nu-mo-kef'-al-us*). Aerocele. Air entering the brain as from an anterior fracture of the base of the skull.
pneumococci (*nu-mo-kok'-i*). *Diplococcus pneumoniae.* Bacteria that may cause lobar or bronchopneumonia, meningitis or otitis media. They can be

divided into over thirty serological types by agglutination tests.

pneumoconiosis (*nu-mo-ko-ne-o'-sis*). Any fibrosis of lung due to inhalation of dust particles. *See* Anthracosis, Asbestosis *and* Silicosis.

pneumodynamics (*nu-mo-di-nam'-iks*). The mechanism of respiration. *See* Appendix 3.

pneumoencephalography (*nu-mo-en-kef-al-og'-raf-e*). *See* Encephalography.

pneumogastric (*nu-mo-gas'-trik*). Pertaining to lungs and stomach. *P. nerve.* The tenth cranial nerve to the lungs, stomach, etc. The vagus nerve.

pneumolysis (*nu-mol'-is-is*). The operation of detaching the pleura from the chest wall in order to collapse the lung when the two pleural layers are adherent.

pneumomycosis (*nu-mo-mi-ko'-sis*). Infection of the lung by microfungi. *See* Bronchomycosis *and* Mycosis.

pneumonectomy (*nu-mon-ek'-to-me*). Removal of a lung. A treatment for disease when only one lung is affected, such as by bronchiectasis or new growth.

pneumonia (*nu-mo'-ne-ah*). Inflammation of the lung. *Aspiration p.* One arising from inhaled material from another infected lesion or, following operation, of vomitus. *Broncho-p.* A descending infection of the bronchi. Widespread and patchy in distribution. *Pneumococcal p.* A specific p. caused by the *Klebsiella pneumoniae. Specific p.* One caused by a particular organism, affecting one or more lobes. *Virus p.* The causative organism is a virus.

pneumonitis (*nu-mon-i'-tis*). An imprecise term denoting any inflammatory condition of the lung.

pneumoperitoneum (*nu-mo-per-it-o-ne'-um*). Air in the peritoneal cavity. It can be introduced into the upper part of the cavity to limit movement of the diaphragm, and was a treatment for pulmonary tuberculosis affecting the base of the lung. It may be performed prior to peritoneal dialysis or peritoneoscopy.

pneumopyothorax (*nu-mo-pi-o-thor'-aks*). *See* Pyo-pneumothorax.

pneumoradiography (*nu-mo-*

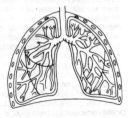

bronchopneumonia

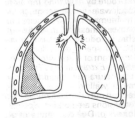

specific pneumonia

PNEUMONIA

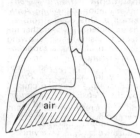

PNEUMOPERITONEUM

ra-de-og'-raf-e). X-ray of a cavity or part after air has been injected into it.

pneumotaxic centre (*nu-mo-taks'-ik*). The centre in the pons (*q.v.*) that influences inspiratory effort during respiration.

pneumothorax (*nu-mo-thor'-aks*). Air in the pleural cavity, caused by perforation of the chest wall or of the lung pleura in which case air enters via the bronchi. Both cause the lung to collapse. The signs may be slight or of a rapidly increasing dyspnoea as the intrapleural pressure rises. Immediate steps must be taken to relieve the pressure by aspirating the air or by a 'water seal'drainage. If due to trauma a petroleum jelly pad will seal the air inlet. *Artificial p.* The introduction of air into the pleural space. A seldom used treatment of collapsing the lung tissue. *Extrapleural p.* The parietal pleura is stripped from the chest wall to enable air to be placed outside the pleura when adhesions are present. *Spontaneous p.* Due to rupture of an over-dilated air-sac as in emphysema which causes the air passages to communicate with the pleura.

pneumoventriculography (*nu-mo-ven-trik-u-log'-raf-e*). *See* Ventriculography.

pock. The pustule of smallpox, or other eruptive fever.

podagra (*pod-ag'-rah*). Gout, particularly of the joint of the foot or the big toe.

podarthritis (*pod-ar-thri'-tis*). Inflammation of joints of the foot.

podopompholyx (*pod-o-pom'-fol-iks*). Eczema of the feet, between the toes and midsole where the sweat glands are most prolific.

poikilocyte (*poi'-kil-o-site*). An irregularly shaped red blood cell.

poikilocythaemia (*poi-kil-o-si-the'-me-ah*). Poikilocytosis. The presence in the blood of red cells irregular in shape and size. The condition indicates excessive activity of the bone marrow.

poikilothermic (*poi-kil-o-ther'-mik*). Cold-blooded. With a body temperature which varies widely with the environment.

poison. Any substance which applied to the body externally or taken internally causes injury to any part or the whole. *Carbon monoxide p. See* Carbon monoxide. *Corrosive p.* One which corrodes or destroys tissues with which it comes in contact. *Irritant p.* One which causes inflammation, as caustic alkalis and mineral acids. *Narcotic p.* One which causes extreme narcosis. *See* Appendix 1.

polar body (*po'-lah*). The small body containing half the chromosomes when the ovum undergoes reduction division (*q.v.*) as it matures.

polio-encephalitis (*pol-e-o-en-kef-al-i'-tis*). Inflammation of the cortex of the brain.

poliomyelitis (*pol-e-o-mi-el-i'-tis*). Inflammation of the grey matter of the spinal cord. *Acute anterior p.* An acute specific fever, due to a virus. It mainly attacks young adults and children, and the inflammation of the anterior horn cells of the spinal cord may result in paralysis and wasting of muscle groups. *Bulbar p.* This may only affect the swallowing reflex, requiring great care in feeding the patient. *Bulbospinal p.* A severe form in which the medulla and spinal cord are affected; the respiratory and swallowing reflexes are lost and artificial respiration is essential.

Politzer's bag (*A. Politzer, Austrian otologist, 1835–1920*). A rubber bag attached to a eustachian catheter, for forcing air into the eustachian tube to clear it.

politzerization (*pol-it-zer-i-za'-shun*). Insufflation of the pharyngotympanic (eustachian) tube to restore patency.

pollen antigen (*pol'-en ant'-e-jen*). See Antigen.

pollution (*pol-u'-shun*). The act of destroying the purity of or contaminating. *Air p.* The discharge of smoke containing impurities into the atmosphere. *Water p.* The discharge of untreated sewage or factory waste into rivers or streams.

poly- (*pol'-e*). Prefix meaning 'many'.

polyarteritis (*pol-e-ar-ter-i'-tis*). Inflammatory changes in the walls of the small arteries likely to lead to hypertension or renal disease.

polyarthralgia (*pol-e-ar-thral'-je-ah*). Pain of a neuralgic type in several joints at a time.

polyarthritis (*pol-e-ar-thri'-tis*). Inflammation of several joints at the same time, as seen in rheumatoid arthritis and Still's disease.

polycystic (*pol-e-sist'-ik*). With many cysts. *P. disease of kidneys.* A congenital disease. The kidneys are much enlarged with many cysts. There is a slowly developing renal failure and hypertension.

polycythaemia (*pol-e-si-the'-me-ah*). Erythrocythaemia. *P. vera.* A rare disease in which there is a greatly increased production of red blood cells. Many cases have been satisfactorily treated by injections of radioactive phosphorus.

polydactylism (*pol-e-dak'-til-izm*). The condition of having more than the normal number of fingers or toes.

polydipsia (*pol-e-dip'-se-ah*). Abnormal thirst.

polymorphonuclear (*pol-e-morf-o-nu'-kle-ar*). (1) Having nuclei of many different shapes. (2) Phagocytic blood cells. See Leucocyte.

polymorphous (*pol-e-morf'-us*). Occurring in several or many different forms.

polymyalgia rheumatica (*pol-e-mi-al'-je-ah ru-mat'-ik-ah*). Persistent aching pain in the muscles often involving the shoulder or pelvic girdle.

polymyositis (*pol-e-mi-o-si'-tis*). Insidious wasting and weakness of muscles.

polyneuritis (*pol-e-nu-ri'-tis*). Multiple neuritis.

polyneuropathy (*pol-e-nu-rop'-ath-e*). A number of disease conditions of the nervous system. There may be polyneuritis, abdominal pain, and mental disturbance.

polypeptides (*pol-e-pep'-tides*). Proteins.

polyposis (*pol-e-po'-sis*). The condition of many polyps in an organ. *P. coli.* Familial polyposis. A hereditary condition in which there are thousands of polyps in the large bowel. Develops in childhood and eventually leads to carcinoma of colon if not excised.

polypus (*pol'-e-pus*). Polyp. A small pedunculated tumour arising from any mucous surface. *Cervical p.* In the cervical canal. *Fibroid p.* Occurs in the uterus and contains fibrous tissue. *Nasal p.* A very vascular one arising in the nose.

polysaccharides (*pol-e-sak'-ar-ides*). Starches.

polyserositis (*pol-e-ser-o-si'-tis*). General inflammation of serous membranes. *See* Pick's disease.

polythene (*pol'-e-theen*). A general term for synthetic resins forming plastic material that can be used for many different purposes. In medicine, largely replacing rubber and mackintosh and used for many utensils.

polyuria (*pol-e-u'-re-ah*). Excessive increase in the discharge of urine, due for example to diuretics (*q.v.*) or diabetes (*q.v.*).

polyvalent (*pol-e-va'-lent*). Having several valencies. Pertaining to sera which are active against several strains of one organism.

pompholyx (*pom'-fo-liks*). An eczematous condition involving the sweat glands.

pons. A bridge of tissue connecting two parts of an organ. *P. varolii.* The part of the brain which connects the cerebrum, cerebellum and medulla oblongata.

pontine hemiplegia (*pon'-tin*). The lesion is in the pons. *See* Hemiplegia.

popliteal (*pop-lit-e'-al*). Relating to the posterior part of the knee.

pore (*por*). A minute circular opening on a surface, such as of a sweat gland.

porphyria (*por-fi'-re-ah*). An inherited abnormality in red blood cell formation. *Acute p.* That precipitated by taking barbiturates or alcohol. *Congenital p.* There is photosensitivity and the child cannot be exposed to sunlight.

porphyrins (*por'-fir-ins*). Substances used in the production of the haem portion of haemoglobin.

porphyrinuria (*por-fir-in-u'-re-ah*). A minor metabolic disorder when urinary porphyrins are present. They are present in lead intoxication in lead workers.

port wine stain. A birth mark which resembles a stain made by port wine.

portacaval anastomosis (*por-tah-ka'-val an-as-tom-o'-sis*). The joining of the portal vein to the inferior vena cava so that much of the blood bypasses the liver. A successful operation in selected cases of Banti's syndrome.

portal circulation. *See* Circulation.

portal hypertension. *See* Hypertension.

position. Attitude or posture. *Dorsal p.* Lying flat on the back. *Genupectoral* or *knee-chest p.* Resting on the knees and chest with arms crossed above the head. *Left lateral p.* On the left side. *Lithotomy p.* Lying on the back with thighs raised and knees supported and held widely apart. *Prone p.* On the face, with pillows under the head and chest or abdomen, to prevent pressure on the toes. *Recumbent p.* Lying on the back. *Sims's p.* or *semi-prone p.* An exaggerated *left lateral p.* with the right knee well flexed

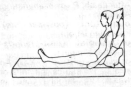

upright

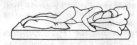

semi-prone

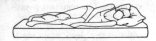

lateral

NURSING POSITIONS

and the left arm drawn back over the edge of the bed. *Trendelenburg p.* Lying down on a tilted plane (usually an operating table at an angle of 45 degrees to the floor), with the head lowermost and the legs hanging over the raised end of the table.

positive pressure ventilator. (*pos'-it-iv pres'-shur ven'-til-a-tor*). Machine designed to assist ventilation by delivering air to the lungs under pressure. *See* Ventilator.

posology (*pos-ol'-o-je*). The science of the dosage of drugs.

posseting (*pos'-et-ing*). Regurgitation of foods in infants.

Possum. Patient-Operated Selector Mechanism. A machine that can be operated with a very slight degree of pressure or suction, using the mouth, if no other muscle movement is possible. It may transmit messages

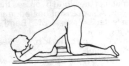

genupectoral

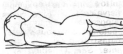

left lateral

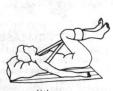

lithotomy

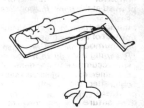

Trendelenburg

GYNAECOLOGICAL POSITIONS

from a lighted panel or be adapted for typing, telephoning, or working certain machinery.

post-. A prefix meaning 'after' or 'behind'.

post-anaesthetic (*post-an-es-thet'-ik*). Occurring after anaesthesia. *P.-a. pneumonia.* See Pneumonia.

postclimacteric (*post-kli-mak-ter'-ik*). Postmenopausal.

post-concussional syndrome (*post-kon-kush'-un-al sin'-drome*). Constant headaches with mental fatigue, difficulty in concentration and insomnia that may persist after head injury.

post-epileptic (*post-ep-e-lep'-tik*). Occurring after an epileptic fit. *P.-e. automatism.* A period sometimes following epileptic attacks, of which the patient has no memory, and during which he cannot be held responsible for his behaviour.

postganglionic (*post-gang-le-on'-ik*). Situated posterior or distal to a ganglion (a collection of nerve cells). *P. fibre.* Nerve fibre posterior to a ganglion of the autonomic nervous system.

post-gastrectomy syndrome. See 'Dumping syndrome'.

posterior (*pos-te'-re-or*). Placed at the back. *P. root.* See Root.

posthitis (*pos-thi'-tis*). Inflammation of the prepuce.

posthumous (*post'-hu-mus*). Occurring after death. *P. birth.* One occurring after the death of the father, or by caesarean section after the death of the mother.

postmature (*post'-mat-ure*). Applied to a fetus before or a baby after birth when it has remained in the uterus longer than 280 days.

post mortem (*post mor'-tem*).

After death. *P.-m. examination.* Autopsy.

postpartum (*post-par'-tum*). Following labour.

postprandial (*post-pran'-de-al*). After a meal.

potassium (*pot-as'-se-um*). An alkaline substance the salts of which are largely used in medicine.

potential (*po-ten'-shal*). Ready for action. *P. energy.* That stored up but not in actual use. The opposite of kinetic.

Pott's disease (*P. Pott, British surgeon, 1714–88*). Caries of the vertebrae, usually due to tuberculosis of one or more of the vertebrae. The resultant necrosis causes kyphosis of the spine.

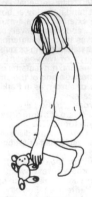

POTT'S DISEASE
A child picking up toy from the floor keeps the spine rigid but flexes the knees

Pott's fracture (*P. Pott, British surgeon, 1714–88*). A fracture-dislocation of the ankle, involving the fibula, internal malleolus of the tibia and displacement of the talus.

pouch. A pocket-like space or cavity. *P. of Douglas.* The lowest fold of the peritoneum between the uterus and rectum. *Morison's p.* A fold of peritoneum below the liver. *Uterovesical p.* The fold of peritoneum between the uterus and bladder.

poultice (*pole'-tis*). Cataplasm. A local application used to improve circulation and relieve pain as in the use of kaolin or linseed. *Starch p.* A cold gelatinous mass to soften and remove crusts from skin lesions.

Poupart's ligament (*F. Poupart, French anatomist, 1616–1708*). The inguinal ligament. The tendinous lower border of the external oblique muscle of the abdominal wall, which passes from the anterior spine of the ilium to the os pubis.

poverty of movement. When the natural movements of facial expression and of the limbs are few or absent as in Parkinson's disease.

powder (*pow'-der*). Fine dry particles, e.g. a drug or medicine in this form.

pox (*poks*). Any disease characterized by an eruption on the skin.

poxvirus (*poks'-vi-rus*). Group of large viruses, two of which cause smallpox and cowpox.

PR. Per rectum. Rectally.

pre-. A prefix meaning 'before'.

precancerous (*pre-kan'-ser-us*). Applied to conditions or histological changes that may precede cancer.

precipitins (*pre-sip'-e-tins*). Substances present in blood, causing precipitation. Produced by antigens.

precocious (*pre-ko'-shus*). Medically applied to premature

development so that puberty arises at an early age.

precognition (*pre-kog-nish'-un*). A direct perception of a future event which is beyond the reach of inference and which is not brought about to fulfil the prediction.

precordial (*pre-kor'-de-al*). Relating to the area over the heart.

precursor (*pre-kurs'-or*). A forerunner, e.g. prothrombin (*q.v.*).

predigestion (*pre-di-jest'-shun*). Partial digestion of food by artificial means before it is taken into the body.

predisposition (*pre-dis-pos-ish'-un*). Implies susceptibility to a specific disease.

prednisolone (*pred-nis'-o-lone*). A synthetic compound that is similar in structure and action to hydrocortisone. It can be given orally and is effective in smaller doses and is less likely to result in salt and water retention.

prednisone (*pred'-ne-sone*). A synthetic cortisone-like drug that is five times as potent and may be given in preference to cortisone (*q.v.*).

pre-eclamptic (*pre-e-klam'-tik*). The symptoms that precede eclampsia: albuminuria, hypertension and oedema.

prefrontal leucotomy. See Leucotomy.

pregnancy (*preg'-nan-se*). Being with child; the condition from conception to the expulsion of the fetus. The normal period is 280 days or nine calendar months. *Ectopic* or *extrauterine p.* Occurs in the uterine tube (*tubal p.*) or very rarely in the abdominal cavity. *P. tests.* These are possible because the pregnant woman secretes chorionic gonadotrophic hormones which not only stimulate the human gonads but also those of mice, rabbits, and toads. *See* Aschheim-Zondek, Friedman, *and* Hogben.

premature (*prem'-at-ure*). Occurring before the anticipated time. *P. infant.* A child weighing 2500 g (5½ lb) or less at birth is considered premature. *P. contraction.* A form of cardiac irregularity in which the ventricle contracts before its anticipated time. *See* Systole.

premedication (*pre-med-ik-a'-shun*). Narcotic drugs given prior to a general anaesthetic. Basal narcosis.

premenstrual (*pre-men'-stru-al*). Preceding menstruation. *P. endometrium.* The hypertrophied and vascular mucous lining of the uterus immediately before the menstrual flow starts.

premolar (*pre-mo'-lar*). A bicuspid tooth in front of the molars.

preoperative (*pre-op'-er-a-tiv*). Before operation. Usually referring to drugs, investigations, and treatment.

prepatellar (*pre-pat-el'-lar*). In front of the patella. *P. bursitis.* *See* Housemaid's knee.

prepuce (*pre'-puse*). Foreskin; a loose fold of skin covering the glans penis.

presbycusis (*pres-be-ku'-sis*). Deafness in old age.

presbyopia (*pres-be-o'-pe-ah*). Impairment of vision with long sight occurring in old age, due to loss of accommodating power of the lens, so that the near point of distinct vision is removed farther from the eye.

prescription (*pre-skrip'-shun*). A formula written by a physician, directing the pharmacist to prepare a remedy.

presenile dementia (*pre-se'-nile de-men'-she-ah*). *See* Dementia.

presentation. That portion of the fetus felt at the os uteri by the examining finger in the vagina. The presenting parts may be: *vertex, face, brow, breech* or *shoulder. See* diagram, p. 284.

pressor (*pres'-or*). A substance that stimulates the vasomotor centre causing vasoconstriction and a rise in the blood pressure.

pressure areas. Areas of the body where the tissues may be compressed between the bed and the underlying bone, especially the sacrum, greater trochanters and heels; so that the tissues become ischaemic.

pressure point. The point at which an artery can be compressed against a bone in order to stop bleeding.

pressure sore. A break in the surface skin due to pressure, which causes interference with the blood supply to the area. Formerly termed *bedsores.*

presystolic (*pre-sis-tol'-ik*). Occurring just before systole.

prevesical (*pre-ves'-ik-al*). In front of the bladder.

priapism (*pre'-ap-izm*). Persistent erection of the penis usually without sexual desire. It may be caused by local or spinal cord injury.

Price precipitation reaction (PPR) (*I. N. O. Price, contemporary British physician*). A serological test for syphilis.

prickle cell. One possessing delicate rod-shaped processes, by which it is connected to other cells. *P.c. layer.* The lowest stratum of the epidermis.

prickly heat. A skin eruption characterized by minute red spots with central vesicles. *See* Miliaria.

primary complex. The combination of Ghon's focus (*q.v.*) in lung tissue with caseous infec-

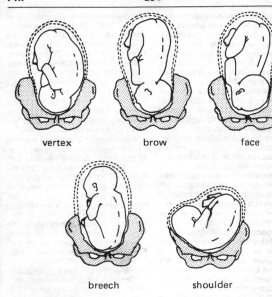

vertex   brow   face

breech   shoulder

PRESENTATION

tion of the associated hilar lymph nodes. Often occurs without general signs of infection, the lesion becoming calcified.

primigravida (*pri-me-grav´-id-ah*). A woman who is pregnant for the first time.

primipara (*pri-mip´-ar-ah*). A woman giving birth to her first child.

primordium (*pri-mor´-de-um*). The earliest discernible sign during embryonic development of an organ or part.

pro-. A prefix meaning 'before'.

probe. A slender metal rod for exploration of a wound or cavity. *Lacrimal p.* One for use in the tear ducts.

probenecid (*pro-ben´-es-id*). A drug which increases the excretion of uric acid and is used between attacks of gout to prevent their occurrence.

procainamide (*pro-kane´-am-ide*). A cardiac depressant drug that may be used in ventricular tachycardia.

procaine (*pro´-kane*). A local anaesthetic.

process (*pro´-ses*). A prominence or outgrowth of any part.

procidentia (*pro-se-den'-she-ah*). Complete prolapse of the uterus so that it extrudes through the vagina.

proctalgia (*prok-tal'-je-ah*). Pain in the rectum.

proctatresia (*prok-tat-re'-se-ah*). Imperforate anus.

proctectomy (*prok-tek'-to-me*). Excision of the rectum.

proctitis (*prok-ti'-tis*). Inflammation of the anus or rectum.

proctocele (*prok'-to-seel*). Hernia or prolapse of the rectum.

proctoclysis (*prok-tok'-lis-is*). Irrigation of the rectum.

proctocolectomy (*prok-to-kol-ek'-to-me*). The surgical removal of the rectum and colon.

proctorrhaphy (*prok-tor'-raf-e*). Suture of a wound in the rectum.

proctoscope (*prok'-to-skope*). An instrument for examination of the rectum. *Tuttle's p.* is a speculum illuminated by an electric bulb, combined with an arrangement by which the rectum can be dilated with air.

proctosigmoiditis (*prok-to-sig-moid-i'-tis*). Inflammation of the rectum and sigmoid colon.

proctotomy (*prok-tot'-o-me*). Incision of the rectum to relieve stricture.

procyclidine (*pro-sik'-le-deen*). A drug used in Parkinson's disease as it reduces rigidity. Kemadrin is a proprietary preparation.

prodromal (*pro-dro'-mal*). Preceding. *P. rash.* One which comes out before the true rash, e.g. in measles. *P. period.* That between the onset of symptoms until the diagnostic signs appear.

proflavine (*pro-fla'-vin*). An antiseptic effective against the *Staphylococcus aureus* and non-harmful to body tissues.

progeria (*pro-je'-re-ah*). Premature senility.

progesterone (*pro-jes'-ter-one*). Formerly known as progestin. A hormone of the corpus luteum, which plays an important part in the regulation of the menstrual cycle and in pregnancy. *See* diagram p. 286.

progestogens (*pro-jes'-to-jens*). Steroids or chemical substances that have an action like progesterone.

proglottis (*pro-glot'-tis*). A mature segment of a tapeworm.

prognathism (*prog'-nath-izm*). Enlargement and protrusion of the lower jaw.

prognathous (*prog-na'-thus*). Having projecting jaws.

prognosis (*prog-no'-sis*). A forecast of the course and duration of a disease.

projectile vomiting. *See* Vomiting.

projection (*pro-jek'-shun*). An unconscious process by which painful thoughts or impulses are made acceptable by transferring them on to another person or object in the environment.

prolactin (*pro-lak'-tin*). A milk-producing hormone of the anterior lobe of the pituitary body, that stimulates the mammary gland. Now termed luteotrophin as it also stimulates the continued secretion of the corpus luteum.

prolapse (*pro'-laps*). Sinking, or falling down. *P. of the cord.* When the umbilical cord is expelled first during labour. *P. of intervertebral disc* (*PID*). Displacement of part of an intervertebral disc, 'slipped disc'. *P. of iris.* Protrusion of a part of the iris through a wound in the cornea. *P. of rectum.* Protrusion of the mucous membrane, and

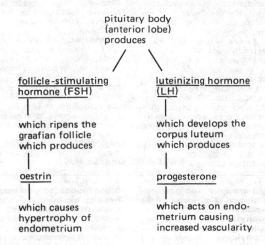

pituitary body
(anterior lobe)
produces

follicle-stimulating
hormone (FSH)

which ripens the
graafian follicle
which produces

oestrin

which causes
hypertrophy of
endometrium

luteinizing hormone
(LH)

which develops the
corpus luteum
which produces

progesterone

which acts on endo-
metrium causing
increased vascularity

HORMONE INFLUENCE ON OVARIAN FUNCTION

sometimes of the muscle coat also, through the anal canal to the exterior. Normally due to general weakness, or straining. *P. of uterus.* In which it protrudes into the vagina, as the result of weakening of its supports.

proliferation (*pro-lif-er-a'-shun*). Rapid multiplication of cells, as may occur in a malignant growth.

proline (*pro-leen*). One of the 22 amino acids formed by the digestion of dietary protein.

promazine (*pro'-maz-een*). A tranquillizing drug used in psychiatry. Sparine is the proprietary preparation.

promethazine (*pro-meth'-az-*

een). An antihistamine drug used in conditions of hypersensitivity, e.g. *hay fever, contact dermatitis, drug rashes* etc. Phenergan is a proprietary preparation of it. *P. theoclate.* Avomine, a similar preparation.

pronation (*pro-na'-shun*). Turning the palm of the hand downward.

prone (*pro-n*). Lying face downward.

proof puncture. An exploratory puncture of the maxillary sinus to assess the necessity for further treatment.

propantheline (*pro-pan'-the-leen*). An antispasmodic drug that blocks the impulses from the vagus nerve to the stomach

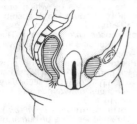

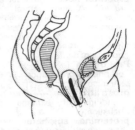

early stage | complete procidentia

PROLAPSE OF UTERUS

and may be used to inhibit gastric secretion and motility in peptic ulceration.

prophylactic (*pro-fil-ak'-tik*). Relating to prophylaxis.

prophylaxis (*pro-fil-ak'-sis*). Measures taken to prevent a disease, e.g. inoculation with TAB vaccine to prevent *typhoid fever*; regular administration of quinine to prevent *malaria.*

proprietary name (*pro-pri'-e-tar-e*). The name assigned to a drug by the firm which made it. A drug may have several different proprietary names.

proprioception (*pro-pre-o-sep'-shun*). Awareness of the position of parts of the body in space without looking at them.

proprioceptors (*pro-pre-o-sep'-tors*). The sensory end-organs that provide information about movements and position of the body. They occur chiefly in the muscles, tendons, joint capsules and labyrinth.

proptosis (*prop-to'-sis*). Projecting forward, e.g. of the eyeball.

prostaglandins (*pros-tah-gland'-ins*). Hormone substances produced in the seminal vesicles of males and also in many other tissues. They fall into the category of fatty acids.

prostate (*pros'-tate*) The gland surrounding the male urethra at its junction with the bladder and associated with the genital organs. It often becomes enlarged after middle age and may require removal, if it causes obstruction to the outflow of urine.

prostatectomy (*pros-tat-ek'-to-me*). Excision of the prostate gland. *Harris p.* and *Freyer's p.* are both suprapubic operations in which the gland is removed after the bladder has been incised. *Millin's p.* or *retropubic p.* The bladder is not opened and the gland is enucleated from around the bladder neck. *Transurethral p.* Removal of the gland via the urethra, by means of a diathermy knife and a cystoscope.

prostatitis (*pros-tat-i'-tis*). Inflammation of the prostate gland.

prostatocystitis (*pros-tat-o-sis-ti'-tis*). Inflammation of the prostate and urinary bladder.

prostatorrhoea (*pros-tat-or-re'-ah*). A thin urethral discharge from the prostate gland in prostatitis.

prosthesis (*pros-the'-sis*). The fitting of artificial parts to the body; e.g. dentures.

Prostigmin (*pro-stig'-min*). A proprietary preparation of neostigmine (*q.v.*).

prostration (*pros-tra'-shun*). A condition of extreme exhaustion.

protamine sulphate (*pro'-tam-een sul'-fate*). A sterile solution of protein from fish sperm that neutralizes circulating heparin should haemorrhage arise during anticoagulant therapy.

protamine zinc insulin (*pro'-tam-een zink*). See Insulin.

protanopia (*pro-tan-o'-pe-ah*). Partial colour blindness (*q.v.*) for red hues.

protein (*pro'-teen*). A complex compound of varying combinations of amino acids (*q.v.*). Man's only source of nitrogen which is necessary for body cells. *First class p.* Provides the essential amino acids. Sources are meat, poultry, fish, cheese, eggs, and milk. *Second class p.* The source is vegetable: peas, beans and whole cereal, but these cannot supply all the body's needs.

protein-bound iodine. The iodine in the plasma which is combined with protein. Measurement of this is made when assessing thyroid function.

protein-losing enteropathy. A condition in which protein is lost from the lumen of the intestine. This causes hypoproteinaemia and oedema.

proteinuria (*pro-teen-u'-re-ah*). A condition in which plasma proteins are present in the urine, often due to increased permeability of the tubules.

proteolysis (*pro-te-ol'-is-is*). The processes by which proteins are reduced to an absorbable form.

proteoses (*pro'-te-o-ses*). The first products in the breakdown of proteins.

Proteus vulgaris (*pro-te-us vul-gar'-is*). A bacillus that commonly occurs in secondary infections of wounds and the urinary tract.

prothrombin (*pro-throm'-bin*). Thrombogen. The precursor of thrombin which is formed in the presence of calcium salts and thrombokinase when blood is shed.

protoplasm (*pro'-to-plazm*). The essential chemical compound of which living cells are made.

prototype (*pro'-to-tipe*). Original from which copies are made.

Protozoa (*pro-to-zo'-ah*). The most primitive class of animal organisms, some of which are pathogenic, e.g. *Entamoeba histolytica* of amoebic dysentery, and *Plasmodium vivax* of malaria.

proud flesh (*prowd flesh*). Excess of granulation tissue in a wound.

provitamin (*pro-vi'-tam-in*). A precursor of a vitamin. *P. 'A'* is carotene. *P. 'D'* is said to be ergosterol.

proximal (*proks'-im-al*). Nearest that point which is considered the centre of a system. The opposite to distal.

prune belly. Congenital absence of abdominal muscles which cause the walls to be of an abnormal shape.

prurigo (*pru-ri'-go*). A chronic skin disease with an irritating papular eruption.

pruritus (*pru-ri'-tus*). Great irritation of the skin. It may affect the whole surface of the body, as in certain skin diseases and nervous disorders, or it may be limited in area.

prussic acid (*prus'-sik*). Hydrocyanic acid (*q.v.*).

pseudo- (*su'-do-*). A prefix meaning 'false'.

pseudo-angina (*su-do-an-ji'-nah*). False angina. Precordial pain occurring in anxious individuals without evidence of organic heart disease. May be part of effort syndrome (*q.v.*).

pseudo-arthrosis (*su-do-arthro'-sis*). A false joint.

pseudocrisis (*su-do-kri'-sis*). A false crisis which is sometimes accompanied by the symptoms of true crisis, but the temperature rises again almost at once, and there is continuation of the disease.

pseudocroup (*su-do-kroop'*). False croup. Laryngismus stridulus.

pseudocyesis (*su-do-si-e'-sis*). A false pregnancy in which subjective signs may be present; amenorrhoea, enlarged abdomen and breast changes, but no fetus.

pseudogynaecomastia (*su-do-gi-ne-ko-mas'-te-ah*). The deposition of adipose tissue in the male breast that may give the appearance of enlarged mammary glands.

pseudohermaphroditism (*su-do-hur-maf'-ro-di-tizm*). Due to a hormone imbalance some of the characteristics of the opposite sex are present and confusion may arise as to the true sex of the individual.

pseudoisochromatic charts (*su-do-i-so-kro-mat'-ik*). Charts of coloured dots for testing colour blindness.

pseudomeningitis (*su-do-men-in-ji'-tis*). *See* Meningism.

Pseudomonas pyocyanea
(*su-do-mo'-nas pi-o-si-a'-ne-ah*). A motile, rod-shaped bacillus normally present in the colon that may infect the urinary tract or wounds.

pseudomucinous (*su-do-mu'-sin-us*). Allied to mucin. *P. cyst. See* Cyst.

pseudomyopia (*su-du-mi-o'-pe-ah*). Spasm of the ciliary muscle causing the same focusing defect as in myopia (*q.v.*).

pseudoplegia (*su-do-ple'-je-ah*). Apparent loss of muscle power but not true paralysis. It may be hysterical in origin.

pseudopodium (*su-do-po'-de-um*). Protrusion of part of cell serving as a method of locomotion or phagocytosis.

psittacosis (*sit-a-ko'-sis*). A virus disease of parrots communicable to man. Conveyed by the budgerigar variety. The symptoms resemble paratyphoid fever with bronchopneumonia.

psoas (*so'-as*). A long strap muscle originating from the lumbar spine with insertion into the lesser trochanter of the femur. It flexes the thigh on the abdomen. *P. abscess.* Arises in the lumbar region and is due to spinal caries as a result of tuberculous infection. It may track down the muscle and point in the region of its insertion in the groin.

psoriasis (*sor-i'-as-is*). A chronic skin disesase characterized by reddish marginated patches with profuse silvery scaling on extensor surfaces like the knees and elbows, but may be widespread. It is non-infectious and the cause is unknown. *See* Goeckerman regimen.

psyche (*si'-ke*). The mind, both conscious and unconscious.

psychiatrist (*si-ki'-at-rist*). A doctor who has devoted himself to the study of mental disorders and their treatment.

psychiatry (si-ki'-at-re). The branch of medicine which deals with mental disorders and their treatment.

psychoanalysis (si'-ko-an-al'-is-is). A prolonged and intensive method of psychotherapy (q.v.) developed by Freud in which the patient is encouraged to speak freely concerning anything on his mind. Repressed material may be brought into consciousness. This may be helpful in partially or completely solving emotional problems and thus helping patients with neurotic traits or symptoms. See Association and Transference.

psychoanalyst (si-ko-an'-al-ist). One who specializes in psychoanalysis. He may or may not be medically qualified.

psychodrama (si-ko-drah'-mah). A form of group psychotherapy in which the patient with other group members acts out past incidents in his life. This is followed by group discussion, and under guidance of the psychiatrist an effort is made to give the patient a greater awareness of his behaviour and to try to solve the problem or conflict presented.

psychodynamic (si-ko-di-nam'-ik). The understanding and interpretation of psychiatric symptoms or abnormal behaviour in terms of unconscious mental mechanisms.

psychogenic (si-ko-jen'-ik). Originating in the mind. P. illness. A disorder having a psychological origin as opposed to an organic basis.

psychogeriatrics (si-ko-jer-e-at'-riks). The study and treatment of the psychological and psychiatric problems of the aged.

psychologist (si-kol'-o-jist). One who studies normal and abnormal mental processes, development and behaviour.

psychology (si-kol'-o-je). The study of the mind and mental processes.

psychometric (si-ko-met'-rik). Related to the measurement of mental characteristics.

psychomimetics (si-ko-mi-met'-iks). A group of drugs that produce an abnormal mental state that may resemble schizophrenia.

psychomotor (si-ko-mo'-tor). Related to the motor effects of mental activity.

psychoneurosis (si-ko-nu-ro'-sis). See Neurosis.

psychopath (si'-ko-path). A term used to describe a person with a defect in his personality. His actions will vary, he may be asocial, withdrawn, inadequate, and unable to take responsibility for himself or others. He may be anti-social, a criminal psychopath or he may have long-standing sexual perversions.

psychopathic disorder (si-ko-path'-ik). Mental Health Act 1959: A persistent disorder or disability of the mind which results in abnormally aggressive or seriously irresponsible conduct on the part of the patient, and requires or is susceptible to medical treatment.

psychopathology (si-ko-path-ol'-o-je). The study of the nature of mental diseases.

psychosexual development (si-ko-seks'-u-al). The stages through which an individual passes from birth to full maturity, especially in regard to sexual urges, in the total development of the person.

psychosis (si-ko'-sis). A severe mental illness affecting the whole personality. *Manic-depressive p.* Mild or severe attacks of elation or depression or both alternating. *Organic p.* This may be due to trauma, new growth or degenerative changes. *Senile p.* That occurring in the aged. *Syphilitic p.* A manifestation of the third stage of syphilis. *Toxic p.* This may be due to alcohol or metallic poisoning.

psychosomatic (*si-ko-so-mat'-ik*). Relating to the mind and the body. *P. disorders.* Those illnesses in which emotional factors have a profound influence. Some better-known examples are migraine, asthma and ulcerative colitis.

psychotherapy (*si-ko-ther'-ap-e*). The treatment of disease by psychological methods. This may be by suggestion, persuasion, hypnosis or by psychoanalytical methods. *See* Group psychotherapy.

psychotomimetics (*si-kot-o-mi-met'-iks*). Hallucinatory drugs that produce an abnormal mental state, mood changes, and delusions.

psychotropic drugs (*si-ko-tro'-pik*). Drugs that have an effect on the psyche. These include anti-depressants and tranquillizers.

pterygium (*te-rij'-e-um*). A patch of thickened conjunctiva which may develop over part of the cornea.

pterylglutamic acid (*ter-il-glu-tam'-ik*). Folic acid (*q.v.*).

ptomaines (*to'-manes*). Alkaloid compounds formed by putrefaction of animal or vegetable tissue.

ptosis (*to'-sis*). (1) Dropping of the upper eyelid due to loss of control by the third cranial nerve. (2) Prolapse of an organ; e.g. *gastroptosis*.

ptyalin (*ti'-al-in*). The enzyme (amylase) in saliva which splits starches.

ptyalism (*ti'-al-izm*). Salivation.

ptyalolith (*ti'-al-o-lith*). Salivary calculus.

puberty (*pu'-ber-te*). The age at which the reproductive organs become functionally active. Generally between the 12th and 17th year.

pubes (*pu'-beez*). The region over the os pubis.

pudence valve (*pu'-dense val-v*). Valve used to alleviate the symptoms of hydrocephalus in children. The accumulated cerebrospinal fluid is drained into the right atrium.

pudenda (*pu-den'-dah*). The external genitals.

pudendal block (*pu-den'-dal*). Infiltration of the sacral nerves that supply the perineum and clitoris, with a local anaesthetic.

puerperal (*pu-er'-per-al*). Pertaining to childbirth. *P. fever* or sepsis. Infection of the genital tract following childbirth.

puerperium (*pu-er-pe'-re-um*). A period of about six weeks following childbirth when the reproductive organs are returning to their normal state.

puking (*pu'-king*). Vomiting.

Pulex (*pu'-leks*). The flea. *P. irritans.* That parasitic on man. The type which infests rats may transmit plague to man.

pulmonary (*pul'-mon-ar-e*). Pertaining to or affecting the lungs. *P. circulation. See* Circulation. *P. embolism. See* Embolism. *P. hypertension.* An increase of pressure in the lungs due to an excessive flow of blood. *P. infarction.* Due to the occlusion of a small blood vessel in the lung by a clot, which causes death of the tissue sup-

plied by that vessel. *P. oedema.*
An excess of fluid in the lungs.
P. stenosis. A narrowing of the
pulmonary valve. *P. tuberculosis.* See Tuberculosis. *P. valve.*
The valve at the point where the
pulmonary artery leaves the
heart.

pulp. Any soft, juicy animal or
vegetable tissue. *P. cavity.* The
centre of a tooth containing
blood tissue and nerves. *Digital
p.* The soft pads at the ends of
the digits. *Splenic p.* The red-
dish-brown tissue of the spleen.

pulsation (*pul-sa'-shun*). A
beating or throbbing.

pulse (*puls*). The local rhythmic
expansion of an artery, which
can be felt with the finger,
corresponding to each contraction of the left ventricle of the
heart. It may be felt in any artery
sufficiently near the surface of
the body, and the normal adult
rate is about 72 per minute. In
childhood it is more rapid, varying from 130 in infants to 80 in
older children. *P. deficit.* When
the pulse rate is slower than the
apex beat. A sign of atrial fibrillation. *Dicrotic p.* See Dicrotic.
High-tension p. The duration of
the impulse in the artery is long,
and the artery feels firm and like
a cord between the beats. *Low-
tension p.* One easily obliterated
by pressure. *P. pressure.* The
difference between diastolic
and systolic blood pressures, as
measured by the sphygmomanometer. *Running p.* Little dis-
tinction between the beats. It
occurs in haemorrhage.
Thready p. Thin and almost
imperceptible. *Venous p.* That
felt in a vein—it is usually taken
in the right jugular vein. *Water-
hammer p.* (Corrigan's pulse).
A full volume, but rapidly collapsing pulse occurring in aortic
regurgitation.

pulsus alternans (*pul'-sus al'-
ter-nans*). Strong and weak
pulse beats alternate.

pulsus paradoxus (*pul'-sus
par-ah-doks'-us*). The pulse
rate slows on inspiration and
quickens on expiration. It may
occur in pericarditis.

pulvis (*pul'-vis*). A powder
(Latin).

pump oxygenator. A heart–
lung machine in which the
blood by-passes the heart and
lungs. The blood is removed
from both venae cavae, oxygenated and returned into the femoral artery so that it runs into
the aorta and so to the rest of
the body, e.g. Melrose machine.

puncta (*punk'-tah*). Openings
of the lacrimal ducts at the inner
canthus of the eye.

punctate (*punk'-tate*). Dotted.
P. erythema. A rash of very fine
spots.

puncture (*punk'-chur*). To
pierce. *Cisternal p.* To withdraw
fluid from the cisterna magna
(*q.v.*). *Exploratory p.* To pierce
where fluid is suspected, and
withdraw it for examination.
Lumbar p. To remove cerebrospinal fluid by puncture between the third and fourth lumbar vertebra. *Sternal p.* Into the
manubrium of the sternum to
withdraw bone marrow for examination. *Ventricular p.* Into a
cerebral ventricle to withdraw
fluid.

pupil (*pu'-pil*). The circular aperture in the centre of the iris,
through which light passes into
the eye. *Argyll Robertson p.*
Absence of response to light
but not to accommodation,
characteristic of locomotor
ataxia. *Artificial p.* One made by
cutting a piece out of the iris.

pupillary (*pu'-pil-lar-re*). Referring to the pupil.

purgative (*pur'-gat-iv*). A drug

which provides evacuation of the bowels. Purgatives may be: (1) Irritants like cascara, senna, rhubarb and castor oil. (2) Lubricants like paraffin emulsion. (3) Mechanical agents that increase bulk like saline aperients and agar preparations.

purines (*pu'-reens*). Compounds containing nitrogen which are essential for the formation of deoxyribonucleic acid. Metabolism of these results in the formation of uric acid.

Purkinje cells (*J. E. Purkinje, Bohemian physiologist, 1787– 1869*). A layer of cells with an extensive dendritic network that are connector neurones in the cerebellar cortex.

Purkinje fibres (*J. E. Purkinje, Bohemian physiologist, 1787– 1869*). Fibres found in cardiac muscle.

purpura (*pur'-pu-rah*). A condition characterized by extravasation of blood in the skin and mucous membranes, causing purple spots and patches. It may be a *primary* disease, most probably an auto-immune process, or a *secondary* sign in other diseases where there is failure of platelet production. (1) *P. haemorrhagica* or *thrombocytopenic p.* A severe form with profuse haemorrhage, especially from the mucous membranes, any of which may be involved. (2) *Non-thrombocytopenic p., Henoch's p.* Occurs in children and is characterized by purpura within the intestinal canal and the passage of blood and mucus in the stools. *Schonlein's p.* Occurs in young adults. Crops of purpuric spots, haemorrhages into joints causing painful swellings.

purulent (*pu'-ru-lent*). Containing or resembling pus.

pus. A thick, yellow semi-liquid substance consisting of dead leucocytes and bacteria, debris of cells, and tissue fluids. It results from inflammation caused by invading bacteria which have destroyed the phagocytes and set up local suppuration. The chief of these pus-forming bacteria are *Streptococcus pyogenes* and *Staphylococcus pyogenes*. *Blue p.* Produced by infection with *Pseudomonas pyocyanea*.

pustule (*pus'-tule*). A small pimple or elevation of the skin, containing pus. *Malignant p.* See Anthrax.

putrefaction (*pu-tre-fak'-shun*). Decomposition of animal or vegetable matter under the influence of micro-organisms, usually accompanied by an offensive odour due to gas formation.

pyaemia (*pi-e'-me-ah*). A condition resulting from the circulation of particles of blood clot from some focus of infection. Blockage of small blood vessels occurs with resultant formation of abscesses, the development of which causes rigor and high fever. *Portal p.* Pylephlebitis (*q.v.*). See Embolism and Thrombophlebitis.

pyarthrosis (*pi-ar-thro'-sis*). Suppuration in a joint.

pyelitis (*pi-el-i'-tis*). A seldom used term as infection affects not only the pelvis of the kidney but also the renal substance. See Pyelonephritis.

pyelography (*pi-el-og'-raf-e*). A method of X-ray examination of the kidney. *Intravenous p.* The dye is inserted into a vein and within 10 minutes is being excreted by the renal tubules. *Retrograde p.* The dye is inserted via cytoscope and ureteric catheters.

pyelolithotomy (*pi-el-o-lith-ot'-o-me*). Removal of a stone from the renal pelvis.

pyelonephritis (*pi-el-o-nef-ri'-tis*). Inflammation of the renal pelvis and renal substance characterized by fever, acute loin pain, frequency of micturition with pus and albumin in the urine. Due to an ascending infection from the ureters and below (urinary stasis or urinary obstruction being important contributory factors) or from the blood stream. Treatment is according to the causative organism, either sulphonamides or penicillin are used. Recurrent acute attacks may lead to chronic infection and eventual renal failure.

pyknic (*pik'-nik*). A type of physique, a stocky rounded figure with a good chest and abdominal capacity and a tendency to put on fat, that is said to go with the cheerful extroverted type of personality. One of the Kretschmer types whereby potential psychopathic tendencies are related to physical characteristics.

pyknolepsy (*pik'-no-lep-se*). Slight and frequent fits which may occur in children. A form of minor epilepsy which ceases as the child grows up.

pylephlebitis (*pi-le-fleb-i'-tis*). Inflammation of the portal vein which gives rise to severe symptoms of septicaemia or pyaemia.

pylethrombosis (*pi-le-thrombo'-sis*). Thrombosis of the portal vein.

pyloric stenosis (*pi-lor'-ik*). Stricture of the pyloric orifice. It may be: (1) Hypertrophic, when there is thickening of normal tissue. This is congenital and occurs in infants from 4 to 7 weeks old, usually males and first babies. (2) Due to scarring from ulceration. (3) Due to carcinoma.

pyloromyotomy (*pi-lor-o-mi-ot'-o-me*). Ramstedt's operation. An incision of the pylorus.

pyloroplasty (*pi-lor'-o-plas-te*). Plastic operation on the pylorus to enlarge the outlet. A longitudinal incision is made and it is resutured transversely.

pylorospasm (*pi-lor'-o-spazm*). Forceful muscle contraction of the pylorus that delays emptying of the stomach.

pylorus (*pi-lor'-us*). The sphincter muscle which guards the opening of the stomach into the duodenum.

pyocolpos (*pi-o-kol'-pos*). Accumulated pus in the vagina.

pyocyanic (*pi-o-si-an'-ik*). Re-

longitudinal incision

resutured transversely

A   B   C

PYLOROPLASTY

lating to blue pus produced by infection with *Pseudomonas pyocyanea*.

pyogenic (*pi-o-jen'-ik*). Producing pus.

pyometra (*pi-o-me'-trah*). Pus in the uterus.

pyonephrosis (*pi-o-nef-ro'-sis*). Obstruction and infection of the pelvis of the kidney. The calyces and pelvis are dilated, contain pus and usually calculi.

pyopericarditis (*pi-o-per-e-kard-i'-tis*). Suppurative infection of the pericardium.

pyopneumothorax (*pi-o-nu-mo-thor'-aks*). Air and pus in the pleural cavity, as may result from rupture of an abscess on the surface of the lung.

pyorrhoea (*pi-or-re'-ah*). A discharge of pus. *P. alveolaris*. Pus in the sockets of the teeth.

pyosalpinx (*pi-o-sal'-pinks*). Pus in the fallopian tube.

pyosis (*pi-o'-sis*). Suppuration.

pyothorax (*pi-o-thor'-aks*). Pus in the pleural cavity. Empyema (*q.v.*).

pyramidal (*pir-am'-id-al*). Of pyramid shape. *P. cells*. Cortical cells from which originate nerve impulses to voluntary muscle. *P. tract*. The nerve fibres which transmit impulses from pyramidal cells through brain and spinal cord.

pyretic (*pi-ret'-ik*). Pertaining to fever.

pyrexia (*pi-rek'-se-ah*). Fever; a rise of body temperature to any point between 37·5 and 40°C; above this is hyperpyrexia. *Continuous p.* The temperature is high and does not vary more than one degree in 24 hours. *Intermittent p.* Rising very high and falling below normal each day. *Remittent p.* The temperature varies more than one degree but never reaches normal.

pyridostigmine (*pir-e-do-stig'-meen*). A drug that prevents destruction of acetylcholine at the neuromuscular junctions and is used in treating myasthenia gravis. It is less powerful than neostigmine but has a more prolonged action. Mestinon is a proprietary preparation.

pyridoxine (*pir-e-doks'-een*). Vitamin B$_6$. This vitamin is concerned with protein metabolism and blood formation.

pyrimidines (*pi-rim'-id-eens*). Compounds containing nitrogen, essential for the formation of deoxyribonucleic acid.

pyrogen (*pi'-ro-jen*). A substance that can produce fever.

pyrogenic (*pi-ro-jen'-ik*). Producing fever.

pyromania (*pi-ro-ma'-ne-ah*). An irresistible desire to set things on fire.

pyrosis (*pi-ro'-sis*). Heartburn, a symptom of dyspepsia, marked by a burning sensation in the stomach and oesophagus with eructation of acid fluid.

pyuria (*pi-u'-re-ah*). Pus in the urine. It is visible as a whitish sediment, which becomes thick and ropy on the addition of liquor potassae; pus cells can be seen on microscopic examination. *See* Appendix 11.

Q

Q fever. Fever caused by *Rickettsia burneti*. It resembles pneumonia.

quack (*kwak*). One who pretends to have medical knowledge and skills that he does not possess.

quadrant (*kwod'-rant*). A quarter of a circle or a fourth part.

quadriceps (*kwod'-re-seps*). Four-headed. *Q. extensor mus-*

cle. The principal extensor of the thigh.

quadriplegia (*kwod-re-ple'-je-ah*). Paralysis in which all four limbs are affected.

quadruple vaccine (*kwod'-ru-pl vak'-seen*). A vaccine to immunize against diphtheria, pertussis, poliomyelitis and tetanus.

qualitative (*kwal-e-ta'-tif*). Referring to or concerned with quality.

quantitative (*kwan-te-ta'-tif*). Referring to the amount or quantity.

quarantine (*kwor'-an-teen*). The period of isolation of an infectious or suspected case, to prevent the spread of disease. For contacts, this is the longest incubation period known for the specific disease.

quartan (*kwor'-tan*). An intermittent fever recurring every third day, i.e. 1st, 4th, 7th, etc. In malaria each attack corresponds with a fresh invasion of red corpuscles by the malarial parasites.

quartz (*kwor'-tz*). Rock crystal. Ultra-violet rays can penetrate it. *Q. lamp.* That used for treatment by artificial sunlight.

quaternary ammonium compounds (*kwot-ern'-ar-e*). A group of bactericidal agents. Examples are cetrimide (Cetavlon), benzalkonium (Roccal), and domiphen (Bradosol).

Queckenstedt's test (*H. H. G. Queckenstedt, German physician, 1876–1918*). A test carried out during lumbar puncture by compression of the jugular veins. When normal there is a sharp rise in pressure, followed by a fall as the compression is released. Blockage of the spinal canal or thrombosis of the jugular vein will result in an ab-

sence of rise, or only a sluggish rise and fall.

'quickening' (*kwik-en-ing*). The first perceptible fetal movement, felt by the mother between the fourth and fifth months of pregnancy.

quicklime (*kwik-lime*). Calcium oxide.

quiescent (*kwi-es'-ent*). Inactive or at rest. Periods when the symptoms of a disease are not evident.

quinalbarbitone (*kwin-al-bar'-be-tone*). A short-acting, quickly absorbed analgesic. Seconal is a proprietary preparation.

quinidine (*kwin'-id-een*). An alkaloid from cinchona. It restores normal rhythm in cases of atrial fibrillation, for which purpose it is given in selected cases.

quinine (*kwin'-een*). An alkaloid obtained from cinchona bark. In small doses it is tonic and antipyretic. In larger doses it is used in the treatment of malaria as a prophylactic and curative. It is also stimulative to uterine contractions. *Q. urethane* is used for injection treatment of varicose veins to cause sclerosis of the vessels.

quininism (*kwin'-in-izm*). Cinchonism (*q.v.*).

quinsy (*kwin'-ze*). Peritonsillar abscess. Acute inflammation of the tonsil and surrounding cellular tissue with suppuration. It is characterized by fever, abscess formation, and great pain and difficulty in swallowing. Antibiotic treatment may abort the attack but if suppuration occurs incision is necessary.

quotient (*kwo'-shent*). A number obtained by division. *Intelligence q.* The degree of intelligence estimated by dividing the mental age reckoned from standard tests by the age in years. *Respiratory q.* The ratio between the CO_2 expired and the O_2 inspired during a specified time.

R

rabid (*rab'-id*). Infected with rabies.

rabies (*ra'-beez*). An acute infectious disease of animals, especially the dog, cat and wolf. The virus is found in the saliva of infected animals, and if transmitted to man produces hydrophobia.

racemose (*rase'-moze*). Grapelike. *R. glands* are compound lobulated in structure, e.g. salivary glands.

rachis (*rak'-is*). The vertebral column.

rad. A unit for measuring radiation dosage. It is a measure of the amount of energy absorbed from a radioactive source.

radial (*ra'-de-al*). Relating to the radius. *R. artery.* The artery at the wrist. *R. pulse.* Pulse of the radial artery felt at the wrist.

radiant (*ra'-de-ant*). Emitting rays. *R. heat bath.* Exposure of the whole or part of the body to heat rays generated by electricity.

radiation (*ra-de-a'-shun*). The emanation of energy from a source. The most usual form of this is that of photons. These vary in their frequency of emission and are called radio waves, light, X-rays or gamma rays. Radiation causes damage to living tissues. *R. pneumonitis.* Inflammatory changes in the alveoli and interstitial tissue due to radiation which may lead to fibrosis later. *R. sickness.* The reaction of the body to radiation. Any or all of the following may be present; anorexia, nausea, vomiting, and diarrhoea.

radical (*rad'-ik-al*). Dealing with the root or cause of a disease. *R. cure.* One which cures by complete removal of the cause.

radioactive (*ra-de-o-ak'-tiv*). Having the power of radioactivity. *See* Isotope. *R. gold* has been used in treating malignant disease. *R. iodine. See* Iodine. *R. phosphorus.* Used to check polycythaemia.

radioactivity (*ra-de-o-ak-tiv'-e-te*). Some elements of high atomic weight have the power of emitting α and β particles and some γ-rays. This results in disintegration of the element to one of lower atomic weight. *Induced r.* Can be produced in certain elements as in an atomic pile by bombarding the nuclei with neutrons.

radio-autography (*ra-de-o-aw-tog'-raf-e*). A form of photography in which molecules labelled with radioactive atoms reveal themselves in photographic emulsion.

radiobiology (*ra-de-o-bi-ol'-o-je*). The branch of medical science that studies the effect of radiation on live animal and human tissues.

radiodermatitis (*ra-de-o-dermat-i'-tis*) A late skin complication of radiotherapy in which

RADIATION HAZARD

there is atrophy, scarring, pigmentation and telangiectases of the skin.

radiograph (ra'-de-o-graf). Skiagram. The picture obtained on a sensitive plate by X-rays passing through the body.

radiographer (ra-de-og'-rafer). One who is trained to take X-ray pictures.

radiography (ra-de-og'-raf-e). The method of making X-ray photographic records. Some substances are less easily penetrated than others and therefore throw a shadow on the film. Bone and many diseased tissues are semi-opaque. X-ray will not penetrate metal and some types of adhesive plaster, which must be remembered when fractured bones are photographed. For diagnosis, drugs opaque to the rays are introduced into the body. *See* Barium, Bismuth.

radiologist (ra-de-ol'-o-jist). One who is skilled in the science of radiology.

radiology (ra-de-ol'-o-je). The science of radiant energy. In medicine the term refers to its use in the diagnosis and treatment of disease.

radiosensitive (ra-de-o-sen'-se-tif). Those structures that respond well to radiotherapy.

radiotherapy (ra-de-o-ther'-ap-e). Treatment of disease by radium, X-rays and radioactive isotopes.

radium (ra'-de-um). A radioactive element obtained from pitchblende and other uranium ores, which gives off emanations of great radioactive power. Usually used in the form of radium bromide, a yellow crystalline powder. It emits three distinct rays:—*alpha* (α); *beta* (β); *gamma* (γ). The last are similar to X-rays but shorter, and it is these which are de-

structive to malignant cells. Used in the treatment of malignant growth, for rodent ulcer and to induce artificial menopause.

radius (ra'-de-us). The smaller bone of the forearm.

radon seeds (ra'-don). A method of treatment by which the emanations from radium are collected, sealed in a container, and inserted into places from which it would be inconvenient to remove radium itself. These emanations lose their effect after a few days; the containers remain harmlessly in the tissues.

râle (rahl). An abnormal rattling sound, heard on auscultation of the chest during respiration in cases of bronchitis.

rami (ra'-mi). Branches, as of arteries, veins and nerves. *R. communicantes.* The nerve fibres which connect the sympathetic ganglia with the spinal cord. *Sing.* ramus.

Ramstedt's operation (*W. C. Ramstedt, German surgeon, 1867–*). For congenital stricture of the pylorus in which the fibres of the sphincter muscle are divided but the mucous lining is left intact.

ranula (ran'-u-lah). A retention cyst usually under the tongue when blockage occurs in a submaxillary or sublingual duct, or in a mucous gland.

Ranvier's node (*L. A. Ranvier, French pathologist, 1835–1922). See* Node.

raphe (raf'-e). A seam or ridge of tissue indicating the juncture of two parts.

rapid eye movement (REM). Movement of the eyes which occurs during dreaming in sleep.

rapport (rap-port'). A psychiatric term used to describe a satisfactory relationship between two persons, either the doctor and patient or nurse and patient, or the patient with any other person significant to him.

rarefaction (*rair-e-fak'-shun*). Thinning. *R. of bone*. Thinning as occurs in tuberculous infection of bone.

rash. A superficial eruption on the skin, frequently characteristic of some specific fever. Desquamation follows it. *Nettle r.* Urticaria (*q.v.*). *Serum r.* An irritating urticaria which may appear 8 to 10 days after an injection of serum. *See* Anaphylaxis.

Rashkind catheter (*W. J. Rashkind, American paediatric cardiologist, 1922–). A balloon catheter used to increase the size of the atrial septal defect in children who have transposition of the great vessels.

raspatory (*ras'-pat-or-e*). An instrument used to strip the periosteum from bone.

rat-bite fever. *See* Weil's disease.

Rastelli's operation (*G. C. Rastelli, American thoracic surgeon, 1933–). Surgical procedure used in the treatment of transposition of the great vessels. The circulation of blood through the heart is diverted to effect adequate oxygenation.

Rathke's pouch (*M. H. Rathke, German anatomist, 1793–1860*). Diverticulum in the roof of the embryonic mouth which becomes part of the pituitary gland.

rationalization (*rash-un-al-i-za'-shun*). The mental process by which an individual explains his behaviour, giving reasons that are advantageous to himself or are socially acceptable. It may be a conscious or an unconscious act.

Raynaud's disease (*M. Ray-naud, French physician, 1834–81*). Spasm of the arterioles of the extremities causing numbness, tingling and discoloration. The treatment is protection from cold and vasodilator drugs. Sympathectomy may prove beneficial, but the condition is progressive.

Raynaud's phenomenon (*M. Raynaud, French physician, 1834–81*). Spasm of the digital arteries in response to cold. *Secondary R. p.* May arise as an occupational hazard in those who work with vibrating tools—pneumatic drills, etc.

rays. Lines of light or heat. Various ones are used in medical treatment. Light from the sun when divided up has colours ranging from red, through orange, yellow, green, blue and indigo, to violet: this is the *visible spectrum*. It extends much farther at each end, and these rays can be made apparent by photography or fluorescence. Those below the red rays (*infra-red*) include Hertzian or radio waves, while the invisible ones beyond the violet are extremely short, i.e. *X-ray* and *ultra-violet ray*. According to their intensity these cause ordinary sunburn, the burns of ultra-violet light, or destruction of malignant growths.

re-. A prefix meaning 'back' or 'again'.

reaction (*re-ak'-shun*). Counteraction; a response to the application of a stimulus. *Acid r.* A test for the presence of acids; blue litmus paper turns red. *Alkaline r.* An indication of the presence of alkalis; red litmus paper turns blue.

reactive (*re-ak'-tiv*). In psychiatry, the response of an individual to adverse external circumstances causing an exogenous depression.

reagent (re-a´-jent). A substance employed to produce a chemical reaction. *Esbach's r.* A solution of picric acid used in Esbach's albuminometer. *See* Appendix 11.

reamer (re´-mur). An instrument for reshaping the head of the femur during arthroplasty and for enlarging root canals in dentistry.

recall (re´-kawl). To bring back to consciousness. Memory consists of registering, retaining, and recall.

receptaculum chyli (re-septak´-u-lum ki´-li). The pouchlike lower end of the thoracic duct, into which the fat passes when absorbed from the intestine.

receptors (re-sep´-tors). The sensory nerve endings that receive stimuli for transmission. *Alpha r.* Nerve receptors associated with the contraction of smooth muscle. *Beta r.* Nerve receptors associated with the relaxation of smooth muscle.

recessive (re-cess´-if). The opposite to dominant. *R. genes.* A gene which will produce its characteristics only when present in a homozygous state, that is when both parents possess this gene. Then the child has only a 1 in 4 chance of inheriting it.

recipient (re-sip´-e-ent). (1) One who receives blood from another by transfusion. (2) One who receives an organ or tissue from another by transplantation. *Universal r.* A person who can receive blood from all groups of donors without harmful effect. *See* Blood grouping.

von Recklinghausen's disease (F. D. von Recklinghausen, German pathologist, 1833–

1910). (1) *Neurofibromatosis.* A rare disease of skin pigmentation and multiple painless fibromata along the course of the peripheral nerves. (2) *Osteitis fibrosa cystica* or hyperparathyroidism of the bones in which the blood calcium is raised but there is decalcification of bone tissue.

recrudescence (re-kru-des´-sense). Renewed aggravation of symptoms following an interval of abatement.

rectal (rek´-tal). Relating to the rectum. *R. anaesthesia. See* Anaesthesia. *R. examination.* By insertion of a glove-covered finger or with the aid of a proctoscope.

rectified spirit (rek´-te-fide). Alcohol having 10 per cent of water in it.

rectocele (rek´-to-seel). Hernia of the rectum, caused by overstretching of the vaginal wall at childbirth. Treated by posterior colporrhaphy.

rectoperineorrhaphy (rek-toper-in-e-or´-raf-e). The operation for repair of the perineum and rectal wall.

rectopexy (rek´-to-peks-e). The operation for fixation of a prolapsed rectum.

rectoscope (rek´-to-skope). *See* Proctoscope.

rectovaginal (rek-to-vaj-i´-nal). Concerning the rectum and vagina. *R. fistula. See* Fistula.

rectovesical (rek-to-ves´-ik-al). Concerning the rectum and bladder. *R. fistula. See* Fistula.

rectum (rek´-tum). The lower end of the large intestine from the sigmoid flexure to the anus.

rectus (rek´-tus). Straight. *R. abdominis.* The straight muscle passing up the front of the abdomen from the pubis to the ribs. *R. femoris.* The straight muscle of the thigh; part of the quadriceps extensor. *R. muscle of the eye.* The four straight muscles which move the eyeball.

recumbent (*re-kum'-bent*). Lying down in the dorsal position.

recuperation (*re-ku-per-a'-shun*). Convalescence.

recurrent (*re-kur'-rent*). Occurring again. *R. fever.* Relapsing fever (*q.v.*). *R. haemorrhage. See* Haemorrhage. *R. bandage.* A pattern used for stumps of limbs, fingers, etc., when the bandage is made to turn back over itself in order to cover in the part.

red cells (*red sells*). Cells in the blood which carry haemoglobin (*q.v.*).

red lotion (*red lo'-shun*). A cleansing astringent lotion containing zinc sulphate.

reduce (*re-duse'*). To restore to normal position, e.g. a hernia or dislocation.

reduction division (*re-duk'-shun di-vi-shun*). Type of multiplication of sex cells in which the chromosomes separate into two duplicate strands, instead of splitting into two as they do in other cells.

reduction en masse (*re-duk'-shun on mass*). Describes an attempt to reduce a strangulated hernia, but the sac is pushed back intact, so that the bowel remains strangulated and the condition is not relieved.

re-education (*re-ed-u-ka'-shun*). The training of the physically or mentally disabled handicapped person; so that he may completely, or in some degree, regain his former powers.

reef knot (*reef not*). A knot used in surgery which does not slip.

referred pain (*re-furd pane*).

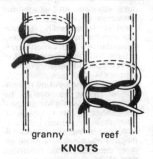

granny   reef

KNOTS

That which occurs at a distance from the place of origin due to the sensory nerves entering the cord at the same level, i.e. the phrenic nerve supplying the diaphragm enters the cord in the cervical region as do the nerves from the shoulder.

reflex (*re'-fleks*). Reflected or thrown back. *R. action.* An involuntary action following immediately upon some stimulus, e.g. the knee jerk, or the withdrawal of a limb from a pinprick. *R. arc.* The sensory and motor neurones together with the connector neurone which carry

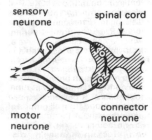

sensory neurone   spinal cord

motor neurone   connector neurone

REFLEX ARC

out a reflex action. *R. of accommodation.* When the size of the pupil alters according to the distance of the image viewed. *Conditioned r.* That which is not natural, but is developed by association and frequent repetition until it appears natural. *Corneal r.* Light pressure on the cornea causes the eyelids to close. This is a test for unconsciousness which is absolute when there is no response. *Deep r.* A muscle reflex elicited by tapping the tendon or bone of attachment. *R. to light.* Alteration of the size of the pupil in response to exposure to light. *Spinal r.* That which takes place through centres in the spinal cord. *Swallowing r.* Initiated by stimulation of the palate. *R. vomiting. See* Vomiting.

reflux (*re'-fluks*). A backward flow.

refraction (*re-frak'-shun*). The bending or deviation of rays of light, as they pass obliquely through one medium and penetrate another of different density.

refractive (*re-frak'-tiv*). Relating to refraction. *R. error.* A defect that prevents light rays from converging on a single focus on the retina.

refractory (*re-frak'-tor-e*). Not yielding to, or resistant to, treatment. *R. period.* Period during which a nerve cannot receive a fresh impulse. It is inexcitable.

refrigeration (*re-frij-er-a'-shun*). The cooling of a part to reduce the metabolic requirements, May be used to aid the formation of a collateral circulation or as a form of anaesthesia.

regeneration (*re-jen-er-a'-shun*). Renewing again, e.g. new growth of tissue in its specific form after injury.

regional ileitis (*re'-jun-al il-e-i'-tis*). Crohn's disease. A localized area of inflammation of the small intestine. The cause is unknown.

regression (*re-gresh'-un*). A tendency to return to primitive or child-like modes of behaviour. This may be done as a means of solving a problem when under emotional stress.

regurgitation (*re-gur-jit-a'-shun*). Backward flow, e.g. of food into the stomach. Fluids regurgitate through the nose in paralysis affecting the soft palate. *Aortic r.* Backward flow of blood into the left ventricle when the aortic valve is incompetent. *Mitral r. See* Mitral.

rehabilitation (*re-hab-il-it-a'-shun*). Re-education. *R. centre* One which provides for organized employment within the capacity of the patient, and with especial regard to the psychical influence of the work.

Reiter protein complement fixation (*H. Reiter, German bacteriologist, 1881–1969*). RPCF. A serological test used to aid the diagnosis of syphilis.

Reiter's syndrome (*H. Reiter, German physician, 1881–1969*). A non-specific urethritis in which there is also arthritis and conjuctivitis.

relapse (*re-laps'*). The return of a disease, after an interval of convalescence.

relapsing fevers. Certain louse- or tick-borne tropical fevers. The fever lasts a few days, but relapses are common. Tetracycline has proved successful in treatment.

relaxant (*re-laks'-ant*). A drug or other agent that brings about muscle relaxation or relieves tension.

relaxin (*re-laks'-in*). Polypeptides that are produced by the ovary and soften the cervix and loosen the ligaments of the symphysis pubis to aid the birth of the baby.

releasing factors. Substances produced in the hypothalamus which cause the anterior pituitary gland to release hormones.

remission (re-mish'-un). Subsidence of the symptoms of a disease for a time.

remittent (re-mit'-tent). Returning at intervals. *R. fever. See* Fever *and* Pyrexia.

renal (re'-nal). Relating to the kidney. *R. asthma. See* Asthma. *R. calculus.* Stone in the kidney. *R. threshold.* The level of the blood sugar, beyond which it is excreted in the urine. Normally 0·18 per cent. *R. rickets, dwarfism,* or *infantilism.* A form of interstitial nephritis, sometimes occurring in children, associated with delayed growth and marked rickets.

renin (re'-nin). A proteolytic enzyme released into the blood stream when the kidneys are ischaemic. It causes vasoconstriction.

rennin (ren'-in). An enzyme in the gastric secretion that curdles milk.

renography (re-nog'-raf-e). Radiography of the kidney. *Arterial r.* A radio-opaque dye is inserted via the femoral artery or aorta to outline the blood supply in the kidney. This may reveal a non-vascular area indicating a tumour.

reorganization (re-or-gan-i-za'-shun). Healing by formation of new tissue, or by operative reconstruction. *See* Arthroplasty.

repolarization (re-po-lar-i-za'-shun). The reforming of an electric charge at the neuromuscular junction (q.v.) after its dispersal by the passage of a nerve impulse.

repositor (re-pos'-it-or). An instrument for replacing a prolapsed organ. *Iris r.* An instrument for replacing the iris following an intra-ocular operation.

repression (re-presh'-un). The inability of an individual to recognize motives and feelings which are unacceptable to him. It is a defence mechanism by which painful experiences are forced out into and kept in the unconscious.

resection (re-sek'-shun). Removal of a part. *Submucous r.* Removal of part of a deflected nasal septum, from beneath a flap of mucous membrane which is then replaced. *Transurethral r.* A method of removing portions of an enlarged prostate gland via the urethra.

resectoscope (re-sek'-to-skope). A telescopic instrument by which pieces of tissue can also be removed. Used for transurethral prostatectomy.

reserpine (res'-er-peen). An alkaloid from *Rauwolfia*, a drug used to reduce the blood pressure in hypertension. It may be used in conjuction with mecamylamine (q.v.) or with the diuretic hydrochlorothiazide in the trade preparation of Salupres.

residual (re-zid'-u-al). Remaining. *R. air. See* Air. *R. juice.* Gastric juice withdrawn from the stomach by a syringe and through a Ryle's tube, before a test meal is given. *R. urine. See* Urine.

resilient (re-zil'-e-ent). Having the power to return to normal shape after stretching or compressing.

resistance. (1) In *electricity,* the opposition made by a non-conducting substance to the passage of a current. (2) In *psychology*, the opposition, stemming from the unconscious, to repressed ideas being brought to consciousness. *Cross r.* Resistance developed by micro-organisms to a certain antibiotic and to other antibiotics in the same group. *R. to infection.* The natural power of the body to withstand the toxins of disease. It can be maintained and increased by conserving the patient's strength by good diet, fresh air, rest, and freedom from mental worries. Artificially, it is increased by injection of vaccines and antitoxic sera. *Peripheral r.* is that offered to the passage of blood through small vessels and capillaries.

resolution (*rez-o-lu'-shun*). The process of returning to normal. It sometimes occurs in inflammatory conditions without the formation of pus.

resonance (*rez'-on-ans*). the reverberating sound obtained on percussing over a cavity or hollow organ, such as the lung.

resonium-A (*re-zo'-ne-um*). Resin used to effect cation exchange. Administered in powdered form to patients.

resorcinol (*res-or'-sin-ol*). Resorcin. A phenol compound used as an ointment in skin diseases, and sometimes as an antiseptic.

resorption (*re-sorp'-shun*). (1) The absorption of morbid deposits, such as the products of inflammation. (2) The absorption of excreted materials.

respiration (*res-pir-a'-shun*). The gaseous interchange between the tissue cells and the atmosphere. *External r.* In man consists of *inspiration*, when the external intercostal muscles and the diaphragm contract and air is drawn into the lungs, and *expiration* or breathing out. *Artificial r.* is the production of respiratory movements by external effort. *See* Appendix 2. *Internal* or *tissue r.* The interchange of gases which occurs between tissues and blood through the walls of capillaries. *Inverse r.* Causes a grunting sound and the sequence is *expiration, inspiration, pause.* Noticeably present in bronchopneumonia, especially in young children. *Laboured r.* That which is difficult and distressed. *Stertorous r.* Snoring. A noisy breathing. *See* Cheyne–Stokes respiration.

respirator (*res'-pir-a-tor*). A device to aid respiration. (1) *A face mask* for giving oxygen or a drug or for removing impurities or poison gases. (2) *Tank r.* The iron lung into which the patient is put except for the head and respiration is brought about by intermittent negative pressure, drawing air into the lungs. (3) *Cuirass r.* The negative pressure created by an appliance strapped to the chest leaving the limbs free. (4) A *positive pressure r.* The patient is attached to a machine which blows air into the lungs via an intratracheal tube or tracheostomy. (5) *Pump r.* The heartlung machine, by which the blood can be removed from the body, oxygenated, and returned into circulation.

respiratory distress syndrome. Dyspnoea occurring between soon after birth and the third day of life. Associated with prematurity it is characterized by severe retraction of the chest wall with expiratory grunting and cyanosis. *Syn.* Hyaline membrane disease.

resuscitation (*re-sus-sit-a'-*

shun). Bringing back to life one who is apparently dead. *See* Appendix 2.

retardation (*re-tard-a'-shun*). Late or delayed activity. *Mental r.* A state of arrested development of the mind, that has existed from birth or from an early age. *Syn.* Subnormality (*q.v.*). *Psychomotor r.* A slowing down of mental processes and of bodily movement.

retching (*ret'-ching*). An involuntary, spasmodic, but ineffectual effort to vomit.

retention (*re-ten'-shun*). Holding back. *R. of urine.* Inability to pass urine from the bladder, which may be due to obstruction or of nervous origin. *R. cyst. See* Cyst. *R. defect.* A term used in psychiatry to describe a defect of memory. Inability to retain material in the mind so that it can be recalled when required. *R. enema. See* Enema.

reticular (*re-tik'-u-lar*). Resembling a network. May be applied to tissues. *R. formation.* Area in the brain stem from which nerve fibres extend to the cerebral cortex. Associated with sleep and the state of consciousness.

reticulocyte (*re-tik'-u-lo-site*). A red blood cell that is not fully mature, it still retains strands of nucleus material.

reticulocytosis (*re-tik'-u-lo-si-to'-sis*). The presence of an increased number of immature red cells in the blood, indicating over-activity of the bone marrow.

reticulo-endothelial system (*re-tik'-u-lo en-do-the'-le-al*). Consists of endothelial cells in the liver, spleen, bone marrow and lymph glands that produce large mononuclear cells or macrophages. These are phagocytic, they destroy red blood cells and have the power of making some antibodies.

reticuloses (*re-tik-u-lo'-seez*). A group of rare malignant diseases of the reticulo-endothelial system. These include Hodgkin's disease, lymphosarcoma and reticulum-cell sarcoma.

reticulosarcoma (*re-tik-u-lo-sar-ko'-mah*). A malignant disease of the blood in which the liver and spleen are involved. It is one of the reticuloses.

retina (*ret'-in-ah*). The innermost coat of the eyeball, formed of nerve cells and fibres, and from which the optic nerve leaves the eyeball and passes to the visual area of the cerebrum. The impression of the image is focused upon it.

retinal (*ret'-in-al*). Relating to the retina. *R. detachment.* When the retina becomes partially detached from the underlying choroid layer, resulting in loss of vision.

retinene (*ret'-in-een*). The component of rhodopsin which can be converted into vitamin A in the light and resynthesized into rhodopsin in the dark, allowing maximum vision in a dim light.

retinitis (*ret-in-i'-tis*). Inflammation of the retina.

retinoblastoma (*ret-in-o-blas-to'-mah*). A malignant growth of nerve cells of the retina that have failed to develop normally. It is congenital and may affect several members of one family.

retinopathy (*ret-in-op'-ath-e*). Degenerative changes occurring in the retinal blood vessels leading to loss of vision. *Diabetic r.* A complication occurring in diabetes.

retinotoxic (*ret-in-o-toks'-ik*). Drugs which may result in damage to the retina in susceptible persons.

retractile (*re-trak'-tile*). Capable of being drawn back.

retraction (*re-trak'-shun*). Drawing back. (1) The process of retraction of the uterus during labour to expel the fetus. (2) Drawing back of the ends of a cut blood vessel before a clot forms in the lumen. *R. ring.* A ridge sometimes felt above the pubes between the upper contracting part of the uterus and the lower dilatable part.

retractor (*re-trak'-tor*). A surgical instrument for drawing apart the edges of a wound to allow the deeper structures to be more accessible.

retro- (*ret'-ro*). A prefix meaning 'backward'.

retrobulbar neuritis (*ret-ro-bul'-bar nu-ri'-tis*). Dimness of vision due to inflammation of the optic nerve. This may be temporary or permanent in some cases of disseminated sclerosis.

retroflexion (*ret-ro-flek'-shun*). Bent backward; applied to the uterus when it is bent backward at an acute angle, the cervix being in its normal position.

retrograde (*ret'-ro-grade*). Going backwards. *R. pyelography.* X-ray of the kidney by injecting an opaque substance into the renal pelvis via the urethra and ureteric catheters.

retrogression (*ret-ro-gres'-shun*). Going backwards. Reverting to primitive type.

retrolental fibroplasia (*ret-ro-len'-tal fi-bro-pla'-ze-ah*). A fibrous condition of the anterior vitreous body which develops when a premature infant is kept in too high an oxygen saturation for too long. Both eyes are affected and it may cause blindness.

retro-ocular (*ret-ro-ok'-u-lar*). Behind the eyeball.

retroperitoneal (*ret-ro-per-it-o-ne'-al*). Behind the peritoneum.

retropharyngeal abscess (*ret-ro-far-in'-je-al*). One between the pharynx and the spine. It may occur in caries of the cervical vertebrae, or in glandular affections.

retropubic (*ret-ro-pu'-bik*). Behind the pubic bone.

retrospection (*ret-ro-spek'-shun*). Morbid dwelling on memories.

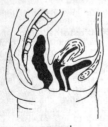

normal

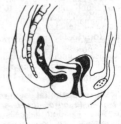

acute retroversion

RETROVERSION OF UTERUS

retrosternal (*ret-ro-ster'-nal*). Behind the sternum.

retroversion (*ret-ro-ver'-shun*). A turning back; applied to the uterus when the whole organ is tilted backward. *See* Retroflexion.

Reverdin's graft (*J. L. Reverdin, Swiss surgeon, 1842–1929*). A form of skin graft in which pieces of skin are placed as islands over the area. *See* Thiersch's graft.

Reye's syndrome (*R. D. K. Reye, contemporary Australian pathologist*). Acute disease occurring in children in which there is fatty degeneration of the liver and other organs, accompanied by vomiting, convulsions and coma. Death usually follows within a few days. Probably caused by a virus.

rhabdomyosarcoma (*rab-do-mi-o-sar-ko'-mah*). A rare malignant growth of skeletal muscle. It grows rapidly and metastasizes early.

rhagades (*rag'-ad-eez*). Cracks or fissures in the skin.

rheostat (*re'-o-stat*). An instrument for regulating the force of resistance against an electric current.

rhesus factor (*re'-sus fak'-tor*). Rh factor. The red blood cells of most humans contain the rhesus factor. Those that do not are said to be rhesus-negative. This is of importance as a probable cause of anaemia and jaundice in the newly born when the infant is rhesus-positive and the mother rhesus-negative. The result of this incompatibility is the formation of an antibody which causes excessive haemolysis in the child's blood. Treatment is by blood transfusion, but not with the mother's blood. *See* Antirhesus serum.

rheum (*room*). Any watery discharge.

rheumatic (*ru-mat'-ik*). Relating to rheumatism. *R. fever. See* Rheumatism. *R. gout.* The same as rheumatoid arthritis. *R. nodules.* Specific lesions of acute rheumatism appearing as small fibrous swellings under the skin, especially over bony ridges, e.g. elbow, spine, occiput, etc. Their presence is a strong indication of active endocarditis.

rheumatism (*ru'-mat-izm*). (1) *Acute r.* or *rheumatic fever.* An acute fever associated with previous streptococcal infection and occurring most commonly in children. The onset is usually sudden with pain, swelling and stiffness in one or more joints. There is fever, sweating, and tachycardia, and carditis is present in most cases. Recurrences are likely and this disease is the commonest cause of mitral stenosis in later life as scar tissue results from the inflammation. In a subacute attack there may be no fever but fatigue, malaise and loss of weight. (2) The term may be loosely applied to any pain of unknown cause in the joints or muscles.

rheumatoid (*ru'-mat-oid*). Resembling rheumatism. *R. arthritis. See* Arthritis.

rheumatology (*ru-mat-ol'-o-je*). The study of rheumatic disease.

Rh factor. *See* Rhesus factor.

rhinitis (*ri-ni'-tis*). Inflammation of the mucous membrane of the nose. *Allergic r.* Hay fever. *Atrophic r.* Ozaena. A degenerative condition of the nasal mucous membrane and inferior turbinate bones.

rhino- (*ri'-no-*). A prefix meaning 'nose'.

rhinoplasty (*ri'-no-plas-te*). Plastic operation on the nose;

repairing a part or forming an entirely new nose.

rhinorrhoea (*ri-nor-re'-ah*). Nasal discharge.

rhinoscope (*ri'-no-skope*). A speculum used to examine nasal cavities.

rhinoscopy (*ri-nos'-kop-e*). Examination of the nose anteriorly by means of a head mirror and speculum. *Posterior r.* Examination of the nasopharynx by means of a post-nasal mirror.

rhinoviruses (*ri-no vi'-rus-ez*). One of several groups of viruses that can cause the common cold.

rhizodontropy (*ri-zo-don'-tro-pe*). Fixing an artificial crown on to a natural tooth root.

rhizoid (*ri'-zoid*). Like a root.

rhizotomy (*ri-zot'-o-me*). Division of a spinal nerve root for the relief of pain.

rhodopsin (*rod-op'-sin*). The visual purple of the retina, the formation of which is dependent upon vitamin A in the diet.

rhonchus (*rong'-kus*). A wheezing sound produced in the bronchial tubes and heard on auscultation.

rhubarb (*ru'-barb*). The root of the rheum plant. In small doses it is highly stimulative to the stomach and liver, in large ones it acts as a purgative.

rhythm (*rithm*). A regular recurring action. *Cardiac r.* The smooth action of the heart when systole is followed by diastole.

riboflavine (*rib-o-flav'-in*). A chemical factor in vitamin B complex. *See* Appendix 10.

ribonuclease (*ri-bo-nu'-kle-aze*). An enzyme from the pancreas which is responsible for the breakdown of nucleic acid.

ribonucleic acid (*ri-bo-nu'-kle-ik*). RNA. A complex chemical found in the cytoplasm of animal cells and thought to be concerned with protein synthesis.

ribs. The twelve pairs of long, flat curved bones of the thorax, each united by cartilage to the spinal vertebrae at the back, and to the sternum in front. *Cervical r.* Elongation of the cervical processes towards the front of the chest. Pressure of this may cause impairment of nerve or vascular function. *See* Scalenus syndrome. *False r.* The last five pairs, the upper three of which are attached by cartilage to each other. *Floating r.* The last two pairs connected only to the vertebra. *True r.* The seven pairs attached directly to the sternum.

rice-water stools. Watery stools which occur in patients who have contracted cholera.

Richter's hernia (*A. G. Richter, German surgeon, 1742–1812*). One in which only a portion of the circumference of the intestine is contained within the hernial sac.

rickets (*rik'-ets*). A deficiency disease of young children from 6 months to 2 years of age. It is caused by a lack of vitamin D which results in a failure of calcium and phosphorus absorption from the diet. This leads to softening and irregular growth of the bones resulting in deformity, such as bowing of the long bones and enlargement of the epiphyses. The disease is preventable, and can be treated by giving adequate vitamin D (*see* Appendix 10) and by exposure to sunlight or ultra-violet light.

Rickettsia (*rik-et'-se-ah*). A group of micro-organisms which are parasitic in lice and similar insects. The bite of the host is thus the means of transmitting the organism, some of which are disease producing. *R.*

prowazeki. Inhabits the digestive tract of lice and is the cause of epidemic typhus fever. *R. tsutsugamushi*. The cause of scrub typhus.

rifamycin (*rif-ah-mi'-sin*). Antibiotic used in the treatment of tuberculosis.

rigor (*ri'-gor*). An attack of intense shivering occurring when the heat regulation is disturbed. The temperature rises rapidly and may either stay elevated or fall rapidly as profuse sweating occurs. *R. mortis* is a name given to the stiffening of the body, occurring soon after death owing to coagulation of the muscle plasma. It begins in the muscles of the neck and jaw, then proceeds to those of the chest and upper extremities, finally reaching those of the lower limbs. The time of its appearance varies (1 to 24 hours after death) and its duration may be from a few minutes to several days.

rima (*ri'-mah*). A narrow fissure or crack. *R. glottidis*. The chink between the vocal cords.

Ringer's solution (*S. Ringer, English physiologist, 1835–1910*). A physiological solution of salt to which small amounts of calcium and potassium salts have been added.

ringworm. A contagious skin disease, characterized by circular patches, pinkish in colour, with a desquamating surface, and due to a parasitic fungus. When affecting the scalp it is called *tinea capitis* or *tinea tonsurans*. See Tinea.

Rinne's test (*H. A. Rinne, German biologist, 1819–1868*). For hearing, in which the degree of conductivity through bone is tested, by holding a vibrating tuning fork alternately in front of the ear and over the mastoid bone.

risus sardonicus (*ri'-sus sardon'-ik-us*). A peculiar grin caused by muscle spasm around the mouth, seen in tetanus and strychnine poisoning.

Ritalin (*rit'-a-lin*). A proprietary preparation of methylphenidate. Stimulant drug sometimes used in the treatment of enuresis in children.

RNA. Ribonucleic acid (*q.v.*) *RNA viruses*. Viruses which contain ribonucleic acid as their genetic material.

ROA. Right occipitoanterior. Pertaining to the postion of the fetus in the uterus.

rocking. A repetitive action the child of 10 months starts when in its cot. It may only last a few weeks but may become habitual and be difficult to stop.

Rocky Mountain spotted fever. Tick fever. Caused by a *Rickettsia* (*q.v.*), common in the United States of America. Causes a rose-red rash to appear, with fever, muscle pain and often an enlarged liver. The disease lasts about three weeks.

rodent ulcer (*ro'-dent*). See Ulcer.

rods. Receptor end-organs in the retina that are sensitive to light and responsible for night vision.

Romberg's sign (*M. H. Romberg, German physician, 1795–1853*). Inability to stand erect without swaying if the eyes are closed. A sign of tabes dorsalis.

Röntgen (*W. K. von Röntgen, German physicist, 1845–1923*). A unit of measurement for X and gamma radiation. It is a measure of exposure to the beam. For dosage received, *see* Rad.

rooting reflex. Reflex seen in newborn infants. The child will respond to a touch on the cheek by turning towards the hand as if seeking the mother's breast.

ROP. Right occipitoposterior. Pertaining to the position of the fetus in the uterus.

Rorschach test (*H. Rorschach, Swiss psychiatrist, 1884–1922*). An intelligence test that consists of ten ink blot designs, some in colours and some in black and white. The patient is asked to look at the cards and tell what he sees. This test also measures some aspects of personality.

rosacea (*ro-za'-se-ah*). See Acne rosacea.

rose bengal (*rose ben'-gal*). A staining agent used in the eye to detect mucous threads in kerato-conjunctivitis.

roseola (*ro-ze-o'-lah*). A rose-coloured rash. *R. infantum.* Acute disease of infancy in which a high temperature which has persisted for several days falls as soon as the rash appears.

rotator (*ro-ta'-tor*). A muscle which causes rotation of a part.

Roth spots (*M. Roth, Swiss physician, 1839–1915*). Small white spots in the retina which may be surrounded by haemorrhages. Seen in bacterial endocarditis.

Rothera's test (*A. C. H. Rothera, Australian biochemist, 1880–1915*). Test for the presence of acetone in urine. *See* Appendix 11.

roughage (*ruf'-faj*). Coarse vegetable fibres and cellulose that give bulk to the diet and stimulate peristalsis.

rouleau formation (*ru'-lo*). The piling of red cells which occurs when blood is removed from the body.

round ligament. See Ligament.

round window. Window which separates the basilar membrane of the inner ear from the middle ear. *See* Ear.

roundworm. See Ascaris.

Rous' sarcoma virus (RSV) (*F. P. Rous, American virologist, 1879– *). A virus which cannot form a protein coat or reproduce itself unless associated with Rous-associated virus (RAV).

Roysing's sign (*N. T. Roysing, Danish surgeon, 1868–1927*). A test for acute appendicitis in which pressure in the left iliac fossa causes pain in the right iliac fossa.

RPCF. See Reiter.

rubefacient (*ru-be-fa'-shent*). An agent causing redness of the skin.

rubella (*ru-bel'-lah*). German measles. A mild contagious disease of short duration in which there is slight pyrexia, enlarged cervical lymph glands and a rash. The greatest risk from this disease is to the offspring of mothers who contract it during the early weeks of pregnancy. The child may be born blind, be a deaf mute or have other congenital defects.

rugae (*ru'-ge*). Ridges or creases, e.g. of the mucosa of the stomach.

rumination (*ru-min-a'-shun*). Recurring thoughts. *Obsessional r.* Thoughts which persistently recur against the patient's will and from which he cannot rid himself.

rupture (*rup'-chur*). (1) Tearing or bursting of a part, as in rupture of an aneurysm; of the membranes during labour; or of a tubal pregnancy. (2) A term commonly applied to hernia.

Russell traction (*R. H. Russell, contemporary Australian surgeon*). A form of extension by use of skin traction and sling supports without the use of a splint. Suitable for some cases of fractured femur. *See* Traction.

Ryle's tube (*J. A. Ryle. British physician 1882– *). A thin,

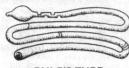

RYLE'S TUBE

weighted rubber or plastic tube used for giving a test meal or for aspirating the stomach contents. A modified tube of larger bore can be used for milk feeds.

S

Sabin vaccine (*A. B. Sabin, American biologist, 1906– *). Against poliomyelitis. *See* Vaccine.

sac (*sak*). A pouch-like cavity. *Air s.* Alveolus. The pouch-like dilatation terminating the bronchioles. *Conjunctival s.* The space between the conjunctiva covering the eyeball, and that lining the eye-lid. *Hernial s.* The pouch of peritoneum containing the loop of intestine. *Lacrimal s.* The dilatation at the top of the lacrimal duct.

saccharides (*sak'-ar-ides*). A series of carbohydrates, including the sugars.

saccharin (*sak'-ar-in*). Gluside. A crystalline substance used as a substitute for sugar.

Saccharomyces (*sak-ar-o-mi'-sez*). A genus of fungi, of which yeast is an example.

sacculated (*sak'-u-la-ted*). Divided into small sacs.

sacral (*sa'-kral*). Relating to the sacrum.

sacroiliac (*sa-kro-il'-e-ak*). Relating to the sacrum and the ilium.

sacrum (*sa'-krum*). A triangular bone composed of five united vertebrae, situated between the lowest lumbar vertebra and the coccyx. It forms the back of the pelvis.

saddle-nose. Flattening of the bridge of the nose, which may occur in congenital syphilis from infection of the nasal bones.

sadism (*sa'-dizm*). A form of sexual perversion in which the individual takes pleasure in inflicting mental and physical pain.

sagittal (*saj-it'-tal*). Arrowshaped. *S. suture.* The junction of the parietal bones.

St Anthony's fire. A term applied to erysipelas (*q.v.*) or to gangrene resulting from ergotism.

St Vitus's dance. Chorea (*q.v.*).

sal. Salt. *S. volatile.* Aromatic ammonium carbonate. Diluted with water it may be given in cases of syncope.

salicylate (*sal-is'-il-ate*). A salt of salicylic acid. *Methyl s.* is the active ingredient in ointments and lotions for joint pains and sprains. *Sodium s.* is the specific drug used for rheumatic fever. It reduces the pyrexia and relieves the pain but does not prevent cardiac complications. Where there is intolerance aspirin or calcium aspirin may be substituted.

saline (*sa'-line*). (1) A solution of sodium chloride and water. *Hypertonic s.* A stronger than normal strength. *Hypotonic s.* A weaker than normal, usually $\frac{1}{5}$ strength is used. *Normal or physiological s.* An 0·9 per cent solution which is isotonic with blood. *See* Appendix 8. (2) Salts of alkalis which are aperient, owing to their hygroscopic action, e.g. magnesium sulphate.

saliva (*sal-i'-vah*). The secretion of the salivary glands which is poured into the mouth when food is taken. It moistens and dissolves certain substances, and partially digests carbohydrates by the action of its enzyme, ptyalin (or amylase).

salivary (*sal'-iv-ar-e*). Relating to saliva. *S. glands.* The parotid, submaxillary and sublingual glands. *S. calculus.* A stony concretion in a salivary duct. *S. fistula.* An unnatural opening into a salivary duct or gland.

salivation (*sal-iv-a'-shun*). Ptyalism, an excessive flow of saliva. A symptom of overdose of mercury.

Salk vaccine (*J. E. Salk, American virologist, 1914–). See* Vaccine.

Salmonella (*sal-mon-el'-lah*). A genus of bacteria that are parasites of the intestinal tract of man and animals. *S. typhi* and *S. paratyphi* are exclusively human pathogens which cause typhoid and paratyphoid fevers (*q.v.*). Other strains, e.g. *S. typhimurium*, can give rise to acute gastroenteritis (food poisoning).

salmonellosis (*sal-mon-el-lo'-sis*). Infection with salmonellae, especially paratyphoid fever and food poisoning; caused by the ingestion of food containing the organisms or their products.

salpingectomy (*sal-pin-jek'-to-me*). Excision of one or both of the fallopian tubes.

salpingemphraxis (*sal-pin-jem-fraks'-is*). Closure of a fallopian tube.

salpingitis (*sal-pin-ji'-tis*). (1) Inflammation of the fallopian tubes. *Acute s.* Most often a bilateral ascending infection due to the streptococcus or gonococcus. One tube may be infected from adjacent structure like the appendix. *Chronic s.* A less acute form that may be blood borne and may be due to the tubercle bacillus. (2) Inflammation of the pharyngotympanic (eustachian) tube.

salpingography (*sal-pin-gog'-raf-e*). Radiography of fallopian tubes after injection of a radioopaque substance to determine their patency.

salpingo-oophorectomy (*sal-pin'-go-o-off-or-ek'-to-me*). Removal of fallopian tube and ovary.

salpingostomy (*sal-pin-gos'-to-me*). Making a surgical opening in the tube near the uterus to restore patency.

salpinx (*sal'-pinks*). A tube— applied to the fallopian or pharyngotympanic (eustachian) tubes.

salt. (1) Sodium chloride, common salt, used in solution as a cleansing lotion, a stimulating bath, or for infusion into the blood, etc. (2) Any compound of an acid with an alkali or base. (3) A saline purgative such as Epsom salts. *Smelling s.* Aromatic ammonium carbonate. A restorative in fainting. *S. depletion.* A loss of salt from the body without water depletion. Only likely to arise where there is profuse sweating and replacement by water only.

salve (*salv*). An ointment.

sanatorium (*san-at-or'-e-um*). A building used for restoring to health, usually used for the treatment of long-term illness like tuberculosis.

sandfly fever. A fever transmitted by the bites of sandflies, and common in Mediterranean countries. Similar to *dengue* (*q.v.*) and sometimes known as *three-day fever*.

sanguineous (*san-gwin'-e-us*). Pertaining to or containing blood.

sanguis (*san'-gwis*). The blood.

sanies (*sa'-ne-eez*). A fetid discharge from a wound consisting of serum, pus and blood.

sanitary (*san'-it-ar-e*). Relating to or promoting health.

saphena (*saf-e'-nah*). Several veins, chiefly superficial, that carry blood from the toes upwards.

saphenous (*saf-e'-nus*). Relating to the saphena.

sapo (*sa'-po*). Soap.

saponaceous (*sap-on-a'-she-us*). Soapy; having the nature of soap.

saponify (*sap-on'-if-i*). To make into soap by combining a fat and an alkali.

sapraemia (*sap-re'-me-ah*). Similar to toxaemia. The toxins are produced by saphrophytes and circulate in the blood.

sapro- (*sap'-ro*). A prefix signifying 'putrefaction'.

saprophyte (*sap'-ro-fite*). An organism bred in and living on putrefying matter.

sarco- (*sar'-ko-*). A prefix denoting 'flesh'.

sarcocele (*sar'-ko-seel*). A tumour of the testicle.

sarcoidosis (*sar-koi-do'-sis*). A rare disease in some ways similar to tuberculosis. It chiefly affects the skin, the lymphatic glands and the lungs.

sarcolemma (*sar-ko-lem'-mah*). A delicate membrane enveloping each striated muscle fibre.

sarcoma (*sar-ko'-mah*). A malignant tumour developed from connective tissue cells, and their stroma. The cells may be round, spindle-shaped, or large like those of bone marrow. *Chondrosarcoma*. One arising in cartilage. *Fibrosarcoma*. One containing much fibrous tissue; this may arise in the fibrous sheath of a muscle. *Melanotic s.* A very malignant type, pigmented with melanin. *Round-celled s.* A very malignant growth, composed of a primitive type of cell. *See* Carcinoma.

sarcomatosis (*sar-ko-mat-o'-sis*). Multiple sarcomatous growths in various parts of the body.

Sarcoptes (*sar-kop'-tes*). A genus of acarids. *S. scabiei*. The cause of scabies (*q.v.*).

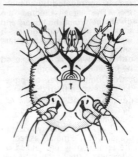

SARCOPTES SCABIEI

sardonic grin. *See* Risus sardonicus.

sartorius (*sar-tor'-e-us*). A long muscle of the thigh, which flexes the leg and bends it inwards.

saturated solution (*sat'-u-ra-ted*). A liquid containing the largest amount of a solid which can be dissolved in it without forming a precipitate.

Sayre's jacket (*L. A. Sayre,*

American surgeon, 1820–1900). A jacket made of plaster of Paris used to support the back in cases of spinal caries.

Sayre's sling (*L. A. Sayre, American surgeon, 1820–1900).* A suspension apparatus for the head, used for the correction of torticollis.

scab. The crust on a superficial wound consisting of dried lymph, etc. *See* Scale.

scabies (*ska'-beez*). 'The itch'. A contagious skin disease caused by the itch mite (*Sarcoptes scabiei*), the female of which burrows beneath the skin and deposits eggs at intervals. It is intensely irritating, and the rash is aggravated by scratching. The sites affected are chiefly between the fingers and toes, the axillae, and groins. It is treated with benzyl benzoate emulsion.

scald (*skawld*). A burn caused by hot liquid or vapour.

scale. Compact layers of epithelial tissue shed from the skin.

scalenus syndrome (*ska-le'-nus sin'-drome).* Symptoms of pain and tenderness in the shoulder, with sensory loss and wasting of the medial aspect of the arm. It may be caused by pressure on the brachial plexus, by spasm of the scalenus anticus muscle or by a cervical rib.

scalp (*skalp*). The hairy skin which covers the cranium.

scalpel (*skal'-pel*). A small pointed surgical knife.

scanner. *See* EMI scanner.

scanning speech (*skan'-ing*). The syllables are separated from each other. A speech disorder that may be present in cerebellar disease.

scaphocephaly (*skaf-o-kef'-al-e*). Abnormal boat-shape of the head due to premature clo-

sure of the sagittal suture of the skull.

scaphoid (*ska'-foid*). Boat-shaped. A term applied to the sunken abdomen seen in cases of meningitis and severe emaciation. *S. bone.* A boat-shaped bone of the carpus and the tarsus.

scapula (*skap'-u-lah*). The large flat triangular bone forming the shoulder-blade.

scar. The fibrous tissue by which a wound heals. *Contracted s.* results if much tissue has been lost, e.g. in a burn. *Keloid s.* An over-growth of scar tissue. *See* Keloid.

scarfskin. The epidermis.

scarlet fever (*skar'-let*). Scarlatina. An acute infectious disease which of latter years has much decreased in severity. It is caused by a haemolytic streptococcus. There is sore throat, high fever and a punctate rash. Now it is readily treated by penicillin or the sulpha drugs, and the complications of nephritis and middle ear infection are less common.

Scarpa's triangle (*A. Scarpa, Italian anatomist and surgeon, 1747–1832).* The triangular area on the inner side of the thigh, bounded above by Poupart's ligament, and on one side by the sartorius and on the other the adductor longus muscle. The femoral artery and vein, with nerves of the thigh, are superficial in this position.

SCAT (sheep cell agglutination test). A serum test for rheumatoid arthritis.

Schafer's method (*Sir E. A. S. Schafer, British physiologist, 1850–1935).* A method of artificial respiration. The patient lies prone, and the rescuer kneels alongside him and exerts pressure on the chest with his hands by leaning forward, and releases it by returning to the original position.

schematic eye (*ske'-mat-ik*). A model of an eye that enables a student to practise examination of the retina and fundus by an ophthalmoscope (*q.v.*).

Scheuermann's disease (*H. W. Scheuermann, Danish surgeon, 1877–1960*). Disease of adolescents in which there is vertebral osteochondritis (*q.v.*). It affects the rings of cartilage and bone around the margin of the superior and inferior surfaces of the vertebral body.

Schick test (*B. Schick, Austrian paediatrician, 1877– *). To test susceptibility to diphtheria. See Test.

Schilling test (*R. F. Schilling, contemporary American haematologist*). One used to confirm the diagnosis of pernicious anaemia by estimating the absorption of ingested radioactive vitamin B_{12}.

Schistosoma (*skis-to-so'-mah*). A genus of minute leaf-shaped worms or flukes, some of which are parasitic in man.

schistosomiasis (*skis-to-so-mi'-as-is*). A parasitic infection of the intestinal or urinary tract, common in Egypt. The parasite enters the skin from contaminated water, and causes diarrhoea, haematuria, and anaemia. The treatment is by the administration of antimony or lucanthone. Bilharziasis.

Schizomycetes (*skiz-o-mi-se'-tes*). A class of minute vegetable organisms that reproduce themselves by fission; bacteria and yeasts are of this type.

schizophrenia (*skiz-o-fre'-ne-ah*). A psychosis of unknown cause but showing hereditary links. Characteristically the patient feels himself to be influenced in a strange way by external forces and suffers delusions and hallucinations; his thought processes are disordered. *Paranoid s.* Predominance of delusions of a persecutory nature. *Simple s.* A progressive deterioration of the patient's efficiency. See Hebephrenia and Catatonia.

schizosis (*skiz-o'-sis*). A mental state with marked tendency to avoid contact with the outside world, and to shun social responsibilities.

Schlatter's disease (*C. Schlatter, Swiss surgeon, 1864–1934*). Osteochondrosis of the tibial tuberosity.

Schlemm's canal (*F. Schlemm, German anatomist, 1795–1858*). A venous channel at the junction of the cornea and sclera.

Schönlein–Henoch syndrome (*J. L. Schönlein, German physician, 1793–1864: E. H. Henoch, German paediatrician, 1820–1910*). See Purpura.

Schultz–Charlton blanching test (*W. Schultz, German physician, 1878–1947: W. Charlton, German physician 1889– *). By this an intradermal injection of scarlet fever antitoxin is made into an area of rash. An area of blanching will arise and persist if the patient has scarlet fever.

Schwartze's operation (*H. H. R. Schwartze, German otologist, 1837–1910*). Opening the mastoid cells, without involvement of the middle ear, in order to drain a mastoid abscess.

sciatic (*si-at'-ik*). Relating to the sciatic nerve which runs down the back of the thigh.

sciatica (*si-at'-ik-ah*). Pain down the back of the leg in the area supplied by the sciatic nerve. It may be owing to pressure on the nerve roots; by a protrusion of intervertebral disc; by a spinal tumour; by tuberculosis of the spine or by malignant disease of the pelvis.

scilla (*sil'-lah*). Squill, an extract from the root of a plant. In large doses it is irritant; in small ones expectorant and diuretic.

scintillography (*sin-til-og'-raf-e*). The method of examination by means of α-rays on a fluorescent screen.

scirrhous (*skir'-rus*). Hard; resembling a scirrhus.

scirrhus (*skir'-rus*). A hard cancer, containing much connective tissue.

scissor-leg deformity. The legs are crossed in walking, as sometimes occurs in disease of both hip joints. *See* Little's disease.

sclera (*skler'-ah*). The fibrous coat of the eyeball—the white of the eye, which covers the posterior part and in front becomes the cornea.

scleritis (*skler-i'-tis*). Inflammation of the sclerotic coat.

scleroderma (*skler-o-der'-mah*). A disease marked by progressive hardening of the skin in patches or diffusely, with rigidity of the underlying tissues. It is often a chronic condition.

scleroma (*skler-o'-mah*). A patch of hardened tissue.

sclerosis (*skler-o'-sis*). The hardening of any part from an overgrowth of fibrous and connective tissue, often due to chronic inflammation. *Amyotrophic lateral s.* Rapid degeneration of the pyramidal (motor nerves) tract and anterior horn cells in the spinal cord. Characterized by weakness and spasm of limb muscles with wasting of the muscle, difficulty with talking and swallowing. *Arterio-s.* The changes occurring in walls of arteries which cause hardening and loss of elasticity. *Athero-s.* The deposition of fatty plaques and hardening and fibrosis of the artery lining. *Disseminated s. See* Multiple s. *Mönckeberg's s.* Extensive degeneration with atrophy and calcareous deposits in the middle muscle coat of arteries, especially of the small ones. *Multiple s.* Scattered (disseminated) patches of degeneration in the nerve sheaths in the brain and spinal cord. Characterized by relapses and remissions. Symptoms include disturbances of speech, vision and micturition and muscular weakness of a limb or limbs.

sclerotherapy (*skler-o-ther'-ap-e*). Treatment by the artificial production of fibrosis by the injection of sclerosant solutions.

sclerotic (*skler-ot'-ik*). Hard. *S. coat.* The tough membrane forming the outer covering of the eyeball, excepting in front of the iris, where it becomes the clear horny cornea.

sclerotomy (*skler-ot'-o-me*). Incision of the sclerotic coat, usually for the relief of glaucoma.

scolex (*sko'-leks*). The head of a tapeworm.

scoliosis (*skol-e-o'-sis*). Abnormal curvature of the spine, but most commonly applied to a lateral deviation. *See* Lordosis and Kyphosis.

scopolamine (*sko-pol'-am-een*). Hyoscine (*q.v.*).

scorbutus (*skor-bu'-tus*). Scurvy (*q.v.*).

scotoma (*sko-to'-mah*). A blind area in the field of vision, due to some lesion of the retina.

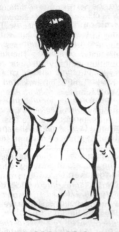

SCOLIOSIS

scrotum (skro'-tum). The pouch of skin and soft tissues containing the testicles.

scurf (skerf). Dandruff (q.v.).

scurvy (sker'-ve). A deficiency disease due to incorrect diet, i.e. one lacking in raw fruits and vegetables and therefore in vitamin C. It rapidly improves with adequate diet. *Infantile s.* This may occur in artificially fed infants as milk is a poor source of vitamin C. To prevent it such children should be given orange, tomato or rose hip juice daily. *See* Appendix 10.

scybalum (sib'-al-um). A mass of abnormally hard faecal matter. *Pl.* Scybala.

sebaceous (se-ba'-shus). Fatty, or pertaining to the sebum. *S. glands* are found in the skin, communicating with the hair follicles and secreting sebum. *S. cyst. See* Cyst.

seborrhoea (se-bor-re'-ah). A disease of the sebaceous glands, marked by an excessive secretion of sebum which collects on the skin in oily scales. It is usually asssociated with itching and burning.

sebum (se'-bum). The fatty secretion of the sebaceous glands.

secondary (sek'-on-dar-e). Second in order of time or importance. *S. disease See under* Disease. *S. haemorrhage. See* Haemorrhage. *S. deposits. See* Metastases.

secretagogue (se-kre'-ta-gog). Any agent that stimulates the secretion of a gland.

secrete (se-kreet'). The action of cells in producing a new substance which either passes into the blood stream or by ducts to where it is required.

secretin (se-kre'-tin). The hormone originating in the duodenum which, in the presence of bile salts, is absorbed into the blood stream and stimulates the secretion of pancreatic juice. *S. test.* A complicated test, both qualitative and quantitative, carried out to estimate external pancreatic secretion.

secretions (se-kre'-shuns). Various substances separated from the blood by glands. They are: (a) used for special purposes in the body, as the digestive juices, or hormones made by endocrine glands, (b) excreted as urine and sweat.

section (sek'-shun). (1) The act of cutting. (2) A portion which has been cut through. *Frozen s.* A thin slice that has been cut from frozen tissue for examination under a microscope. *Caesarean s. See* Caesarean.

sedative (sed'-at-iv). An agent which lessens excitement or functional activity.

sedentary (sed'-en-ter-e). Pertaining to sitting, physically inactive.

sedimentation (*sed-e-men-ta'-shun*). Deposition of solids in a fluid to form a sediment. *Erythrocyte s. rate* (ESR). *See* Erythrocyte.

segment (*seg'-ment*). A small piece separated from any part by an actual or imaginary line.

segregation (*seg-re-ga'-shun*). Separation of a number of people from others, e.g. infectious patients in a fever hospital; or those mentally affected, tuberculous, etc., in special communities.

Seidlitz powder (*sed'-lits*). A saline purgative. Named after a mineral spring in Bohemia.

sella turcica (*sel-lah ter'-sik-ah*). The fossa in the sphenoid body which protects the pituitary gland.

semen (*se'-men*). The secretion of the testicles containing spermatozoa.

semi- (*sem'-e*). A prefix meaning 'half'.

semicircular canals (*sem-e-ser'-ku-lar*). Part of the labyrinth of the internal ear, consisting of three canals in the form of arches which contain fluid, and by their nerve supply are connected with the cerebellum. Impressions of change of position of the body are registered in these canals by oscillation of the fluid, and are conveyed by the nerves to the cerebellum—the balancing organ of the brain.

semicomatose (*sem-e-ko'-mat-ose*). In a condition of unconsciousness from which one can be roused by painful stimuli.

semilunar (*sem-e-lu'-nar*). Shaped like a half-moon. *S. cartilages.* Two crescent-shaped cartilages in the knee-joint. *S valves. See* Valve.

seminal (*sem'-in-al*). Relating

to the semen. *S. vesicles. See* Vesicle.

seminoma (*se-min-o'-mah*). A malignant tumour of the testis.

semipermeable (*sem-e-per'-me-a-bl*). Used to describe a membrane that permits the passage of some substances in solution and hinders that of others.

semiprone (*sem-e-pro'-n*). Partly prone. *See* Sims's p. *under* Position.

senega (*sen'-e-gah*). An expectorant vegetable drug. In large doses it is emetic.

senescence (*sen-es'-ense*). The process of growing old.

Sengstaken's tube (*R. W. Sengstaken, American neurosurgeon, 1923– *). An oesophageal compression tube for the treatment of bleeding oesophageal varices.

senile (*se'-nile*). Related to the involutional changes associated with old age. *S. delirium.* The patient is disorientated, restless and unable to sleep and often there are visual or auditory hallucinations. *S. dementia.* Deterioration of mental activity in the elderly associated with impaired blood supply to the brain.

senility (*sen-il'-it-e*). The condition of being senile.

senna (*sen'-nah*). A laxative derived from the cassia plant, given in the form of an infusion of the pods in water. Proprietary standardized preparations, e.g. Senokot, are available as tablets or granules.

sense. The power by which conditions and properties of things are perceived, e.g. hunger or pain. *Special s.* Any one of the faculties of sight, hearing, touch, smell, taste, and muscle sense, through which the consciousness receives impressions from the external world. *S.*

organ. One which receives a sensory stimulus.

sensible (*sen-sib-l*). Perceptible to the senses. *S. perspiration*. That obvious on the skin as moisture.

sensitive (*sens'-it-iv*). Reacting to a stimulus. *See also* Hypersensitive.

sensitization (*sen-sit-i-za'-shun*). Rendering susceptible. *Protein s.* The condition occurring in an individual when a foreign protein is absorbed into the body, e.g. shell fish causing urticaria when eaten. *See* Desensitization.

sensitized. Rendered sensitive.

sensory (*sen'-sor-e*). Relating to sensation. *S. nerve*. A nerve conveying impressions from the periphery to the brain or spinal cord.

sentiment (*sen'-te-ment*). An organized system of tendencies directed towards some object or person. Sentiments are acquired and profoundly influence a person's actions.

sepsis (*sep'-sis*). Describes the condition of infection of the body by pus-forming bacteria. *Oral s.* Infection of the mouth which causes general ill-health by absorption of toxins. *Puerperal s.* That occurring during the puerperium. *See* Asepsis.

septal (*sep'-tal*). Relating to a septum. *S. defect*. Usually refers to a congenital defect when there is either an opening between the two atria or two ventricles of the heart.

septic (*sep'-tik*). Relating to sepsis. (1) *S. wound*. One infected by pus-forming bacteria. (2) *S. tank*. One in which sewage is liquefied and purified by anaerobic organisms.

septicaemia (*sep-tis-e'-me-ah*). The presence in the blood of bacteria and their toxins. The symptoms are: a rapid rise of temperature, which is later intermittent, rigors, sweating, and all signs of acute fever. It is treated by antibiotic drugs which have to a great extent reduced the development of this condition.

septum (*sep'-tum*). A division or partition. (1) That between the right and left ventricles of the heart. (2) The structure made of bone and cartilage which separates the nasal cavities.

sequelae (*se-kwe'-le*). Morbid conditions following a disease and resulting from it.

sequestrectomy (*se-kwes-trek'-to-me*). The removal of a sequestrum.

sequestrum (*se-kwes'-trum*). *Pl.* Sequestra. A piece of dead bone. Inflammation in bone leads to pressure and thrombosis of blood vessels resulting in necrosis of the affected part, which separates from the living structure.

serological (*se-ro-loj'-ik-al*). Relating to serum. *S. tests*. Those that are dependent on the formation of anitbodies in the blood as a response to specific organisms or proteins.

serology (*se-rol'-o-je*). The scientific study of sera, their actions and reactions. A branch of medicine particularly concerned with diagnosis and immunity.

serosa (*se-ro'-sah*). A serous membrane. It consists of two layers—the *visceral*, in close contact with the organ, and the *parietal*, lining the cavity. The serum exudes, and lubricates between the layers giving a smooth movement without friction.

serotonin (*se-ro-to'-nin*). An amine present in blood platelets, the intestine and the brain. It is derived from the amino acid tryptophan and inactivated by monoamine oxidase.

serous (*se'-rus*). Related to serum. *S. effusion.* Increase of serous exudate. *S. inflammation.* Inflammation of a serous membrane. *See* Serosa.

serpiginous (*ser-pij'-in-us*). Creeping from one place to another.

serrated (*ser-a'-ted*). With saw-like edge.

serum (*se'-rum*). The clear, fluid residue of blood, from which the corpuscles and fibrin have been removed. *Antidiphtheritic s.* Contains antibodies to neutralize the toxins of diphtheria. *Antitetanic s.* That which contains antibodies to neutralize toxins of tetanus *Antitoxic s.* One which contains the antibodies to some specific infection. *S. sickness.* An allergic reaction usually 8 to 10 days after a serum injection. It may be manifest by an irritating urticaria, pyrexia and painful joints. It readily responds to adrenaline and antihistaminic drugs. *See* Anaphylaxis. *S. therapy.* The treatment of infectious diseases by injection of antitoxic serum made by inoculation of animals (usually the horse) with the virus of the disease. It produces passive immunity (*q.v.*).

serum alkaline phosphatase. *See* Alkaline phosphatase.

sesamoid (*ses'-am-oid*). Resembling a sesame seed. *S. bone.* One roughly this shape and developed in a tendon, e.g. the patella and pisiform.

sessile tumour (*ses'-ile*). A tumour without a peduncle. *See* Tumour.

sex. The fundamental differences between men and women. Often taken to mean the emotions and pleasures associated with a relationship between the two.

sex chromatin (*seks kro'-mat-in*). An extra bit of *c.* found in the nuclei of cells in women who possess two X chromosomes and not in men.

sex chromosomes (*seks kro'-mo-somes*). The chromosomes in the human cell that decide the sex. Women have two X *c.* and men one X and one Y *c.*

sex-linked (*seks-linkt'*). Transmitted by genes that are located on the sex chromosomes, e.g. haemophilia.

SGOT. Serum glutamic oxalacetic transaminase, an enzyme excreted by damaged heart muscle. A raised serum level occurs in cardiac infarction.

SGPT. Serum glutamic pyruvic transaminase. An enzyme excreted by the parenchymal cells of the liver. There is a raised blood level in infectious hepatitis.

Sheehan's syndrome (*H. L. Sheehan, British pathologist, 1900–).* Hypopituitarism caused by thrombosis of the pituitary blood supply. It occurs in association with post-partum haemorrhage.

shelf operation. A type of arthroplasty in which the acetabulum is deepened by splitting the ilium and drawing the split portion down.

Shigella (*shig-el'-ah*). A genus of bacilli containing a number of species that cause dysentery. *S. sonnei.* Commonest in the West. *S. flexneri* and *S. shigae.* Common in the East.

Shiga's dysentery (*K. Shiga, Japanese bacteriologist, 1870–1957*). A severe bacillary dysentery caused by *Shigella shi-*

gae. Not applied to the *Shigella* infections as a rule.

shingles (*shing'-gls*). Herpes zoster (*q.v.*).

Shirodkar's operation (*Shirodkar, contemporary Indian obstetrician*). A suture is placed round an incompetent cervix during pregnancy to prevent abortion. It is removed at the thirty-eighth week.

shock. A condition in which there is a sudden fall in blood pressure; this, untreated, will lead to lack of oxygen in the tissues and greater permeability of the capillary walls, so increasing the degree of shock, by greater loss of fluid. *Primary s., neurogenic s.* or *vasovagal s.* Arises at the time from pain, fear or unpleasant sight as in a faint. *Hypovolaemic s.* A state of shock in which there is loss of fluid from circulation as in haemorrhage or burns. *Normovolaemic s.* Shock arising when there is no reduction in blood volume, as in coronary thrombosis. *Anaphylactic s.* The severe reaction produced by the injection of a protein to which the person is sensitive. *Electric s.* Caused by the passage of an electric current through the body. *See* Appendix 1. *Protein s.* A little-used method of producing a severe reaction with fever by introducing a foreign protein, e.g. boiled milk.

short-circuit. A term applied to intestinal anastomosis.

short sight. Myopia (*q.v.*).

'show'. A term used to denote the blood-stained discharge at the onset of labour.

shunt. A diversion, particularly of blood, due to congenital defect, disease or surgery. *Atrioventricular s. See* Atrioventricular.

SI units. Système International

d'Unités. The metric system of measurement now adopted by all hospitals in Britain. *See* Appendix 6.

sialogogue (*si-al'-o-gog*). A drug increasing the flow of saliva.

sialogram (*si-al'-o-gram*). An X-ray of the salivary ducts following the insertion of a radio-opaque dye.

sialolith (*si-al'-o-lith*). A salivary calculus.

sibilus (*sib'-il-us*). A high-pitched sound heard on auscultation.

sibling (*sib'-ling*). One of a family of children having the same parents. Applied in psychology to one of two or more children of the same parent or substitute parent figure. *S. rivalry.* Jealousy, compounded of love and hate of one child for its sibling.

sick headache. Migraine (*q.v.*).

sickle-cell anaemia (*sik'-l-sell an-e'-me-ah*). An inherited disease of Negro races in which the red blood cells are crescent-shaped and very friable.

siderosis (*sid-er-o'-sis*). Chronic inflammation of the lung due to inhalation of particles of iron.

sigmoid (*sig'-moid*). Shaped like the Greek letter Σ. *S. flexure.* That part of the colon in the left iliac fossa just above the rectum.

sigmoidoscope (*sig-moid'-o-skope*). An instrument, by which the interior of the rectum and sigmoid flexure can be seen.

sidmoidostomy (*sig-moid-os'-to-me*). An artificial opening into the sigmoid flexure.

sign (*sine*). An indication of the presence of disease that can be seen or elicited.

silicones (*sil'-ik-ones*). A group of organic compounds which have silica as part of their molecule and when used on the skin, on glass or on metals, are repellent to water.

silicosis (*sil-ik-o'-sis*). A fibrosis of lung due to the inhalation of silica dust particles. It occurs in miners, stone masons and quarry workers and is often complicated by tuberculosis.

silk ligature. Thread silk used for deep sutures. Non-absorbable.

silver nitrate (*ni'-trate*). AgNO₃. A crystalline salt. In solid form it is used as a caustic for reducing excessive granulation tissue. In solution it is antiseptic and astringent.

Simmonds's disease (*M. Simmonds, German physician, 1855–1925*). A condition of anterior pituitary deficiency, causing arrest of growth and premature senility.

Sims's position (*J. M. Sims, American gynaecologist, 1813–83*). See Position.

sinapis (*sin-a'-pis*). Mustard.

sinew (*sin'-u*). A tendon.

sino-atrial node (*si'-no a'-tre-al*). See Node.

sinogram (*si'-no-gram*). Outlining the extent of a sinus by means of a radio-opaque dye.

sinus (*si'-nus*). (1) A cavity in a bone. (2) A venous channel, especially within the cranium. (3) An unhealed passage leading from an abscess or internal lesion to the surface. *Air s.* A cavity in a bone containing air. *Cavernous s.* A venous sinus which lies along the body of the sphenoid bone. *Coronary s.* The vein which returns the blood from the heart muscle into the right atrium. *Ethmoid s.* Air spaces in the ethmoid bone. *Frontal s.* Air spaces in the frontal bone. *Sphenoid s.* Air spaces in the sphenoid bone. *S. arrhythmia.* See Arrhythmia. *S. thrombosis.* Clotting of blood in

a cranial venous channel. In the lateral sinus it is a complication of mastoiditis.

sinusitis (*si-nu-si'-tis*). Inflammation of a sinus, especially applied to the bony cavities of the face.

sinusoid (*si'-nu-soid*). Like a sinus. Used to describe the irregular channels by which blood vessels anastomose in certain organs, as the liver, suprarenal glands, heart, etc.

siphonage (*si'-fon-aj*). A method of drawing a liquid from one vessel into another.

situs inversus (*si'-tus in-ver'-sus*). Condition in which the positions of the body organs are reversed.

sitz-bath (*sits*). A hip bath.

skatole (*skat'-ole*). A product of protein decomposition in the intestine.

skeleton (*skel'-e-ton*). The bony framework of the body, supporting and protecting the organs and soft tissues.

skiagram (*ski'-ah-gram*). An X-ray photograph.

skiagraphy (*ski-ag'-raf-e*). Photography by X-rays.

skin. The outer protective covering of the body. It consists of the *epidermis* or cuticle, and the *dermis* or corium, which is known as 'true skin'. The skin and nervous system are developed from the same primitive layer of cells in the embryo, and keep this deep-rooted relation through life, as is often seen in disease. *Scarf s.* The cuticle. *S. grafting.* Transplantation of pieces of healthy skin to an area where loss of surface tissue has occurred.

skull. The bony framework of the head, consisting of the cranium and facial bones.

sleeping pulse. The rate of the pulse while sleeping. Can be recorded in patients who have diseases which may damage the heart, i.e. thyrotoxicosis.

sleeping sickness. Trypanosomiasis. A tropical fever occurring in parts of Africa, caused by a protozoal parasite (*Trypanosoma*) which is conveyed by the tsetse fly.

sling. A bandage for support of the upper limb.

slit lamp. A special light source so arranged with a microscope that examination of the eyelids and eye can be carried out at the level of each layer. Such an examination is also termed biomicroscopy.

slough (*sluf*). Local death of soft tissues due to injury or thrombosis in small veins of the part. It is ultimately washed away by exuded serum, leaving a granulating surface.

SMA. Scientific milk adaptation. Milk powder for infant feeding. Although made from cows' milk it has been modified to resemble human milk as closely as possible.

smallpox. See Variola.

smear. A specimen for microscopic examination that has been prepared by spreading a thin film of the material across a glass slide.

smegma (*smeg'-mah*). The secretion of sebaceous glands of the clitoris and prepuce.

Smith-Petersen nail (*Y. N. Smith-Petersen, American surgeon, 1886–1953*). A metal nail used to fix the fragments of bone in intracapsular fracture of the head of the femur.

snail track ulcers. Lesions occurring in the mouth in patients who have secondary syphilis.

snake venom antitoxin (*ven'-om*). Made from a horse serum, it is specific against cobra bites but may be given in all cases of

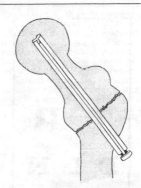

SMITH-PETERSEN NAIL

snake bite since individual antitoxins are not available.

Snellen's test types (*H. Snellen, Dutch ophthalmologist, 1834–1908*). Square-shaped letters on a chart, used for sight testing. See diagram p. 324.

snow. Frozen water vapour. *Carbon dioxide s.* Solidified frozen carbon dioxide, used in the treatment of warts and naevi. *S. blindness.* Photophobia due to the glare of snow.

snuffles (*snuf'-fls*). A chronic discharge from the nose occurring in congenital syphilis, due to infection of the nasal mucous membrane.

sociology (*so-se-ol'-o-je*). The scientific study of the development of man's social relationships and organization, i.e. interpersonal and intergroup behaviour as distinct from the behaviour of an individual.

sodium (*so'-de-um*). A metallic alkaline element widely distributed in nature, and forming an

SNELLEN'S TEST LETTERS

E
T B
D L N
P T E R
F Z B D E
O E L Z T G
L P O R F D Z

**SNELLEN'S TEST
LETTERS**

important constituent of animal tissue. *S. aminosalicylate.* An antituberculous drug used in conjunction with streptomycin and isoniazid (*q.v.*). *S. bicarbonate* is an antacid but its use is inadvisable as it stimulates the gastric mucosa and later increases acidity. Repeated use can cause alkalosis. *S. chloride* (common salt) is widely used for the cleansing of wounds, irrigation of body cavities and for intravenous therapy. *S. cit-*

rate is used to prevent clotting of blood during blood transfusions. *S. cromoglycate.* A drug commonly used in the treatment of asthma. It is administered through a spinhaler, which ensures that only a carefully measured dose is inhaled. *S. morrhuate.* Used for injection in the treatment of varicose veins. *S. phosphate* and *S. sulphate* are purgatives.

soft chancre (*shan'-ker*). *See* Chancroid.

soft soap. A mixture of oil and potash.

solapsone (*sol-ap'-zone*). A sulphone drug used in the treatment of leprosy.

solar plexus (*so'-lar pleks'-us*). A network of sympathetic nerve ganglia in the abdomen; the nerve supply to abdominal organs under the diaphragm.

solarium (*sol-ar'-e-um*). A room designed to admit as much sunlight as possible.

solution (*so-lu'-shun*). (1) A liquid in which a substance has been dissolved. (2) A break in continuity, e.g. a fracture.

solvent (*sol'-vent*). A liquid which dissolves or has power to dissolve.

somatic (*so-mat'-ik*). Relating to the body as opposed to the mind.

somnambulism (*som-nam'-bu-lizm*). Walking and carrying out other complex activities during a state of sleep. It is a state of dissociation and may occur in hysteria, in epilepsy and in a condition of low blood sugar.

Sonne dysentery (*C. O. Sonne, Danish bacteriologist, 1882–1948*). *See* Dysentery.

sonograph (*so'-no-graf*). A tracing of sounds heard by use of a sonometer (*q.v.*).

sonometer (*so-nom'-e-ter*). An

instrument for measuring the acuity of hearing or the frequency and pitch of sound waves.

sopor (*so'-por*). Profound sleep.

soporific (*sop-or-if'-ik*). Causing sleep.

sorbitol (*sor'-bit-ol*). A sweetening agent which is converted into sugar in the body though it is slowly absorbed from the intestine. It is used in some diabetic foods but as it has the same calorific value as sugar it should not be used in reducing diets.

Sorbo (*sor'-bo*). A foam or aerated rubber used for the manufacture of air rings, mattresses, and pillows.

sordes (*sor'-dez*). Brown crusts which form on the teeth and lips of unconscious patients, or those suffering from acute or prolonged fevers. The result of neglect of mouth hygiene.

sore. A general term for any ulcer or open skin lesion. *Cold s.* Herpes (*q.v.*). *Pressure s.* One due to impaired blood supply due to pressure.

souffle (*soo'-fl*). A blowing sound heard on auscultation.

sound. An instrument shaped like a probe for exploring cavities and detecting the presence of foreign bodies. Also for dilatation of a canal.

Sourdille's operation (*M. L. J. M. Sourdille, French otologist, 1885–1961*). *See* Fenestration.

South African tick-bite fever. A disease occurring in southern Africa, caused by *Rickettsia conori*, transmitted by ticks. Boutonneuse fever.

Southey's tubes (*R. Southey, English physician, 1835–99*). Small perforated metal tubes with trocar, for drainage of fluid from subcutaneous tissues, and from the peritoneal cavity.

soya bean (*soi-ah*). Bean which has a high protein content. May be made into infant 'milk' powder for babies who have an allergy to cows' milk. Also sold generally in certain 'meat' preparations as an alternative and cheaper form of protein.

Spanish fly. A species of beetle from which cantharidin, a blistering agent, is derived.

spansule (*span'-sule*). A drug made up in a capsule in such a way that there is slow release of its contents.

spasm (*spazm*). A sudden involuntary muscle contraction. *Carpopedal s.* Of the hands and feet. A sign of tetany. *Clonic s.* Alternate muscle rigidity and relaxation. *Habit s.* A tic. *Nictitating s.* Spasmodic twitching of the eyelid. *Tetanic s.* Violent muscle spasms, including opisthotonos. *Tonic s.* Muscle rigidity.

spasmolytic (*spaz-mo-lit'-ik*). A drug which reduces spasm, such as propantheline.

spastic (*spas'-tik*). Characterized by spasm. *S. paralysis.* One associated with lesions of the upper motor neurone as in cerebral vascular accidents and characterized by increased muscle tone and rigidity.

spasticity (*spas-tis'-it-e*). Marked rigidity of muscle.

spastics (*spas'-tiks*). A term applied to persons suffering from congenital paralysis due to some cerebral lesion or impairment.

spatial (*spa'-shal*). Pertaining to space.

spatula (*spat'-u-lah*). (1) A flexible blunt blade used for spreading ointment. (2) A rigid blade-shaped instrument for depressing the tongue in throat examination, etc.

spatulated (*spat'-u-la-ted*). Flattened like a spatula.

Special Hospitals. Under the Mental Health Act, 1959, those for the detention of mentally disordered persons who in the opinion of the Minister require treatment under conditions of special security on account of their dangerous, violent or criminal propensities.

species (*spe'-sheez*). A subdivision of genus.

specific (*spes-if'-ik*). (1) Relating to a species. (2) The special remedy for a particlar disease. *S. medicine.* A remedy which has a distinct curative influence on a particular disease, e.g. quinine in malaria. *S. disease.* A disease produced by a specified micro-organism and running a definite course. *S. gravity.* The density of fluid compared with that of an equal volume of water.

spectacles (*spek'-tak-ls*). A frame containing lenses worn in front of the eyes to correct errors of vision.

spectrum. The division of light into its component colours by a prism which separates the colours. *See* Rays.

speculum (*spek'-u-lum*). *Pl.* Specula. An instrument for dilating and holding open the orifice of a body cavity to assist examination of the interior.

speech. The utterance of vocal sounds. *Clipped s.* The words are incomplete. It may be a sign of general paresis. *Incoherent s.* Due to disturbance of the sequence of thought. *Staccato s.* Each syllable is separately pronounced. It may occur in disseminated sclerosis.

Spencer Wells forceps (*Sir T. Spencer Wells, British surgeon, 1818–97*). *See* Forceps.

sperm. Abbreviation for spermatozoon, the male sex cell.

spermatic (*sper-mat'-ik*). Pertaining to the semen. *S. cord. See* Cord.

spermatorrhoea (*sper-mat-or-re'-ah*). Involuntary discharge of semen.

spermatozoa (*sper-mat-o-zo'-ah*). The generative cells which form the essential part of semen. *Sing.* spermatozoon.

spermicide (*sper'-mis-ide*). Any agent which will destroy the reproductive cell.

sphenoid (*sfen'-oid*). Wedge-shaped. *S. bone.* Forms part of the base of the skull. Its shape resembles that of a bat.

spherocytosis (*sfer-o-si-to'-sis*). When the erythrocytes are more nearly spherical than biconcave. A feature of acholuric jaundice also known as *hereditary s.*

sphincter (*sfink'-ter*). A ring-shaped muscle, contraction of which closes a natural orifice.

sphincterotomy (*sfink-ter-ot'-o-me*). Cutting a sphincter to relieve constriction.

sphygmic (*sfig'-mik*). Relating to the pulse.

sphygmocardiograph (*sfig-mo-kard'-e-o-graf*). An instrument that records both the pulse and heart beat.

sphygmograph (*sfig'-mo-graf*). An instrument which, when applied to the wrist, registers graphically the force and character of the pulse beats.

sphygmomanometer (*sfig-mo-man-om'-e-ter*). An instrument for measuring the force of the arterial blood pressure.

spica (*spi'-kah*). A bandage applied to a joint in a series of 'figures of eight'.

spicule (*spi'-kul*). A splinter-like fragment of bone.

spider naevus (*spi-der ne'-*

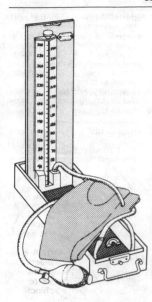

SPHYGMOMANOMETER

vus). Dilatation of small blood vessels in the skin giving the appearance of a spider. Happens during pregnancy or as a result of stimulation by oestrogen. Also seen after liver damage.

Spigelius' lobe (*A. van Spieghel (Spigelius), Flemish anatomist, 1578–1625*). The small lobe on the under surface of the liver.

spigot (*spig'-ot*). A small wooden or plastic peg to close the opening of a tube.

spina (*spi'-nah*). (1) Any sharp projection. (2) The vertebral column. *S. bifida.* A congenital defect of non-union of one or more vertebral arches, allowing protrusion of the meninges and possibly their contents. *See* Meningocele *and* Meningomyelocele.

spinal (*spi'-nal*). Relating to the spine. *S. anaesthesia. See* Anaesthesia. *S. bed* is made of plaster of Paris. It is a cast of the back of the head and trunk of the patient, and is so designed that he may rest in it and maintain complete immobility of the spine. Used in spinal caries or following operation on the vertebrae. *S. canal.* The hollow in the spine formed by the neural arches of the vertebrae. It contains the spinal cord, meninges, and cerebrospinal fluid. *S. caries.* Disease of the vertebra, usually tuberculous. *See* Pott's disease. *S. column.* The backbone, composed of thirty-three vertebrae, separated by pads of cartilage, and enclosing the spinal canal. *S. cord. See* Cord. *S. curvature.* Abnormal curving of the spine. If associated with caries, it is known as Pott's disease. (*See* Kyphosis, Lordosis, *and* Scoliosis.) *S. jacket.* A support for the spine, made of plaster of Paris, or other material, and used to give rest in caries of spine, or after injury to it. *S. nerves.* The thirty-one pairs of nerves which leave the spinal cord at regular intervals throughout its length. They pass out in pairs one on either side between each of the vertebra, and are distributed to the periphery.

spine. (1) The backbone or vertebral column. (2) A sharp process of bone.

spiral (*spi'-ral*). Winding, as the method of applying a roller bandage. *S. fracture.* One that is usually due to a rotational strain.

Spirillum (*spi-ril'-um*). A genus of spiral-shaped bacteria.

spirit. An alcoholic solution of a volatile substance. *See* Rectified spirit.

spiritus (*spir'-it-us*). Latin for spirit. *S. frumenti.* Whisky. *S. vini gallici.* Brandy.

spirochaetes (*spi'-ro-keets*). Micro-organisms in the form of a spiral. They are motile. An example is *Treponema pallidum*, the causative organism of syphilis.

spirograph (*spi'-ro-graf*). An instrument for registering respiratory movements.

spirometer (*spi-rom'-e-ter*). An instrument for measuring the air capacity of the lungs.

spironolactone (*spi-ron-o-lak'-tone*). A diuretic drug used when there is excess secretion of aldosterone. It promotes the excretion of sodium and water but retention of potassium.

Spitz–Holter valve (*Spitz, engineer; J. W. Holter, contemporary American engineer*). This is used in the treatment of hydrocephalus to drain the cerebrospinal fluid from the ventricles into the superior vena cava or right atrium.

splanchnic (*splank'-nik*). Pertaining to the viscera. *S. nerves.* Sympathetic nerves to the viscera. *S. sympathectomy.* An operation performed with the object of giving relief in some cases of high blood pressure. *See* Sympathectomy.

spleen (*splee-n*). A very vascular lymphoid organ, situated in the left hypochondrium under the border of the stomach. It manufactures lymphocytes and breaks down red blood corpuscles.

splenectomy (*splen-ek'-to-me*). Excision of the spleen.

spleneolus (*splen-e-o'-lus*). An accessory spleen.

splenic anaemia (*splen'-ik ane'-me-ah*). *See* Anaemia.

splenitis (*splen-i'-tis*). Inflammation of the spleen.

splenomegaly (*splen-o-meg'-al-e*). Enlargement of the spleen.

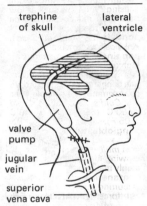

trephine of skull — lateral ventricle — valve pump — jugular vein — superior vena cava

SPITZ-HOLTER VALVE

splenorenal (*splen-o-re'-nal*). Applied to the spleen and the kidney. *S. anastomosis.* The spleen is excised and the splenic vein is inserted into the renal vein.

splenovenography (*splen-o-ven-og'-raf-e*). An X-ray of the spleen and its blood vessels following the insertion of a radio-opaque dye.

splint. An appliance used to support or immobilize a part while healing takes place or to correct or prevent deformity.

spondylitis (*spon-dil-i'-tis*). Inflammation of a vertebra. *Ankylosing s.* A disease chiefly of young males in which there is abnormal ossification with pain and rigidity of the intervertebral, hip and sacroiliac joints.

spondylolisthesis (*spon-dil-o-lis-the'-sis*). A sliding forwards or displacement of one vertebra over another. Usually the fifth lumbar over the sacrum, causing symptoms such as low back pain due to pressure on the nerve roots.

spondylosis (*spon-dil-o'-sis*). Ankylosis of vertebral joints.

sponging. A method of reducing high temperature by encouraging evaporation from the skin. The temperatures suggested are approximate, but suitable ones are: *Cold s.* 20°C (65°F), *Tepid s.* 30°C (85°F), *Hot s.* 40°C (105°F).

spongioblastoma multiforme (*spon-je-o-blas-to'-mah mult-e-for'-me*). A rapidly growing brain tumour that is highly malignant.

spontaneous (*spon-ta'-ne-us*). Occurring suddenly and without force. Applies to certain cases of fracture or pneumothorax (*q.v.*).

sporadic (*spor-ad'-ik*). A term applied to isolated cases of a disease which occurs in various and scattered places.

spore (*spor*). (1) A reproductive stage of some of the lowest forms of vegetable life, e.g. moulds. (2) A protective state which some of the bacilli are able to assume in adverse conditions, such as lack of moisture, food, or heat. In this form the organism can remain alive, but inert, for years.

spotted fever. A name given both to cerebrospinal fever and typhus on account of the pur-

puric rash which may be present in either disease.

sprain. Wrenching of a joint, producing laceration of the capsule or stretching of the ligaments, with consequent swelling, which is due to effusion of fluid into the affected part. Firm bandaging at once will prevent swelling and lessen disability. If there is effusion, applications of heat or cold can be made and support by a firm bandage or splint will be needed to ensure rest. Exercises are started early.

Sprengel's shoulder deformity (*O. G. K. Sprengel, German surgeon, 1852–1915*). A congenital condition in which one scapula is higher than the other, causing some limitation of abduction power.

sprue (*sproo*). A disease of malabsorption in the intestine, associated with the tropics; there is steatorrhoea, diarrhoea, glossitis, and anaemia. Lack of absorption of vitamin K leads to easy bleeding. Treatment is by giving vitamin B, particularly B_{12} and folic acid, vitamin K, iron and calcium. A gluten-free diet does not usually help these patients.

spurious labour (*spu'-re-us*). See Labour.

sputum (*spu'-tum*). Excess of secretions from the air-passages. It consists chiefly of mucus and saliva, but in diseased conditions of the air-passages it may be purulent, blood-stained, frothy, and contain many bacteria. *Rusty s.* Having altered blood permeating the mucus. Characteristic of acute lobar pneumonia. Sputum should always be regarded as highly infectious and should be expectorated wherever possible into disposable containers and incinerated.

squamous (*skwa'-mus*). Scaly. *S. bone.* The thin part of the temporal bone which articulates with the parietal and frontal bones.

squill (*skwill*). Scilla (*q.v.*).

squint (*skwint*). See Strabismus.

staccato speech (*stak-ah'-to*). A form of hesitation of speech between words and syllables followed by the sound uttered sharply.

Stacke's operation (*L. Stacke, German otolgist, 1859–1918*). Removal of bony structures between the mastoid cells and middle ear so that one cavity is made. An operation for chronic infection in this area.

stadium (*sta'-de-um*). The stage of a disease. *S. decrementi.* The period of decline in severity. Defervescence (*q.v.*). *S. incrementi.* The stage of advance when symptoms are developing.

staghorn calculus (*stag'-horn kal'-ku-lus*). A stone occurring in the urinary tract which is large, with branches giving the appearance of stag's horns.

stammering (*stam'-mer-ing*). A speech disturbance with repetition of syllables.

stapedectomy (*sta-pe-dek'-to-me*). Removal of the stapes and insertion of a vein graft or other device to re-establish conduction of sound waves in otosclerosis.

stapediolysis (*sta-pe-di-ol'-is-is*). An operation of mobilizing the footpiece of the stapes to aid conduction deafness from otosclerosis.

stapes (*sta'-pez*). The stirrup-shaped bone of the middle ear.

staphylectomy (*staf-il-ek'-to-me*). Removal of the uvula.

Staphylococcus (*staf-il-o-kok'-kus*). A species of pyogenic bacteria which, under the microscope, appear grouped together in small masses like bunches of grapes. This organism is especially responsible for the formation of boils and carbuncles. *S. pyogenes* or *S. aureus.* A type which grows as yellow colonies on artificial media, and is pus-producing.

staphyloma (*staf-il-o'-mah*). A protrusion of the cornea or sclerotic coat of the eyeball as the result of inflammation or wound.

staphyloptosis (*staf-il-op-to'-sis*). Elongation of the uvula.

staphylorrhaphy (*staf-il-or'-raf-e*). The operation for suture of a cleft soft palate of the uvula.

starch. A carbohydrate occurring in many vegetable tissues. *S. bath.* An emollient bath for skin diseases. 1 kg (2lb) of starch tied in a muslin bag is fixed to the hot water tap, and the water allowed to run through it into the bath. *S. powder* is often used with zinc powder as a soothing external application. *S. poultice* is a stiff mucilage of starch spread on old linen and applied cool to remove scabs; e.g. in skin diseases.

startle reflex. See Moro reflex.

starve. To deprive of or to suffer from a lack of food.

stasis (*sta'-sis*). Stagnation or stoppage. *Intestinal s.* Sluggish movement of the muscles of the bowel wall, which may be due to simple causes as unsuitable diet or lack of exercise. More seriously it may be caused by paralysis of the muscle wall or to obstruction. See Ileus. *Venous s.* Congestion of blood in the veins.

static (*stat'-ik*). Stationary, at rest. *S. electricity.* The term applied to a build-up of an electrical charge which may cause an explosion. *See* Appendix 4.

stationary air. *See* Air.

status (*stat'-us*). Condition. *S. asthmaticus.* A severe and prolonged attack of asthma. *S. epilepticus.* A condition in which there is rapid succession of epileptic fits. *S. lymphaticus.* A condition in which all lymphatic tissues are hypertrophied, especially the thymus gland. This may be found at post-mortem following sudden death.

steapsin (*ste-ap'-sin*). *See* Lipase.

steatoma (*ste-at-o'-mah*). A sebaceous cyst or a fatty tumour.

steatopygia (*ste-at-o-pi'-je-ah*). Excessive deposit of fat in the buttocks.

steatorrhoea (*ste-at-or-re'-ah*). The presence of undigested fat in the stools. A sign of pancreatic deficiency and occurring in coeliac disease.

steatosis (*ste-at-o'-sis*). (1) Fatty degeneration. (2) Disease of sebaceous glands.

Stein–Leventhal syndrome (*I. F. Stein, American gynaecologist, 1887– ; M. L. Leventhal, American gynaecologist, 1901–).* Condition affecting females in which obesity, hirsutism and sterility are associated with polycystic ovaries and menstrual irregularities.

Steinmann's pin (*F. Steinmann, Swiss surgeon, 1872–1932).* A fine metal rod passed through bone, by which extension is applied to overcome muscle contraction in certain fractures. *See* Kirschner's wire.

stellate (*stel'-ate*). Starlike. *S. ganglion.* The sympathetic ganglion of the first dorsal region.

S. fracture. A radiating fracture of the patella.

Stellwag's sign (*C. Stellwag von Carion, Austrian ophthalmologist, 1823–1904).* Infrequent blinking as may occur in exophthalmos.

stenocardia (*sten-o-kar'-de-ah*). Angina pectoris.

stenosis (*sten-o'-sis*). Narrowing or contraction of a channel or opening. *Aortic s.* Narrowing of the aortic valve as the aorta leaves the heart, due to scar tissue formation, as the result of inflammation. *Mitral s.* Of the mitral orifice from the same cause. *Pyloric s.* Of the stomach due to scar tissue, new growth, or congenital hypertrophy.

Stensen's duct (*H. Stensen, Danish physician, 1638–86).* The duct of the parotid gland, opening into the mouth at the level of the first upper molar.

stent (*stent*). An impression of the shape of the jaws taken on a plastic material which sets very hard. Used in dentistry when an artificial denture has to be made.

stepping reflex. Reflex seen in newborn infants. One foot is placed in front of the other when the child is held in the standing position on a hard surface. Also known as primary walking.

stercobilin (*ster-ko-bil'-in*). The colouring matter of the faeces; derived from bile.

stercolith (*ster'-ko-lith*). A faecal concretion which sometimes blocks the lumen of the vermiform appendix. Faecalith (*q.v.*).

stercoraceous (*ster-kor-a'-shus*). Faecal, or resembling faeces. *S. vomit.* Faecal vomit. *See* Vomiting.

stereognosis (*ster-e-og-no'-sis*). The identification of objects through the sense of touch.

stereostatics (*ster-e-o-stat'-iks*). The science relating to weight and its mechanical effects.

stereotaxy (*ster-e-o-taks'-e*). A manipulative operation for replacing displaced parts as in hernia reduction. The precise direction of an instrument into the brain tissue.

stereotypy (*ster-e-o-ti'-pe*). Term used to describe repetitive actions carried out or maintained for long periods in a monotonous fashion.

sterile (*ster'-ile*). (1) Barren; incapable of producing young. (2) Aseptic; free from micro-organisms.

sterility (*ster-il'-it-e*). The inability of a woman to become pregnant or of a man to produce sperm.

sterilization (*ster-il-i-za'-shun*). (1) Rendering incapable of reproduction by any means, e.g. removal of ovaries in the female, or bilateral severing of the vas deferens in the male. (2) Rendering dressings, instruments, etc., aseptic by destroying or removing all microbial life. *See* Appendix 5. *High pressure steam s. See* Autoclave.

sterilizer (*ster'-il-i-zer*). An apparatus in which objects can be sterilized. A term previously applied to a water boiler.

sternal (*ster'-nal*). Relating to the sternum. *S. puncture. See under* Puncture. *S. transfusion.* A method of introducing blood into the circulation via the bone marrow.

sternocleidomastoid (*ster-no-kli-do-mas'-toid*). A muscle group stretching from the mastoid process to the sternum and clavicle.

sternotomy (*ster-not'-o-me*). The operation in which the sternum is cut through.

sternum (*ster'-num*). The breast-bone; the flat narrow bone in the centre of the anterior wall of the thorax.

sternutator (*stern'-u-ta-tor*). A substance which causes sneezing. Nose gas.

steroids (*ster'-oids*). Hormones whose chemical structure is closely related to sterols. They include oestrogens, progestins, androgens, and hormones of the adrenal cortex. They may be naturally occurring or they may be synthetized.

sterol (*ster'-ol*). Non-saponifiable fats. Cholesterol is one.

stertorous (*ster'-tor-us*). Snoring; applied to a snoring sound produced in breathing in cases of cerebral compression, apoplexy, etc.

stethometer (*steth-om'-e-ter*). An instrument for measuring the expansion of the chest.

stethoscope (*steth'-o-skope*). The instrument used in mediate auscultation. It consists of a hollow tube, one end of which is placed over the part to be examined and the other at the ear of the examiner. *Binaural s.* branches into two flexible tubes, one for each ear of the examiner.

Stevens–Johnson syndrome (*A. M. Stevens, American paediatrician, 1884–1945: F. C. Johnson, American paediatrician, 1894–1934*). Febrile illness in which ulcers appear in the mouth and on the conjunctiva followed by bullous eruptions over the body. It may be treated with prednisolone.

sthenic (*sthen'-ik*). Strong, active. *S. fever* is marked by high temperature, rapid strong pulse, and highly coloured urine.

stibophen (*stib'-o-fen*). A preparation of antimony given intramuscularly. Used in the treatment of schistosomiasis.

stigma (*stig'-mah*). (1) A small haemorrhagic spot or mark on the skin. (2) Any mark or sign characteristic of a condition or defect, or of a disease, e.g. the *stigmata* of congenital syphilis—the depressed bridge of nose, radiating scars round the mouth, Hutchinson's teeth, etc. It refers to visible signs rather than symptoms.

stilboestrol (*stil-be'-strol*). A synthetic oestrogen preparation.

stilette (*stil-et'*). A wire or rod for keeping the lumen of tubes clear, e.g. of catheters, hollow needles, and cannulae.

stillbirth. As defined by the Central Midwives Board; a fetus, born after the twenty-eighth week of pregnancy, which, after complete expulsion, has not breathed or shown any sign of life.

Still's disease (*Sir G. F. Still, English paediatrician, 1868–1941*). A form of rheumatoid arthritis in children, associated with enlargement of lymph glands. The cause is unknown.

stimulant (*stim'-u-lant*). An agent which causes temporary increased energy or functional activity of any organ. *Alcoholic s.* Wines, brandy, whisky and malt liquors. *Cardiac s.* One which increases the action of the heart, as nikethamide.

stimulus (*stim'-u-lus*). An impulse causing stimulation. *Chemical s.* One which produces chemical change in a tissue. *Electric s.* Galvanic or other form of electric current applied to muscle tissue. *Thermal s.* Application of heat to produce a response.

stirrup bone (*stir'-rup*). See Stapes.

stitch. (1) A sudden sharp pain. (2) A suture. *S. abscess.* Pus formation where a stitch is inserted.

stock culture. A growth of specific organisms on culture media from which fresh growths can be made. *Stock vaccines* are made from such a culture.

Stockholm technique (*stok'-ho-lm tek-neek'*). A treatment of carcinoma of the uterine cervix by radium. Radium applicators are inserted in the cervical canal and fornices for 22 hours. The treatment is repeated one week later and again after two weeks.

Stokes-Adams syndrome (*Sir W. Stokes, Irish surgeon, 1804–78: R. Adams, Irish physician, 1791–1875*). Attacks of syncope or fainting due to cerebral anaemia in some cases of complete heart block. The heart stops, but breathing continues. Convulsions or death occur if the heart does not establish its own ventricular beat. See Myogenic.

stoma (*sto'-mah*). An orifice or opening to a free surface.

stomach (*stum'-ak*). The dilated portion of the alimentary canal between the oesophagus and the duodenum, just below the diaphragm. *Hourglass s.* Describes the shape of the organ in a type of deformity resulting from scar-tissue formation. *Leather bottle s.* Induration and thickening of the gastric wall, usually the result of cancer. *Senoran's s. pump.* Removes the contents of the stomach by suction. *S. tube* is a tube used for washing out the stomach, or for the administration of liquid food.

stomachic (*stum-ak'-ik*). (1)

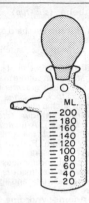

SENORAN'S STOMACH PUMP

Pertaining to the stomach. (2) A gastric tonic. A drug which stimulates and improves gastric function.

stomatitis (*sto-mat-i'-tis*). Inflammation of the mouth, either simple or with ulceration. The latter condition is accompanied by copious salivation, fetid breath, slight fever, and at times great prostration. Disinfectant mouthwashes, gentian violet and nystatin are used in treatment. It occurs in scurvy, acute leukaemia, and in infections of the mouth, as in thrush. *Aphthous s.* Characterized by small, white, superficial ulcers on the mucous membrane. *Ulcerative s.* shows painful shallow ulcers on the tongue, cheeks and lips. A severe type having serious constitutional effects.

stomatonoma (*sto-mat-o-*no'-mah*). Gangrene of the mouth. Noma.

-stomy (*sto'-me*). A suffix meaning 'to make an opening' or 'mouth'. *See* '-ectomy.

stool. A motion or discharge from the bowels. *Fatty s.* That which contains undigested fat. *Hunger s.* Stool passed by underfed infants; frequent, small and green in colour.

stop-needle. A needle with an enlargement on the shank to prevent deep penetration, e.g. sternal marrow puncture needle.

strabismus (*strab-iz'-mus*). Squint. A fixed deviation of either eye from its normal direction. It is called *convergent* when the eye turns in toward the nose, and *divergent* when it turns outward.

strain. (1) Over-use or stretching of a part, e.g. muscle or tendon. (2) To pass a liquid through a filter.

stramonium (*stra-mo'-ne-um*). A vegetable drug containing the alkaloid hyoscyamine, which in its action resembles belladonna. It may be used in paralysis agitans.

strangulated (*strang'-gu-la-ted*). Compressed or constricted, e.g. so that the circulation of the blood is arrested. *S. hernia. See* Hernia.

strangulation (*strang-gu-la'-shun*). (1) Choking caused by compression of the air passages. (2) Arrested circulation to a part, which will result in gangrene.

strangury (*strang'-gu-re*). A frequent desire to micturate, but only a few drops of urine are passed with difficulty and pain. It results from local inflammatory conditions and muscle spasm. It may also occur in fracture of the pelvis, when it indicates rupture of the bladder or urethra.

stratified tissue (*strat'-e-fide tis'-u*). A covering tissue in which the cells are arranged in layers. The germinating cells are the lowest and as surface cells are shed there is continual replacement.

stratum (*strah'-tum*). A layer; applied to structures such as the skin and mucous membranes. *S. corneum*. The outer, horny layer of epidermis. *Pl.* strata.

Streptococcus (*strep-to-kok'-kus*). A genus of bacteria occurring in chain-like formation. *S. faecalis*. A type which inhabits the intestines. *S. haemolyticus*. This may be the cause of acute tonsillitis, cellulitis, otitis media, scarlet fever, septicaemia, and puerperal fever. Its toxins cause haemolysis of red blood cells. It may be divided into Lancefield Groups of which A is most important to man and this can be further divided into serological Griffith types, by which the source of infection can be more easily traced. *S. viridans* is commonly found in the mouth and may enter the blood stream during dental extraction. It is the possible cause of some forms of non-suppurative arthritis which sometimes follow teeth extraction.

streptokinase (*strep-to-kin'-aze*). An enzyme derived from a streptococcal culture and used to liquefy clotted blood and pus. Vasidase contains it.

streptomycin (*strep-to-mi'-sin*). An antibiotic drug derived from a mould used particularly in the treatment of tuberculosis, and then usually given in conjunction with calcium or sodium aminosalicylate or isoniazid.

Streptothrix (*strep'-to-thriks*). Former name for some species of *Actinomyces* (*q.v.*) and *Fusiformis* (*q.v.*).

stress. The reaction, both physical and mental, to the demands made upon a person. *S. disorders*. Those associated with the individual's inability to meet these demands.

striae gravidarum (*stri'-e-grav-id-ar'-um*). The lines which appear on the abdomen of pregnant women. They are red in first pregnancy, but white subsequently and are due to stretching and rupture of the elastic fibres.

stricture (*strik'-chur*). A narrowing or local contraction of a canal. It may be caused by muscle spasm, new growth, or scar tissue formation following inflammation.

stridor (*stri'-dor*). A harsh, vibrating, shrill sound, produced during respiration.

stridulous (*strid'-u-lus*). Accompanied by stridor. *See* Laryngismus.

stroke. A popular term to describe the sudden onset of symptoms especially those of cerebral origin. *Apoplectic s*. Cerebral haemorrhage. *Heat s*. A hyperpyrexia accompanied by cerebral symptoms. It may occur in someone newly arrived in a very hot climate.

stroma (*stro'-mah*). The tissue forming the foundation and framework of an organ which supports the functioning cells. Disease may attack either the stroma or the specialized cells.

strontium 90 (*stron'-te-um*). A radioactive isotope with a half-life of 28 years, it is a fission product of atomic explosions. The danger lies in its power to replace calcium in the skeleton, especially in young growing bones.

strychnine (*strik'-neen*). A

highly poisonous alkaloid, the active principle of *Strychnos nux vomica.* In small doses it may be given as a nerve and muscle stimulant.

stupor (*stu'-por*). A state occurring in the course of many varieties of mental illness where the patient does not move, speak, and makes no response to stimuli, but consciousness is intact. *Depressive s.* Stupor occurring in the course of endogenous depression. *See* Catatonia.

stuporous (*stu'-por-us*). In a drowsy or semi-conscious state.

Sturge–Weber syndrome (*W. A. Sturge, British physician, 1850–1919; Sir H. D. Weber, British physician, 1824–1918*). Congenital abnormality in which there is a port wine stain apparent on the face over the trigeminal nerve. An angioma of the meninges is present on the same side as the port wine stain and this causes pressure on the underlying brain.

'STYCAR' developmental charts. Charts designed to show the 'norms' of childhood development, against which the progress of individual children may be measured.

stye. *See* Hordeolum.

styloid (*sti'-loid*). Like a pen. *S. process.* A sharp point on the temporal and ulna bones.

styptic (*strip'-tik*). An astringent which, applied locally, arrests haemorrhage, e.g. alum and tannic acid.

sub-. A prefix denoting 'under' or 'near'.

subacute (*sub'-ak-ute*). Moderately acute. *S. bacterial endocarditis.* A condition in which damaged heart valves become colonized by bacteria causing a severe febrile illness. *S. com-* *bined degeneration of the spinal cord.* See Degeneration.

subarachnoid (*sub-ar-ak'-noid*). Below the arachnoid. *S. space.* Between the arachnoid and pia mater of the brain and spinal cord, and containing cerebrospinal fluid.

subclavian (*sub-kla'-ve-an*). Beneath the clavicle. *S. artery.* The main vessel of supply to the upper limb.

subclinical (*sub-klin'-ik-al*). An infection in which the signs are so mild that a diagnosis is not made.

subconjunctival (*sub-kon-junk-ti'-val*). Occurring below the conjunctiva as in a haemorrhage.

subconscious (*sub-kon'-shus*). The condition in which memories are not within the consciousness but can be recalled to it with greater or less effort, sometimes called the preconscious.

subcutaneous (*sub-ku-ta'-ne-us*). Beneath the skin. *S. injection.* One given hypodermically.

subdural (*sub-du'-ral*). Below the dura mater. *S. haematoma.* A blood clot between the arachnoid and dura mater. It may be acute or arise slowly from a minor injury.

subinvolution (*sub-in-vo-lu'-shun*). Incomplete contraction of the uterus after labour.

subjective (*sub-jek'-tiv*). Related to the individual. *S. symptoms.* Those of which the patient is aware by sensory stimulation, but which cannot easily be seen by others. *Cf.* Objective.

sublimate (*sub'-lim-ate*). A substance obtained by vaporization of a solid and condensation of the vapour.

sublimation (*sub-lim-a'-shun*). A redirecting of energy at an unconscious level. The transference into socially acceptable channels of tendencies that cannot be expressed. An important aspect of maturity.

subliminal (*sub-lim'-in-al*). Below the threshold of perception.

sublingual (*sub-lin'-gwal*). Beneath the tongue. *S. glands.* Two salivary glands in the floor of the mouth.

sublobular (*sub-lob'-u-lar*). Beneath the lobules. *S. veins.* Convey the blood from the liver lobules.

subluxation (*sub-luks-a'-shun*). Partial dislocation.

submaxillary (*sub-maks-il'-lar-e*). Beneath the lower jaw. *S. glands.* Two salivary glands on the floor of the mouth.

submucous (*sub-mu'-kus*). Beneath mucous membrane. *S. resection.* An operation to correct a deflated nasal septum.

subnormality (*sub-nor-mal'-it-e*). Mental Health Act 1959. A state of arrested or incomplete development of the mind and is of a nature or degree which requires or is susceptible to medical treatment or other special care or training. *Severe s.* The degree of arrested or incomplete development is of such a nature that the patient is incapable of living an independent life or of guarding himself against serious exploitation.

subperiosteal (*sub-per-e-os'-te-al*). Beneath the periosteum.

subphrenic (*sub-fren'-ik*). Beneath the diaphragm. *S. abscess.* One which develops below the diaphragm and may point into the pleural cavity.

substitution (*sub-ste-tu'-shun*). The acceptance of an alternative. In psychology this may be the nurse or foster mother for the child's own mother. In psychotherapy the nurse or therapist may be substituted for someone in the patient's background.

subtertian (*sub-ter'-shun*). The term applied to the more continuous fever present in malaria due to infection by *Plasmodium falciparum.*

subtotal hysterectomy (*sub-to'-tal his-ter-ek'-to-me*). *See* Hysterectomy.

succinylsulphathiazole (*suk-sin-il-sul-fah-thi'-az-ole*). A sulphonamide preparation used for intestinal infections. It is not absorbed from the tract. Especially successful in infantile epidemic diarrhoea.

succus (*suk'-kus*). A juice. *S. citri.* Lime juice. *S. entericus.* A clear alkaline digestive fluid secreted by intestinal glands.

succussion splash (*suk-kush'-un*). The sound made by shaking the patient when free fluid is present in a cavity in the body.

sucrose (*su'-krose*). Cane or beet sugar.

suction (*suk'-shun*). The removal of air or fluid from a container by decreasing the pressure. *Hydraulic s.* Removing fluid from a body cavity by an attachment to a water tap or by the three bottle method.

sudamina (*su-dam'-in-ah*). An eruption of whitish vesicles associated with retention of sweat, and sometimes occurring in febrile conditions.

sudor (*su'-dor*). Sweat.

sudorific (*su-dor-if'-ik*). Diaphoretic; an agent causing sweating.

suffusion (*suf-fu'-zhun*). A sudden flushing of the skin, as in blushing.

sugar. A class of carbohydrates which include the following: (1) *Fermentable s.* (a) *Cane s.,* from the sugar-cane; (b) *Glucose* or *grape-s.*, from fruits, honey, etc. (2) *Lactose*, a nonfermentable sugar of milk. (3) *Muscle s.*: *Inositol.* Found in muscle and other tissues, and in the juice of asparagus and various vegetables.

suggestibility (*suj-es-ti-bil'-it-e*). A condition in which there is a greater susceptibility to suggestion.

suggestion (*suj-est'-shun*). A tool of psychotherapy in which an idea is presented to a patient and accepted by him. *Post-hypnotic s.* This influence lasts after his return to normal condition.

sulcus (*sul'-kus*). A furrow or fissure; applied especially to those of the brain.

sulphacetamide (*sul-fah-set'-am-ide*). A soluble sulphonamide useful for treating urinary infection and as drops or ointment for eye infections.

sulphadiazine (*sul-fah-di'-az-een*). A useful sulphonamide drug which is relatively nontoxic.

sulphadimidine (*sul-fah-di'-mid-een*). A sulphonamide in which a high blood level can be obtained but toxic effects are rare.

sulphaemoglobinaemia (*sulf-heem-o-glob-in-e'-me-ah*). A condition of cyanosis that used to arise during the administration of the earlier sulphonamides. Now rarely seen but should it arise it can be treated by giving methylene blue.

sulphafurazole (*sul-fah-fur'-az-ole*). A soluble, rapidly excreted sulphonamide useful in treating renal tract infections.

sulphaguanidine (*sul-fah-gwan'-id-in*). A sulphonamide preparation having specific action on organisms causing bacillary dysentery.

sulphamethizole (*sul-fah-meth'-e-zole*). A sulphonamide used in urinary infection as it is rapidly excreted in an active form.

sulphanilamide (*sul-fan-il'-am-ide*). A simple sulphonamide compound, less active than sulphadimidine.

sulphasalazine (*sul-fah-sal'-az-een*). A sulphonamide that has been used with some success in treating ulcerative colitis.

sulphate (*sul'-fate*). A salt of sulphuric acid.

sulphathiazole (*sul-fah-thi'-az-ole*). A very active but less used preparation; liable to give rise to rashes and drug fever; very rapidly excreted from the body.

sulphmethaemoglobin (*sulf-met-hem-o-glo'-bin*). The substance produced in the blood by excess of sulphur which gives rise to sulphaemoglobinaemia (*q.v.*).

sulphonamide (*sul-fon'-am-ide*). The generic term for all aminobenzine-sulphonamide preparations.

sulphones (*sul'-fones*). A group of drugs which with prolonged use have been successful in treating leprosy.

sulphonylureas (*sul-fon-il-ur-e'-ahs*). Oral hypoglycaemic drugs that may be used in milder forms of diabetes. Examples are tolbutamide and chlorpropamide.

sulphuric acid (*sul-fu'-rik*). Oil of vitriol. A heavy colourless liquid and corrosive poison, which burns any organic substance with which it comes into contact.

sunburn. A dermatitis due to exposure to the sun's rays, causing burning and redness.

sunstroke. Overwhelming prostration caused by exposure to excessive heat from the sun. See Heat stroke.

super- (*su'-per*). A prefix meaning 'over'.

superciliary (*su-per-sil'-e-are*). Relating to the eyebrow.

supercilium (*su-per-sil'-e-um*). The eye-brow.

superego (*su-per-e'-go*). That part of the personality that is concerned with moral standards and ideals that are derived unconsciously from the parents, teachers and environment, and influence the person's whole mental make-up acting as a control on impulses of the ego.

superfatted (*su-per-fat'-ted*). Having in it more fat than can combine with the alkali present.

superficial (*su-per-fish'-al*). On or near the surface. Often applied to those blood vessels near the skin.

superior (*su-per'-e-or*). Above; the upper of two parts.

superstition (*su-per-stish'-un*). A belief or practice which is unnatural and not based on reason. See Fetishism.

supination (*su-pi-na'-shun*). Turning upwards. *S. of hand.* The palm is upward. *Cf.* Pronation.

supine (*su'-pine*). Lying on the back, with the face upward.

suppository (*sup-pos'-it-or-e*). A method of introducing a drug in solid form into a body cavity so that it will dissolve at body temperature. *Rectal s.* May be used to evacuate the bowels (glycerin or bisacodyl) or to relieve muscle spasm (aminophylline). *Vaginal s.* See Pessary.

suppressant (*sup-pres'-ant*). A drug which will prevent a disease from developing, e.g. quinine suppresses malaria.

suppression (*sup-presh'-un*).

(1) Complete cessation of a secretion. *S. of urine.* No secretion of urine by the kidneys. (2) In psychology, *conscious* inhibition as distinct from *repression* which is *unconscious*.

suppuration (*sup-pu-ra'-shun*). The formation of pus.

supra- (*su'-pra*). A prefix meaning 'above'.

suprapubic (*su-prah-pu'-bik*). Above the pubic bone. *S. catheters.* Those used for drainage following cystostomy. *S. cystotomy.* Opening the bladder above the pubis. *S. drainage.* A method of draining the bladder after cystotomy, with or without prostactectomy.

supracondylar (*su-prah-kon'-de-lah*). Above the condyles. *S. fracture.* Usually refers to one above the lower end of the humerus.

suprarenal (*su-prah-re'-nal*). Above the kidney. *S. capsule.* A small triangular, endocrine gland, one above each kidney. See Adrenal and Cortin.

surdity (*sur'-dit-e*). Deafness.

surgery (*sur'-je-re*). The branch of medicine that treats disease by operative measures.

surgical (*sur'-jik-al*). Pertaining to surgery. *S. neck.* The narrower part of the humerus, just below the tuberosities.

surrogate (*sur'-o-gate*). In psychology, an imagined person by which the patient conceals the real individual from his consciousness.

susceptibility (to disease) (*sus-sep-tib-il'-it-e*). Lack of resistance to infection.

suspensory bandage (*sus-pen'-sor-e*). A bandage worn to support the scrotum.

suture (*su'-chur*). (1) A stitch or series of stitches used to close a wound. (2) The jagged line of junction of the bones of the

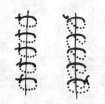

interrupted   continuous

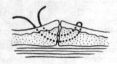

mattress

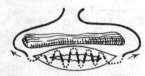

subcuticular

SUTURES

cranium. *Atraumatic s.* A suture fused to the needle, to obtain a single thickness through each puncture of the needle. *Continuous s.* A form of oversewing with one length of suture. *Blanket s.* A continuous blanket stitch. *Everting s.* A type of mattress s. that turns the edges outwards to give a closer approximation. *Fascial s.* A strip of fascia taken from the patient. *Interrupted s.* A series of sepa-

rate sutures. *Mattress s.* Each suture taken twice through the wound giving a loop one side and a knot the other. *Purse-string s.* A circular continuous suture round a small wound or appendix stump. *Subcuticular s.* A continuous suture placed just below the skin. *Tension s.* One taking a large bite and relieving the tension on the true stitch line.

suxamethonium chloride (*suks-a-meth-o'-ne-um*). A short-acting muscle-relaxant drug that may be used to get good muscle relaxation during operation. Scoline is a proprietary preparation.

swab. (1) A small piece of wool or gauze. (2) In pathology a dressed stick used in taking bacteriological specimens.

swallowing (*swal'-lo-ing*). The act of deglutition in which food is passed from the mouth to the oesophagus.

sweat (*swet*). A clear watery fluid secreted by the sudoriferous glands. *S. test.* Pilocarpine is passed through the epidermis by means of an electrode and stimulates the sweat glands. The sweat is collected and tested for sodium chloride, of which there is an excessive secretion in fibrocystic disease of the pancreas.

sweetbread. The pancreas.

sycosis (*si-ko'-sis*). Staphylococcal inflammation of the hair-follicles, especially those of the beard. It is characterized by pustules which form into scabs. *S. barbae.* That affecting the beard. Barber's itch.

Sydenham's chorea (*T. Sydenham, British physician, 1624–1689*). Disease, chiefly affecting children, in which there is inability to control movement. Its cause is similar to that of acute rheumatism (*q.v.*).

symbiosis (*sim-bi-o'-sis*). When a parasite and its host are of mutual benefit to each other.

symblepharon (*sim-blef'-ar-on*). Adhesion of an eyelid to the eyeball.

symbolism (*sim'-bol-izm*). An abnormal mental condition in which events or objects are interpreted as symbols of the patient's own thoughts. In psychiatry, when repressed material re-enters consciousness in another form though it was previously unacceptable. A child's play may be symbolic, as may the painting of an emotionally disturbed patient.

symbols (*sim'-bols*). (1) Letters or marks used by convention to denote a substance or process. (2) Objects or activities representing and substituting for something else.

Syme's amputation (*J. Syme, Scottish surgeon, 1799–1870*). Amputation of the foot, at the ankle-joint.

sympathectomy (*sim-path-ek'-to-me*). Division of the pre- or post-ganglionic fibres which control specific involuntary muscles. An operation performed for many conditions, e.g. Raynaud's disease, severe spasmodic dysmenorrhoea or megacolon.

sympathetic (*sim-path-et'-ik*). (1) Exhibiting sympathy. (2) A division of the autonomic nervous system. *S. anuria.* Suppression of urine, which may occur in the remaining kidney if the other has been removed, or is temporarily out of action. *S. ganglionectomy.* An operation performed for the same reasons as sympathectomy, but with removal of the ganglion concerned. *S. nervous system.* A branch of the automatic nervous system which supplies involuntary muscle and glands. It stimulates the ductless glands and the circulatory and respiratory systems but inhibits the digestive system. *S. ophthalmia.* Inflammation leading to loss of sight in the opposite eye following a perforating injury in the ciliary region.

sympathin (*sim'-path-in*). A substance released into the blood stream when sympathetic nerve fibres are stimulated. It is similar to adrenaline in action.

sympathomimetic (*sim-path-o-mim-et'-ik*). Drugs that mimic or act in the same way as the sympathetic nerves.

symphysis (*sim'-fis-is*). The line of union of two bones which originally were separate. *S. pubis.* The cartilaginous junction of the two pubic bones.

symptom (*simp'-tum*). Any evidence as to the nature and location of a disease. It is *subjective*, i.e. noted by the patient; *signs* are noted by the observer and are therefore *objective*. Thus the phrase 'signs and symptoms'. *Withdrawal s.* Those arising when a drug or alcohol is withheld from an individual who is dependent on it.

symptomatology (*simp-to-mat-ol'-o-je*). The study of the symptoms of disease.

syn-. A prefix meaning 'together'.

synalgia (*sin-al'-je-ah*). Pain felt in one part of the body but caused by inflammation or of injury to another part.

synapse (*sin'-aps*). The termination of an axon with the dendrites of another nerve cell. Chemical transmitters pass the impulse across the space.

synarthrosis (*sin-ar-thro'-sis*).

A form of articulation, in which the bones are wedged immovably together with no intervening synovial membrane, e.g. cranial sutures.

synchondrosis (*sin-kon-dro'-sis*). The junction of bones by means of cartilage.

synchysis (*sin'-kis-is*). Softening of the vitreous humour of the eye.

syncope (*sin'-ko-pe*). A simple faint or temporary loss of consciousness due to cerebral anaemia; often caused by dilatation of the peripheral blood vessels and a sudden fall in blood pressure. *Cardiac s. See* Stokes-Adams syndrome.

syncytium (*sin-sit'-e-um*). The superficial layer of cells covering the chorionic villi.

syndactylism (*sin-dak'-til-izm*). Webbed fingers or toes.

syndrome (*sin'-drome*). A group of symptoms typical of a distinctive disease or frequently occurring together and so labelled collectively. *See* Stokes-Adams *s. and* Fröhlich's *s.*

synechia (*sin-ek'-e-ah*). Adhesion of the iris to the cornea in front (*anterior s.*) or capsule of the lens behind (*posterior s.*).

synergy (*sin'-er-je*). The harmonious action of two agents or muscles working together.

synovectomy (*si-no-vek'-to-me*). Excision of a diseased synovial membrane to restore movement.

synovial membrane (*si-no'-ve-al*). A serous membrane lining the articular capsule of a movable joint, and terminating at the edge of the articular cartilage. It secretes a lubricating fluid—*synovia.*

synovitis (*si-no-vi'-tis*). Inflammation of a synovial membrane. It may be suppurative and result in ankylosis.

synthesis (*sin'-thes-is*). The building up of a more complex structure from simple components. This may apply to drugs or to plant or animal tissues.

synthetic (*sin-thet'-ik*). Artificial. Made by synthesis.

syphilide (*sif'-il-id*). Any disease of the skin due to syphilis. It may be erythematous, vesicular, pustular, etc.

syphilis (*sif'-il-is*). A specific, contagious venereal disease, caused by the *Treponema pallidum. Acquired s.* Commonly transmitted by sexual intercourse; there is an early infectious stage, followed by a latent period of many years before the non-infectious late stage when serious disorders of the nervous and vascular systems arise. *Congenital s.* This is transmitted by the mother to her child but is preventable if the mother receives a full course of penicillin during her pregnancy.

syringe. An instrument for injecting fluids or for aspirating or irrigating body cavities. *Aural s.* one for ear irrigation. *Bladder s.* for bladder irrigation or for aspiration of blood clots. *Eccentric s.* The needle mount is placed on the circumference, making intravenous injection easier. *Luer Lok s.* A syringe used for chest aspiration that is fitted with a simple locking device so that the needle will not be accidentally displaced.

syringing (*sir'-in-jing*). The act of using a syringe to wash out a cavity.

syringobulbia (*sir-in-go-bul'-be-ah*). The formation of cavities in the brain stem.

syringomyelia (*sir-in-go-mi-e'-le-ah*). A disease of the nervous system causing the formation of cavities filled with fluid, inside the spinal cord. Impairment of muscle function and sensation result. Painless injury may be the first symptom.

syringomyelitis (*sir-in-go-mi-el-i'-tis*). Inflammation of the spinal cord, as the result of which cavities are formed in it.

syringomyelocele (*sir-in-go-mi'-el-o-seel*). A type of spina bifida in which the protruded sac of fluid communicates with the central canal of the spinal cord.

syrup (*sir'-up*). An aqueous solution of refined sugar to which drugs may be added. *Easton's s.* A tonic containing iron, quinine, strychnine, and phosphates. *S. of figs* or *senna.* Pleasant-tasting aperients for children. *S. of codeine.* Soothing for cough.

system (*sis'-tem*). A combination of organs in the performance of a common function, e.g. the organs of digestion = the digestive system.

systemic (*sis-tem'-ik*). Pertaining to a whole system or collection of systems. *S. circulation.* Circulation of the blood throughout the whole body. *S. lupus erythematosus.* Acute systemic disease occurring in young females in which there is disordered immunity.

systole (*sis'-to-le*). The contraction of the heart. *See also* Diastole. *Extra-s.* A premature contraction of the atrium or ventricle, without alteration of the fundamental rhythm of the pacemaker. *Ventricular s.* The contraction of the heart by which the blood is pumped into the aorta and pulmonary artery.

systolic murmur (*sis-tol'-ik*). An abnormal sound produced during systole, in heart affections.

T

T cells (*te-sels*). Lymphocytes which have the ability to produce antibodies as a result of being produced and controlled by the thymus gland.

TAB. A vaccine of the killed organisms that cause typhoid fever and paratyphoid A and B. Used as a preventive against these diseases giving an active immunity.

tabes (*ta'-beez*). Wasting away. *T. dorsalis.* Locomotor ataxia. A slowly progressive disease of the nervous system affecting the posterior nerve roots and spinal cord. It is a late manifestation of syphilis (*q.v.*).

tabetic (*ta-bet'-ic*). Affected with tabes.

taboparesis (*ta-bo-par-e'-sis*). When the symptoms of both tabes dorsalis and general paralysis of the insane are present in a patient suffering from late syphilis.

tablet (*tab'-let*). A solid dosage form consisting of compressed powder.

tachy-. A prefix meaning 'rapid'.

tachycardia (*tak-e-kar'-de-ah*). Abnormally rapid action of the heart and consequent increase in pulse rate. (*See also* Bradycardia.) *Paroxysmal t.* Spasmodic increase in cardiac contractions of sudden onset lasting a variable time from a few seconds to hours. Sometimes a sign of ailing heart muscle, but in young people especially it may be of nervous origin.

tachylalia (*tak-e-la'-le-ah*). Extreme rapidity of speech.

tachyphrasia (*tak-e-fra'-ze-ah*). Extreme volubility of speech. It may be a sign of mental disorder.

tachyphrenia (*tak-e-fre'-ne-*

ah). Hyperactivity of the mental processes.

tachypnoea (*tak-e-pne′-ah*). Rapid, shallow respirations; a reflex response to stimulation of the vagus nerve endings in the pulmonary vessels.

tactile (*tak′-tile*). Relating to the sense of touch.

T-bandage. Used to retain a perineal dressing in position.

Taenia (*te′-ne-ah*). A genus of tapeworms. *T. saginata.* The common type of tapeworm found in the human intestine. *T. solium.* The pork tapeworm. Can also be parasitic in man.

taeniafuge (*te′-ne-ah-fuj*). A drug which expels tapeworms, e.g. filix mas.

TAF. Toxoid-antitoxin flocules. A preparation used for diphtheria immunization. *See* Toxoid.

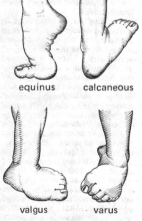

equinus   calcaneous

valgus   varus

TALIPES

talcum (*tal′-kum*). A preparation of magnesium silicate, used as a dusting powder.

talipes (*tal′-ip-eez*). Clubfoot. Deformity caused by congenital or acquired contraction of muscles or tendons of the foot. *T. calcaneous.* The heel alone touches the ground on standing. *T. equinus.* Walking on the toes only. *T. valgus.* The inner edge of the foot only is in contact with the ground. *T. varus.* The person walks on the outer edge of the foot.

talus (*ta′-lus*). The astragalus or ankle bone.

tampon (*tam′-pon*). An absorbent wool plug with long thread attached by which it can be anchored. Used to restrain haemorrhage or absorb secretion.

tamponade (*tam-pon-ade′*). The surgical use of tampons. *Cardiac t.* Impairment of heart action by haemorrhage into the pericardium. This may be owing to a stab wound or following surgery.

tannin (*tan′-nin*). Tannic acid. A yellowish powder prepared from vegetable substances, e.g. from tea. A powerful astringent and haemostatic, which on contact with any mucous membrane causes contraction and diminishes secretions.

tantalum (*tan′-tal-um*). A metal used for prosthesis and wire sutures. *Radioactive t.* ([182]Ta) emits γ- and β-rays. It is a flexible wire and can be used to treat carcinoma in difficult situations such as the mouth and the bladder.

tantrum (*tan′-trum*). An outburst of ill-temper. *Temper t.* A behaviour disorder of childhood. A display of bad temper in which the child performs

uncontrolled actions in a state of emotional stress.

tap water. Water direct from the main supply. It is sometimes given as a rectal injection in dehydration in preference to saline solution as it is more readily absorbed. *See* Enema.

tapeworm. *Taenia* (*q.v.*). A genus of cestode worms parasitic in the intestines of man and many animals. The adult consists of a round head with suckers or hooklets for attachment. From this numerous segments arise, each of which produces ova capable of independent existence for a considerable length of time. Treatment is by drugs to expel the parasite, and cure is not complete until the *head* is discharged or destroyed as from this growth takes place.

tapotement (*tap-ote-mon'*). A tapping movement used in massage.

tapping (*tap'-ping*). *See* Paracentesis.

tar. A dark brown or black viscid fluid, derived from the bark of various species of pine. Used externally in certain skin diseases. *Coal t.* Obtained from coal or petroleum. The source of phenol, creosol, xylene, benzene, etc.

tarsal (*tar'-sal*). Relating to the tarsus. *T. bones.* The seven irregular bones of the foot. *T. cyst.* Chalazion (*q.v.*). *T. plates.* Small cartilages in the upper eyelids.

tarsalgia (*tar-sal'-je-ah*). Pain in the foot, with flattening of the arch.

tarsoplasty (*tar'-so-plas-te*). Plastic surgery of the eyelid.

tarsorrhaphy (*tar-sor'-raf-e*). Stitching the eyelids together to protect the cornea or to allow healing of an abrasion.

tarsus (*tar'-sus*). (1) The seven small bones of the instep. (2) The connective tissue which forms the firm supporting tissue of the eyelid.

tartar (*tar'-tar*). (1) Potassium bitartrate (*cream of t.*). (2) A hard incrustation deposited on neglected teeth.

taste (*ta'-st*). The sense by which it is possible to identify what is eaten and drunk. Taste receptors (buds) lie in the posterior part of the tongue and give the sensations of sweet, sour, salt and bitter.

taurocholate of sodium (*tor-o-ko'-late*). One of the bile salts. Used as a cholagogue.

Taussig's operation (*Helen B. Taussig, American paediatrician, 1889–*). Block dissection of the pelvic lymphatic glands for carcinoma of the uterus.

Tawara's node (*S. Tawara, Japanese pathologist, 1873–*). The atrioventricular node. *See* Node.

taxis (*taks'-is*). Manipulation by hand to restore any part to its normal position. It can be used to reduce a hernia.

taxonomy (*taks-on-o-me*). Classification, e.g. of bacteria.

Tay–Sachs disease (*W. Tay, English physician, 1843–1927; B. Sachs, American neurologist, 1858–1944*). *See* Amaurotic familial idiocy.

TDS (*ter die sumendum*). Order on a prescription meaning 'to be taken three times a day'.

technetium (*tek-ne'-te-um*). A metallic element. *Radioactive t.* (*99Tc*) is used in a number of diagnostic tracer tests.

technique (*tek-neek'*). The details of a method or procedure. *Aseptic t.* That by which a wound is kept surgically clean.

teeth. *See* Tooth.

teething. Dentition (*q.v.*).

Teflon. A synthetic woven fabric that is used in cardiovascular surgery for heart valves, patches and blood vessel grafts.

Tegretol (*teg'-ret-ol*). Proprietary preparation of carbamazepine. Used in the treatment of trigeminal neuralgia.

tegument (*teg'-u-ment*). The skin.

tela (*te'-lah*). A web-like tissue. *T. choroidea.* The fold of pia mater containing a network of blood vessels found in the ventricles of the brain from which the cerebrospinal fluid originates.

telangiectasis (*tel-an-je-ek'-tasis*). A group of dilated capillaries, web-like or radiating in form, seen chiefly on the face in certain disorders of the circulation.

telangioma (*tel-an-je-o'-mah*). A tumour of dilated blood capillaries.

teleceptors (*tel-e-sep'-tors*). Nerve receptors concerned with events at a distance. Telereceptors.

teletherapy (*tel-e-ther'-ap-e*). Treatment with a γ-ray beam unit in which the source of radiation is housed in a well-protected chamber and only brought to the aperture head when the patient is in position and the personnel have left the area. Radium, cobalt and caesium may be used.

telophase (*tel'-o-faze*). The stage in the division of cells when the chromosomes have been reconstituted in the nuclei at either end of the cell and the cell cytoplasm divides forming two new cells.

temper tantrums. *See* Tantrum.

temperature (*tem'-per-at-chur*). The degree of heat of a substance or body as measured by a thermometer. *Inverse t.* One which is lower in the evening than the morning. *Normal t.* of the human body is 36·9°C (98·4°F) with a slight decrease in the early morning, and a slight increase at night. It indicates the balance between heat production and heat loss. A thermometer inserted under the tongue or into the rectum will register slightly higher than one placed in the axilla or groin. *Subnormal t.* is below the normal. A sign of shock. *See* Pyrexia *and* Fever.

temporal (*tem'-por-al*). Pertaining to the side of the head. *T. bone.* That at the side of the skull and containing the organ of hearing. *T. arteritis.* Giant cell arteritis. An inflammatory condition of the carotid arteries and their branches. *T. lobe epilepsy.* Form of epilepsy in which only the temporal lobe of the brain is affected. Patients may perform stereotyped movements or experience flushing, sweating or abdominal pain. It may be limited to frightening hallucinatory experiences.

temporomandibular (*tempor-o-man-dib'-u-lar*). Relating to the temporal region or bone and the mandible.

tenacious (*ten-a'-shus*). Thick and viscid, a term applied to sputum or other body fluids.

tenaculum (*ten-ak'-u-lum*). A hook-shaped instrument.

tendinous (*ten'-din-us*). Having the nature of a tendon.

tendon (*ten'-don*). A band of fibrous tissue, forming the termination of a muscle and attaching it to a bone. *T. of Achilles.* That inserted into the calcaneum. *T. grafting.* An operation which repairs a defect in one tendon by a graft from another. *T. of insertion.* The attachment of a muscle to a bone which it moves. *Kangaroo t.* A form of suture derived from the tail of a kangaroo. *T. of origin.* The beginning of a muscle at its attachment to the more fixed bone. *T. reflex.* The muscle action produced on percussing a tendon.

tenesmus (*ten-ez'-mus*). A painful ineffectual straining to empty the bowel or bladder.

tennis elbow. Painful disorder which affects the extensor muscles of the forearm at their attachment to the external epicondyle.

Tenon's capsule (*J. R. Tenon, French surgeon, 1724–1816*). The fibrous tissue in which the eyeball is situated.

tenoplasty (*ten'-o-plas-te*). Plastic operation on a tendon.

tenorrhaphy (*ten-or'-raf-e*). The suturing together of the ends of a divided tendon.

tenosynovitis (*ten-o-si-no-vi'-tis*). Inflammation of a tendon and its synovial sheath.

tenotomy (*ten-ot'-o-me*). Cutting a tendon.

tension (*ten'-shun*). The act of stretching or the state of being stretched. *Arterial t.* The pressure of blood on the vessel wall during cardiac contraction. *Intraocular t.* Pressure of the contents of the eye on its walls, measured by a tonometer. *Premenstrual t.* Symptoms of abdominal distension, headache, emotional lability and depression occurring a few days before the onset of menstruation. *See* Cyclical syndrome. *Surface t.* The resistance offered by a liquid to another substance in contact with it. *T. suture. See* Suture.

tensor (*ten'-sor*). A muscle which stretches a part.

tent. (1) A small cone-shaped plug of compressed seaweed which swells considerably on the absorption of moisture. It may be used to dilate the cervix. *See* Laminaria. (2) *Steam t.* A contrivance by which the head of the bed is surrounded by screens and the top covered over to form a tent. A long-spouted kettle projects steam into this enclosure to moisten and warm the air. Used with benefit for upper respiratory diseases such as laryngitis.

tentorium (*ten-tor'-e-um*). The dividing wall of dura mater between the cerebrum and the cerebellum.

tepid (*tep'-id*). Slightly warm: 32–37°C (89.6–98.6°F).

teratogenesis (*ter-at-o-jen'-e-sis*). The development and birth of a monster or a child with gross congenital abnormalities.

teratoma (*ter-at-o'-mah*). A solid tumour of the ovary containing tissues similar to those of a dermoid cyst. 80 per cent of these tumours are malignant.

teres (*ter'-ez*). Round. *Ligamentum t.* Round ligament.

terminal (*ter'-min-al*). Placed at or forming the extremity. The ends of the conducting wires of an electric battery. *T. infection.* An added infection which is fatal.

terminology (*ter-min-ol'-o-je*). The science of nomenclature (*q.v.*) of scientific and technical subjects.

tertian (*ter'-she-an*). Recurring every 48 hours. *See* Malaria.

tertiary (*ter'-she-ar-e*). Third. *T. syphilis.* The non-infectious stage of neurosyphilis.

test. (1) A trial. (2) Analysis of the composition of a substance, by the use of chemical reagents. *Colloidal gold t.* Carried out on the cerebrospinal fluid, it aids in the diagnosis of neurosyphilis.

Hippuric acid t. One for liver efficiency, when sodium benzolate given by mouth is excreted in the urine. *Hogben t.* A test for pregnancy in which urine of the patient is injected into the Xenopus toad; if positive, eggs are voided by the toad 8 hours later. *Papanicolaou t.* A cervical smear is examined for cell changes indicating a pre-cancerous phase of the cervix. *Schick t.* An intradermal test for susceptibility to diphtheria which has proved invaluable in preventing the disease, as those without resistance can be immunized. *T. meal.* A procedure used to test the digestive powers of the gastric juice. *Fractional t. meal.* Designed to estimate the activity of the gastric glands in producing hydrochloric acid. Alcohol, histamine or pentagastrin may be used and successive specimens taken to estimate the acid content. *T. tube.* A thin glass tube closed at one end, used for carrying out chemical tests on fluids. *T. type.* A card of letters of varying size for testing the acuity of sight. For *renal function*, and *urine t.s, see* Appendix 11.

testamentary capacity (*test-am-ent'-ar-e kap-as'-it-e*). The ability of a person to understand fully what he is doing when he wishes to make a will.

testicles or **testes** (*test'-ik-kls, tes'-teez*). The two glands in the scrotum which produce spermatozoa. *Undescended t.* When the organ remains in the pelvis or inguinal canal.

testosterone (*tes-tos'-ter-one*). The hormone produced by the testes which stimulates the development of sex characteristics. Now made synthetically. It is used medicinally in cases of failure of sex function

and in some cases of female cancer.

tetanic (*tet-an'-ik*). Relating to tetanus. *T. spasms* occur also in strychnine poisoning.

tetanus (*tet'-an-us*). A disease due to *Clostridium tetani,* an anaerobe found in cultivated soil and manure, and therefore likely to infect accidental wounds. The incubation period is 3 to 10 days but may be much longer. *Signs.* Stiffness of muscles around the wound, followed by rigidity of face and neck muscles; hence 'lockjaw'. All muscles are then affected and opisthotonos may occur. *T. vaccine* or *toxoid* will give an active immunity. *T. antitoxin.* A serum that gives a short-term passive immunity and may be used for treatment of a case of tetanus.

tetany (*tet'-an-e*). An increased excitability of the nerves due to a lack of available calcium, accompanied by painful muscle spasm (*carpopedal spasm*). The cause may be hypothyroidism or alkalosis owing to excessive vomiting or hypoventilation (*q.v.*).

tetracycline (*tet-rah-si'-kleen*). An antibiotic drug belonging to the group known as the tetracyclines which are used to combat organisms that are resistant to penicillin. Achromycin is a proprietary preparation.

tetradactylous (*tet-rah-dak'-til-us*). Having four digits on each limb.

tetralogy of Fallot (*E.-L. A. Fallot, French physician, 1850–1911*). *See* Fallot's tetralogy.

tetraparalysis (*tet-rah-par-al'-is-is*). Paralysis of all four limbs. Quadriplegia.

tetraparesis (*tet-rah-par-e'-*

sis). Partial paralysis of all four limbs.

thalamotomy (*thal-am-ot'-o-me*). The destruction of the nucleus in the thalamus by diathermy. The area needs to be carefully localized first.

thalamus (*thal'-am-us*). A mass of nerve cells at the base of the cerebrum. Most sensory impulses from the body pass to this area and are transmitted to the cortex.

thalassaemia (*thal-as-e'-me-ah*). A group of disorders mostly found in the Mediterranean region, caused by the inheritance of an abnormal haemoglobin. *T. minor.* Moderate to mild anaemia. *T. major.* Cooley's anaemia; the severest form of thalassaemia with death usually occurring before adolescence.

Thalidomide (*thal-id'-o-mide*). Drug used in the late 1950s and early 1960s as a sedative. Many pregnant women took the drug during the first trimester of pregnancy and gave birth to children with abnormalities of the limbs. Approximately 4000 such children were born in Britain and Germany.

theca (*the'-kah*). A sheath, such as the covering of a tendon. *T. vertebralis.* The membranes enclosing the spinal cord.

theine (*the'-een*). The alkaloid found in tea.

theinism (*the'-in-izm*). Chronic poisoning resulting from excessive tea drinking.

thenar (*the'-nar*). The palm of the hand.

Theobroma (*the-o-bro'-mah*). A genus of plants, the oil of which is cacao butter used as a base for suppositories and ointments.

theobromine (*the-o-bro'-min*). An alkaloid from *Theobroma*

whose action is similar to that of caffeine.

theophylline (*the-off'-il'-een*). An alkaloid from tea leaves. Used as a diuretic as is aminophylline.

therapeutics (*ther-ap-u'-tiks*). The science and art of healing and the treatment of disease.

therapy (*ther'-ap-e*). Treatment. *Curie t.* Treatment with radium. *Group t.* A form of psychotherapy. *See* Group. *Occupational t.* Treatment by providing interesting and congenial work within the limitations of the patient in mental diseases and in order to re-educate and coordinate muscles in physical defects. *See* Rehabilitation. *Oxygen t.* Treatment by inhalations of oxygen. *Rôle t.* A method of psychiatric treatment in which the patient casts the nurse or psychotherapist into the rôle of someone who has had a great influence on his past. The nurse, under guidance of the psychiatrist, assists by behaving in the manner of the object of the patient's emotion. *Solar t.* Heliotherapy (*q.v.*).

therm (*ther'-m*). A unit of heat. *See* Unit.

thermal (*ther'-mal*). Relating to heat.

thermocautery (*ther-mo-kaw'-ter-e*). The 'actual' cautery. *See* Cautery.

thermodilution (*ther-mo-di-lu'-shun*). A method of measuring the volume of blood in the ventricles. A temperature recording head is inserted in a cardiac catheter and ice cold water, which causes a drop in temperature, is introduced. The result is obtained by mathematical formula.

thermogenesis (*ther-mo-jen'-e-sis*). The production of heat.

thermography (*therm-og'-raf-e*). A photographic method of early detection of cancer by means of infra-red rays. It depends on the greater blood supply of a cancerous growth to that of the surrounding tissue.

thermolysis (*ther-mol'-is-is*). The loss of body heat.

thermometer (*ther-mom'-e-ter*). An instrument for measuring temperature. *Centigrade t.* One graduated to the Centigrade (Celsius) scale. Internationally used in industry and increasingly in medicine. *Clinical t.* One used to measure the body temperature. *Fahrenheit t.* One marked in the Fahrenheit scale. *See* Appendix 7.

thermostat (*ther'-mo-stat*). An apparatus which automatically regulates the temperature by cutting out the source of heat.

thermotaxis (*ther-mo-taks'-is*). The regulation of body temperature by maintaining the balance between heat production and heat loss.

thermotherapy (*ther-mo-ther'ap-e*). The treatment of disease by application of heat.

thiamine (*thi'-am-een*). Vitamin B_1, or aneurine. Necessary for healthy nerve and mucous membranes. The source is liver and unrefined cereals.

Thiersch's skin graft (*I. Thiersch, German surgeon, 1822–75*). The transplantation of areas of partial thickness skin. *See* Graft.

thigh (*thi*). The lower limb, from the pelvis to the knee.

thiopentone sodium (*thi-o-pen'-tone*). A basal narcotic of the barbiturate group given intravenously. Pentothal is a proprietary preparation of it.

thiotepa (*thi-o-te'-pah*). An intravenous cytotoxic drug used in the treatment of leukaemia.

thiouracil (*thi-o-u'-ras-il*). A synthetic drug used in the medical treatment of hyperthyroidism or to stabilize a patient before operation. *Methyl-t.* and *propyl-t.* are the forms used and are unlikely to give rise to the toxic effects of fever, rash and agranulocytosis.

thirst. An uncomfortable sensation of dryness of the mouth and throat with a desire for oral fluids.

Thomas' frame (*H. O. Thomas, British orthopaedic surgeon, 1834–91*). A metal frame used in the treatment of tuberculosis of the spine.

Thomas' splint. A useful splint. The limb is supported by cross-pieces of material slung between side rods. It is used for fractured femur, and for injuries to the lower limb.

thoracentesis (*thor-ah-sen-te'-sis*). Aspiration of the pleural cavity.

thoracic (*thor-as'-ik*). Relating to the thorax. *T. duct.* The large lymphatic vessel, situated in the thorax along the spine. It opens into the left subclavian vein.

thoracoplasty (*thor'-ak-o-plas-te*). An operation on the chest, e.g. to produce collapse of the lung or to obliterate an empyema cavity by removing a number of ribs.

thoracoscopy (*thor-ak-os'-ko-pe*). Examination of the pleural cavity by means of an endoscopic instrument.

thoracotomy (*thor-ak-ot'-o-me*). An incision into the thorax, e.g. to break down adhesions or for drainage purposes.

thorax (*thor'-aks*). The chest; a cavity containing the heart, lungs, bronchi and oesophagus. It is bounded by the diaphragm, the sternum, the dorsal vertebrae, and the ribs. *Barrel-*

shaped t. A development in emphysema, when the chest is malformed like a barrel.

thorium X (*thor'-e-um*). Radioactive isotope, particles from which will penetrate about 1 mm of tissue.

threadworm. A species of *Oxyuris*, parasitic in the colon of children.

threonine (*thre'-o-neen*). One of the 22 amino acids formed by the digestion of dietary protein.

thrill. A tremor discerned by palpation.

throat. (1) The anterior surface of the neck. (2) The pharynx. *Sore t.* Pharyngitis. *Clergyman's sore t.* Laryngitis.

thrombectomy (*throm-bek'-to-me*). Excision of a thrombus.

thrombin (*throm'-bin*). An enzyme released in the clotting process from the precursor protherombin.

thrombo-angeitis (*throm-bo-*
an-je-i'-tis). Inflammation of blood vessels with clot formation. *T.-a. obliterans.* Obstruction of the circulation, causing gangrene. Usually, but not invariably, occurs in the lower limb. Buerger's disease.

thrombocytes (*throm'-bo-sites*). Blood platelets (*q.v.*).

thrombocytopenia (*thrombo-si-to-pe'-ne-ah*). A disease in the platelets of the blood. Spontaneous bleeding may occur.

thrombocytopenic purpura (*throm-bo-si-to-pe'-nik pur'-pu-rah*). A severe disease in which there are too few platelets and haemorrhages arise from all mucous surfaces. Purpura haemorrhagica.

thrombocytosis (*throm-bo-si-to'-sis*). Increase in the number of platelets in blood.

thrombo-endarterectomy (*throm'-bo end-art-er-ek'-to-*

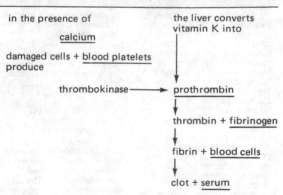

CLOTTING OF BLOOD
Underlined substances are normally present in blood

me). Removal of a clot from a thrombosed vessel.

thrombo-endarteritis (*throm'-bo-end-art-er-i'-tis*). Inflammation in small arteries with clot formation as a result.

thrombogen (*throm'-bo-jen*). Prothrombin. The precursor of thrombin.

thrombokinase (*throm-bo-kin'-aze*). Thromboplastin. A lipid containing protein activated by blood platelets and injured tissues, which is capable of activating prothrombin to form thrombin.

thrombolysis (*throm-bol'-is-is*). The disintegration or disolving of a clot.

thrombophlebitis (*throm-bo-fle-bi'-tis*). A term applied to blood clot formation in a vein with inflammation of the vessel lining.

thromboplastin (*throm-bo-plas'-tin*). *See* Thrombokinase.

thrombosis (*throm-bo'-sis*). The formation of a thrombus. *Cavernous sinus t.* This may be a result of infection of the face, when the veins in the sinus are affected via ophthalmic vessels. *Coronary t.* The occlusion of a coronary vessel, by which the heart muscle is deprived of blood according to the size of the vessel blocked. *Lateral sinus t.* A complication of mastoiditis when infection of the sinus occurs and there is clot formation.

thrombotest (*throm'-bo-test*). A test used to measure factors IX and X in the blood, which may be affected by anticoagulants, and where deficiency may lead to bleeding.

thrombus (*throm'-bus*). A stationary blood clot caused by coagulation of the blood, usually in a vein, and often the result of stasis.

thrush. An infection of the mucous membrane of the mouth by a fungus, the *Candida albicans*. It arises in undernourished infants when unclean teats and bottles are used, also in older persons suffering from debilitating disease where there is lack of oral hygiene. Thus it is a preventable disease. It can be treated by application of nystatin. *See* Stomatitis.

thymectomy (*thi-mek'-to-me*). Removal of the thymus gland. A treatment for myasthenia gravis.

thymine (*thi'-meen*). One of the nucleic bases found in deoxyribonucleic acid.

thymokesis (*thi-mo-ke'-sis*). Persistence of the thymus gland in an adult.

thymol (*thi'-mol*). An aromatic antiseptic used in solution as a mouth wash.

thymoma (*thi-mo'-mah*). A benign new growth that originates in thymus tissue and is found to be present in a number of patients suffering from myasthenia gravis.

thymus (*thi'-mus*). A gland-like structure situated in the upper thorax and neck. Present in early life, it reaches its maximum size at 10 to 12 years and then slowly regresses. Its only known function is the formation of lymphocytes. The gland is often enlarged in myasthenia gravis and its removal has benefited a number of patients.

thyrocricotomy (*thi-ro-kri-kot'-o-me*). An opening made between the thyroid and cricoid cartilages.

thyroglobin (*thi-ro-glo'-bin*). The protein in thyroxine, the endocrine secretion of the thyroid.

thyroglossal (*thi-ro-glos'-al*).

Relating to the thyroid and the tongue. *T. cyst.* See Cyst.

thyroid (*thi'-roid*). Shaped like a shield. *T. crisis.* A serious complication of partial thyroidectomy in which there is hyperpyrexia, tachycardia and extreme restlessness. Now less common because it is possible to stabilize the patient before operation by the use of an antithyroid drug. *T. cartilage* is the largest of the laryngeal cartilages. *T. extract* is a preparation from the thyroid gland of animals, used to treat cretinism and myxoedema (*q.v.*). *T. gland* is a bilobed endocrine gland situated in front of the trachea. *Retrosternal t.* when the gland is wholly or in part behind the sternum.

thyroid-stimulating hormone (TSH). Hormone produced by the anterior pituitary gland which controls the activity of the thyroid gland.

thyroidectomy (*thi-roid-ek'-to-me*). Partial or complete removal of the thyroid gland.

thyroparathyroidectomy (*thi'-ro-par-ah-thi-roid-ek'-to-me*). Removal of the thyroid and parathyroid glands.

thyrotomy (*thi-rot'-o-me*). Division of the thyroid cartilage.

thyrotoxicosis (*thi-ro-toks-e-ko'-sis*). Hyperthyroidism. The symptoms arising when there is overactivity of the thyroid gland. The metabolism is speeded up and there is enlargement of the gland and exophthalmos.

thyrotrophin (*thi-ro-tro'-fin*). The hormone secreted by the pituitary that stimulates the thyroid gland.

thyroxine (*thi-roks'-een*). The iodine-containing hormone secreted by the thyroid gland. Now prepared synthetically.

tibia (*tib'-e-ah*). The shin bone. The larger of the two bones of the leg, extending from knee to ankle.

tic. Spasmodic twitching of certain muscles, usually of the face or neck. *T. douloureux.* Spasmodic facial neuralgia.

tick. A blood-sucking parasite, which may transmit the organisms of disease.

tidal air. See Air.

tincture (*tink'-chur*). An alcoholic solution of a drug.

tine test. Form of tuberculin testing in which a skin puncture by several short needles allows tuberculin solution to be injected from a single dose container.

tinea (*tin'-e-ah*). A skin disease caused by parasitic fungi of the genus *Trichophyton.* Named after the area of the body affected; *T. barbae*—the beard; *T. capitis*—the head; *T. circinata* or *T. corporis*—the body; and *T. cruris*, the groin. See Ringworm.

tinnitus (*tin'-it-us*). A ringing or roaring sound in the ears.

tintometer (*tin-tom'-e-ter*). An instrument by which changes in colour can be measured.

tissue (*tis'-u*). A mass of cells or fibres forming one of the structures of which the body is composed. *Adipose t.* Fatty tissue. *Areolar t.* Connective tissue of bundles of white fibres, elastic fibres and connective tissue cells. *Cancellous t.* The honeycomb arrangement of bone cells beneath the compact layer, especially at the ends of long bones, and in the centre of such bones as the clavicle, sternum, ribs, cranium and vertebra. It contains red bone marrow. *Compact t.* The close arrangement of bone cells which forms the outer layer of all bones and is especially thick in the shafts. *Connective t.* A general term for all those tissues of the body which support and connect the various organs and other structures. *Fibrous t.* Connective tissue composed of bundles of white fibres. *Elastic t.* Connective tissue chiefly composed of yellow elastic fibres. *Gamgee t.* A layer of wool completely enclosed in gauze. Used as a surgical dressing. *Interstitial t.* The stroma (*q.v.*). *Homologous t.* One similar in structure to another. *Parenchymatous t.* The essential functioning cells of an organ, as distinct from its supporting tissues. *Trophoblastic t.* The lining cells of the chorionic villi. *T. culture.* The growing of animal and human tissues in a test-tube. Tissues have been used as a medium for cultivating the virus of poliomyelitis.

titrate (*ti'-trate*). To estimate by titration.

titration (*ti-tra'-shun*). A method of estimating the weight of a solute in solution by dropping a measured amount of a reagent into a measured quantity of solution and the expected colour change or reaction occurs.

tocopherol (*tok-off'-er-ol*). Vitamin E present in wheat germ, green leaves and vegetables.

tolazoline (*tol-az'-ol-een*). A vasodilator drug of the peripheral blood vessels. It may be used in treating Raynaud's disease. Priscol is a proprietary preparation.

tolbutamide (*tol-bu'-tam-ide*). An oral drug that appears to stimulate the release of insulin from the pancreas and may be used in some cases of diabetes.

tolerance (*tol'-er-anse*). The capacity for assimilating large amounts of a drug or food without harmful effects. *Sugar t.* The amount of sugar which a diabetic can metabolize as shown by the blood sugar curve, or by the appearance of sugar in the urine.

tolu (*tol-oo*). An aromatic balsam. An ingredient in linctus preparations.

tomograph (*to'-mo-graf*). An X-ray apparatus so designed that a photograph can be taken at any depth of tissue. A clear picture is thus obtained.

-tomy (*to'-me*). A suffix meaning 'to cut'.

tone. The normal degree of tension, e.g. in a muscle.

tongue (*tung*). The movable muscular organ attached to the floor of the mouth and concerned in taste, mastication and speech. It is covered by mucous membrane from which project numerous papillae. *Strawberry t.* Typical of scarlet fever. It is first thickly furred but dotted with protruding red papillae. In a day or two the fur peels off leaving the characteristic bright red appearance.

tonic (*ton'-ik*). (1) A term popularly applied to drugs supposed to brace or tone up the body or any particular part or organ. (2) In a state of contraction, e.g. muscles. *T. spasm.* A prolonged contraction of one or several muscles. *See* Clonic.

tonicity (*ton-is'-it-e*). A term applied to the effective osmotic pressure of a fluid in relation to plasma.

tonography (*to-nog'-raf-e*). A tracing made by an electric tonometer recording the intra-ocular pressure and so indirectly the drainage of aqueous humour from the eye.

tonometer (*to-nom'-e-ter*). An

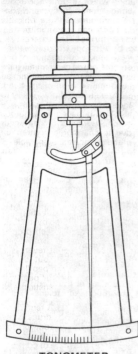

TONOMETER

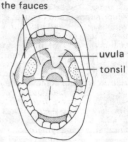

pillars of
the fauces

uvula

tonsil

TONSIL

instrument for measuring intraocular pressure.

tonsil (*ton'-sil*). One of two small almond-shaped bodies, situated one on each side between the pillars of the fauces. It is composed of lymphoid tissue covered by mucous membrane, and its surface is pitted with follicles. *Pharyngeal t.* The lymphadenoid tissue of

the pharynx between the eustachian tubes.

tonsillectomy (*ton-sil-ek'-to-me*). Excision of one or both tonsils.

tonsillitis (*ton-sil-i'-tis*). Inflammation of the tonsils. *Follicular t.* Affects chiefly the follicles, and causes purulent patches on the tonsils, which are pus exuded from the follicles *Vincent's t.* Due to infection by Vincent's organism. *See* Vincent's angina.

tonsillotome (*ton-sil'-o-tome*). An instrument for excising tonsils.

tonsillotomy (*ton-sil-ot'-o-me*). Cutting off the hypertrophied tonsil without enucleating it.

tonus (*ton'-us*). A state of partial contraction, e.g. muscles.

tooth. A structure in the mouth designed for the mastication of food. Each is composed of a crown, neck and root with one or more fangs. The main bulk is of dentine enclosing a central pulp; the crown is covered with a hard white substance called enamel. *See* Dentition. *Deci-*

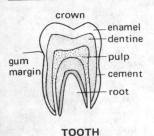

crown — enamel
— dentine
— pulp
gum
margin — cement
— root

TOOTH

duous (*milk*) *t.* One of the first set, later replaced by the permanent dentition. *Eye t.* A canine. *Hutchinson's t.* Ones with notched and irregular edges, indicative of congenital syphilis. *Impacted t.* One which is unable to erupt owing to its position in the jaw. *Wisdom t.* One of the last molars to appear, at either end of each jaw. *Pl.* Teeth.

topectomy (to-pek'-to-me). Gyrectomy. The cutting of part of the frontal lobe of the cerebral cortex. A method of cerebral surgery in mental illness.

tophus (to'-fus). A small, hard, chalky deposit occurring in gout, and sometimes appearing on the auricle of the ear. It is composed of urate of sodium.

topical (top'-ik-al). Relating to a particular spot; local. *T. fluid.* One for local or external application.

topography (to-pog'-raf-e). Mapping out the surface of the body in reference to the underlying structures.

torpor (tor'-por). A sluggish condition, in which response to stimuli is absent or very slow.

torsion (tor'-shun). Twisting. (1) Of an artery to arrest haemorrhage. (2) Of the pedicle of a

cyst which produces venous congestion in the cyst and consequent gangrene—a possible complication of ovarian cyst.

torso (tor'-so). The trunk.

torticollis (tor-te-kol'-lis). Wry-neck, a contraction of one or more of the cervical muscles on one side only, resulting in an abnormal position of the head. *Congenital t.* is due to injury to the sternocleidomastoid muscle at birth. It becomes a fibrous cord. *Spasmodic t.* May occur due to spasmodic contraction of the sternomastoid muscle.

tourniquet (toor'-ne-ka). Any constrictive band applied to a limb to arrest arterial haemorrhage. When available an inflated sphygmomanometer cuff is the safest type to apply. If in an emergency an improvised or rubber tourniquet is applied there is a grave risk of permanent damage to muscles or nerve supply.

tow (to). The coarse part of flax used for padding splints.

toxaemia (toks-e'-me-ah). Poisoning of the blood by the absorption of toxins. *T. of pregnancy.* Characterized by albuminuria, hypertension and oedema, with the possibility of eclampsia developing if untreated.

toxic (toks'-ik). Poisonous, relating to a poison. May refer to substances produced in the body by infection or metabolic disturbance.

toxicity (toks-is'-it-e). The degree of virulence of a poison.

toxicology (toks-e-kol'-o-je). The science dealing with poisons.

toxicosis (toks-e-ko'-sis). The state of poisoning by toxins.

toxin (toks'-in). Any poisonous nitrogenous compound, usually referring to that produced by bacteria.

toxoid (*toks'-oid*). A toxin which has been deprived of some of its harmful properties but is still capable of producing immunity. *Diphtheria t.* Toxin which has been treated with formaldehyde. Used for immunization against diphtheria. *See* TAF *and* APT. *T.–antitoxin.* A mixture of a toxoid and its antitoxin.

toxoplasmosis (*toks-o-plaz-mo'-sis*). A condition of enlarged glands and fever caused by a protozoon, the *Toxoplasma.* May cause hydrocephalus and other disorders in infants born of infected mothers.

trabecula (*trab-ek'-u-lah*). A dividing band or septum, extending from the capsule of an organ into its interior and holding the functioning cells in position.

tracer. A substance or instrument that can be used to gain information, e.g. *t.* doses of radioactive iodine are used to investigate disease of the thyroid gland.

trachea (*trak-e'-ah*). The windpipe: a cartilaginous tube lined with ciliated mucous membrane, extending from the lower part of the larynx to the commencement of the bronchi.

tracheitis (*trak-e-i'-tis*). Inflammation of the trachea.

trachelorrhaphy (*trak-el-or'-raf-e*). Operation for suturing lacerations of the cervix of the uterus.

tracheobronchitis (*trak-e-o-brong-ki'-tis*). Acute infection of the trachea and bronchi due to viruses or bacteria.

tracheostomy (*trak-e-os'-to-me*). Making an opening or stoma into the trachea. *T. tubes.* Those used to maintain an airway following this operation until the normal use of the air-passages is regained. The tube must be kept clear, the inner one being removed frequently and cleaned in bicarbonate of soda solution. The operation is used to maintain respiration and to treat excessive bronchial secretions in many surgical and medical conditions. It is usually a temporary measure. *Inferior t.* The opening is made below the thyroid isthmus. *Superior t.* The opening is made above the thyroid isthmus.

tracheotomy (*trak-e-ot'-o-me*). Cutting into the trachea.

trachoma (*trak-o'-mah*). A contagious conjuctivitis marked by granulations on the membrane and contractions of the lids to scar tissue formation.

traction (*trak'-shun*). The act of pulling or drawing. *Skeleton t.* A method of keeping the fractured ends of bone in position by actual pull on the bone. A metal pin or wire is passed through the distal fragment or adjacent bone to overcome muscle contraction. *Russell t.* A

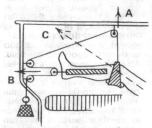

RUSSELL TRACTION
Traction at A and B exerts force in direction C

form of movable traction in which there is an upward pull over a beam and the cord is continuous with a series of three pulleys attached to the limb by skin traction horizontally. The combined direction of pull on the femur is between the two at 45°. *Skin t. See* Extension.

tragacanth (*trag´-ak-anth*). A substance resembling *gum arabic.* Used in pharmacy for suspending insoluble powders. A demulcent. *T. powder.* A useful skin application around an ileostomy.

tragus (*tra´-gus*). (1) The small prominence of cartilage at the external meatus of the ear. (2) One of the hairs at the external auditory meatus. *Pl.* Tragi.

trait (*tra*). An inherited physical or mental characteristic.

trance (*trahnse*). A condition of unnatural sleep of hysterical, cataleptic or hypnotic origin. It is not due to organic disease.

tranquillizers (*tran´-kwil-i-zers*). Drugs that allay anxiety and have a calming effect on the patient, and appear to render him indifferent to pain, e.g. chlorpromazine and promethazine.

trans-. A prefix meaning 'through' or 'across'.

transaminase test (*trans-am´-in-ase*). A diagnostic test for cardiac infarction and infective hepatitis. The *serum glutamic oxalacetic t.* (SGOT) is raised in cardiac infarction; it is an enzyme excreted by damaged heart muscle. The *serum glutamic pyruvic t.* (SGPT) is raised in infective hepatitis as it is excreted by damaged parenchymal cells of the liver.

transducers (*trans-du´-sers*). The data sources or electrodes attached to the patient to enable recordings to be made. *See* Monitoring.

transection (*trans-sek´-shun*). Section across the long axis of a part, e.g. *t. of stomach,* which is performed in partial gastrectomy.

transfer RNA (*trans-fer*). Molecules of ribonucleic acid which are important in the formation of protein in that they attach the amino acids in the correct order.

transference (*trans´-fer-ense*). A term used in psychiatry whereby the patient unconsciously transfers on to the psychiatrist feelings which belong to other people significant to him, both past and present.

transfusion (*trans-fu´-zhun*). The introduction of whole blood or plasma into a vein, performed in cases of severe loss of blood, shock, septicaemia, etc. It is used to supply actual volume of blood, or to introduce constituents as clotting factors, or antibodies, which are deficient in the patient. *Exchange* or *Exsanguination t.* Performed on newly born infants for complete replacement of the baby's blood. *See* Rhesus factor. *Intra-arterial t.* Blood is passed into an artery under positive pressure in cases where large quantities are required rapidly as in cardiovascular surgery. *Intra-medullary t.* The needle or special cannula is passed into the bone marrow either of the sternum or tibia. *Plasma t.* The fluid is transfused after the cell content has been removed.

transillumination (*trans-il-lu-min-a´-shun*). The illumination of a cavity by means of an electric light, as an aid to diagnosis.

translocation (*trans-lo-ka´-shun*). In morphology the transfer of a segment of a chromosome to a different site on the same chromosome or to a different chromosome. It can be a cause of congenital abnormality.

translumbar (*trans-lum'-bar*). Via the lumbar area, often used in aortography.

transmigration (*trans-mi-gra'-shun*). Wandering. The passage of blood cells through the walls of the capillaries. Diapedesis. *External t.* The passage of an ovum from its ovary to the fallopian tube on the opposite side.

transplacental (*trans-plas-ent'-al*). Across the placenta. Movement may be from mother to fetus or *vice versa*. *T. infection* may affect the unborn child. *See* Rubella.

transplantation (*trans-plant-a'-shun*). The removal of a section of tissue from one part to another, or to another body. *Tendon t.* The transfer of a strip of tendon from a healthy muscle to a paralysed one. *T. of ureters.* A necessary accompaniment to excision of the bladder. The ureters are usually implanted in the colon or loop of ileum.

transposition (*trans-po-sish'-un*). (1) Displacement of any of the viscera to the opposite side of the body. (2) The operation which partially removes a piece of tissue from one part of the body to another, the complete severance being delayed until it has become established in its new position.

transudate (*trans'-u-date*). Any fluid which passes through a membrane. *T. pleurisy.* When fluid oozes into the pleural sac, as may occur in oedematous conditions, e.g. chronic nephritis or congestive heart failure.

transurethral (*trans-u-re'-thral*). Via the urethra. *T. prostatectomy. See* Prostatectomy.

transverse (*trans-verse'*). Oblique, cross-wise. *T. presentation.* The child lies across the pelvis, which position must be corrected before normal birth can take place. *T. ligaments.* Those stretching from the pelvis to the cervix and supporting the uterus.

transvestitism (*trans-vest'-it-izm*). Condition in which the patient dresses as a member of the opposite sex, and may identify completely with that sex.

tranylcypromine (*tran-il-si'-pro-meen*). A drug used in psychiatry for the treatment of depression. Parnate is a proprietary preparation.

trapezium (*trap-e'-ze-um*). A bone in the distal row of the carpus.

trapezius (*trap-e'-ze-us*). One of two large muscles situated between the shoulders; its action is to draw the head backward.

Trasylol (*tra'-se-lol*). A non-toxic inhibitor of proteolytic enzymes that may be given intravenously in acute pancreatitis.

trauma (*traw'-mah*). A wound or injury. *Psychic t.* A mental or physical injury which can lead to mental illness.

traumatic (*traw-mat'-ik*). Caused by injury. *T. automatism.* As the result of injury, the patient responds normally to his environment, but has no memory of such actions. *T. fever.* That following an operation or injury when no bacterial infection is present. It is due to absorption of injured tissues, especially blood. Also known as *aseptic* fever.

treatment. Mode of dealing with a patient or disease. *Active t.* is vigorously applied. *Ante-*

natal t. Deals with the care of the mother during pregnancy to maintain her health and ensure normal delivery of the child. *Conservative t.* That which aims at preserving and restoring injured parts by natural means, e.g. rest, fluid replacement, etc., as opposed to radical or surgical methods. *Empirical t.* Treatment based on observation of symptoms and not on science. *Expectant t.* Symptoms only are treated, leaving nature to cure. *Palliative t.* Relieves symptoms but does not cure disease. *Prophylactic t.* Aims at the prevention of disease.

Trematoda (*trem-a-to'-dah*). Fluke-worms.

tremor (*trem'-or*). An involuntary, muscular quivering which may be due to fatigue, emotion, or disease. *Fine t.* One which occurs with 10 to 12 vibrations per second. *Intention t.* One which occurs on attempting a movement, as in disseminated sclerosis.

Trendelenburg's operation (*F. Trendelenburg, German surgeon, 1844–1924*). Section and ligature of the long saphenous vein in the treatment of varicose veins.

Trendelenburg position. *See* Position.

Trendelenburg's sign. An aid in diagnosis of congenital dislocation of the hip. The patient stands on the affected leg and flexes the other knee and hip. If there is dislocation the pelvis is lower on the side of the flexed leg which is the reverse of normal.

trephine (*tre-fine'*). An instrument for cutting out a circular piece of bone, usually from the skull; employed in certain cases of cerebral compression.

Treponema carateum (*trep-o-*ne'-mah ca-ra-te'-um*). The spirochaete causing pinta (*q.v.*).

Treponema pallidum (*trep-o-ne'-mah- pal'-id-um*). The parasite of syphilis. Formerly known as the *Spirochaeta pallida. T. p. immobilization.* A complement fixation test for syphilis.

Treponema pertenue (*trep-o-ne'-mah per-ten'-u*). The spirochaete causing yaws (*q.v.*).

tretamine (*tre'-tam-een*). TEM. A cytotoxic drug related to nitrogen mustard. It interferes with division of the cell nucleus. The drug can be administered orally or intravenously.

triamcinolone (*tri-am-sin'-o-lone*). A glucocorticoid steroid which is less likely to cause salt and water retention.

triamterine (*tri-am'-ter-een*). A diuretic that acts by antagonizing aldosterone and does not cause potassium loss.

triangular bandage (*tri-an'-gu-lar band'-aj*). A triangle of unbleached calico, useful for various emergencies. A large folded scarf or handkerchief is a substitute.

triceps (*tri'-seps*). Having three heads. The muscle which extends the forearm.

trichiasis (*trik-i'-as-is*). Friction and irritation of the cornea due to abnormal position of the eyelashes.

trichinosis (*trik-in-o'-sis*). A disease caused by eating underdone pork containing a parasite—*Trichinella spiralis.* This becomes deposited in muscle, and causes stiffness and painful swelling. There may also be nausea, diarrhoea, fever, and in severe cases, prostration.

trichloroethylene (*tri-klor-o-eth'-e-leen*). An anaesthetic, the fumes of which are inhaled to produce a light anaesthesia with freedom from pain. Useful in midwifery, for painful dressings and in general anaesthesia as it is non-explosive.

Trichomonas (*trik-o-mo'-nas*). A ciliated protozoon which normally inhabits the bowel and may give rise to vaginitis.

trichomoniasis (*trik-o-mon-i'-as-is*). Infestation of the genital tract with a parasite of the genus *Trichomonas*.

trichophytosis (*trik-o-fi-to'-sis*). Disease of the hair produced by a fungus, the *Trichophyton*. It may attack many areas of the body. Griseofulvin is an effective treatment. *See* Tinea.

trichorrhoea (*trik-o-re'-ah*). Premature loss of hair.

trichosis (*trik-o'-sis*). Any abnormal growth of hair.

Trichuris (*trik-u'-ris*). A genus of whipworms, which sometimes infects the colon of man and causes diarrhoea.

trichuriasis (*trik-u-ri'-as-is*). Infestation by the whipworm.

tricuspid (*tri-kus'-pid*). Having three flaps or cusps. *T. valve*. That at the opening between the right auricle and the right ventricle of the heart.

tricyclic antidepressants (*tri-si'-klik ant-e-de-press'-ants*). Drugs used to treat depression.

trifluoperazine (*tri-flu-o-per'-az-een*). A potent tranquillizing drug that is used in psychiatry. Stelazine is a proprietary preparation.

trigeminal nerve (*tri-jem'-in-al*). The fifth pair of cranial nerves, each of which is divided into three main branches and supplies one side of the face.

trigeminal neuralgia (*tri-jem'-in-al nu-ral'-je-ah*). Pain in the face which is confined

to branches of the trigeminal nerve.

trigeminus (*tri-jem'-in-us*). Triple. *Pulsus t.* The type of pulse in which there are three beats and then a missed beat. A regular irregularity. *See* Bigeminus.

trigger finger. A stenosing of the tendon sheath at the metacarpophalangeal joint allowing flexion of the finger but not extension without assistance when it 'clicks' into position.

trigone (*tri'-gone*). A triangular area. *T. of the bladder*. The triangular space on the floor of the bladder, between the ureteric openings and the urethral orifice.

triglycerides (*tri-glis'-er-ides*). Esters of glycerol and the fatty acids; palmitic, oleic and stearic.

Trilene (*tri'-leen*). A triangular preparation of trichloroethylene (*q.v.*).

trimeprazine (*tri-mep'-raz-een*). An antihistamine drug with a sedative action. It is supplied in syrup or tablet form and may be used for premedication. Vallergan is a proprietary preparation.

trimester (*tre-mes'-ter*). A third part. *First t. of pregnancy*. The first 3 months during which rapid development is taking place.

trinitrin (*tri-ni'-trin*). Nitroglycerin. A vasodilatant drug used in the treatment of angina pectoris.

tri-iodothyronine (*tri-i-o-do-thi'-ro-neen*). Hormone produced by the thyroid gland which circulates mainly in the free state.

trismus (*triz'-mus*). Lock-jaw. A tonic spasm of the muscles of the jaw either caused by tetanus or resulting from caries of the jaw.

trisomy (*tri'-so-me*). The cause of mongolism, namely the presence of three chromosomes 21, an abnormality of chromosome division.

tritium (*trit'-e-um*). An isotope of hydrogen (H_3) that is used as a tracer in studies of metabolism.

trocar (*tro'-kar*). A pointed instrument used with a canula for performing paracentesis.

trochanter (*tro-kan'-ter*). Two prominences, below the neck of the femur. *Large* or *Great t*. That on the outer side forming the bony prominence of the hip. *Minor* or *Lesser t*. On the inner side at the neck of the femur.

troche (*tro'-ke*). A medicated tablet.

trochlea (*trok'-le-ah*). Any pulley-shaped structure; but particularly the fibrocartilage near the inner angular process of the frontal bone through which passes the tendon of the superior oblique muscle of the eye.

trochlear nerves. The fourth pair of cranial nerves.

trophic (*trof'-ik*). Relating to nutrition. *T. nerves*. Those which control the nutrition of a part. *T. ulcer. See* Ulcer. *T. hormones*. The hormones of the anterior pituitary that stimulate the secretion of other endocrine glands.

trophoblast (*trof'-o-blast*). The layer of cells surrounding the embryro at the time of and responsible for implantation.

trophoneurosis (*trof-o-nu-ro'-sis*). Malnutrition of a part, due to disturbance of the trophic nerves.

tropical (*trop'-ik-al*). Relating to the areas north and south of the equator termed the tropics. *T. medicine*. That concerned

with diseases that are more prevalent in hot climates.

Trousseau's sign (*A. Trousseau, French physician, 1801–67*). Sign indicating increased excitability of nerves caused by a lowered plasma calcium level. It is demonstrated by placing a tourniquet around the upper arm. This stimulates the underlying nerves and causes carpospasm.

truancy (*tru'-an-se*). When a child stays away from school without leave. A disorder of conduct which may result from emotional insecurity or a feeling of unfairness.

truncus arteriosus (*trunk'-us ar-ter-e-o'-sus*). The arterial trunk connected to the fetal heart which develops into the aortic and pulmonary arteries. *Persistent t.a.* A rare congenital deformity in which this persists causing a mixing of the systemic and pulmonary circulation.

truss (*trus*). An apparatus in the form of a belt with a pressure pad, for retaining a hernia in place after reduction.

Trypanosoma (*trip-an-o-so'-mah*). A genus of parasites, which may pass one half of their life cycle in the blood of man. *T. gambiense* and *T. rhodensiense*. Transmitted by the bite of the tsetse fly, and the cause of sleeping sickness.

trypanosomiasis (*trip-an-o-so-mi'-as-is*). *See* Sleeping sickness.

trypsin (*trip'-sin*). A digestive enzyme converting protein into amino acids.

trypsinogen (*trip-sin'-o-jen*). The precursor of trypsin. It is secreted in the pancreatic juice, and activated by the enterokinase of the succus entericus into trypsin.

tryptophan (*trip'-to-fan*). One of the essential amino acids.

tsetse fly (*tset'-se*). The insect which transmits the parasite *Trypanosoma* to man.

tsutsugamushi disease (*tsu-tsu-gah-mu'-shi*). Scrub typhus that occurs in Japan and is transmitted by the bite of a mite.

tubal. Relating to a tube. *T. pregnancy.* Extra-uterine pregnancy where the embryo develops in the Fallopian tube.

tubectomy (*tu-bek'-to-me*). Excision of a portion of a Fallopian tube.

tubercle (*tu'-ber-kl*). (1) A small nodule or a rounded prominence on a bone. (2) The specific lesion—a small nodule—produced by the tubercle bacillus.

tuberculides (*tu-ber'-ku-lids*). Eruptions on the skin of tuberculous origin.

tuberculin (*tu-ber'-ku-lin*). The filtrate from a fluid medium in which *Mycobacterium tuberculosis* has been grown and which contains its toxins. *Old t.* or *tuberculin T.* is prepared from the human bacillus. It is used in skin tests in diagnosing tubercolosis. *See* Mantoux test.

tuberculosis (*tu-ber-ku-lo'-sis*). A specific infectious disease produced by the *Mycobacterium tuberculosis*, discovered by Koch. *Bovine t.* A form found in cattle and spread by infected milk. *Miliary t.* A severe form with small tuberculous lesions spread throughout the body with severe toxaemia. *Open t.* Pulmonary tuberculosis in which the organisms are being excreted in the sputum. *Pulmonary t.* That affecting the lungs; also termed phthisis.

tuberculous (*tu-ber'-ku-lus*). Infected with or relating to tuberculosis.

tuberosity (*tu-ber-os'-it-e*). A flat protuberance on a bone. *Radial t.* The surface into which the tendon of the biceps muscle is inserted. *T. of tibia.* A raised and roughened surface on the tibia.

tuberous sclerosis (*tu'-ber-us skler-o'-sis*). *See* Epiloia.

tubocurarine (*tu-bo-ku-rar'-ine*). A preparation of curare (*q.v.*) used to secure muscle relaxation during abdominal surgery or to relieve muscle spasm in tetanus or to prevent convulsions during electroconvulsive therapy.

tubular (*tu'-bu-lar*). Relating to or resembling a tube.

tubules (*tu-bules*). Small tubes. *Renal* or *Uriniferous t.* The essential secreting tubes of the kidney.

tularaemia (*tu-lar-e'-me-ah*). An undulant fever, the cause of which (*Brucella tularensis*) may be transmitted to man by various insects or by rats. The lymph glands are involved and they may supurate.

tulle gras (*tule grah'*). A French preparation of gauze impregnated with petroleum jelly. Other drugs may be added. Most useful on a granulating surface to stop a dressing adhering.

tumefaction (*tu-me-fak'-shun*). A swelling.

tumour (*tu'-mor*). A swelling due to morbid growth of tissue, not resulting from inflammation. *Cystic t.* One which contains fluid. *Innocent, simple,* or *benign t.* is encapsulated, does not infiltrate or cause metastases, and is unlikely to recur if removed. *Malignant t.* One which is not encapsulated and causes metastatic deposits. *Phantom t.* An abdominal swelling, usually of gas. A form of neurosis.

Sessile t. One with a broad base, not pedunculated.

tunica (*tu'-nik-ah*). A coat. *T. adventitia, t. media, t. intima.* The outer, middle and inner coats of an artery.

tuning fork. A metal instrument used for testing hearing by means of the sounds produced by its vibration. *See* Rinne's *and* Weber's tests.

turbinate (*ter'-bin-ate*). Scroll-shaped. *T. bones.* Those in the nose which increase the surface area for warming and moistening the inspired air.

turbinectomy (*ter-bin-ek'-to-me*). Excision of a turbinate bone.

turgescence (*ter-jes'-sense*). Swelling due to congestion of blood as in catarrh.

turgid (*ter'-jid*). Swollen and congested with blood.

turgor (*ter'-gor*). The state of being swollen or distended.

Turner's syndrone (*H. H. Turner, American physician, 1892–*). A condition in which there is absence of one X chromosome. Congenital abnormalities result, commonly ovarian agenesis, infantile sex characteristics and webbing of the neck.

tussis (*tus'-sis*). A cough.

twilight states. Periods of dissociation in which a patient may perform acts of which he is not conscious later on. Though rare, they may follow an epileptic fit. *Hysterical t.s.* The patient shows mild clouding of consciousness giving rise to irrelevant speech or clumsy actions.

twin. One of a pair of individuals who have developed in the uterus together. *Binovular t.* Each has developed from a separate ovum. *Uniovular t.* Both have developed from the same cell. Identical twins.

tylosis (*ti-lo'-sis*). The formation of hard patches of skin. A callosity.

tympanectomy (*tim-pan-ek'-to-me*). Excision of the tympanum of the ear.

tympanic (*tim-pan'-ik*). Relating to the tympanum. *T. membrane.* The drum of the ear.

tympanites (*tim-pan-i'-tez*). Distension of the abdomen by accumulation of gas in the intestines.

tympanitis (*tim-pan-i'-tis*). Inflammation of the middle ear. Otitis media.

tympanoplasty (*tim-pan-o-plas'-te*). An operation to restore conductivity to the middle ear.

tympanosclerosis (*tim-pan-o-skler-o'-sis*). Fibrosis and the formation of calcified deposits in the middle ear that lead to deafness.

tympanum (*tim'-pan-um*). (1) The middle ear. (2) The ear drum or tympanic membrane.

typhlitis (*tif-li'-tis*). Inflammation of the caecum.

typhlon (*tif'-lon*). The caecum.

typhlosis (*tif-lo'-sis*). Blindness.

typhoid fever (*ti'-foid*). Enteric fever. An acute specific infectious disease caused by the *Salmonella typhi;* the incidence of which is rare in Britain although it occurs in areas where the sanitation is poor and the water supplies are contaminated. *T. carrier.* One who harbours the infection and discharges the organisms in the faeces. The gall-bladder is usually the seat of infection.

typhus (*ti'-fus*). An acute infectious fever lasting about 14 days, and then terminating abruptly. It is likely to occur where there is overcrowding, lack of personal cleanliness, and bad hygienic conditions, as the infection is spread solely by bites of infected lice or by rat fleas. The causative organism is *Rickettsia prowazeki*. It is treated by chloramphenicol or the tetracyclines. *Scrub t.* A form spread by mites and widespread in the Far East.

tyramine (*ti'-ram-een*). An enzyme present in cheese, game, broad bean pods, yeast extracts, wine, and strong beer. All these should be avoided when monoamine oxidase inhibitors are used to treat depression.

tyrosine (*ti'-ro-seen*). An amino acid. In some diseases especially of the liver, it is present in the urine.

tyrosinosis (*ti-ro-sin-o'-sis*). An alternative name for phenylketonuria in which there is an error of metabolism and phenylalanine cannot be reduced to tyrosine.

U

ulcer (*ul'-ser*). An erosion or loss of continuity of the skin or of a mucous membrane, often accompanied by suppuration. *Duodenal u.* Occurs in the mucous lining of the first 2 cm of the small intestine. *Gastric u.* One in the lining of the stomach. *Gravitational u.* A varicose ulcer of the leg which is difficult to heal because of its dependent position and the poor venous return. *Gummatous u.* One arising in late non-infective syphilis; it is slow to heal. *Indolent u.* One which heals slowly. *Intractable u.* One which does not respond to treatment. *Peptic u.* Occurs on the mucous membrane of either the stomach or duodenum. *Perforated u.* Erodes through the thickness of

the wall of an organ. *Rodent u.* A slow-growing epithelioma of the face which may cause much local destruction and ulceration, but does not give rise to metastases. *Trophic u.* One due to failure of nutrition. *Varicose u.* Gravitational ulcer. *See above.*

ulcerative (*ul'-ser-a-tiv*). Characterized by ulceration—the formation of ulcers. *U. colitis.* A condition of inflammation and ulceration of the colon of unknown cause.

ulna (*ul'-nah*). The bone on the inner side of the forearm from elbow to wrist.

ulnar (*ul'-nar*). Relating to the ulna. *U. artery, U. nerve.* Those situated near the ulna. *U. paralysis.* That due to injury to the ulnar nerve. The ring and little finger are affected.

ulorrhagia (*u-lor-raj'-e-ah*). Bleeding from the gums.

ultramicroscopic (*ul-trah-mi-kro-skop'-ik*). Too small to be seen by a microscope.

ultrasonic (*ul-trah-son'-ik*). Relating to sound waves having a frequency range beyond the upper limit perceived by the human ear. *U. echo sounding.* Reflected sound waves are used to localize the placental site. This is valuable in the diagnosis of placenta praevia or before amniocentesis (*q.v.*). *U. echo tests.* An aid to the detection of brain tumours by the transmission of very high frequency vibrations that reflect back changes in tissue density.

ultra-violet rays (*ul'-trah vi'-o-let*). Those beyond the violet end of the spectrum. *U.-v. light* is used to promote vitamin D formation and for skin conditions.

umbilical (*um-bil'-i-kal*). Relating to the umbilicus. *U. cord.* See Cord. *U. hernia.* See Hernia.

umbilicated (*um-bil'-ik-a-ted*). Having a depression like that of the navel, as on a small-pox vesicle.

umbilicus (*um-bil-i'-kus*). The navel; the circular depressed scar in the centre of the abdomen.

unciform (*un'-se-form*). Hook-shaped. *U. bone* (*hamate*). A bone of the carpus. *U. process.* A hook-shaped projection on the unciform bones.

uncinate process (*un'-se-nate*). A part of the ethmoid bone.

unconscious (*un-kon'-shus*). Receiving no sensory impulses. Insensible. *U. mind.* A term used in psychology for that part of the mind containing the urges, feelings, and experiences of which the individual is unaware and which he cannot normally recall although they influence his actions.

unconsciousness (*un-kon'-shus-nes*). The state of being in coma (*q.v.*). This may vary in depth. (1) *Deep u.* When no response can be obtained. (2) Lesser degrees of *u.* are seen when the patient can be roused by painful stimuli. (3) When the patient can be roused by speech or non-painful stimuli.

unconjugated bilirubin (*un-kon'-ju-ga-ted bil-e-ru'-bin*). Bilirubin (*q.v.*) which has not passed through the liver and combined with glucuronic acid.

undine irrigator (*un'-dine*). A form of glass flask with long spout used for irrigation of the eye.

undulant fever (*un-'du-lant*). Recurring attacks of fever with enlargement of spleen, swelling of joints, neuralgic pains, and profuse sweating. Repeated attacks cause weakness and an-aemia. The cause is *Brucella abortus* transmitted in cow's milk or *Brucella melitensis* from goat's milk (*Malta fever*). *Syn.* Brucellosis.

unguentum (*ung-gwen'-tum*). An ointment.

unguis (*ung'-gwis*). A finger- or toe-nail.

uni-. A prefix meaning 'one'.

unicellular (*u-ne-sel'-u-lah*). Consisting of one cell.

unilateral (*u-ne-lat'-er-al*). On one side only.

union (*u'-ne-on*). The repair of tissue after separation by incision or fracture. *See* Callus *and* Healing.

uniovular (*u-ne-o'-vu-lar*). From one ovum. *U. twins.* Of the same sex.

unipara (*u-nip'-ar-ah*). A woman who has had only one child.

unit. A standard of measurement. *British Thermal u.* The amount of heat which will raise 1 lb of water through one degree Fahrenheit. *U. of heat.* A calorie (*q.v.*). *U. of insulin.* An international measurement of the pure crystalline insulin arrived at by biological assay. *See* Electromotive force *and* Angström unit.

Unna's zinc gelatin (*P. G. Unna, German dermatologist, 1850–1929*). A useful paste for treating skin conditions and in which other drugs can be incorporated.

unsealed sources. The term applied to radioactive isotopes that are not enclosed in metal containers but used in liquid form either orally or by injection.

unstriated muscle (*un-stri-a'-ted mus'-l*). Involuntary muscle found in the digestive tract, respiratory passages, blood vessels and eye. *See* Muscle.

upper motor neurone. Motor nerve fibres extending from the brain to the anterior horn cell. *See* Neurone.

urachal (*u'-rak-al*). Referring to the urachus. *U. cyst.* A congenital abnormality when a small cyst persists along the course of the urachus. *U. fistula.* When the urachus fails to close and urine may leak from the umbilicus.

urachus (*u'-rak-us*). A tubular canal existing in the fetus, connecting the bladder with the umbilicus. In the adult it persists in the form of a solid fibrous cord.

uracil (*u'-ras-il*). One of the nucleic bases found in ribonucleic acid.

uraemia (*u-re'-me-ah*). A condition of high blood urea, muscle weakness and increasing drowsiness. Renal function is impaired. *Renal u.* The cause lies in disease of kidney structure. *Extrarenal u.* The cause is outside the kidney such as circulatory failure due to shock or haemorrhage. *Haemolytic u.* A disorder where acute nephritis is associated with haemolytic anaemia. Most commonly found in young children.

uraniscorrhaphy (*u-ran-is-kor'-raf-e*). Suture of a cleft palate.

uranium (*u-ra'-ne-um*). The metal from which radium is derived.

urate (*u'-rate*). A salt of uric acid. *Sodium u.* is generally found in concentration around joints in cases of gout.

uraturia (*u-rat-u'-re-ah*). Excess of urates in the urine. Lithuria.

urea (*u-re'-ah*). Carbamide. A white crystalline substance which is the chief nitrogenous constituent of urine. The normal daily output is about 33 g. *Blood u.* That which is present in the blood. Normal 20 to 40 mg per 100 ml. For *U. clearance test, see* Appendix 11.

urecchysis (*u-rek'-is-is*). The extravasation of urine into cellular tissue, e.g. in rupture of the bladder as a complication of fractured pelvis.

uresis (*u-re'-sis*). Urination.

ureter (*u-re'-ter*). One of the two long narrow tubes which convey the urine from the kidney to the bladder.

ureteric (*u-re-ter'-ik*). Relating to the ureter. *U. catheter.* A fine catheter for insertion via the ureter into the pelvis or the kidney, either for drainage or for retrograde pyelography. *See* Renal function tests—Appendix 11. *U. transplantation.* The ureters are divided from the bladder and implanted in the colon or loop of ileum. Congenital defects or malignant growth may make this necessary.

ureteritis (*u-re-ter-i'-tis*). Inflammation of the ureter.

ureterocele (*u-re'-ter-o-seel*). Cystic enlargement of the portion of the ureter which is situated in the bladder wall.

ureterocolostomy (*u-re-ter-o-kol-os'-to-me*). *See* Ureterosigmoidoscopy.

ureterolith (*u-re'-ter-o-lith*). Calculus in a ureter.

ureterolithotomy (*u-re-ter-o-lith-ot'-o-me*). Removal of a stone from the ureter.

ureterosigmoidostomy (*u-re-ter-o-sig-moid-os'-to-me*). Implantation of the ureters into the sigmoid colon.

ureterostomy (*u-re-ter-os'-to-me*). Making a permanent opening through which the ureter discharges urine. *Cutaneous u.* When the ureters are transplanted to open on to the abdominal wall.

ureterovaginal (*u-re'-ter-o-*

vaj-i'-nal). Relating to the ureter and vagina. *U. fistula.* An opening into the ureter by which urine escapes via the vagina. It may be congenital due to erosion, as in carcinoma of the cervix, or to an error in operative technique.

urethane (*u'-re-thane*). Ethyl carbamate used in the treatment of myeloid leukaemia. Also, with quinine, in the injection treatment of varicose veins.

urethra (*u-re'-thrah*). The canal through which the urine is discharged from the bladder. In a man it measures 20 to 23 cm (8 to 9 in) in length; in a woman 4 cm (1·5 in).

urethral (*u-re'-thral*). Relating to the urethra. *U. caruncle. See* Caruncle.

urethritis (*u-re-thri'-tis*). Inflammation of the urethra. *Non-specific u. See* Non-specific urethritis.

urethrocele (*u-re'-thro-seel*). A prolapse of the urethral wall

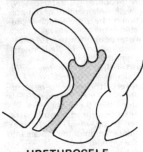

URETHROCELE

which may result from damage to the pelvic floor during childbirth.

urethrogram (*u-re'-thro-gram*). An X-ray examination of

the urethra. The dye may be inserted by catheter which is then removed and X-ray films taken as the urine is voided.

urethroplasty (*u-re'-thro-plaste*). Operation for repair of the urethra.

urethroscope (*u-re'-thro-skope*). An instrument for examining the interior of the urethra.

urethrostenosis (*u-re-thro-sten-o'-sis*). Stricture of the urethra.

urethrotomy (*u-re-throt'-o-me*). Incision of the urethra, to remedy stricture.

uric acid (*u'-rik*). Lithic acid, a normal constituent of urine. Its accumulation in the blood produces uricaemia. Renal calculi are frequently formed of it.

uricosuric (*ur-ik-o-su'-rik*). A drug that promotes the excretion of uric acid in the urine.

uridrosis (*u-rid-ro'-sis*). The presence of urinary constituents, such as urea and uric acid in the perspiration. They may become deposited as crystals upon the skin.

urinalysis (*u-rin-al'-e-sis*). Examination of the urine. *See* Appendix 11.

urinary (*u'-rin-ar-e*). Relating to urine. *U. diversion.* When the ureters are transplanted into either the colon, the ileum (*see* Ileal bladder) or on to the abdominal wall (*see* Ureterostomy).

urination (*u-rin-a'-shun*). Micturition.

urine (*u'-rin*). The fluid secreted by the kidneys and excreted through the bladder and urethra. It is 96 per cent water and 4 per cent solid constituents, the most important being urea and uric acid. *Examination of the u. See* Appendix 11. *Residual u.* That which remains in the bladder after micturition, as in cases of cystocele or enlargement of the prostate gland. *U. tests. See* Appendix 11.

uriniferous (*u-rin-if'-er-us*). Conveying urine. *U. tubule. See* Tubule.

urinometer (*u-rin-om'-e-ter*). A glass instrument consisting of

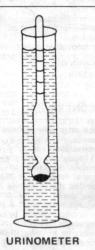

URINOMETER

a graduated stem weighted with a mercury bulb, used for measuring the specific gravity of urine.

urobilin (*u-ro-bi'-lin*). The main pigment of urine, derived from urobilinogen.

urobilinogen (*u-ro-bi-lin'-o-jen*). A pigment derived from bilirubin which on oxidation forms urobilin.

urochrome (*u'-ro-krome*). Colouring matter of urine.

urogenital (*u-ro-jen'-it-al*). Relating to urinary and genital organs.

urography (*u-rog'-raf-e*). Radiography of any part of the urinary tract.

urokinase (*u-ro-kin'-aze*). An enzyme in urine which may be activated by trauma or disease and so retard the normal clotting mechanism and cause bleeding from the kidney.

urolith (*u'-ro-lith*). A calculus passed with the urine.

urologist (*u-rol'-o-jist*). A specialist in urology.

urology (*u-rol'-o-je*). The study of diseases of the urinary tract.

uropathy (*u-rop'-ath-e*). Any disease condition affecting the excretory power of the kidneys.

urticaria (*er-tik-a'-re-ah*). Nettle-rash or hives. A skin condition characterized by the recurrent appearance of an eruption of weals, causing great irritation. The condition is probably due to hypersensitiveness to some form of protein, and is therefore allied to hay fever, asthma, etc. *See* Allergy.

uterine (*u'-ter-ine*). Relating to the uterus.

uterogestation (*u-ter-o-jes-ta'-shun*). Development of a fetus within the uterus. *See* Extrauterine gestation.

uterovesical (*u-ter-o-ves'-ik-al*). Referring to the uterus and bladder. *U. pouch.* The fold of peritoneum between the two organs.

uterus (*u'-ter-us*). The womb; a triangular, hollow, muscle organ situated in the pelvic cavity between the bladder and the rectum. Its function is the nourishment and protection of the fetus during pregnancy and its expulsion at term. *Bicornate u.* One having two horns. A congenital malformation. *U. didelphys.* A double uterus owing to

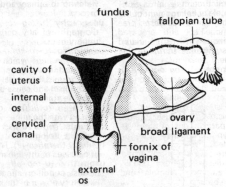

UTERUS AND ADNEXA

the failure of union of the two Müllerian ducts from which it is formed. *Gravid u.* The pregnant uterus.

utricle (*u'-trik-l*). The delicate membranous sac in the bony vestibule of the ear.

uvea (*u'-ve-ah*). Uveal tract. The pigmented layer of the eye, consisting of the iris, ciliary body and choroid.

uveitis (*u-ve-i'-tis*). Inflammation of the iris, ciliary body and choroid coat of the eye.

uvula (*u'-vu-lah*). The small fleshy appendage which is the free edge of the soft palate, hanging from the roof of the mouth.

uvulitis (*u-vu-li'-tis*). Inflammation of the uvula.

uvulotomy (*u-vu-lot'-o-me*). The operation of cutting off a part or the whole of the uvula.

V

vaccinate (*vak'-sin-ate*). To inoculate with a vaccine to produce an active immunity to a disease.

vaccination (*vak-sin-a'-shun*). (1) Inoculation with the virus of cowpox in order to protect against smallpox. It is recommended that it should first be done during the second year and again between 8 and 12 years and every 3 to 5 years afterwards. (2) The injection of a vaccine in order to produce artificial active immunity.

vaccine (*vak'-seen*). A suspension of killed or attenuated organisms in normal saline designed to protect the body against a specific disease by stimulating the formation of antibodies. *Attenuated v.* One prepared from living organisms which through long cultivation have lost their virulence. *Bacille Calmette Guérin v.* An attenuated bovine bacillus to give immunity from tuberculosis. *Quadruple v.* Protects against whooping cough, diphtheria, poliomyelitis, and tetanus.

Triple v. Protects against diphtheria, tetanus, and whooping cough. *V. lymph.* Used to prevent smallpox and prepared from healthy calves inoculated with smallpox. *Sabin v.* An attenuated poliovirus *v.* that can be administered by mouth, in a syrup or on sugar. *Salk v.* One prepared from an inactivated strain of poliomyelitis virus. *TAB v.* A sterile solution of the organisms that cause typhoid and paratyphoid A and B. Paratyphoid C may now be included.

vaccinia (vak-sin'-e-ah). Cowpox, a disease resembling smallpox, affecting animals and human beings.

vaccinotherapy (vak-sin-o-ther'-ap-e). Treatment by means of bacterial vaccines.

vacuole (vak'-u-ole). A clear space in a cell substance.

vacuum (vak'-u-um). A space from which air has been extracted. *V. extractor.* An instrument to assist delivery of the fetus. A suction cup is attached to the head and a vacuum created slowly. Traction is applied during uterine contractions.

vagal (va'-gal). Relating to the vagus nerve.

vagina (vaj-i'-nah). The canal, lined with mucous membrane, which leads from the vulva to the cervix uteri.

vaginismus (vaj-in-iz'-mus). Muscular spasm of the vagina on being touched.

vaginitis (vaj-in-i'-tis). Inflammation of the vagina. *Gonococcal v. See* Gonorrhoea. *Senile v.* That occurring in the aged, causing discharge, and adhesions which may obliterate the canal. *Trichomonas v.* Infection owing to the *Trichomonas*, a protozoan which causes a thin,

yellowish discharge, giving rise to local tenderness and pruritus.

vagotomy (va-got'-o-me). Cutting the vagus nerve. A treatment for peptic ulcer.

vagus (va'-gus). *Pl.* vagi. The tenth cranial nerve arising in the medulla and providing the parasympathetic nerve supply to the organs in the thorax and abdomen. *V. resection.* Operation on the vagus nerve. *See* Vagotomy.

valgus (val'-gus). Turned inwards. *Genu v.* Knock-kneed. *Hallux v.* Big toe displaced towards other toes.

valine (val'-een). One of the 22 amino acids formed by the digestion of dietary protein.

Valium (val'-e-um). Proprietary preparation of diazepam, a tranquillizing drug used to alleviate anxiety.

Vallergan (val-er'-gan). Proprietary preparation of trimeprazine (q.v.).

Valsalva's auto-inflation (*A. M. Valsalva, Italian anatomist, 1666–1723*). Insufflation of the eustachian tubes by closing the nostrils and mouth and blowing out the cheeks to force air back into the nasophraynx.

valve. A fold of membrane in a passage or tube, so placed as to permit passage of fluid in one direction only. They are important structures in veins and lymph vessels, to help the ascent of fluid against gravity. *Auriculoventricular v's.* The bicuspid and tricuspid valves of the heart. *Houston's v's.* Folds of mucous membrane in the rectum. *Ileocaecal v.* Membranous folds at the junction of the ileum and caecum. *Pyloric v.* A fold of mucous membrane at the junction of the stomach and deodenum. *Semilunar v.s.* At the junction of the pulmonary artery and aorta respectively, with the heart. *V. replacement.* A cardiac operation to replace a diseased aortic or mitral valve.

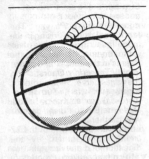

PROSTHETIC HEART VALVE

valvotomy (*val-vot'-o-me*). A surgical operation to increase the lumen of a fibrosed valve, e.g. mitral valvotomy to relieve mitral stenosis.

valvulae (*val'-vu-le*). Small valves. *V. conniventes.* Transverse folds of mucous membrane in the lining of the small intestine.

valvulitis (*val-vu-li'-tis*). Inflammation of a valve, particularly of the heart.

van den Bergh's test (*A. A. H. van den Bergh, Dutch physician, 1869–1943*). A chemical test to aid the diagnosis of jaundice.

Vaquez's disease (*L. H. Vaquez, French physician, 1860–1936*). Polycythaemia vera (*q.v.*).

varicella (*var-e-sel'-lah*). Chickenpox. An infectious disease of childhood having an incubation period of 14 days. There is slight fever and an eruption of transparent vesicles on the chest on the first day of disease, which comes out in successive crops all over the body. The vesicles soon dry up, sometimes leaving shallow pits in the skin. The isolation period is until all scabs have been shed and complications are rare.

varicelliform (*var-e-sel'-e-form*). With vesicles similar to those of varicella.

varices (*var'-e-seez*). *Sing.* varix. Dilated veins. *Oesophageal v.* Those at the lower end of the oesophagus due to portal hypertension. *Rectal v.* Haemorrhoids (*q.v.*).

varicocele (*var'-ik-o-seel*). A dilatation of the veins of the spermatic cord.

varicocelectomy (*var-ik-o-se-lek'-to-me*). Operation for removal of dilated veins from the scrotum.

varicose (*var'-ik-oze*). Swollen or dilated. *V. veins.* A dilated and twisted condition of the veins (usually those of the leg), due to structural changes in the walls or valves of the vessels. *V. ulcer.* See Ulcer.

varicotomy (*var-ik-ot'-o-me*). Excision of a varicose vein.

variola (*var-e-o'-lah*). Smallpox. A highly contagious infection spread by droplets or contaminated articles. Its incidence is controlled by widespread vaccination. It is occasionally introduced into Great Britain from abroad. There is a high mortality in unvaccinated cases. *V. minor.* A modified form of smallpox may arise in a partially immune person who has previously been vaccinated but the rash is sparser and the fever milder. The danger is that a non-immune contact may develop a major attack.

varioloid (*var'-e-o-loid*). Variola minor (*q.v.*).

varix (*var'-iks*). An enlarged or varicose vein. *Pl.* varices (*q.v.*).

varus (*va'-rus*). A bending outwards. *Genu v.* Bow legged. *Talipes v.* The foot is inverted and weight is carried on the outer aspect.

vasa vasorum (*va'-zah vaz-or'-um*). The minute nutrient vessels that supply the walls of the arteries and veins.

vascular (*vas'-ku-lar*). Relating to, or consisting largely of vessels.

vascularization (*vas-ku-lar-i-za'-shun*). The process of becoming vascular.

vasculitis (*vas-ku-li'-tis*). A severe allergic response to drugs or to cold. Arising in small arteries or veins with fibrosis and thrombi formation.

vas deferens (*vas def'-er-ens*). The duct conveying the semen from the epididymis up the spermatic cord to its opening in the prostatic part of the urethra.

vasectomy (*vas-ek'-to-me*). Removal of a part of the vas deferens.

vasoconstrictor (*va-zo-kon-strik'-tor*). A nerve or a drug that causes contraction of a blood vessel wall. Applies to nerves or drugs that decrease the size of the lumen of a blood vessel.

vasodilator (*va-zo-di-la'-tor*). A drug or motor nerve that causes an increase in the lumen of blood vessels.

vasomotor (*va-zo-mo'-tor*). Controlling the muscles of blood vessels, both dilator and constrictor. *V. nerves.* Sympathetic nerves regulating the tension of the blood vessels. *V. centre.* Nerve cells in the medulla oblongata controlling the vasomotor nerves.

vasopressin (*va-zo-press'-in*). A hormone from the posterior lobe of the pituitary gland which causes constriction of plain muscle fibres and reabsorption of water in the renal tubules. It is used to relieve symptoms in diabetes insipidus.

vasovagal attack (*va-zo-va'-gal*). Fainting or syncope from psychogenic causes such as fear or witnessing an unpleasant sight. There is postural hypotension.

vasovesiculitis (*va-zo-ves-ik-u-li'-tis*). Inflammation of the vas deferens and seminal vesicles.

Vater's ampulla (*A. Vater, German anatomist, 1684–1751*). Dilatation at the point where the common bile duct enters the duodenum.

vectis (*vek'-tis*). An instrument used to hasten delivery of the fetal head in parturition.

vector (*vek'-tor*). (1) An animal that carries organisms or parasites from one host to another, either of the same species or to one of another species. (2) A quantity with magnitude and direction. *Electrocardiographic v.* The area of the heart which is monitored during electrocardiographic investigation.

vectorcardiography (*vek'-tor-kar-de-og'-raf-e*). Electrocardiographic investigation of the heart in which individual vectors are monitored.

vegetation (*vej-e-ta'-shun*). An overgrowth. *Adenoid v.* Overgrowth of lymphoid tissue in the nasopharynx.

vehicle (*ve'-e-kul*). A substance or medium in which a drug is administered.

vein (*vane*). A vessel carrying blood from the capillaries back to the heart. It has thin walls and a lining endothelium from which the venous valves are formed.

Velactin (*vel-ak'-tin*). A complete milk substitute when a milk-free diet is required. The protein is from soya beans, the fat arachis oil and the carbohydrate is starch, dextrose dextrin and sucrose.

vena cava (*ve'-nah ka'-vah*). Pl. venae cavae. *Superior* and *inferior v. c.* are the two large veins which return the venous blood to the right atrium of the heart.

venepuncture (*ve-ne-punk'-ture*). The insertion of a needle into a vein usually to obtain a blood specimen.

venereal (*ven-e'-re-al*). Pertaining to or caused by sexual intercourse. *V. diseases.* Syphilis, gonorrhoea, and soft chancre.

venereology (*ven-er'-e-ol-o-je*). The study and treatment of venereal disease.

venesection (*ve-ne-sek'-shun*). Surgical blood-letting by opening a vein or introducing a wide bore needle. Commonly performed on blood donors and occasionally to relieve venous congestion.

venoclysis (*ve-nok'-lis-is*). Introduction of fluids directly into veins.

venofibrosis (*ve-no-fi-bro'-sis*). Sclerosis of veins.

venogram (*ve'-no-gram*). The skiagram or X-ray taken at venography.

venography (*ve-nog'-ra-fe*). The insertion of a dye to trace the pathway of veins.

venom antiserum (*ven'-um an-te-se-rum*). A serum containing antibodies against the bites of poisonous snakes.

venomotor tone (*ve-no-mo'-tor*). Muscle tone in the walls of the veins which can produce changes in the capacity of the circulation without affecting their resistance to blood flow.

venous (*ve'-nus*). Pertaining to the veins. *V. sinus.* A channel in the cranium by which blood leaves the brain.

ventilation (*ven-til-a'-shun*). The process of removing vitiated air (the products of respiration, combustion, or putrefaction), and replacing it with fresh air. *Natural v.* By natural diffusion of gases, controlled by windows, doors, and ventilating devices. *Artificial v.* By propulsion and extraction methods, as is used for large buildings, mines, underground railways, etc.

ventilator (*ven'-til-la-tor*). A machine which inflates the lungs by positive pressure through an endotracheal or tracheostomy tube, in a rhythmic manner.

ventral (*ven'-tral*). Pertaining to a hollow structure or belly. *V. aspect.* That of the belly. *V. root.* Motor nerve pathway. Route along which motor impulses travel from the spinal cord to the muscles.

ventricle (*ven'-trik-l*). A small pouch or cavity; applied especially to the lower chambers of the heart, and to the four cavities of the brain. *Fourth v.* A ventricle in the brain in which cerebrospinal fluid is formed. *Third v.* One of the ventricles of the brain in which cerebrospinal fluid is formed.

ventricular (*ven-trik'-u-lah*). Pertaining to a ventricle. *V. folds.* The outer folds of mucous membrane forming the false vocal cords. *V. septal defect (VSD).* Congenital abnormality in which there is communication between the two ventricles of the heart due to mal-development of the intraventricular septum.

ventriculography (*ven-trik-u-*

log'-raf-e). An aid to diagnosis, by which the ventricles of the brain are filled with air, and an X-ray photograph taken. Used to help locate a cerebral tumour.

ventriculoscope (*ven-trik'-u-lo-skope*). An instrument for viewing the inside of the ventricles of the brain. It may also be used for coagulating blood vessels.

ventrofixation (*ven-tro-fiks-a'-shun*). Stitching a displaced uterus or other abdominal organ to the abdominal wall.

ventrosuspension (*ven-tro-sus-pen'-shun*). An abdominal operation performed to remedy displacement of uterus.

venule (*ven'-ule*). (1) A minute vein. (2) A special type of syringe or evacuated glass phial for collecting blood from a vein.

verbigeration (*ver-bij-er-a'-shun*). The monotonous repetition of phrases. A disturbance of behaviour that may be present in schizophrenia.

vermicide (*ver'-mis-ide*). An agent which destroys intestinal worms.

vermiform (*ver'-me-form*). Worm-shaped. *V. appendix.* The worm-shaped structure attached to the caecum.

vermifuge (*ver'-me-fuj*). An agent which expels intestinal worms; an anthelmintic.

verminous (*ver'-min-us*). Infested with worms or other animal parasites, such as lice.

vermix (*ver'-miks*). The vermiform appendix.

vernix caseosa (*ver'-niks ka-se-o'-sah*). The fatty covering on the skin of the fetus during the last months of pregnancy. It consists of cells and sebaceous material.

verruca (*ver-ru'-kah*). A wart. A localized hypertrophy of the prickle cell layer of the epidermis and thickening of the horny layer. A virus is the causative organism. *V. acuminata.* A venereal wart that appears on the external genitalia and may be associated with gonorrhoea.

version (*ver'-shun*). Turning a part; applied particularly to the turning of a fetus in order to facilitate delivery. *External v.* Manipulation of the uterus through the abdominal wall in order to change the position of the child. *Internal v.* Rotation of the fetus by means of manipulation with one hand in the vagina. *Podalic v.* Turning of the fetus so that the head is uppermost and the feet presenting.

vertebrae (*ver'-te-bre*). The thirty-three irregular bones forming the spinal column. They are divided into: 7 *cervical*, 12 *dorsal*, 5 *lumbar*, 5 *sacral* (sacrum), and 4 *coccygeal* (coccyx). *Sing.* vertebra.

vertebrate (*ver'-te-brate*). Possessing a vertebral column.

vertebrobasilar disease (*ver-te-bro-bas'-il-ar*). Disease affecting the vertebral and basilar arteries which causes recurrent attacks of blindness, diplopia, vertigo, dysarthria and hemiparesis.

vertex (*ver'-teks*). The crown of the head. *V. presentation.* The fetus is so placed that the crown of the head appears in the vagina first.

vertigo (*ver'-tig-o*). A feeling of rotation or of going round, in either oneself or one's surroundings, particularly associated with disease of the cerebellum and vestibular nerve of the ear. It may occur in diplopia or Ménière's syndrome.

vesica (*ves-i'-kah*). A bladder; usually referring to the urinary bladder. *See* Ectopia vesicae.

vesical (*ves'-ik-al*). Relating to the bladder.

vesicant (*ves'-ik-ant*). A blistering agent.

vesicle (*ves'-ik-l*). A blister or small sac usually containing fluid. *Air v.* An alveolus of the lung. *Seminal v.* The sac which arises from the vas deferens near the bladder and contains semen.

vesico-ureteric (*ves-ik-o-u-re-ter'-ik*). Relating to the urinary bladder and the ureters. *V. reflux.* When urine is also passed backwards up the ureter during micturition. A cause of pyelonephritis in children.

vesicovaginal (*ves'-ik-o-vaj-i'-nal*). Relating to the bladder and vagina. *See* Fistula.

vesicular (*ves-ik'-u-lar*). Relating to or containing vesicles. *V. breathing.* The soft murmur of normal respiration, as heard on auscultation. *V. mole.* Hydatidiform mole (*q.v.*).

vesiculitis (*ves-ik-u-li'-tis*). Inflammation of the seminal vesicles.

vesiculopapular (*ves-ik'-u-lo-pap'-u-lar*). An eruption of both vesicles and papules.

vessel (*ves'-sel*). A tube or canal for conveying fluid, usually blood or lymph.

vestibular (*ves-tib'-u-lar*). Relating to a vestibule. *V. glands.* Those in the vestibule of the vagina, including Bartholin's glands. *V. nerve.* A branch of the eighth cranial nerve supplying the semicircular canals and concerned with balance and equilibrium.

vestibule (*ves'-tib-ule*). An entrance, e.g. the cavity at the entrance to the cochlea of the ear.

vestibulocochlear nerve (*ves-tib'-u-lo-kok'-le-ah*). The eighth cranial nerve. Also known as the auditory nerve.

vestigial (*ves-tij'-e-al*). Rudimentary. Referring to the remains of an anatomical structure, which being of no further use has atrophied.

viable (*vi'-ab-l*). Capable of independent life. A term applied to the fetus after 7 months of intra-uterine life.

Vibramycin (*vi-brah-mi'-sin*). Proprietary preparation of doxycycline, a broad spectrum antibiotic.

Vibrio (*vib'-re-o*). A microorganism short, curved, and motile by having flagellae. *Vibrio cholerae,* or *V. comma,* is that which causes cholera.

vicarious (*vi-ka'-re-us*). Substituted for another; a term used when one organ functions instead of another.

villi (*vil'-li*). Finger-like processes from a surface. *Intestinal v.* Those of the mucous membrane of the small intestine, each of which contains a blood capillary and lacteal. *Chorionic v.* The essential structure of the placenta by which the fetus is nourished. *Sing.* villus.

Vincent's angina (*J. H. Vincent, French physician, 1862–1950*). *See* Angina.

vincristine (*vin-cris'-teen*). Drug used in the treatment of acute lymphoblastic leukaemia. Oncovin is a proprietary preparation of it.

vinyl (*vi'-nil*). A plastic material now used extensively for medical equipment.

viraemia (*vi-re'-me-ah*). The presence of viruses in the blood.

virilism (*vir'-il-izm*). Masculine traits exhibited by the female owing to the production of excessive amounts of androgenic hormone either in the adrenal cortex or from an ovarian tumour. *See* Arrhenoblastoma.

virology (*vi-rol'-o-je*). The scientific study of viruses, their growth and diseases caused by them.

virulence (*vir'-u-lense*). The power to produce toxins or poisons. In infection this depends on: (1) The number and power of the bacteria invading. (2) The resistance of the patient.

virulent (*vir'-u-lent*). Malignant; dangerously poisonous. *V. infection.* One which is abnormally severe and dangerous.

virus (*vi'-rus*). A minute living organism smaller than bacteria. Only the largest viruses can be seen with the ordinary microscope. An electron microscope is required to 'see' the majority. Viruses can be grown only in living cells, e.g. chick embryos, tissue cultures (*q.v.*). They cause many diseases such as influenza, measles and poliomyelitis.

viscera (*vis'-er-ah*). Plural of viscus (*q.v.*).

visceroptosis (*vis-ser-op-to'-sis*). A general tendency to prolapse of the abdominal organs.

viscid (*vis'-id*). Sticky and glutinous.

viscosity (*vis-kos'-it-e*). A sticky and glutinous quality.

viscus (*vis'-kus*). A term applied to any one of the organs contained in the body—especially in the abdomen. *Pl.* viscera.

vision (*viz'-shun*). Act or faculty of seeing.

visual (*viz'-u-al*). Relating to sight. *V. acuity.* Acuteness of vision. *V. cells.* The rods and cones of the retina. *V. field.* The area within which objects can be seen. *V. purple.* The pigment in the outer layers of the retina.

vita glass (*ve'-tah*). Quartz glass which is capable of transmitting ultra-violet rays of light.

vital (*vi'-tal*). Relating to life. *V. capacity.* The amount of air which can be expelled from the lungs after a full inspiration. *V. statistics.* The records kept of births and deaths among the population; including the causes of death; and the factors which seem to influence their rise and fall.

vitallium (*vi-tal'-e-um*). A metal alloy used in dentistry and for screws and plates in bone surgery.

vitamins (*vi'-tam-ins*). Accessory food factors. Substances contained in foodstuffs which are essential to life, growth, and reproduction. *See* Appendix 10.

vitellin (*vi-tel'-in*). The chief protein of egg yolk.

vitellus (*vi-tel'-us*). The yolk of an ovum, or egg.

vitiation (*vish-e-a'-shun*). Lessening of efficiency.

vitiligo (*vit-il-i'-go*). A skin disease marked by an absence of pigment, producing white patches on the face and body. Leucoderma.

vitreous (*vit'-re-us*). Glassy. *V. humour.* The transparent jelly-like substance filling the posterior of the eye, from lens to retina.

vivisection (*viv-e-sek'-shun*). The use of living animals for experimental purposes. The procedures are carefully controlled by law and the animals are usually anaesthetized if surgery is being used.

VMA. Vanillylmandelic acid. Metabolite of catecholamines excreted in small amounts in the urine.

vocal (*vo'-kal*). Pertaining to the

organs which produce the voice. *V. cords.* Vocal folds in the larynx formed of fibrous tissue covered with squamous epithelium.

volatile (*vol'-at-ile*). Having a tendency to evaporate readily.

volition (*vo-lish'-un*). The conscious adoption by the individual of a line of action and maintaining it.

volitional (*vo-lish'-un-al*). Being impelled by will power.

Volkmann's ischaemic contracture (*R. von Volkmann, German surgeon, 1830–89*). Atrophy and fibrosis occurring in the muscles owing to an impaired blood supply. Usually applied to the upper limb when the brachial artery is compressed by a fracture of the lower end of the humerus.

volt. The unit of electromotive force (*q.v.*).

volume (*vol'-ume*). The space occupied by a substance; usually expressed in cubic measure. *Minute v.* The total volume of air breathed in or out in 1 min. *Packed cell v.* That occupied by the blood cells after centrifuging, about 45 per cent of the blood sample.

voluntary (*vol'-un-tar-re*). Under the control of the will. *See* Involuntary.

volvulus (*vol'-vu-lus*). Twisting of a part of the intestine, causing obstruction. Most common in the sigmoid colon.

vomer (*vo'-mer*). A thin plate of bone forming the posterior septum of the nose.

vomit (*vom'-it*). Material vomited. *Bilious v.* Bile is mixed with the matter ejected. *Coffeeground v.* Small quantities of altered blood ejected, which have this appearance. *Faecal* or *stercoraceous v.* Arises in intestinal obstruction when the con-

tents of the upper intestine regurgitate back into the stomach. It is dark brown with an unpleasant odour. *See* Vomiting.

vomiting (*vom'-it-ing*). A reflex act of expulsion of the stomach contents via the oesophagus and mouth. It may be preceded by nausea and excess salivation if the cause is local irriation in the stomach. *Cyclical v.* Recurrent attacks of vomiting often occurring in children and associated with acidosis. *Morning v.* Occurs on rising as in pregnancy and chronic gastritis. *Projectile v.* The gastric contents are forcibly ejected, usually without warning. Present in hypertrophic pyloric stenosis, and in cerebral diseases. *Psychogenic v.* That without organic cause.

vulnerability (*vul-ner-ab-il'-i-te*). Susceptibility to injury or infection.

vulva (*vul'-vah*). The external female genital organs.

vulvectomy (*vul-vek'-to-me*). Excision of the vulva.

vulvitis (*vul-vi'-tis*). Inflammation of the vulva.

vulvovaginitis (*vul-vo-vaj-in-i'-tis*). Inflammation of the vulva and vagina.

W

wafer (*wa'-fer*). A thin double layer of flour paste used to enclose a dose of medicinal powder. A cachet.

Waldeyer's ring (*H. W. G. von Waldeyer–Hartz, German anatomist, 1836–1921*). The circle of lymphoid tissue in the pharynx formed by the *lingual, faucial,* and *pharyngeal* tonsils.

Waldeyer's fascia. A portion of the pelvic fascia that sheaths the lower part of the ureter. It contains some plain muscle fibres and kinking may occur here when the bladder is over distended.

Waller's shields (*Waller, contemporary British paediatrician*). Shields placed over the nipples of pregnant women to correct retraction and facilitate breast feeding. Also known as Woolwich shells.

Wangensteen tube (*O. H. Wangensteen, American surgeon, 1898– *). A gastrointestinal aspiration tube with a tip that is opaque to X-rays.

warfarin (*war'-far-in*). An anticoagulant drug that depresses the prothrombin level.

wart (*wawt*). An elevation of the skin, which is often of a brownish colour, caused by hypertrophy of papillae in the dermis. *See* Verruca *and* Condyloma.

Wassermann reaction (*A. P. von Wassermann, German bacteriologist, 1866–1925*). A method of testing the blood serum of a patient to aid in the diagnosis of syphilis. It can also show the progress whilst under treatment.

water balance or fluid balance. That between the fluid intake by all routes (oral, intravenous and rectal) and the fluid lost by all routes (urine, vomit or drainage from any body cavity).

water-borne (*waw-ter born*). Spread by contaminated water.

water-brash. The eructation of dilute acid from the stomach to the pharynx, giving a burning sensation. Pyrosis (*q.v.*).

water-hammer pulse. *See* Pulse.

water-seal drainage. A closed method of drainage from the pleural space allowing the escape of fluid and air but pre-

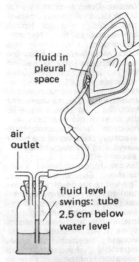

fluid in pleural space

air outlet

fluid level swings: tube 2.5 cm below water level

WATER-SEAL DRAINAGE

venting air entering as the drainage tube discharges under water.

Waterhouse–Friderichsen syndrome (*R. Waterhouse, British physician, 1873–1958: C. Friderichsen, Danish physician, 1886– *). Peripheral vascular collapse which occurs in septicaemia. It is the result of adrenal haemorrhage and is usually seen in children.

Waterston's operation (*D. Waterston, British paediatric surgeon, 1910– *). A palliative operation of anastomosis of the right pulmonary artery to the ascending aorta. Used in the treatment of Fallot's tetralogy in the young child.

Watson–Crick hypothesis (*J. D. Watson, American geneticist, 1928– : F. Crick, British biochemist, 1916– *). Hypothesis proposed by Watson and Crick, who were awarded the Nobel Prize in 1962, to describe the structure of the DNA molecule.

watt. A unit of electric power.

wavelength. The measurement from the crest of one wave to the crest of the next one. Applied to the electromagnetic spectrum, the longest are radio waves and the shortest are X-rays and γ-rays.

waves. Uniform advancing undulation. *Electromagnetic w.* The entire range of waves including light waves in the ether.

wax (*waks*). In pharmacy, *beeswax*, used for making ointments. *Ear w. See* Cerumen. *Bone w.* An antiseptic form for stopping bleeding from bone, especially whilst performing operations on the skull. *Paraffin w.* Hard paraffin prepared from petroleum.

waxy flexibility (*wak'-se fleksib-il'-it-e*). When a patient's limbs are held indefinitely in any position in which they have been placed. *See* Catatonia.

weal (*hweel*). A raised stripe on the skin, as is caused by the lash of a whip. Typical of urticaria (*q.v.*).

weaning (*wee-ning*). The change from breast to normal feeding. It should be effected gradually from about the fourth month.

webbing of neck. Folds of skin in the neck giving the webbed appearance. Occurs in certain congenital conditions, i.e. Turner's syndrome (*q.v.*).

webbing of hands and feet. Congenital abnormality in which the digits are not separated from each other. *See* Syndactyly.

Weber's test (*F. E. Weber-Liel, German otologist, 1832–91*). For hearing. A vibrating tuning fork is held in the centre of the forehead. If the sound is heard best in the affected ear, there is obstruction in the passage of that ear; if in the unaffected, there is disease of the organ of hearing.

Weil's disease (*A. Weil, German physician, 1848–1916*). Spirochaetal jaundice. The organism, *Leptospira icterohaemorrhagiae*, is harboured and excreted by rats and enters through a bite or skin abrasion and infected water.

Weil–Felix reaction (*E. Weil, Austrian physician, 1880–1922; A. Felix, Czech bacteriologist, 1887–1956*). An agglutination test of blood serum used for diagnosis of typhus fever.

Welch's bacillus (*W. H. Welch, American pathologist, 1850–1934*). *Clostridium welchii* or *perfringens*, the organism most usually found in gas gangrene.

wen. A small sebaceous cyst.

Wenckebach's periods (*K. F. Wenckebach, Dutch physician in Austria, 1864–1940*). Abnormal heart rhythm in which the P–R interval gradually increases until a beat is missed.

Werdnig–Hoffmann disease (*G. Werdnig, Austrian neurologist, 1862– : J. E. Hoffmann, German neurologist, 1857–1919*). Disease characterized by progressive lower motor neurone atrophy affecting the shoulder, neck, pelvis and eventually respiratory muscles.

Werner's syndrome (*C. W. O. Werner, German contemporary physician*). Hereditary condition characterized by cataracts, osteoporosis, stunted growth and premature greying of the hair.

Wernicke's encephalopathy (*K. Wernicke, German neurologist, 1848–1905*). A congenital neurological condition due to vitamin B₁ deficiency. Untreated it progresses from double vision to lethargy and coma.

Wertheim's operation (*E. Wertheim, Austrian gynaecologist, 1864–1920*). *See* Hysterectomy.

Wharton's duct (*T. Wharton, British physician, 1614–73*). The duct of the submaxillary gland.

Wharton's jelly (*T. Wharton, British physician, 1614–73*). Connective tissue of the umbilical cord.

Wheelhouse's operation (*C. G. Wheelhouse, British surgeon, 1826–1909*). Perineal incision for the relief of urethral obstruction.

wheeze (*hweez*). To breathe with difficulty, producing a hoarse whistling sound.

Whipple's operation (*A. O. Whipple, American surgeon, 1881–1963*). One performed for carcinoma of the head of the pancreas in which most of the pancreas, the pylorus, duodenum and the common bile duct are excised. Gastrojejunostomy is performed with anastomosis of the tail of the pancreas and gall-bladder to the jejunum.

whipworm. *See* Trichuris.

white cell transfusion (*wite sel trans-fu'-shun*). Intravenous infusion of white blood cells used to treat certain diseases of the blood.

Whitehead's varnish (*W. Whitehead, British surgeon, 1840–1913*). A preparation containing benzoin, iodoform, and ether. It may be used as a protective covering to a wound.

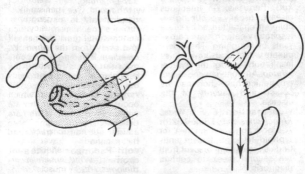

WHIPPLE'S OPERATION

white leg. *See* Phlegmasia.

'white fluids' (*wite flu'-ids*). Coal tar disinfectants which are suitable for linen and unstained wood as they do not cause discoloration.

'whites' (*wites*). A popular term for leucorrhoea.

White's tar paste (*J. C. White, American dermatologist, 1833–1916*). A paste of zinc and starch containing crude coal tar used in the treatment of psoriasis.

Whitfield's ointment (*A. Whitfield, British dermatologist, 1868–1947*). Used for skin diseases. It consists of: *Salicyclic acid*, 3 per cent and *benzoic acid*, 6 per cent, in a petroleum jelly base. Benzoic acid compound ointment.

whitlow (*hwit'-lo*). A suppurating inflammation of a finger near the nail. *Subperiosteal w.* The infection involves the bone covering. *Superficial w.* A pustule between the true skin and cuticle. *See* Paronychia.

whooping cough (*hoop'-ing kof*). Pertussis. An infectious disease usually occurring in children, characterized by acute respiratory catarrh, with paroxysms of coughing. These terminate with a long-drawn noisy inspiration giving the typical *whoop*. Aureomycin and chloramphenicol have shortened the course and severity of the disease.

Widal reaction (*G. F. I. Widal, French physician, 1862–1929*). A blood agglutination test for typhoid fever. Sufficient antibodies are usually present from the second week to confirm diagnosis.

von Willebrand's disease (*E. A. von Willebrand, contemporary Finnish physician*). Inher-

ited disorder in which there is a deficiency in blood clotting.

Wilms' tumour (*M. Wilm, German surgeon, 1867–1918*). A highly malignant congenital tumour of the kidney. An embryoma of kidney. Treated by radiotherapy and nephrectomy.

Wilson's disease (*S. A. K. Wilson, British neurologist, 1878–1937*). Hepatolenticular degeneration. A congenital abnormality in the metabolism of copper leading to neurological degeneration.

wintergreen oil. *See* Methylsalicylate.

wiring (*wi'-ring*). The fixing together of a broken or split bone by the use of a wire. Commonly used for the jaw, the patella and the sternum.

wisdom teeth (*wis-dum teeth*). The back molar teeth, the appearance of which is often delayed until maturity.

wish fulfilment. A desire, not always acknowledged consciously by the person, which is fulfilled through dreams or by day-dreaming.

witch hazel. *See* Hamamelis.

withdrawal. In psychiatry a defence mechanism in which an individual turns into himself and away from the world. *W. bleeding.* Bleeding that occurs from the uterus following the cessation of giving oestrogens for therapeutic reasons. *W. symptoms.* Symptoms which occur when drugs or alcohol are withdrawn from those who are dependent upon them. These may include nausea, tremor and hallucinations.

Wolff–Parkinson–White syndrome (*L. Wolff, American cardiologist, 1898– : Sir J. Parkinson, British physician, 1885– : P. D. White, American cardiologist, 1886–)*. Abnormal heart rhythm caused by an accessory bundle between the atria and ventricles.

wolffian bodies (*K. F. Wolff, German anatomist, 1733–1794*). Two small organs in the embyro, representing the primitive kidneys.

Wood's glass (*R. W. Wood, American physicist, 1868–1955*). Glass containing *nickel oxide*. It produces fluorescence of infected hairs when placed over a scalp affected with ringworm.

woolsorter's disease. Anthrax (*q.v.*).

word blindness. *See* Dyslexia.

word salad (*wurd sal-ad*). Rapid speech in which the words are strung together without meaning.

worms (*wurms*). A group of invertebrate animals. *See* Ascaris; Bilharziasis; Echinococcus; Tapeworm; *and* Oxyuris.

wound (*woond*). A cut or break in continuity of any tissue, caused by injury or operation. It is classified according to its nature: *Abrased w.* The skin is scraped off, but there is no deeper injury. *Aseptic w.* A non-infected one. *Contused w.* With bruising of the surrounding tissue. *Incised w.* Usually the result of operation, and produced by a knife or similar instrument. The edges of the wound can remain in apposition, and it should heal by first intention. *Lacerated w.* One with torn edges and tissues, usually the result of accident or injury. It is often septic, and heals by second intention. *Open w.* One which is draining freely. *Penetrating w.* Often made by gunshot, shrapnel, etc. There may be an inlet and outlet hole and vital organs are often pene-

trated by the missile. *Punctured w.* Made by a pointed or spiked instrument. *Septic w.* Any type into which infection has been introduced, causing suppurative inflammation. It heals by second intention. *See* Healing.

wrist (*rist*). The joint of the carpus and bones of the forearm. *W. drop.* Loss of power in the muscles of the hand. It may be due to nerve or tendon injury, but can result from lack of sufficient support by splint or sling. *See* Palsy.

writer's cramp (*ri'-ters kramp*). Painful spasm of the hand and forearm, caused by excessive writing.

wryneck (*ri'-nek*). *See* Torticollis.

X

xanthelasma (*zan-thel-az'-mah*). A disease marked by the formation of flat or slightly raised yellow patches on the eyelids.

xanthine (*zan'-theen*). A nucleoprotein. Sometimes found in renal calculi. *X. diuretics.* Those that increase the glomerular filtration rate, such as caffeine.

xanthochromia (*zan-tho-kro'-me-ah*). The yellow colouring of cerebrospinal fluid seen in patients who have had a subarachnoid haemorrhage.

xanthoderma (*zan-tho-der'-mah*). Yellowness of the skin.

xanthoma (*zan-tho'-mah*). *Pl.* xanthomata. The presence in the skin of flat areas of yellowish pigmentation due to deposits of lipoids. There are several varieties. *X. palpebrarum,* Xanthelasma.

xanthopsia (*zan-thop'-se-ah*).

Yellow vision, a condition in which all objects appear yellow.

xanthosis (*zan-tho'-sis*). A yellow skin pigmentation, seen in some cases of cancer.

X-chromosome (*eks kro'-mo-some*). The sex chromosome present in all female gametes and only half the male gametes, the rest having a *Y-c.* When union takes place two *X-c.* result in a female child (*XX*) but one of each results in a male child (*XY*).

xenon (*zen'-on*). An inert gaseous element. *Radioactive x.* (^{133}Xe) is used in blood flow clearance tests as it dissolves in the blood but does not form a chemical combination and the gas is excreted as the blood flows through the lungs.

Xenopsylla cheopis (*zen-op-sil'-ah che-o'-pis*). Rat flea that transmits bubonic plague.

Xenopus toad (*zen'-o-pus*). An animal used for early diagnosis of pregnancy. Similar to the Ascheim–Zondek test but more economical as if positive the toad sheds its eggs and it is thus unnecessary to kill it.

xeroderma (*zer-o-der'-mah*). A disease in which there is excessive dryness of the skin. A mild form of ichthyosis (*q.v.*).

xerophthalmia (*zer-off-thal'-me-ah*). A condition in which the cornea becomes horny and necrosed. It is due to the dietary deficiency of vitamin A. A symptom is night blindness.

xerosis (*zer-o'-sis*). A condition in which the conjunctiva appears dry and lustreless. Small white patches of horny epithelium appear on the cornea (*Bitôt's spots*). Mild cases may appear in children during the summer months.

xerostomia (*zer-o-sto'-me-ah*). Dryness of the mouth.

xiphoid (*zif'-oid*). Sword-shaped. *X. cartilage.* That at the lower end of the sternum.

X-rays. Röntgen-rays. Electromagnetic waves of short length which are capable of penetrating many substances and of producing chemical changes and reactions in living matter. They are used to aid diagnosis and to treat disease.

xylol (*zi'-lol*). Xylene. Dimethylbenzene. A clear inflammable liquid resembling benzene. Used as a solvent for rubber and in microscopy.

xylose (*zi'-lose*). A pentose sugar not metabolized in the body. *X. absorption.* An oral dose is given and the urine collected for five hours. The amount of xylose present is proportional to that absorbed through the intestinal wall. It is a test for malabsorption.

XYY syndrome. Condition in males in which there is an extra Y chromosome making a total of 47. Often the affected individuals are very tall and liable to exhibit aggressive and anti-social behavioural patterns.

Y

yawning (*yaw'-ning*). A respiratory act the physiology of which is not understood. It may accompany tiredness and is infectious.

yaws (*yaws*). A skin infection common in tropical countries caused by the *Treponema pertenue*. Associated with dirt and poverty it is not a venereal disease though the Wassermann and Kahn tests are positive. *See* Framboesia.

Y-chromosome (*wi kro'-mo-some*). The chromosome present in some male gametes which determines the sex of the off-spring. *See* X-chromosome.

yeast (*yee-st*). Saccharomyces. A species of vegetable micro-organisms. They produce fermentation in malt, and in sweetened fruit juices, resulting in the formation of alcoholic solutions such as beer and wines. Thrush (*q.v.*) is due to infection by a species of yeast.

yellow fever. An acute, specific, infectious disease of the tropics, spread through the bite of a mosquito (*Aedes aegypti*). The incubation period varies from a few hours to several days, and the onset is marked by rigor, headache, pain in the back and limbs, high fever and black vomit. Haemorrhage from the intestinal mucous membrane may occur. There is a high mortality rate but vaccination with 17D virus vaccine gives active immunity for 7 years.

yellow ointment. *See* Ointment.

yellow spot. Macula lutea (*q.v.*).

yolk sac (*yoke sak*). Part of the chick embryo frequently used for cultivating micro-organisms in the laboratory.

Young's rule (*T. Young, British physician and physicist, 1773–1829*). To determine the dose of a drug suitable for a child from the adult dose.

yttrium (*it'-tre-um*). An element used as radioactive yttrium (^{90}Y) in the treatment of malignant effusions or to destroy remnants of the pituitary gland that cannot be removed by surgery.

Z

Zactirin (*zak'-tir-in*). An anal-gesic. A proprietary preparation of ethoheptazine.

Zarontin (*zar-on'-tin*). A proprietary preparation of ethosuximide, an anticonvulsant drug used in the treatment of petit mal epilepsy (*q.v.*).

Ziehl–Nielsen's stain (*F. Ziehl, German bacteriologist, 1857–1926: F. K. A. Nielsen, 1854–1894*). A method of staining tubercle bacilli for microscopic study.

zein (*ze'-in*). Maise protein.

zero. Nought. Nothing. The point on any scale from which measurements start.

zinc (*zink*). A bluish-white metallic element. *Z. chloride* is used as disinfectant for the treatment of ulcers, and as an astringent. *Z. acetate* is used in ophthalmia. *Z. sulphate* is given as an emetic. *Z. ointment* is an emollient dressing.

zingiber (*zin'-jib-er*). Ginger.

Zollinger–Ellison syndrome (*R. M. Zollinger, American physician, 1903– : E. H. Ellison, American physician, 1903– *). Condition in which a pancreatic tumour causes excessive outpouring of gastric juice.

zona (*zo'-nah*). (1) A zone. (2) Herpes zoster (*q.v.*). Shingles. *Z. facialis*. Herpes of the face. *Z. ophthalmica*. Herpes over the ophthalmic nerve.

Zondek–Aschheim test. *See* Aschheim–Zondek test.

zonular fibres (*zon'-u-lar*). The suspensory ligament that suspends the lens behind the iris. Zonules.

zonulolysis (*zon-u-lol'-is-is*). Dissolving the zonular fibres by zonulysin to aid cataract extraction.

zonulysin (*zon-u-li'-sin*). A proteolytic enzyme that may be used in eye surgery to dissolve the suspensory ligament.

zoology (*zo-ol'-o-je*). The science of animal life.

zoster (*zos'-ter*). *See* Herpes.

zygoma (*zi-go'-mah*). The arch formed by the union of the temporal with the malar bone in front of the ear.

zygote (*zi'-got*). A single fertilized cell formed from two gametes. *Dizygote* twins developed from two fertilized cells termed fraternal twins. *Monozygote* twins developed from the same cell termed identical twins.

zymosis (*zi-mo'-sis*). (1) Fermentation. (2) The development of infectious diseases.

zymotic (*zi-mot'-ik*). Relating to zymosis. *Z. disease*. A general term including all epidemic, contagious, and endemic diseases due to the action of microorganisms.

Z-plasty. A plastic operation for removing and repairing deformity resulting from a contraction scar.

APPENDIX 1

FIRST AID AND BANDAGING

FIRST AID

Nurses are not usually very knowledgeable about first aid, owing mainly to the fact that they rarely have to use the skills involved. In an emergency, however, valuable time can be saved, and further injury to the victim prevented, if the nurse or helper can quickly assess the situation and has a good knowledge of priorities and the most efficient treatment.

Medical assistance should be obtained as soon as possible and the helper should remember that only the minimum of treatment can be administered at the scene of an accident.

Unconsciousness

Unconsciousness may be due to many different causes, such as asphyxia, trauma, shock or poisoning, but in all cases the first two conditions to be treated are cessation of breathing and cessation of heart beat. The helper should note if there is continuing danger from fire, fumes, electric current or traffic and eliminate the source or remove the patient from it.

Next make sure the airway is clear by loosening constrictive clothing and clearing the mouth with the fingers; tilt the head backwards and draw the jaw forward. If breathing is established, place the patient in the semi-prone position (Fig. 1) and continue to observe him closely.

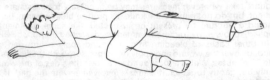

Fig. 1. The semi-prone position. The head is tilted slightly forward and no cushion is used.

Should breathing not resume immediately, expired air artificial respiration must be started without delay. Full details are given and illustrated on pp. 394–7.

After artificial respiration has been started by breathing into the patient's lungs three times, the pulse must be felt (Fig. 2) in order to establish whether the heart is beating and, if it is not, external cardiac massage must be begun. Full details of this is given on p. 397.

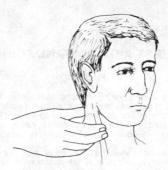

Fig. 2. Taking the carotid pulse.

Once the heart is beating and respiration has been established other measures can be taken.

Haemorrhage

External bleeding. When the bleeding is visible, examine the wound to see whether any cause, such as projecting metal or glass, can be seen. When there is danger that either may still be present in the wound, the area should be lightly covered with a clean cloth or first aid dressing (Fig. 3) while pressure, for not longer than 15 minutes, is applied to the artery proximal to the injury. In the event of a stab wound, take whatever measures may be necessary to resuscitate the patient, but do not remove the knife, as profuse bleeding may occur. Should a fracture be present or suspected, the same treatment is applied, followed by fracture treatment as described on pp. 389–90.

In other cases of bleeding from a wound apply a firm pad and bandage over the wound and apply direct pressure with the fingers for 5 to 15 minutes. With a large wound area press the sides of the wound firmly but gently together. If a limb is involved elevate the part. If the bleeding has been severe or shock is present treat as described below.

Internal bleeding. The signs of haemorrhage are an increasing pulse rate, pallor and deep sighing respirations. The patient will be restless and anxious and may complain of thirst, a feeling of faintness and blurred vision. This patient is in a state of shock due to depletion of circulating blood and the helper must treat this and at the same time send for a doctor.

Whilst waiting for medical aid, reassure and calm the patient, lay him flat with the head low. Cover him, but do not apply heat and give nothing by mouth. Record the pulse and respiration every 15 minutes.

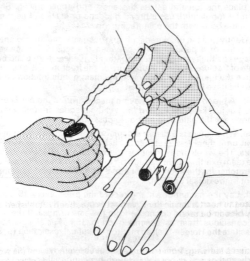

Fig. 3. Applying an improvised dressing to a wound to prevent further damage from an embedded fragment.

Fractures

Fractures may be either closed, simple fractures or compound fractures in which there is communication between the site of the fracture and the air through either the skin or a mucous surface. In the latter case the risk of infection entering the wound must be minimized and in treating any fractures the first aid worker must handle the injured part with great care in order that further damage may not be done.

Suspected fractures should be treated as fractures without trying to elicit signs of fracture such as unnatural mobility and crepitus. Cover any wound with as clean a dressing as is available and if there is much bleeding apply pressure to the arterial pressure point proximal to the wound. Give the treatment for shock.

Immobilize the fracture by moving the injured part as little as is necessary. Untrained workers are advised to use the body and slings for immobilizing the part.

Bandages should be checked every 15 minutes as they may become too tight owing to swelling of the injured tissues.

Arm and shoulder. If the elbow can be flexed without increasing the pain, place the forearm across the chest and apply a sling. Should flexion be too painful, use a broad bandage or scarf and tie the arm against the body with the palm facing inwards.

Leg. Gently pull the uninjured limb to rest against the injured one and place pads or a padded splint between the legs. With scarves or bandages tie the feet and knees together or the legs above and below the site of fracture, putting no pressure on the fracture. If it is necessary to move the injured limb, apply and maintain gentle traction until the two limbs have been tied together.

Pelvis. A broad folded cloth may be placed around the pelvis to give support or just keep the patient flat. As the bladder or urethra may be damaged ask the patient to try not to pass urine.

Spine. When there is a suspected injury to the spine do not move the patient until there is a stretcher available and a sufficient number of helpers. The whole body must be lifted or turned in unison with two of the team exerting slight traction on the head and feet. Place pads on the stretcher for the neck, lumbar curve, and ankles, and transport the patient in the dorsal position.

Skull. Lay the patient down and record the pulse every 15 minutes. Observe the condition of the eyes and pupils and note whether there is any bleeding or fluid discharge from the ears or nose. If the patient is unconscious treat as described on p. 394. Facial injuries may necessitate the Holger–Nielsen method of artifical respiration (p. 396).

Patients suffering from fractures should be removed to hospital as quickly and gently as possible. Rough handling will greatly increase the degree of shock.

Road Accidents

Carry out the following as required in descending order:
   Only remove the injured person (whether in a vehicle or on the roadway) if he is in danger, e.g. from fire or oncoming traffic. Unnecessary movement may worsen the injuries.

Send for help and whilst waiting:

   Treat asphyxia (p. 394)
   Treat cardiac arrest (p. 397)
   Arrest haemorrhage (p. 388)
   Keep the patient calm
   Immobilize fractures (p. 389)
   Cleanse and cover wounds

Poisoning

Take a quick note of the surroundings to establish the cause of the poisoning if possible and send for medical aid, stating the drug if known. If the patient is unconscious, notice whether he is breathing and whether his pulse can be felt. Should these signs be absent, follow the instructions on pp. 394–7. If respiration and circulation are present or restored but the patient is unconscious no attempt must be made to make him vomit and no stomach washout should be carried out until medical aid is present.

Corrosive poisoning. The lips may be stained grey or yellowish and the patient may have a burning pain in the mouth and throat, denoting that a corrosive has been taken. Do not make the patient vomit, but give demulcent drinks such as milk or egg white to soothe and dilute the poison. If an acid has been taken it can be neutralized by magnesium oxide or other alkali and an alkaline poison by giving diluted vinegar 100 ml to 0.5 litre of water.

Non-corrosive poisoning. When the poison taken is non-corrosive and the patient is conscious try to make him vomit by giving him copious amounts of salt and water and placing a finger or spoon handle at the back of the mouth.

Aspirin. Should the cause be aspirin or iron tablets an emetic may be given as a first aid measure before transport to hospital.

Barbiturates. Barbiturates and tranquillizers are commonly consumed poisons and the danger of overdosage is greatly increased if taken at the same time as alcohol. Drowsiness may cause accidental overdosage to be taken if the container is by the bedside.

Inhalation of poisonous gas. Where possible turn off the gas and remove the patient to the fresh air or an open window. Loosen tight clothing and begin artificial respiration and cardiac massage if required (p. 394).

Hospital care. Patients suffering from poisoning need the facilities available in hospital for their treatment and there should be no delay in transporting them there, guarding against shock and respiratory failure in transit.

Poison Information Centres

National Poisons Information Centres have been set up from which a doctor may obtain advice in a case where he is in doubt about the correct treatment for a particular drug. There are five centres altogether and their addresses are as follows:

London
Poisons Reference Service
New Cross Hospital
Avonley Road
London SE14 5ER
Tel. 01–407 7600

Edinburgh
Scottish Poisons Information
  Bureau
The Royal Infirmary
Lauriston Place
Edinburgh EH3 9YW
Tel. 031–229 2477

Cardiff
Poisons Information Centre
c/o Medical Records
  Department
Cardiff Royal Infirmary
Cardiff
South Glamorgan
Tel. 0222 33101

Belfast
Poisons Information Centre
Casualty Department
Royal Victoria Hospital
Grosvenor Road
Belfast BT12 6BA
Tel. 0232 30503

Dublin
Poisons Information Centre
Jarvis Street Hospital
Dublin
Tel. Dublin 745588

Burns

Extinguish burning clothing by smothering the flames with a rug or coat. Reassure and calm the patient and relatives while immersing the burnt part in cold water if feasible. Do not remove adherent burnt clothing but cover the area with a freshly laundered cotton article. Treat the patient for shock and transfer him to hospital as quickly as possible.

Chemical burns. To remove the chemical, wash the burnt area by flooding the part thoroughly with gallons of water to which a neutralizing agent may be added. Use slowly running water, ensuring that it drains away freely and safely. Remove contaminated clothing if possible at the same time. Treat an acid burn with a solution of sodium bicarbonate and a corrosive alkali burn with weak vinegar or lemon juice. Speed in treatment is essential: if obtaining the correct antidote would entail loss of time, the use of plain water is to be preferred; this particularly applies to splash injuries to the eye.

Scalds. Remove clothing if possible as this will retain the heat from the hot liquid. Run cold water over the scalded area in order to minimize the severity of the injury.

BANDAGING

Bandages are being used less but they still have a place in nursing. At the present time a wide choice of bandages is on the market and in deciding which bandage to use the nurse should consider the purpose for which it is to be applied, the comfort of the patient and the cost of the bandage. The following are some examples:

Roller Bandages
White openwove. The traditional bandage, which is used when a light bandage is required, and is normally discarded after use.

Domette. Domette is a mixture of cotton and wool. It is a strong bandage and may be used to apply pressure following an operation on the knee. A pressure bandage in this case consists of alternate layers of wool and bandage. It is a useful material for making up into many-tailed and T bandages, for making a collar and cuff sling and for dressing a Thomas' or Braun's splint.

Crêpe. This is an elasticated cotton bandage which has the advantage of conforming to body contours and giving a measure of support. It is useful as a head bandage following mastoidectomy or enucleation of the eye. It may also be used as a chest bandage following mastectomy or for the legs when a degree of pressure is required to aid venous return or to prevent oedema.

Elastic web. This bandage is often referred to as a blue- or red-line bandage from the coloured line appearing throughout its length. It is a strongly supporting bandage and is used on the lower limb for the treatment of varicose ulcers.

Rayon elastic. This has more elasticity than the plain crêpe and is advocated for application to amputation stumps to aid healing with the formation of a good firm stump by preventing oedema.

Conforming bandage. This is a very light bandage of fine cotton mesh and is particularly useful when a dressing requires supporting with the minimum of material and the avoidance of even slight pressure or the use of adhesive. This applies to the extremities when the blood supply to the area is much reduced.

Tubular Bandages

Tubular gauze. Light-weight bandages knitted in a tubular form that can be applied to any part of the body. In many cases a special applicator is required. The bandages can be applied with varying degrees of tension and they are cool and comfortable to wear. Tubular gauze is particularly recommended for finger and head dressings and where extensive covering is required in the treatment of skin disease.

Elastic net. This is a tubular mesh bandage of cotton and elastic fibres and stretches widely without becoming constrictive. It is a more expensive bandage but this is offset by the comfort to the patient in securing a dressing in an area that is awkward to bandage by the older methods. It can be applied to most areas of the body.

RESUSCITATION

In all conditions of unconsciousness, from whatever cause, the first consideration is maintenance of the airway. In hospital the commonest form of unconsciousness, apart from sleep, is that induced at operation, and every student is instructed at an early stage of her training in the care of these patients. The necessary equipment should always be at hand. This should include a mouth gag, an angled spatula, sponge-holding forceps and swabs and a tongue clip. Equipment for oxygen administration, for suction and for artificial respiration should also be available.

For the sake of safety, unconscious patients are best transported and placed in bed in the lateral or semi-prone position. This enables the tongue to fall forward, preventing blockage of the larynx, and allows the secretions to collect in the lower cheek or run out of the mouth. If this position is not possible, owing to the patient's condition, the angle of the jaw should be drawn forward and supported. The patient must be breathing quietly and adequately and no cyanosis should be present.

ARTIFICIAL RESPIRATION

Obstructed Airway

Should the breathing appear laboured, the nostrils dilated or the soft tissues of the neck and upper thorax be sucked inwards, obstruction of the airway must be suspected. The jaw and tongue should be drawn forward, but if this does not relieve the obstruction, a gag must be inserted, the tongue drawn forward and the back of the throat cleared using swabs and sponge-holding forceps. This emergency is unlikely to arise with good positioning of the patient, but it may occur owing to inhalation of food or foreign bodies. If immediate steps are not taken to dislodge the obstruction, either by sweeping the finger across the back of the throat or, as in the case of a child, holding his head down and giving him a few taps on the back of the chest, asphyxia may easily result.

Cessation of Breathing

If breathing has ceased, artificial respiration must be started at once to supply oxygen to the blood and the blood must reach the brain within 3 minutes or irreparable damage will be done.

Expired Air Artificial Respiration

Mouth-to-nose Respiration (Fig. 4)
(1) Sweep the finger round the back of the patient's mouth to remove any obstructing matter.

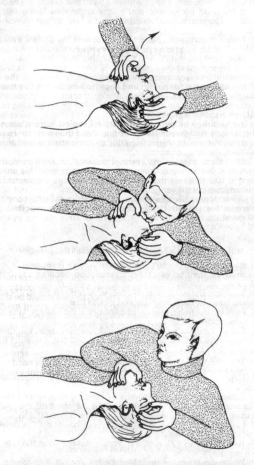

Fig. 4. Expired-air artificial respiration by the mouth-to-nose method.

(2) Grasp the patient's head with one hand and extend his neck by pressing his head backwards and at the same time lifting his jaw upwards and forwards with the other hand. Close his mouth with the thumb.

(3) Take a deep breath, place the mouth over the patient's nostrils and exhale forcibly into his lungs. Chest expansion should be observed.

(4) Withdraw the mouth and take another deep breath while the patient exhales. Repeat the cycle 10 to 12 times a minute. The first six breaths should be given as rapidly as possible.

(5) In a child both his mouth and nose may be covered by the lips and the breaths should be gentler.

Mouth-to-mouth Respiration

This method may be preferred, in which case the patient's nostrils should be closed by pressing with the finger and thumb and the breath exhaled into his mouth. Apart from this the procedure is the same as for mouth-to-nose respiration.

An *artificial mouthpiece and airway*, if available, may be used. Draw the patient's jaw forward, open his mouth and insert the airway, directing it first towards the roof of the mouth and then rotating it downwards behind the tongue.

The stomach may become blown up with air, especially if the head is not properly extended. If this occurs, apply pressure over the upper part of the abdomen.

Holger–Nielsen Method of Artificial Respiration

This method (Fig. 5) may be suitably used when it is impossible to use the expired air method of artificial respiration because the face is smashed.

(1) With the patient prone, flex his arms and rest his forehead on his hands, so as to keep the nose and mouth free.

(2) Kneel at the head, placing one knee near the head and the other foot by the elbow.

(3) Place the hands over the shoulder blades, with the thumbs touching on the midline and the fingers spread out, the arms being kept straight (Fig. 5A).

(4) Bend forward with arms straight, applying light pressure, while counting 'one, two, three' (Fig. 5B). This is expiration.

(5) Release pressure gradually and slide the hands to just above the elbows of the patient. Count 'four'.

(6) Raise the arms and shoulders by bending backwards until you feel resistance and tension, without lifting the chest off the ground, while counting 'five, six, seven' (Fig. 5C). This is inspiration.

(7) Lay the arms down and replace your hands on the patient's back while counting 'eight'.

(8) Repeat (3) to (7) with a rhythmic movement at the rate of 9 times a minute.

(9) When breathing is re-established, carry out arm raising and lowering (6 and 7 above) alone, 12 times a minute. Arm-raising—one, two, three (inspiration). Arm-lowering—four, five, six (expiration).

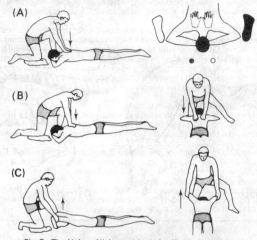

Fig. 5. The Holger–Nielsen method of artificial respiration.

Manual Resuscitators

There are several simple devices that can be manually operated to maintain respiration by blowing air into the lungs. Two examples are the Ambu resuscitator and Oxford inflator (Fig. 6).

Where artificial respiration has to be maintained for a prolonged period, these methods are inadequate and a power-driven mechanical respirator is required.

EXTERNAL CARDIAC MASSAGE

Once the lungs have been inflated several times, the operator must feel for the patient's pulse in the carotid artery, or on the radial or femoral pressure point. Should no pulse be present cardiac arrest has occurred and another helper must start external cardiac massage. If no assistant is present the operator must carry out artificial respiration and cardiac massage alternately.

(1) Place the patient on a firm surface, e.g. the floor, a trolley, or a board placed on a bed.

(2) Place the heel of one hand on the lower third of the patient's sternum and superimpose the other hand upon it.

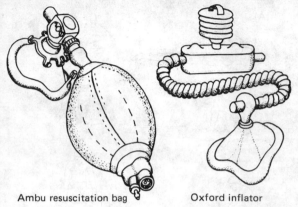

Ambu resuscitation bag   Oxford inflator

Fig. 6. Resuscitators.

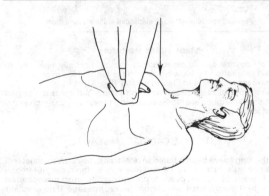

Fig. 7. External cardiac massage.

(3) Depress the sternum rhythmically 3 to 4 cm towards the spine and repeat 50 or 60 times per minute until the patient's circulation becomes re-established.

This procedure entails the risk of fracturing the ribs, a factor which makes practice difficult, and should not be carried out unless necessary. However models are available and the operator can check the success of his efforts, as blood pressure readings can be taken and the lungs can be seen to inflate.

RESPIRATION AND ADMINISTRATION OF OXYGEN

RESPIRATION

The oxygen supply to the tissues depends on many factors. There must be adequate respiratory effort so that sufficient air is inhaled. Alveolar lung tissue must be healthy to enable diffusion of oxygen into the blood and of carbon dioxide from the blood into the alveoli for expiration. Moreover there must be sufficient red blood cells to transport the oxygen to the tissues and adequate cardiac output to propel the blood round the circulation, and the calibre of the blood vessels must be such that the blood can reach the whole body.

This chain of events may be broken at any one of the stages and this will cause oxygen deficiency, with or without carbon dioxide accumulation. For example, when the lung tissue is impaired there is difficulty in oxygenating the blood and in eliminating carbon dioxide; hence the patient will be breathless and cyanosed. In severe anaemia there are insufficient red blood cells to carry the oxygen, but the carbon dioxide is transported in the plasma and does not accumulate in the blood.

Impairment in function of any of the links in the oxygen transport chain may necessitate administration of oxygen. The choice of method will vary with the cause of the oxygen insufficiency.

The air passages are never entirely free from air. At the end of expiration they hold about 150 ml of air which, on inspiration, will be the first to enter the alveoli, followed, in quiet respiration, by 250 ml of fresh air. However, part of the inhaled air never enters the depths of the lungs but remains in the area known as the anatomical dead space where no gas exchange can take place (i.e. the trachea and main bronchi down as far as the bronchioles) (Fig. 8). The volume retained at the end of inspiration is about 150 ml but varies with the depth of breathing. It is referred to as the effective dead space and on expiration it is the first air to be expelled, followed by 200 ml from the alveoli. This still leaves 150 ml in the respiratory passages, the so-called alveolar gas or alveolar air. Coming from the alveoli it has a high carbon dioxide content (5.5 per cent as compared with 0.04 per cent in atmospheric air) and a low oxygen content (14 per cent as compared with 20 per cent in atmospheric air).

ADMINISTRATION OF OXYGEN

There are two groups of patients requiring oxygen therapy. Those who need it in controlled amounts and those who need it in high concentration.

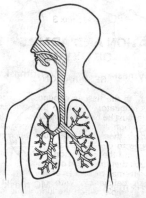

Fig. 8. Pulmonary dead space (hatched area).

Controlled oxygen therapy. Used for patients with a degree of respiratory failure, mainly those with chronic bronchitis. Such patients may need a low arterial oxygen level as a stimulus for them to maintain respiration. Too large an amount of inspired oxygen will raise the blood level and abolish this stimulus, stopping respiration and causing carbon dioxide retention, with resultant coma. These patients should be given only 24 to 28 per cent oxygen, which will raise the blood level without stopping respiration (*see* Ventimask).

High percentage oxygen therapy. Used for patients who have a low arterial oxygen level not due to respiratory failure; such as those with heart failure or low blood pressure and postoperative patients. Oxygen (30 to 60 per cent) is required, but provided it is high enough the percentage does not need to be carefully controlled.

Methods of Administration

Masks

Polymask and Pneumask. These are cheap soft plastic disposable masks in which considerable rebreathing takes place, thus creating a large dead space, so that with flow rates of 10 litres per minute, carbon dioxide retention may occur.

Ventimask. The Ventimask is a plastic disposable mask which gives a consistent alveolar concentration of oxygen and there is no rebreathing. The thin stream of oxygen draws in a good volume of air, which helps to flush out the dead space air. It is the best type of face mask for use where there is serious impairment of lung ventilation.

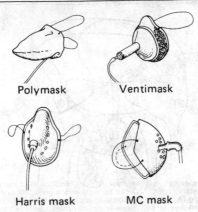

Polymask Ventimask

Harris mask MC mask

Fig. 9. Oxygen masks.

There are three models giving a controlled intake of 24 or 28 per cent at 4 litres of oxygen per minute, or 35 per cent oxygen at a flow rate of 8 litres per minute.

Harris mask. The Harris mask is a stiff transparent plastic disposable mask with good air entry holes. It does not cause rebreathing or increase the dead space air. Where a controlled intake is not necessary it is a cheaper model than the Ventimask.

MC and Edinburgh masks. These are transparent semi-rigid plastic masks, comfortable to wear and very useful if no controlled oxygen percentage is required as the concentration does vary with the lung ventilation. There is some rebreathing but less than with soft plastic masks.

Nasal Catheters
Nasal catheters used with a humidifier have the advantage that there is no rebreathing and oxygen administration can be continued during meals. The percentage of oxygen received is considerably higher if the patient breathes through the nose than through the mouth. The catheters need to be cleaned and lubricated regularly.

Tracheostomy or Endotracheal Tubes
Oxygen may, if required, be given to a patient who has undergone tracheostomy by means of a mask which fits over the tube (Fig. 10).

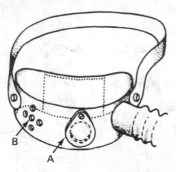

Fig. 10. A Perspex tracheostomy mask (Vickers Medical) to fit round the neck over a tracheostomy opening. It can be used with a humidifier and there is a separate opening (A) to allow suction to be carried out. The holes (B) allow the escape of carbon dioxide and provide an air entry should there be a failure in the oxygen supply.

If oxygen is administered in this way, humidification of the gas is required to prevent the mucous membrane from drying. This can be done by attaching a humidifier (Fig. 11) to the flowmeter on the oxygen cylinder or to a wall supply. The humidifier can also be used as a nebulizer to administer drugs.

Oxygen Tents

In modern oxygen tents every effort has been made to control the oxygen concentration, the carbon dioxide content, the humidity and the temperature. The control of oxygen concentration is not easy as the patient treated in a tent is the very person who requires repeated physiotherapy and nursing attention which necessitates opening the tent. With improved tracheostomy and endotracheal care the tents are used less often than formerly, but are still useful for young children or adults who cannot tolerate a face mask or nasal catheters.

Mechanical Respirators

The intermittent positive-pressure machine. This machine by which air is blown into the lungs is, at present, the most favoured method for maintaining artificial respiration. A tracheostomy is frequently performed first and a cuffed tracheostomy tube inserted. This has the advantage of protecting the bronchi from the entry of secretions and makes removal of normal secretions by suction much easier. The air can be humidified and the oxygen content varied according to the needs of the individual patient. The nurse can then

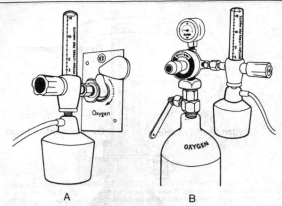

Fig. 11. An oxygen humidifier. A, Attached to the wall supply. B, Attached to an oxygen cylinder.

attend to all the patient's other bodily requirements quite easily and there is no restriction of movement of the limbs.

This type of artificial respiration is used for a great variety of conditions where the patient cannot adequately maintain normal breathing or where the nerve supply to the pharyngeal muscles is impaired and the protective mechanisms of the larynx are lost.

Nursing Observations

During oxygen administration the nurse should observe the rate and depth of respiration, the rate and strength of the pulse and the colour of the skin. A patient who becomes pink, who is difficult to rouse and whose respiration has become shallow and infrequent is likely to be suffering from a serious degree of carbon dioxide retention.

The apparatus used should be checked frequently to ensure that it is working correctly. Precautions must be taken against the risk of fire. No smoking must therefore be allowed in the vicinity and antistatic precautions must be observed. See Appendix 4.

Hyperbaric Oxygen

This is oxygen under increased pressure and allows more oxygen to be carried in the blood. Normally the haemoglobin in the red blood cells is fully oxygenated on leaving the lungs and the amount of oxygen carried can only be increased by increasing the number of red blood cells. If the pressure of oxygen is increased then oxygen is dissolved in the plasma and so transported to the tissues. Raised atmospheric

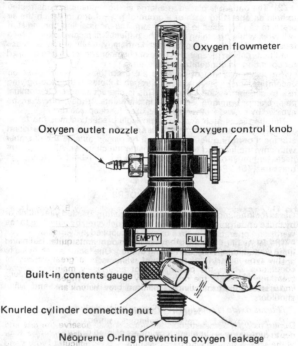

Oxygen flowmeter

Oxygen outlet nozzle

Oxygen control knob

EMPTY FULL

Built-in contents gauge

Knurled cylinder connecting nut

Neoprene O-ring preventing oxygen leakage

Fig. 12. Oxygen safety regulator and flowmeter (Vickers Medical).

pressure increases the partial pressures of the individual gases that comprise it, in proportion to their percentage of the whole. These gases are chiefly oxygen and nitrogen. Hyperbaric oxygen may be administered in two ways:

(1) The patient is placed in an individual chamber or capsule with a transparent canopy in which the oxygen pressure will be raised. He can, however, remain in the chamber for only limited periods since nursing treatment cannot be carried out while he is enclosed. This type of chamber has been used with success for persons suffering from gas gangrene, frostbite and carbon monoxide poisoning.

Radiotherapy may be carried out with the patient in an hyperbaric oxygen capsule. The increased oxygen supply to the tumour cells renders them more susceptible to radiation.

(2) The patient is placed in a large air-tight chamber constructed to hold an operating team or a group of patient and in which the air pressure can be raised to 2, 3 or 4 atm. The medical and nursing staff will work while breathing air but the patient will receive oxygen by a face mask. With the exception of radiotherapy, treatment for all these conditions can be given in this type of chamber and it can also be used for operating on congenital heart lesions.

If more than 2 atm of pressure are used there is serious risk on decompression of the release of nitrogen bubbles in the blood giving rise to decompression sickness. This is characterized by abdominal pain, cramp, vomiting, and pain in the joints. It may, however, be avoided by slow decompression, as used for deep-sea divers.

The fire risk is high and every possible precaution must be taken against a spark discharge. All towels and clothing must be fire-resistant and the monitoring equipment must be placed outside the chamber with only the leads to the patient inside the chamber. All equipment necessary must be tested to ensure that it is suitable for use at high pressures. (See Plate VIII.)

GAS CYLINDERS

Gases for inhalation, either by patients requiring assisted ventilation or by those undergoing anaesthesia, may be delivered by pipe-line to the wards and operating theatres or may be supplied in cylinders.

The safety of patients is always of paramount importance, but never more so than when gases are being utilized. One factor which helps to ensure safety is the colour coding of cylinders:

Oxygen is supplied in cylinders painted black with white shoulders.

Air is supplied in cylinders painted grey with black and white shoulders.

Nitrous oxide is supplied in cylinders painted blue.

Carbon dioxide is supplied in cylinders painted grey.

Cyclopropane is supplied in cylinders painted orange.

APPENDIX 4

STATIC ELECTRICITY AND ANTISTATIC PRECAUTIONS

Static electricity is produced by two different surfaces being in close association or rubbing against each other, so that the objects become electrically charged. This charge may be built up so that a spark discharge of electricity may occur. This may give rise to an unpleasant sensation or cause minor accidents such as the spilling of hot fluids; if it happens in the vicinity of oxygen or other explosive anaesthetic vapours it may cause a serious explosion. Thus the question of static electricity is an important one in the anaesthetic room and operating theatre or where oxygen is being administered.

If the substances charged are good conductors of electricity or are in contact with good conductors the charge will drain away and not be built up. Water is a good conductor so that in a humid atmosphere sparks of static electricity are less likely to occur and an electric charge is unlikely to be built up on a moist surface. Conversely, a dry atmosphere (particularly where there is central heating), dry blankets, mackintoshes and rubber surfaces are poor conductors and an electric spark may easily occur.

When a patient is conveyed to the theatre on a metal trolley with ordinary rubber tyres and rubber sheeting and is covered by blankets, and the attendants are wearing rubber shoes or the floor is of non-conducting material, a powerful charge of static electricity can be built up.

Similarly, nylon in contact with the skin can build up an electric charge, and this can happen as well when garments are of different materials, e.g. wool next to nylon or nylon next to artifical silk. Most nurses will have experienced the crackling that occurs on removing garments that have become electrically charged.

PRECAUTIONS

To minimize the risks attached to a spark discharge, special precautions should be taken:

(1) An antistatic rubber has been manufactured in which carbon particles are impregnated in the rubber and these particles drain away the electric charge. The carbon particles colour the rubber black and in Great Britain this is identified by a bright yellow disc or patch. This yellow may be seen on the wheels of trolleys fitted with antistatic tyres or on the toecaps of antistatic theatre boots. Rubber tubing and fittings for the anaesthetic machine are now made of antistatic rubber and the Langdon Hewer antislip theatre table mattress is of corrugated antistatic rubber.

(2) An earthing chain trailing from trolley to floor is another safeguard, which is effective as long as the floor is a good conductor. It is important that the floors in hospitals should be made of conductive material or incorporate metal strips.

(3) The relative humidity in the air should be kept above 60 per cent since below this hazards are greater. Humidity can be measured by means of a hygrometer.

APPENDIX 5

METHODS OF STERILIZATION

HEAT STERILIZATION

Autoclave

Autoclaving, or sterilization by steam under pressure, is a very effective way of destroying organisms and spores, and is the method of choice for all linen or cotton articles, surgeons' and nurses' gowns and towels. Dressing packs, or any pack incorporating absorbent wool dressing, or absorbent gauze or cotton wool balls, should be sterilized by this method. It is also suitable for glass, metal and rubber articles. Polypropylene, a plastic from which measures, kidney dishes and bowls may be made, can be sterilized in this way but many other plastics are damaged by autoclaving.

The temperature reached inside the autoclave will depend on the efficiency of the vacuum created and the pressure of the steam. The greater the vacuum and the higher the pressure, the higher will be the temperature reached and the shorter the time necessary for sterilization. The nature of the load must be considered so that there is complete penetration by the steam. High-vacuum high-pressure autoclaves are machines in which a high vacuum is rapidly created by an electric pump. For sterilizing dressings, gowns and towels in such a machine, a vacuum of 75 cm is created and steam under pressure is introduced for a preliminary warming, then a second vacuum is drawn and steam at 13.5 kg pressure is let in. This will raise the temperature to 135°C where it is held for 3.5 minutes. A third vacuum draws off the steam and the articles are left to dry. The whole cycle is fully automatic and takes between 20 and 28 minutes.

Small machines can be installed in ward or theatre units to sterilize smooth articles such as instruments. Penetration is not required, so no preliminary warming or drying time is necessary and the whole cycle takes 6 minutes.

Hot Air Oven

Dry heat in a hot air oven may be used for sterilization. Dry heat requires a higher temperature for efficient sterilization than moist heat, and that commonly used is 160°C for 1 hour. This method is suitable for delicate eye instruments and for syringes. The instruments or syringes are thoroughly washed and dried and individually packed in glass tubes or aluminium containers; the latter are labelled or the plastic or tinfoil seal may bear the size or be of a distinctive colour. The plastic seal is applied as the warm tube is removed from the cabinet.

Boiling

Though water at boiling point can kill all non-spore-forming pathogenic bacteria in 2 minutes, spores cannot be killed by this method and boiling in ward boilers (no longer miscalled sterilizers) is open to much abuse. Frequently the articles are not completely immersed in the boiling water and the sterilizing time may have been interrupted by the insertion of contaminated articles. Articles not required tend to be left in the boiler accumulating a coating of lime deposits which will interfere with the sterilizing process. Boilers are still used in wards which cannot yet be supplied by a Central Supply Sterilizing Department.

Boiling is a useful method where speedy decontamination is required for tracheostomy inner tubes or by individuals dealing with their own hypodermic or insulin syringes. In all cases the articles should be completely immersed in the water so that the water can come in contact with all surfaces and the 2 minutes boiling time must be taken after the water has reached boiling point.

Cystoscopes labelled 'boilable' may safely be treated by this method between cases, but those not so labelled are damaged by boiling as the cement used to fix the lens in position cannot withstand so high a temperature, although it can withstand a temperature of 75°C. This temperature is sufficient to kill the organisms with which the cystoscope is likely to be contaminated, and which may be the cause of cross infection from one patient to another. If a thermostat is fitted to the boiler the water can be kept at a constant temperature of 75°C and the cystoscopes can be immersed for 10 minutes between cases. This has proved a very satisfactory method of decontamination during a cystoscopy clinic. It is termed pasteurization.

RADIATION

Infra-red Radiation

This is an alternative method of sterilization for syringes. The packed syringes are placed on a shallow tray and fed on to a conveyor belt and are slowly passed through the source of heat to emerge the other end. If there is a heavy demand for syringes this method can give a more even flow and the infra-red machine can do the work of a number of hot air ovens. In spite of the initial cost this can be a cheaper method than using disposable syringes when there is sufficient demand.

Gamma Radiation

Gamma radiation, released from radioactive cobalt, is used commercially as a method of sterilization. Many plastic disposable articles, syringes, catheters, Ryle's and oesophageal tubes and plastic tracheostomy tubes are prepacked and gamma irradiated for the manufacturers at the Atomic Energy Research Laboratory at Wantage in Berkshire.

CHEMICAL STERILIZATION

To sterilize an article, a chemical must have the power to kill all types of bacteria and the spores that any of them produce. This ability will depend on the type of chemical, the strength used and the time in which it is in contact with the articles to be sterilized. The presence of organic matter such as blood or faeces will prevent effective action by the germicide. Such chemical agents should not harm the tissues or cause deterioration in the articles for which they are used. With the foregoing methods of sterilization available there is little need for chemical sterilization and it is now being used less widely.

Formalin

Formalin cabinets are used in theatre units to sterilize electrical equipment such as flexes and light bulbs, and for the outside of ampoules, but they should not be used if the ampoule contains fluid for intrathecal or intravenous use. Solid formalin is placed in a container in the base of the cabinet and heat causes a rapid sublimation to formalin gas, which will kill bacteria and spores as long as it comes in contact with all surfaces. Silk web catheters and endoscopic instruments may be treated by this method, but two dangers are present: the formalin may not penetrate down the long tube, and it is a very irritating substance to the tissues if rinsing should prove inadequate.

Formalin may be incorporated in an autoclave for decontamination of mattresses and bedding and in instrument solution to prevent the growth of organisms in storage solutions for glass ampoules or tinfoil packs or for handling forceps.

Chlorine and Chlorine Compounds

These are effective in killing bacteria and spores so long as no organic matter is present and in the form of hypochlorite solution may be used for sterilizing clean glassware or for disinfection of baths, basins, lavatory seats, etc. A 0.5 to 1.0 per cent solution of available chlorine is necessary. Deosan is a crude hypochlorite solution suitable for disinfecting purposes, but Milton 1:80 is to be preferred for sterilizing glassware and babies' feeding bottles. Milton may also be used for the irrigation of wounds.

Chlorhexidine (Hibitane)

Chlorhexidine is an antiseptic which is bacteriostatic and bactericidal and is non-injurious to tissues. It may be used for skin cleansing or disinfection in a 1 per cent solution or for bladder irrigation 0.02 per cent (1:5000). It is supplied as a bactericidal cream or added to other disinfectants to enhance their effect. Savlon consists of cetrimide 0.5 per cent and chlorhexidine 0.05 per cent and is popular in midwifery practice.

Cetrimide (Cetavlon)

Cetrimide is a good skin cleansing agent and is effective against many organisms but not the tubercle bacilli or spores. It should not be stored in bottles with corks which in themselves may be a source of contamination.

Hexachlorophene

Hexachlorophene 1.0 per cent in soap causes a great reduction in bacteria recovered from the skin and is being used widely in skin preparation before operation, for the patient, the surgeon and the nurse. pHisoHex solution and Ster-Zac powder both contain hexachlorophene.

Proflavine Hemisulphate

Proflavine is slowly bactericidal and may be used with effect for wound cleansing to prevent sepsis arising.

Alcohol

A 70 per cent solution with water is the most effective strength in killing bacteria but it does not kill spores. Isopropanol is 70 per cent isopropyl alcohol and is the alcohol of choice for skin cleansing. Industrial methylated spirit is a 95 per cent solution and is much less effective as without the water it cannot penetrate the surface to kill the organisms. Though this preparation may be used for individual syringes it is not recommended for ward storage of either instruments or syringes.

Sudol

Sudol is a proprietary coal tar derivative which is less likely to cause burn injuries than Lysol, which it resembles. It is an efficient disinfectant where crude disinfection is required. As a 10 per cent solution it can be mixed with infected excreta for one hour before disposal or for disinfecting bedpans or lavatory brush jars.

Glutaraldehyde

Glutaraldehyde is a potent antimicrobial agent particularly against hepatitis viruses. It is, however, expensive and unstable in the pH range where it is effective. It is used in a 2 per cent solution for soaking bedpans and urinals of patients with hepatitis. The equipment must be soaked for 1 hour.

Ethylene Oxide Gas

Effective sterilization may be achieved when this vapour is used in rigidly controlled conditions of humidity and pressure. Some substances such as rubber absorb the ethylene oxide, so time must be allowed for the gas to disperse. Articles that may be sterilized by this method include embolectomy catheters, cardiac pacemakers, cryothermy electrodes and probes and heart valve prostheses.

Disinfection of bulky equipment such as respirators, incubators and suction machines can be achieved by allowing them to cycle for 24 hours in an atmosphere of 10 per cent ethylene oxide.

CENTRAL SUPPLY STERILIZING DEPARTMENT

From the foregoing it will be seen that the most efficient methods of sterilization are those employing heat or radiation and where the most expensive equipment is required. If this equipment is assembled in a central department under the supervision of a senior member of the staff there should be a more uniform efficiency in the sterilization and the cost of the equipment is more economic. At the same time great advances have been made in the manufacture of disposable equipment to cut down the labour costs and laundry.

In planning a department considerable thought must go into the arrangement of the production line. Non-disposable equipment is received into the dirty area, where it is sorted and mechanically washed, either in a washing machine or in an ultrasonic washer where vibrations loosen the dirt. Then it is rinsed off. From the washers the articles are placed on trays in a drying cabinet before they are packed. The packing area should be so arranged that the articles are readily to hand at a comfortable height for the packers, who must be well drilled in the packing procedure. This must be uniform and reliable so that the user of the pack may know the contents and be able to open it without contaminating the articles it contains.

Some departments favour the method where each article is separately wrapped while others favour standard basic packs with separate packing of additional articles that may be required. Most packs are double-wrapped, first in bonded fibre (strong paper) and then in paper bags. Theatre packs have a third dust wrapping that is removed when the pack is taken from the theatre pack store before it is conveyed to the theatre. The packs are sealed with indicator tape which shows that the pack has been through the autoclave. The prepared packs should be placed directly in perforated containers that will fit into the autoclave.

It is a great advantage if the laundry can work closely with the Central Supply Sterilizing Department particularly residing surgeons' and nurses' gowns and towels and theatre drapes so that after washing they can be inspected, mended and folded before returning to the department for packing.

THE METRIC SYSTEM AND SI UNITS

METRIC SYSTEM

Opinion in favour of adopting the metric system in Great Britain in preference to the older English systems of measurement gradually gained strength during the first half of this century, when it was argued that there would be many advantages to be obtained from using the same methods of measurement as were used in most other countries. This argument has become increasingly valid as closer social, economic and political links have been established between the United Kingdom and western Europe.

There is also much to commend the replacing of lengthy and poorly understood systems by simpler ones, provided there is no loss of efficiency. Such views were held by the rulers of France at the end of the eighteenth century, for it was they who introduced the metric system into Europe in a successful bid to simplify matters. At that time there were not just a few units of measurement which could and did confuse the populace, but no fewer than two hundred standards of weight alone, and no matter how conservative one's views might be, it was obvious that such a state of affairs should not be allowed to continue.

In 1790 an invitation was extended from France to Great Britain to share in a common system of weights and measures, but no action was taken. However, in Europe and elsewhere the metric system gained rapid acceptance. An international treaty, the Metric Convention, was signed in 1875 by seventeen countries and by the United Kingdom in 1884. More than 90 per cent of the world's population are now using the metric system of measurement, although its full implementation in this country has still not been achieved.

In 1965, following a request from the Confederation of British Industries, the Government finally agreed to introduce the metric system. The target date for the completion of the changeover was set at 1975 and, in order to facilitate this, the Metrication Board was set up in 1969. For a variety of reasons, the target was not achieved, although metrication of the pound sterling was effected in 1971, and many prepacked goods have been sold in metric quantities since 1975. In 1978, however, it was decided that the planned legislation to enforce completion of the change by 1981 should not be pursued and so the target date has now been delayed indefinitely.

The National Health Service started the changeover to metrication by introducing the system for the handling of pharmaceutical preparations. Once nurses became accustomed to administering drugs in metric doses they quickly realized that the system was easier to understand than the traditional weights and measures.

There is one basic unit for each property to be measured, such as weight or volume. The size of a unit can be expressed as a multiple of ten or as tenths of a larger amount. This method of expression is much easier than previously used methods as it requires only an adjustment of the decimal point. Furthermore each unit is based on a definite measurable and fixed standard and not as formerly on a variable and ill-defined quantity like the length of an arm from elbow to finger-tip, or the weight of a grain of wheat.

SI UNITS

The Système International d'Unités was introduced to British hospitals on 1 December 1975 despite much protest. The history of this system dates back to the early part of this century. After the introduction of the metric system in western Europe, the original basic units were found to be inadequate. There were three of these for length, mass and time, namely the centimetre, the gram and the second. Accordingly, three more units were added and these were the metre, the kilogram and the ampere.

Fifty years later the system was again found to be inadequate to deal with the vast amount of scientific knowledge which had been acquired during this century, probably a greater increase than at any time in our history. It was therefore decided that a system was required which would encompass present and, it was hoped, future needs: so, in the 1960s, an international organization was established which was named the General Conference on Weights and Measures. This body revised and extended the existing system and called it the Système International d'Unités. This system is now used by scientists throughout the world, but its use in hospitals in the UK has come very late. The generally accepted name for the system is SI units.

Basic Units

The SI system comprises seven basic units from which calculations can be made. The definitions of these are as follows:

Kilogram (kg). The kilogram is based on the weight of a cylinder of platinum iridium which is kept in France at Sèvres, near Paris. The use of this was adopted in 1875.

Metre (m). The international metre was adopted for use in 1962 and is based on the wavelength of an orange line in the krypton spectrum.

Second (s). The unit is now based on the frequency of radiation of the caesium atom.

Ampere (A). This unit is based on the attractive force produced when an electric current flows through two straight and parallel conductors which are 1 metre apart.

Degree Kelvin (K). The degree Kelvin is described in relation to degrees Celsius (centigrade). Absolute zero $0°K = -273.15°C$. For practical purposes degrees Celsius will continue to be used. Body temperature $38°C$ is equal to $311°K$.

Candela (cd). A candela is described as 1/60th of the luminous intensity per square metre of platinum at 1773°C.

Mole (mol). A mole is described as the amount of substance which contains the same number of elementary units as there are atoms to be found in 12 g of carbon 12. In practical terms a mole is the molecular weight of a substance expressed in grams. As this unit is of great importance in medicine, further explanation will be given later.

Derived Units

In addition to the seven basic units there are a number which have been obtained or derived from a combination of these. They are as follows:

Newton (N). The newton is the force which will accelerate a mass of 1 kilogram by 1 metre a second per second.

Pascal (Pa). The pascal is a unit of pressure which is derived by relating force to area, and results from the application of 1 newton per square metre. This should be the unit for the recording of blood pressure, but the old method of using mmHg will still continue as the expense of changing every sphygmomanometer is at the moment prohibitive. Blood gas estimations will, however, be expressed in kilopascals (kPa).

Joule (J). The joule is described as the potential energy which is released when 1 kg weight falls through 1 m by the force of gravity. The joule is the alternative unit to the calorie as the measure of nutritional energy. The Metrication Board have, however, decided to retain the calorie for the present, which means that two units are now being used because hospitals had already effected the change by the time that this decision was taken.

As the joule is smaller than the calorie, dieticians (who have long been using the Calorie, or kilocalorie) are using the kilojoule which is one thousand times greater than the joule. While the change over is being effected there will be a period during which there may be considerable confusion. In order to ameliorate this situation the conversion from calories to joules is given below:

$$1 \text{ calorie} = 4.184 \text{ joules}$$
$$1000 \text{ Calories} = 1 \text{ Calorie or kilocalorie}$$
$$1 \text{ Calorie} = 4184 \text{ joules or } 4.184 \text{ kilojoules}$$
$$1000 \text{ Calories} = 4184 \text{ kilojoules}$$

Litre (l). The unit of volume is the cubic metre (m^3). This, however, is too large for use in biochemistry and so the cubic decimetre (1000 cubic centimetres) has been substituted. The universally accepted term for this is the litre, and it will continue to be used in medicine. Most nurses have been familiar with the litre for a considerable time since it has been common practice to measure the fluid intake and output of patients in this way. In common usage litre is best not abbreviated, to avoid confusion with the numeral 1.

Millimole (mmol). Since the introduction of SI units, the majority of biochemical results have been expressed in millimoles per litre, and it is the unit which causes the greatest confusion.

It is useful at this point to return to the definition of the mole. A mole is the molecular weight of a substance expressed in grams. For example sodium chloride comprises one atom of sodium and one of chlorine. The molecular weight of sodium is 23 and that of chlorine 35.5, and so molecular weight of sodium chloride is $23 + 35.5 = 58.5$. A mole of sodium chloride is therefore 58.5 g.

The mole is a very large unit and is impractical for use in biochemistry. As a result, the unit that is most commonly used in medicine is the millimole, which is one thousand times smaller. It is used for substances, such as potassium chloride, which are added to intravenous infusions, as well as for the results of laboratory investigations. Concentrations are given in millimoles per litre (mmol/litre).

If the exact molecular weight of a substance is uncertain, the molar system cannot be used. This means that the concentration of a substance has still to be expressed in grams or milligrams per litre. One such substance is serum protein, which instead of being expressed in grams per 100 ml (g%) is now expressed in grams per litre. For example, a reading of serum protein at 7 g/100 ml will now be recorded as 70 g/litre. Haemoglobin, which is a complex molecule, will be expressed, as hitherto, in grams per 100 millilitres (g/100 ml).

Many of the electrolyte readings will appear to be the same in the new units as in the old. This is due to their chemical structure, for they are monovalent, which means that the atoms concerned have the power to combine with only one other atom. This means that the figures for the normal values of these remain unchanged, but it must be remembered that the units in which they are being expressed have altered. For example the normal range of plasma sodium was previously expressed as 135–143 milliequivalents but is now 135–143 millimoles per litre.

Rules for Use of SI Units

In order to reduce the margin of error, the General Conference on Weights and Measures stipulated the way in which the symbols should be abbreviated and written down. It was decided that the abbreviations should not alter in the plural.

Therefore when describing weight:

> One kilogram = 1 kg
> Ten kilograms = 10 kg

It is *incorrect* to add an 's' to the symbol.

Multiples and Submultiples

Multiples and submultiples are formed by using prefixes, e.g.

> 1 milligram = 1/1000th of 1 gram
> 1 kilogram = 1 gram × 1000

Time

Time is always expressed in seconds and is not converted into minutes and hours.

Decimal Points

The decimal point is shown as a full stop on the line. A raised point now indicates a multiplication sign. In addition, in western Europe, it is acceptable to use a comma as a decimal point. Thus, two and a half might be written as 2.5 or 2,5 but not as 2·5, as this means two times five and equals ten.

When writing large numbers the figures should be grouped in threes with a space between the figure groups. Four figure units are usually written without space. This means that five million five hundred thousand should be written in the following way: 5500 000. The number can be expressed more shortly as 5.5×10^6 or $5,5 \times 10^6$.

The tables below show the basic and derived units for the SI system with their abbreviations, and also the prefixes which are commonly used when denoting multiplication or division of units.

Units

Physical quantity	Name of unit	Symbol
Basic units		
Mass	kilogram	kg
Length	metre	m
Time	second	s
Electric current	ampere	A
Temperature	kelvin	°K
Luminous intensity	candela	cd
Amount of substance	mole	mol
Derived units		
Force	newton	N
Pressure	pascal	Pa
Energy (work)	joule	J
Volume	litre	l

Prefixes

Prefix	Factor	Symbol
deci	10^{-1}	d
centi	10^{-2}	c
milli	10^{-3}	m
micro	10^{-6}	μ
nano	10^{-9}	n
pico	10^{-12}	p
femto	10^{-15}	f
atto	10^{-18}	a
deca	10^{1}	da
hecto	10^{2}	h
kilo	10^{3}	k
mega	10^{6}	M
giga	10^{9}	G

COMPARATIVE WEIGHTS, MEASURES AND TEMPERATURES

COMPARATIVE WEIGHTS AND MEASURES

Measures of Length

1 kilometre	= 1000 metres
1 metre	= 1000 millimetres
	100 centimetres
1 centimetre	= 10 millimetres
1 millimetre	= 1000 micrometres
1 mile	= 1.6 kilometres
1 yard	= 0.9 metre
1 foot	= 0.3 metre
1 inch	= 25.4 millimetres

Measures of Capacity

1 litre	= 1000 millilitres
1 gallon	= 4.5 litres
1 pint	= 0.57 litres
	568.37 millilitres
1 fluid ounce	= 28.42 millilitres

Measures of Weight

1 kilogram	= 1000 grams
1 gram	= 1000 milligrams
1 milligram	= 1000 micrograms
1 ton	= 1016 kilograms
1 pound	= 0.454 kilogram
	454 grams
1 ounce	= 28.35 grams

AVERAGE WEIGHTS AND HEIGHTS

Children from Birth to Eighteen Years

Boys		Age	Girls	
Weight (kg)	Height (cm)		Weight (kg)	Height (cm)
3.4	50.6	Birth	3.34	50.2
10.07	75.2	1 year	9.75	74.2
12.56	87.5	2 years	12.29	86.6
14.61	96.2	3 years	14.42	95.7
16.51	103.4	4 years	16.42	103.2
18.89	110.0	5 years	18.58	109.4
21.91	117.5	6 years	21.09	115.9
24.54	124.1	7 years	23.68	122.3
27.26	130.0	8 years	26.25	128.0
29.94	135.5	9 years	28.94	132.9
32.61	140.3	10 years	31.89	138.6
35.2	144.2	11 years	35.74	144.7
38.28	148.6	12 years	39.74	151.9
42.18	155.0	13 years	44.95	157.1
48.81	162.7	14 years	49.17	159.6
54.48	167.8	15 years	51.48	161.1
58.83	171.6	16 years	53.07	162.2
61.78	172.7	17 years	54.02	162.5
63.05	174.5	18 years	54.39	162.8

These figures only represent average heights and weights. Many children will therefore not conform to them. There are a number of factors which influence growth and which can cause a child to be considerably below or above average.

Adults Aged Thirty Years

Height (cm)	Weight (kg)		
	Small build	Medium build	Large build
Women			
152.5	48.5	53.9	60.7
157.5	51.2	56.6	63.9
162.5	53.9	59.8	67.5
167.5	57.1	63.4	71.6
172.5	60.2	67.0	75.7
178.0	63.4	70.2	78.9
Men			
167.5	58.4	64.8	72.9
172.5	61.6	68.4	77.0
177.5	65.7	72.9	82.0
183.0	70.7	78.4	87.9
188.0	75.7	83.8	94.2

COMPARATIVE TEMPERATURES

Celsius °C		Fahrenheit °F	Celsius °C		Fahrenheit °F
100	Boiling point	212	38.5		101.3
			38		100.4
95		203	37.5		99.5
90		194	37		98.6
85		185	36.5		97.7
80		176	36		96.8
75		167	35.5		95.9
70		158	35		95
65		149	34		93.2
60		140	33		91.4
55		131	32		89.6
50		122	31		87.8
45		113	30		86
44		112.2	25		77
43		109.4	20		68
42		107.6	15		59
41		105.8	10		50
40		104	5		41
39.5		103.1	0	Freezing point	32
39		102.2			

To convert readings of the Fahrenheit scale into Celsius degrees subtract 32, multiply by 5, and divide by 9, as follows:

$98 - 32 = 66 \times 5 = 330 \div 9 = 36.6$. Therefore 98°F = 36.6°C.

To convert readings of the Celsius scale into Fahrenheit degrees multiply by 9, divide by 5, and add 32, as follows:

$36.6 \times 9 = 330 \div 5 = 66 + 32 = 98$. Therefore 36.6°C = 98°F.

The term 'Celsius' (from the name of the Swede who invented the scale in 1742) is now being internationally used instead of 'Centigrade', which term is employed in some countries to denote fractions of an angle.

FLUIDS, ELECTROLYTES AND TRANSFUSION FLUIDS

FLUID

An average-sized man has some 45 litres of water in his body, and this water accounts for approximately 70 per cent of his weight. The quantity present remains relatively constant and the balance between the quantities of water and of electrolytes present in the body fluids is controlled by a most delicate mechanism. To understand how this balance can be upset during disease or surgical procedures it is necessary to have some knowledge of the normal functioning of the salt and water balance in the body.

Fluid is normally lost by the body:

(1) In the urine.
(2) Through the skin in sweat and in sensible loss.
(3) In expired air.
(4) In the faeces.

The body normally obtains its fluid from:

(1) The fluids taken in in liquid form.
(2) The high fluid content of most foods eaten.
(3) The metabolism of food and cell activity. Much of the latter is a process of oxidation in which water is released.

This can be illustrated by an example:

1 molecule glucose + 6 molecules oxygen
= 6 molecules carbon dioxide + 6 molecules water + energy
$$C_6H_{12}O_6 + 6O_2 = 6CO_2 + 6H_2O + energy$$

In health the balance between fluid intake and fluid output depends mainly on the kidneys, which are able to excrete large amounts of dilute urine when the fluid intake is high and excrete only small quantities of concentrated urine when less fluid is available. The latter condition may be the result of a lessened fluid intake or of an increased fluid loss from the body.

The skin is primarily concerned with the regulation of body temperature; the amount of fluid evaporated from the skin depends on the body's need either to lose or to conserve heat. If the body is warm or the atmospheric temperature is high, much sweat will be excreted and evaporated in an attempt to cool the body. Under cool conditions the sweat glands will be less active in an endeavour to retain more heat within the body, although some loss occurs all the time.

The fluid in the body is present in three different compartments:

(1) The smallest quantity is the circulating fluid or blood plasma. This constitutes 3 litres.

(2) The fluid in the tissues or interstitial spaces constitutes 12 litres. These two together are termed the extracellular fluid.

(3) The fluid within the cell walls forms the greatest proportion of the body fluid, amounting to 30 litres. This is termed intracellular fluid.

Different factors help in maintaining the level of fluid in these three compartments. The plasma proteins, serum albumin, serum globulin, and fibrinogen are the chief factors that maintain the osmotic pressure within the capillaries and so keep the circulating fluid within the vessels. The salt content chiefly influences the tissue fluid and intracellular fluid.

Salts and Electrolytes

Within the body fluids are inorganic elements, or salts, which are in solution. Many of these carry an electrical charge. They are known as electrolytes and carry ions, which are atoms that have lost or gained one or two electrons and as a result have become electrically charged. They are able to take part in chemical changes and the way in which they do so depends on the type of charge which they have.

There are two types of electrolytes: those carrying negative charges, known as anions, and those carrying positive charges, known as cations. Cations unite chemically with anions to form molecules and herein lies the secret of electrolyte balance within the body.

The main salt of extracellular fluid is sodium chloride. This contains sodium (Na) which has a positive charge and chloride (Cl) which has a negative charge. It is not only essential for health that these two elements are present and able to combine, but there must also be a balance between them. This fact is true of all other electrolytes. The balance is maintained by the action of both the respiratory system and the kidneys, which themselves are influenced by the nervous system and by hormones.

Hormones

The pituitary and adrenal glands both have an influence on the salt and water balance in the body. The antidiuretic hormone from the posterior lobe of the pituitary gland controls the final reabsorption of water in the renal tubules. If the hormone is lacking there is excessive diuresis. Aldosterone from the adrenal cortex increases the reabsorption of sodium by the renal tubules and reduces the sodium content of sweat.

Disturbance of the Fluid and Electrolyte Balance

Upset of the fluid and electrolyte balance may occur in many ways:

Water Depletion
(1) When there is lack of intake.
(2) When there is excessive loss from vomiting, diarrhoea, sweating or haemorrhage.

There is loss of fluid from the subcutaneous tissues and the skin becomes hot and dry and loses its elasticity. The circulating fl becomes less, the capillary walls suffer from lack of oxygen and become more permeable, and further leakage from the vessels occurs, giving rise to the condition of shock.

Sodium Depletion
(1) In excessive sweating.
(2) In diarrhoea or where there is much faecal loss from a fistula or ileostomy.
(3) In pathological conditions, such as Addison's disease or hypo-pituitarism, where the kidneys are unable to conserve sodium.

Chloride Depletion
(1) Persistent vomiting where heavy loss of chlorides from the hydrochloric acid will lead to the condition of alkalosis.
(2) Prolonged gastric aspiration.

Potassium Depletion
This may arise whenever there is prolonged diarrhoea, vomiting, condition of shock, or lack of intake, and where there is excessive diuresis or continued use of diuretics such as chlorothiazide.

In prolonged loss of sodium and chloride, potassium migrates from the cells to replace extracellular salt. Potassium is slow to leave the cells but also is slow to permeate back into the cells when replacement is being carried out. Its lack leads to muscular weakness, apathy and mental confusion. The kidneys still excrete potassium, making the condition worse.

Protein Depletion
(1) Where there is inadequate intake, malnutrition or starvation.
(2) Where there is excessive protein loss in renal disease or severe burns.
There is loss of osmotic pressure in the blood and great loss of fluid into the tissues.
(3) In severe haemorrhage where the only satisfactory replacement is by blood of the correct group.

It is seldom that any one of these depletions occurs alone. Fluid, sodium, and chloride are all lost together, but in severe diarrhoea more sodium is lost and in persistent vomiting it is the heavy loss of chlorides which upsets the acid–base balance.

Normally a diet containing an adequate protein and fluid content will also supply the necessary sodium, chloride and potassium.

Replacement of Fluid Loss

Oral fluids. Where there is a fluid lack, replacement is best by the oral route. It is unlikely there will be a lack of water only, and for excessive sweating a one-fifth strength normal saline may be taken by mouth. Most of the other conditions will not benefit from oral fluids and another route will have to be chosen.

Rectal fluids. These may be given for temporary relief of dehydration but their administration cannot be maintained over a period of days.

Subcutaneous infusion. Normal saline (a 0.9 per cent solution of sodium chloride) may be given to replace salt and water loss. The use of hyaluronidase, the spreading factor, aids absorption. This is not now used when facilities for intravenous infusion are available.

Intravenous infusion. This is the commonest way of combating water and salt depletion and if due regard is paid to the electrolyte balance it can be maintained over long periods. It is most usual to give a 4 per cent dextrose solution in one-fifth strength normal saline (0.18 per cent solution). Hartmann's solution may also be used. This is an isotonic solution containing salts of sodium, potassium and calcium with lactic acid.

In any condition in which there is likely to be a depletion of water, salts or protein, or whenever parenteral fluids are given, there must be close observation of the patient with careful measurement and recording of all sources of fluid loss and fluid intake. Analysis of the blood chemistry will be carried out in all severe or prolonged cases.

Other Parenteral Fluids

Dextran Infusion

Dextrans are polysaccharides produced by the action of bacteria on the disaccharide sucrose. They are plasma substitutes which increase the osmotic pressure in the circulation and have a combining power with water, so increasing the circulating volume of fluid. They are useful in treating hypovolaemic shock, moderate blood loss and severe burns.

Dextraven and *Intradex* have an average molecular weight of 110 000. Before infusion a sample of blood should be removed for blood grouping and cross-matching.

Macrodex has an average molecular weight of 70 000 and may be given in normal saline or dextrose solution.

Rheomacrodex has an average molecular weight of 40 000. This lower weight increases capillary blood flow and renal excretion, giving advantages if used during vascular or cardiac surgery. There is no interference with blood typing or cross-matching.

Intravenous Nutrition

Carbohydrate. *Sorbitol* 30 per cent solution is a sugar alcohol and supplies calories in a small volume of fluid (1 litre supplies 1200 calories). Sorbitol is metabolized into fructose and then utilized or stored in the liver as glycogen. It is not re-absorbed by the renal tubules and thus produces diuresis; but it is well utilized and the excretion rate is low. Sorbitol metabolism is not dependent on insulin.

Protein. *Aminosol-Vitrum* is an amino acid solution prepared from casein and dialysed to remove pyrogens and the large molecules that might cause allergy. It may be used alone as a 10 per cent solution (50 g amino acids and 165 cal in 500 ml) or in combination with glucose or fructose and ethanol. Aminosol–fructose–ethanol solution provides 875 calories per litre.

Trophysan is a colourless solution of pure crystalline amino acids a preparation containing vitamins and mineral salts. It may be given alone or with sorbitol to increase the calorie value.

Fat emulsions. These may be used in conjunction with protein solutions and provide a high calorie value in a small volume of fluid.

Intralipid is prepared from soya bean oil. A 20 per cent solution provides 2000 calories per litre.

Lipiphysan is an isotonic solution of either 10 or 15 per cent emulsion of cotton-seed oil with sorbitol and yields 1240 and 1780 calories per litre respectively.

BLOOD TRANSFUSION

Blood Groups

It is frequently necessary to replace blood when a patient has lost a large amount as the result of accidental haemorrhage or major surgery. Although this practice is common, it is not without its dangers. Thus it is of vital importance for the medical and nursing staff to make sure that blood of the correct group is given to each patient. Elaborate precautions are taken to ensure that errors do not occur, because the administration of blood which is not compatible with that of the recipient may well prove fatal.

All blood for transfusion is compared with that of the recipient in a procedure known as cross-matching. There are four major groups, A, B, AB and O. Fig. 13 shows their compatibility. Group O blood may be donated to a person of any group and for this reason a person with group O blood is known as a universal donor. Group AB can receive blood from any group and is therefore known as the universal recipient group.

		A	B	AB	O
	A	O	X	O	X
Donor	B	X	O	O	X
	AB	X	X	O	X
	O	O	O	O	O

Recipient

X = Incompatible   **O** = Compatible

Fig. 13. Compatibility of the four main blood groups.

One other factor to be considered when cross-matching is the Rhesus factor, so named because it was discovered in the blood of Rhesus monkeys in 1940. Some 85 per cent of Caucasians possess this factor and are described as Rhesus-positive (Rh +ve). The 15 per cent that do not possess it are termed Rhesus-negative (Rh −ve). A Rhesus-positive person may be transfused with positive or negative blood, but a Rhesus-negative person must receive blood which is also negative, or else he will produce antibodies to the factor.

If a Rhesus-negative woman has a child by a Rhesus-positive man, there is a danger that some of the fetus's positive cells may cross the placental barrier and cause the mother to develop Rhesus antibodies. However nowadays it is possible, immediately after the birth of the child, to give the mother serum which will destroy the antibodies and so eliminate the danger of a later child being harmed by exposure to them while he is still unborn.

Blood Donors

A large body of public-spirited men and women offer themselves as blood donors at regular intervals and, often at inconvenience to themselves, attend at the required time. It is the duty of the nursing and medical staff to treat them with courtesy and not to keep them waiting. This service allows a blood bank to be maintained for the regular supply of stored blood and plasma. The Red Cross Society keeps a roll of donors who are available when fresh blood is required, but, where possible, relatives of the patient should be asked to give blood if these can provide the right group. The donor's ABO and Rhesus group must be ascertained and Wassermann and Kahn tests carried out. No person with a history of malaria or infective jaundice is permitted to be a blood donor in the United Kingdom.

Blood Transfusion Fluids

Fresh blood. This is particularly useful in cases of active sepsis or haemolytic disease because the cells will not have undergone change.

Stored blood. This is stored at 4°C and may be kept for up to 3 weeks. A slight reaction is likely if the blood has been kept for 3 weeks. It is particularly useful for all emergency cases of haemorrhage, and as a pre- or postoperative measure or during operation when special hazards are encountered.

Frozen blood. Liquid nitrogen held at a temperature of −79°C enables blood to be stored indefinitely. Several hours are needed to prepare it for use, by a process of washing and centrifugation.

Packed red cells. Part of the plasma is removed from whole blood. Using the closed sterile system (transfer unit attached to blood-pack unit) the packed red cells can be stored for 21 days, whereas bottled red cells must be used within 12 to 24 hours. It is used to increase the number of cells without overloading the circulation with fluids, as in some cases of anaemia.

Platelet rich blood. This may be collected with silicone-treated equipment or in a disposable bag in which there is 50 ml of EDTA solution (a di-sodium salt of ethylene diamine tetra-acetic acid), an anticoagulant which is preferable to acid citrate dextrose solution in preserving the platelet content of blood. Platelets are required in controlling haemorrhage in haemolytic disease.

White cells. In certain diseases transfusions of white cells only are required. These can be prepared and infused in a similar manner to other fluids.

APPENDIX 9

NORMAL VALUES

	SI units	Old units
Blood		
Bleeding time	1–6 min	1–6 min
Clotting time	4–10 min	4–10 min
Haemoglobin	12–18 g/dl	12–18 mg/100 ml
pH	7.35–7.45	7.35–7.45
$P\text{CO}_2$	5–6 kPa	38–45 mmHg
$P\text{O}_2$	11–15 kPa	80–100 mmHg
Platelets	$150–400 \times 10^9$/litre	150 000–400 000/mm³
Red cells	$4–6 \times 10^{12}$/litre	4–6 million/mm³
White cells	$4–11 \times 10^9$/litre	4000–11 000/mm³
Plasma		
Bicarbonate	21–28 mmol/litre	21–28 mEq/litre
Chloride	98–107 mmol/litre	98–107 mEq/litre
Glucose (fasting)	2.5–4.7 mmol/litre	48–80 mg/100 ml
Potassium	3.6–5.0 mmol/litre	3.6–5.0 mEq/litre
Sodium	135–145 mmol/litre	135–143 mEq/litre
Urea	3–7 mmol/litre	20–40 mg/100 ml
Urine		
Creatinine	10.0–15.0 mmol/litre	1.1–1.7 g/24 hours
Urea	170–580 mmol/litre	1.0–3.5 g/100 ml
Specific gravity	1002–1040	1002–1040
Cerebrospinal fluid		
Glucose	2.8–3.9 mmol/litre	45–70 mg/100 ml
Protein	150–300 mg/litre	15–30 mg/100 ml

DIETETICS

ENERGY REQUIREMENTS

The unit of energy by which the heat-producing power of foods is measured was known until the introduction of SI units as the **Calorie** or kilocalorie. Since that time there has been indecision as to whether or not the joule, which is the SI unit of energy, should be used. In view of this, both units will be quoted in the following paragraphs. It should be remembered that 1 Calorie = 4.184 kilojoules (4.2 is the number used for convenience).

Definition of Calories and Joules

A *Calorie* is the amount of heat required to raise the temperature of 1 litre of water by 1 degree celsius. A *joule* represents the potential energy which is released when 1 kilogram in weight falls through 1 metre in height by the force of gravity.

Heat-producing Foods

The food materials which produce heat are carbohydrates, proteins, fats and alcohol:

> 1 gram of carbohydrate = 4 Calories = 17 kilojoules
> 1 gram of protein = 4 Calories = 17 kilojoules
> 1 gram of fat = 9 Calories = 38 kilojoules
> 1 gram of alcohol = 7 Calories = 29 kilojoules

Basal Metabolic Rate

The basal metabolic rate is the energy requirement of the body under basal conditions, i.e. when the body is at complete rest, in a room at a comfortable temperature, 12 to 18 hours after having eaten any food.

Fever increases basal metabolism by about 14 per cent for every 1°C rise in temperature.

The basal requirement is 40 Calories (170 kJ) per square metre of body surface area for a man and 37 Calories (155 kJ) for a woman. When estimating energy requirements, add the basal amount to that required for all the activities undertaken in the course of the day. The following table shows the amounts required for various activities.

Energy Requirements for Various Activities

	Activity	Energy required	
		Cal	kJ
Men			
18–35 years	No work (lying in bed)	1750	7350
	Sedentary	2700	11 340
	Moderately active	3000	12 606
	Very active	3600	15 120
35–65 years	As above, subtract	100	420
65–75 years	Sedentary life	2350	9870
75 years +	Sedentary life	2100	8820
Women			
18–55 years	No work (lying in bed)	1500	6300
	Most occupations	2200	9200
	Very active	2500	10 500
55–75 years	Sedentary life	2050	8610
75 years +	Sedentary life	1900	7980

Based on Report No. 120 of the Department of Health and Social Security

Energy requirements vary with the age, sex and build of the individual. In everyday practice it is best to ensure that the essential foods are supplied and then allow the remaining calories in carbohydrate foods, provided the person does not become overweight, in which case it is the carbohydrate foods that should first be reduced.

The components of a normal diet are carbohydrates, proteins, fats, mineral salts and vitamins. Water is an essential to life and at least 1 litre should be taken daily, but it supplies no calorie or nutrient value.

Carbohydrate is utilized by the body for energy. If excess to immediate needs is taken in, some is stored in the liver and muscles as glycogen and the surplus is converted into fat and stored in the fat depots. Sugar is an easily absorbed carbohydrate but the body's main requirements are consumed in the form of starch, a more complex carbohydrate which is found in bread and potatoes.

Protein is used in the body for growth and repair of tissue and must be taken in regularly as it cannot be stored for use later. Excess protein can be utilized only in the same way as carbohydrate and fat after the nitrogen portion of the molecule has been removed by the liver. The waste products are then excreted by the kidneys. Protein is made up of numerous amino acids, many of which can be converted from one kind to another in the body, but ten cannot be manufactured and are termed essential amino acids. Animal sources of protein are rich in essential amino acids but in vegetable sources some of them are lacking. In a vegetarian diet a greater variety of different vegetable proteins must be taken than if the body's requirements are supplied from animal and vegetable sources combined.

Fats are the richest heat-producing foods.

MINERAL REQUIREMENTS

The following are the principal minerals essential to health in adults and children and for growth in children: calcium, phosphorus, iron, sodium, potassium, iodine, copper, magnesium, sulphur and manganese. In a varied diet the only two which may not be supplied in sufficient quantities are calcium and iron.

Approximate Daily Requirements

	Adults	Children
Calcium	0.5 g	0.5–1.4 g
Iron	10–15 mg	6–15 mg

The richest sources of **calcium** are milk, cheese, sardines, herrings, watercress, bread and flour: 0.5 litre of milk supplies 0.6 g of calcium.

The richest sources of **iron** are liver, kidney, meat (particularly beef), egg yolk, baked beans, wholemeal bread, raisins and watercress: 30 g of beef supplies 1.1 mg of iron and 30 g of wholemeal bread supplies 0.6 mg.

FOOD VALUES

Since Calories are still in general use by those involved in dietetics, the amounts in the following dietary information have been given in Calories only.

The weight in grams needed to supply 100 Calories is given in the table below.

Protein		Fats		Carbohydrate	
Streaky		Olive oil	10	Sugar	30
bacon	20	Butter	15	Cream crackers	20
Cheese	22	Margarine	15	Syrup	30
Beef (lean)	30	Dripping	10	Shredded	
Ham	45	Cream	30	wheat (1)	30
Mutton	30			Bread	45
1 Egg				Potatoes	120
Corned beef	45			Apples	270
Liver	45			Oranges	300
Chicken	60			Carrots	600
Herring	60			Milk	150
Kipper	60				
Rabbit	60				
Tinned salmon	75				
Tripe	105				
White fish	120				

In order to take in 7 grams of protein, it is necessary to consume the amount in grams shown in the table below.

Animal sources		Vegetable sources	
Meat	30	Soya flour	15
Cheese	30	Bread (Hovis)	90
Poultry	30	Bread (white)	90
Bacon	30	Chocolate (milk)	90
Fish	45	Beans (baked)	120
Milk (dried, skimmed)	22	Beans (dry boiled)	105
Milk (evaporated)	90	Peas (boiled)	150
Milk (fresh)	210	Lentils (boiled)	120

VITAMIN REQUIREMENTS

The vitamins are a group of accessory factors present in various foodstuffs and essential for many bodily processes. Their functions and the symptoms and signs produced by specific vitamin deficiencies are described in the table on pp. 434–436, which also gives details of the main sources and average daily requirements.

SPECIAL DIETS

1000 Calorie Diet

A reducing diet for those who are overweight and particularly those suffering from heart failure, hypertension and osteoarthritis.

This diet is achieved by allowing the patient in each 24 hours:

5 × 100-Calorie portions of protein foods	500 Cal
60 g only of bread	150 Cal
15 g of butter	100 Cal
150 g of milk	100 Cal
3 helpings of fruit (except those listed below)	150 Cal

Green vegetables and salad can be taken as much as desired.
Avoid:

Potatoes, peas, beans or beetroot
Bananas, grapes, prunes, figs or dried fruits
Sugar, pastry, cake or confectionery

Saccharin must be used for sweetening.
Unsugared fruit drinks, Marmite, Oxo and Bovril may be taken as desired.

High-calorie Diet

Designed for those who are underweight or have had a debilitating illness. A full general diet can be taken with the addition of extra milk and milk reinforced by the addition of dried milk powder. Reinforced milk can be used in the cooking of milk puddings, creamed soup and

Vitamins

Vitamin	Functions	Deficiency	Chemical properties	Sources	Average daily requirements*
Fat-soluble A (retinol)	For normal growth in children. To maintain a healthy condition of the skin and mucous membranes, particularly of the respiratory tract and conjunctiva. Aids night vision	Roughened and dry skin. More liable to infection where mucous membranes in poor condition. Inability to see in dim light. Xerophthalmia leading to blindness	Can be synthesized in the body from carotene present in coloured fruits and vegetables. May be stored in the liver	Halibut- and cod-liver oil, liver, butter, margarine, cheese and egg yolk. Carrots, spinach, water-cress, dried apricots and tomatoes	750 μg (retinol equivalents)
D (calciferol)	Necessary for the absorption and metabolism of calcium and phosphorus in the body	Rickets. Osteomalacia. Defective deposition of enamel leading to dental caries	Can be formed by the action of ultra-violet light on the ergosterol in the skin	Halibut- and cod-liver oil. Fat fish. Egg yolk. Butter, margarine, cheese and milk	2.5 μg cholecalciferol
E (tocopherol)	Related to reproduction in rats but no conclusive evidence that it plays any part in fertility in human beings	—	—	Wheat-germ, lettuce, green leaves and milk	—

Vitamin	Essential for	Deficiency	Notes	Sources	Daily requirement*
K	Essential for the proper clotting of blood	Deficiency only temporary due to jaundice or sterilization of the gut by chemotherapy	Not absorbed from the gut if bile missing. Can be synthesized in the bowel	Green plants, cabbage and green peas	—
Water-soluble B1 (thiamine)	To obtain a steady and continuous release of energy from carbohydrate.	Check in growth of children. Neuritis. Beri-beri	Easily destroyed by high temperatures and baking soda	Brewers' yeast, bacon, liver. Wholemeal and national bread. Vegetables	1.2 mg
B2 (riboflavine)		Checks growth. Cracks and soreness at corner of the mouth and of the tongue. Opacity of the cornea	Little lost during normal cooking	Yeast, dairy produce, eggs and liver	1.7 mg
Nicotinic acid or niacin		Skin becomes rough and red. Diarrhoea and digestive upsets. Mental symptoms. Pellagra		Yeast, meat extracts, meat, offal. Wholemeal bread	18 mg
B6 (pyridoxine)	Concerned with protein metabolism	Unlikely	May be usefully given during radiotherapy treatment	Present in most foods	—

*For a moderately active man (excludes infants, pregnancy, lactation). Based on Report No. 120 of the Department of Health and Social Security 1969 (HMSO).

Vitamin	Functions	Deficiency	Chemical properties	Sources	Average daily requirements*
Folic acid	Aids in formation of red blood corpuscles	Some cases of macrocytic anaemia		Liver and green vegetables	—
B12 (cyano-cobal amin, cytamen)	Necessary for development of red blood corpuscles	Pernicious anaemia	Cannot be absorbed unless the intrinsic factor is present in the stomach	Liver and other sources, as above. Prepared from streptomycin cultures	—
Biotin, choline, inositol, pantothenic acid and *para*-aminobenzoic acid are also members of the vitamin B complex					
C (ascorbic acid)	Necessary for the proper formation of collagen in connective tissue and for formation of intercellular cement. Also for the formation of bones and teeth	Checks growth in children. Delays wound healing. Soreness of the mouth and gums. Capillary bleeding. Scurvy	Lost by long storage of fruit and vegetables. By cooking in the presence of air. By plant enzymes released by grating and chopping	Rose hip syrup, blackcurrants, oranges and lemons. Green leaf vegetables and potatoes. High content in new potatoes, decreasing with age	30 mg

*For a moderately active man (excludes infants, pregnancy, lactation). Based on Report No. 120 of the Department of Health and Social Security 1969 (HMSO).

porridge. Glucose and lactose may be added. Biscuits should be served with the mid-morning and late night drink and mayonnaise with a sardine, salmon or cheese salad at teatime.

Low-protein Diet

Various levels of protein restriction may be ordered for patients with renal or hepatic disorders. The following constitutes 40 g of protein:

Bread is limited to 180 g a day, or 150 g and 1 helping of cereal
Milk is limited to 300 g a day
One 7-g portion of protein is allowed at breakfast, lunch and supper
Fruit and vegetables may be taken freely except peas, beans and lentils
Butter, sugar, jam, boiled sweets and treacle should be taken liberally to prevent breakdown of body protein for energy purposes

High-protein Diet

Over 100 g of protein a day should be taken by patients suffering from burns, certain renal conditions, and where much repair of body tissue is required. The diet should include 1 litre of milk and eight 7-g portions of protein divided throughout the day's meals, e.g.

Breakfast	1 egg and 30 g bacon
Lunch	60 g meat
Tea	30 g cheese or sardine
Supper	135 g fish

There is no restriction on the amount of bread, cake, fruit and vegetables consumed, from all of which a portion of the day's protein requirements will be obtained. Where there is a still greater requirement of protein or where a patient is not eating well, protein supplements can be added to the milk or in the cooking. Casilan contains 90 per cent, Complan 31 per cent and skimmed milk powder 34.5 per cent of protein.

Low-fat Diet

This is useful in cases of jaundice or cholecystitis and in certain malabsorption syndromes.

Skimmed milk should be used. Give white fish, lean meat and a plentiful supply of fruit, vegetables and green salad; honey, jam, syrup or Marmite spread on bread. Boiled sweets and barley sugar may be taken.

Avoid the following:

Butter, margarine and dripping
Fat meats, salmon, herrings and sardines
All fried foods
Nuts, egg yolk, salad cream and olive oil
Pastries, puddings and cakes, in the making of which suet, cooking fat or margarine has been used.

Low-residue or Gastric Diet

The diet for patients with ulceration or inflammation of the gastrointestinal tract is much less restrictive than that used formerly. The diet should consist of small helpings taken at regular intervals with a short rest before and after meals. The meal should be eaten slowly and the food well chewed. These points are considered more important than the content of the diet and within certain limits the patient can have the food he enjoys, but should avoid those foods he finds disagree with him.

Fried foods are best avoided and those containing tough fibres, skins and pips, also highly seasoned foods and pickles. In the acute stages alcohol and smoking should be avoided and even later these should not be indulged in when the stomach is empty.

High-residue Diet

This is suitable for those suffering from diverticulosis. The aim is to increase the bulk of the diet to stimulate peristalsis. It is recommended that a plentiful supply of the following be included in the normal diet and that more refined cereals be avoided.

Wholemeal or brown bread
Wholemeal biscuits
Wholemeal flour in cooking
Oatmeal, Ryvita and All Bran
All fruits including the peel of apples and pears
Vegetables, particularly green vegetables, salads, peas and beans

Recent research has shown that this type of diet should be eaten by everyone. The refined foods which constitute much of the diet in western society have a tendency to cause many of the problems which are common nowadays, but which were not known until fairly recent times and are not seen in underdeveloped countries.

Low-salt Diet

This may be ordered for patients with congestive heart failure and severe hypertension where there is much tissue oedema.

(1) A moderate restriction of sodium (5 g of sodium chloride giving 1.5 g of sodium) can be achieved by:

Using no table salt or salt in the cooking
Avoiding all foods containing bicarbonate of soda or baking powder
Avoiding salty foods like bacon, smoked haddock, and kippers, tinned and frozen meat, fish and vegetables
No chocolate or syrup is allowed

(2) A greater restriction (1.5 g of sodium chloride containing 0.5 g of sodium can be achieved only by obtaining low-salt bread and butter and restricting the milk and protein foods.

Gluten-free Diet

This diet is essential for all patients with coeliac disease and dermatitis herpetiformis. Medical opinion at the present time favours total exclusion of gluten throughout life. Patients with coeliac disease are unable to absorb gluten, which is the protein present in wheat, rye, barley and possibly oats. Therefore a major dietary change is necessary; that of excluding ordinary flour from the diet.

In the initial stages of severe coeliac disease it is usual to give 2- to 3-hourly feeds of skimmed milk, Prosol (Trufood Ltd) and glucose, gradually increasing the diet by adding gluten-free cereals, fruit, animal protein and fat. When a full gluten-free diet is given Prosol can be omitted.

Certain foods are prescribed on form EC10 for coeliac patients. These are (a) gluten-free flour, (b) gluten-free bread, (c) gluten-free biscuits and (d) gluten-free pasta. There are several manufacturers of these products. Further information may be obtained from *The Coeliac Society*, P.O. Box No. 181, London NW2 2Q7. The aim of the society is to promote the welfare of those with the disease and to help them in as many ways as possible. Cooking with gluten-free flour is different from cooking with ordinary flour. Manufacturers of the above products supply recipes for use with their products. Further details can be obtained from the *Coeliac Handbook*, edited by Bee Nilson (The Coeliac Society); also *Diets for Sick Children* by Francis (Oxford: Blackwell Scientific).

The following is a brief guide to foods to be excluded because they contain gluten. If there is doubt about any food it should not be eaten.

Baking powder—unless certified gluten-free

Bread made from wheat or rye flour

Biscuits, cakes and pastry

Breakfast cereals—puffed wheat, Weetabix, Grapenuts, Bemax, Farex, Farley's rusks, oatmeal

'Compound' condiments (pure pepper and pure mustard only permitted)

Drinks—Bengers, Horlicks, malted milks, Ovaltine

Flour—wheat and rye and products made from flour such as pasta, semolina. Barley

Meats containing 'cereal binder' or rusk, e.g. sausages, certain cooked meats

Preserves such as mincemeat and lemon curd unless known to be gluten-free

Sauces and soups unless guaranteed gluten-free

Sweets—caution with all sweets, especially unwrapped sweets and filled chocolates

Vegetables, e.g. frozen potato croquettes

Many manufactured foods contain gluten and the Coeliac Society's current list of gluten-free manufactured foods gives more detail. Nevertheless always check the ingredients panel.

Some foods carry this symbol which is the manufacturer's guarantee of a gluten-free food:

Cereals which do not contain gluten are:

Pure cornflour and custard powder—if guaranteed gluten-free
Potato starch—potato flour or farina
Rice flour
Soya flour
Rice Krispies, cornflakes
Rice, sago, tapioca

DIABETIC DIET

Protein Foods

Average helpings of the following foods may be eaten; but if the patient has to lose weight care must be taken with the foods in the left-hand column.

Cheese (not cream cheese)	Eggs	Crab meat
Grilled lean bacon	Corned beef	Bloaters
Lean ham	Boiled beef	Fish roes
Lean mutton chop	Liver	Salmon
Duck (small portion)	Chicken	Rabbit
Goose (small portion)	Grouse	Tripe
Lean roast beef	Kidneys	White fish
Lean roast lamb	Herring	Kipper
Lean roast mutton		Smoked haddock
Lean roast pork		
Sardines (drain off the oil)		

Fat Foods

Those patients who require to lose weight should avoid fried foods and take only very little, and certainly no more than the stated amount, of the following:

Butter	Dripping
Margarine	Olive oil
Cooking fat	Cream

Many mild diabetics are overweight and for them a 1000 Calorie-reducing diet will be suitable, as this automatically restricts carbohydrates.

Carbohydrate (CHO) includes sugar, glucose, sweets, chocolate, jams, marmalade, syrup, sweet biscuits, cakes and pastries, sweetened minerals. In general all these should be avoided by all diabetics as they are concentrated sources of CHO. In addition, bread, potatoes, plain biscuits are moderate sources of carbohydrate and may be taken in controlled amounts.

For this purpose carbohydrate-containing foods are classified according to the amount of that food which yield one 10-g carbohydrate exchange, e.g. a diet of 150 g CHO = 15 × 10 g carbohydrate exchanges from the following list (in grams except where otherwise stated):

Carbohydrate Foods in 10-g Portions

Cereals, etc.		Fruits	
		(weighed with stones and juice, but no peel)	
Biscuits, plain	15		
Bread	20	Apple, raw	120
Breakfast cereal	15	Apple, stewed	150
Oatmeal, dry	15	Apricots, fresh	180
Rice, semolina, tapioca,		Apricots, dried, stewed	60
cornflour, etc.	15	Banana, raw	60
Milk, fresh	200 ml	Cherries, raw	120
Milk, evaporated	90 ml	Cherries, stewed	120
Bournvita, etc.	15	Damsons, stewed	180
Cocoa powder		Gooseberries, raw, ripe	120
(unsweetened)	30	Grapes	80
		Greengages, raw	120
Vegetables		Greengages, stewed	120
Beans, baked	60	Melon	210
Beans, broad	150	Orange	120
Beans, haricot	60	Peaches, fresh	120
Beetroot	120	Pears, raw	120
Parsnips	90	Pears, stewed	150
Peas, fresh or frozen	120	Plums, stewed	240
Peas, dried	60	Prunes, stewed	60
Potatoes	60	Raspberries, raw	180
Potato, chips	30	Strawberries, raw	180

The following contain little or no carbohydrate and need not be weighed:

Vegetables	Salads	Fruits
Artichokes, green	Cucumber	Blackcurrants
Asparagus	Lettuce	Gooseberries, stewed
Beans, french	Mustard and cress	Grapefruit
Beans, runner	Radishes	Loganberries
Broccoli	Watercress	Rhubarb
Brussels sprouts		
Cabbage	Beverages	Condiments
Cauliflower	Tea	Salt
Celery	Coffee	Pepper
Marrow	Soda water	Mustard
Mushrooms	Clear meat or chicken	Vinegar
Onions	soup	Saccharine
Spinach	Marmite	Vanilla
Tomatoes	Oxo, Bovril	Lemon juice
	Diabetic squash	Salad oil

Supplements

One tablespoon of the following may be given once a day.

Artichokes (Jerusalem), cooked
Carrots, raw or cooked
Leeks, boiled

Swedes, boiled
Turnips, boiled

Sample Diet

Sample of a 150-g carbohydrate diet when the patient is having soluble insulin morning and evening.

		CHO (g)	Exchanges
Milk for tea throughout day = 200 ml over and above that indicated		10	1
Early morning	Tea—milk from allowance		
Breakfast 45 g or 4½ exchanges	Tea or coffee Milk for cereal 100 ml 15 g cereal or porridge oats Protein as required 60 g bread Butter as required	5 10 30	½ 1 3
Mid-morning 10 g or 1 exchange	Milk for coffee 100 ml 1 plain biscuit	5	½
Lunch 30 g or 3 exchanges	60 g bread for sandwich Meat, fish, cheese, egg as required Tea—milk from allowance	30	3
Tea 5 g or ½ exchange	Tea—milk from allowance 2 plain biscuits	10	1½
Evening meal 40 g or 4 exchanges	Meat, fish, egg Vegetables, salad as required 120 g potato Fruit—1 exchange 2 cream crackers cheese, butter as required	 20 10 10	 2 1 1
Bedtime 10 g or 1 exchange	Tea—milk from allowance 2 plain biscuits	10	1
		150	15

Emergencies

Diabetics on insulin must never stop their insulin. In sickness it may be necessary to take CHO in a simple form:

10 g 2 tsp sugar or glucose or 3
   small sugar lumps
120 ml fresh fruit juice
15 ml Ribena   } = 10 g CHO
60 ml Lucozade
198 g milk

INFANT FEEDING

Infant feeds require careful calculation, particularly when the infant concerned is sick. The healthy baby will, on the whole, dictate his needs in a fairly lusty and determined manner, but when he is not well he is unable to do so.

In order to calculate such feeds accurately, it is essential to know two basic facts before commencing:

(1) The birth weight of the baby.
(2) The age of the baby in weeks.

This is necessary in order to obtain the expected weight on which the feed will be calculated. A baby should regain his birth weight by the time he is 2 weeks old, having initially lost anything up to 10 per cent in the first few days of life. The first fortnight is therefore ignored when making the calculation since a baby of twelve weeks of age will have actually been gaining for only ten of them. From two to twelve weeks a baby should gain about 200 g each week. Therefore a baby of 12 weeks who weighed 3000 g (3 kg) at birth would have his expected weight calculated as follows:

$$\text{Birth weight} = 3000 \text{ g}$$
$$\text{Age} = 12 \text{ weeks} - 2 \text{ weeks} = 10 \text{ weeks}$$
$$\text{Expected gain} = 200 \text{ g/week}$$

Thus

$$200 \times 10 = 2000 \text{ g gained}$$

This is then added to the original weight

$$2000 + 3000 = 5000$$

resulting in an expected weight of 5000 g (5 kg).

Having ascertained the expected weight of the baby, it is then compared with the actual weight. If he is sick, his weight is probably less than it should be, then it is necessary to feed him to a level somewhere between his actual and his expected weight. Two more factors have now to be considered:

    (1) Fluid requirements.
    (2) Energy requirements.

Fluid requirements. The normal infant requires 150 to 200 ml/kg body weight per day. If a baby weighs 4 kg he therefore requires 4×150 ml to 4×200 ml/kg/day = 600 to 800 ml/kg/day.

Energy requirements. The normal infant requires 420 to 540 kJ (100 to 130 Cal)/kg body weight per day. If a baby weighs 4 kg he thus requires 420 kJ $\times 4$ to 540 kJ $\times 4$/day = 1680 to 2160 kJ (400 to 520 Cal)/day.

The calculated amount is then divided into evenly spaced feeds of equal amount, e.g. 120 ml four-hourly for five feeds.

After three months of age, the baby usually gains weight less rapidly, and the following table gives the approximate gains for the first two years of life. As the growth rate slows down, the fluid and energy requirements per kilogram become less. However the total amount required continues to increase as the child grows.

Approximate Weight Gain for Infants up to 24 Months

Age (months)	Weight gain (g/week)
0–3	200
3–6	150
6–9	100
9–12	50–75
12–24	2500

URINE TESTING

Fresh specimens of urine should be tested whenever possible as changes in composition occur when urine is allowed to stand. Specimens should always be collected in dry, clean containers.

The Ames tests for abnormal constituents in urine are quickly and easily carried out, but should they not be available the student should remember to acidify alkaline urine by the addition of acetic acid before carrying out chemical tests.

In all cases the equipment must be clean and the pipettes well rinsed immediately after use.

The findings should be recorded at once. In carrying out a routine examination first note the colour, appearance, reaction and specific gravity.

When using Ames Reagents always replace the cap tightly immediately after use and store away from excessive heat and moisture. Reagent strips should not be used if there is any brownish discoloration of the test areas. Remember: (a) Specimen containers must be absolutely clean. (b) Do not acidify the urine prior to testing. (c) Reagent strips should be dipped into the urine and immediately removed, and where applicable they *must* be compared with the colour charts provided *at the times stated*.

Multistix (Ames). One reagent strip combines six urine tests. The tests are for the reaction of the urine (pH) and abnormalities of protein, glucose, ketones, bilirubin, blood and urobilinogen. After dipping the strip in freshly mixed urine tap the edge of the strip on the container to remove excess urine. The colour reaction of the test areas is compared with a colour chart provided.

As with all laboratory tests, definitive diagnostic or therapeutic decisions should not be based on any single result or method.

Chemical Urine Tests

Test	Reagent	Method	Reaction+
For albumin Albustix	Reagent strips	Dip the strip in urine and remove it immediately. Compare it with colour scale	Turns green at once
Hot	Acetic acid	Heat over a methylated spirits lamp the top of a test tube three parts full of urine, turning the tube in the fingers at the same time. When boiling, add a few drops of the acid	Urates will disappear on heating, phosphates when the acid is added. Any cloud left is due to the presence of coagulated albumin
Salicyl-sul-phonic acid	Salicyl-sul-phonic acid (saturated solution)	To 2 cm of the urine in a test tube add a few drops of the reagent	An opalescent cloud
Quantitative (Esbach's)	Esbach's solution of picric acid	In the special graduated tube place urine up to the marking 'U'. Add solution to 'R'. Cork and shake thoroughly. Allow to stand in special holder for 24 hours	The albumin will be seen as a sediment at the bottom of the tube. The graduations at the bottom give the amount of albumin in grams per 1000 ml of urine. This divided by 10 gives the percentage

N.B. The specific gravity must be 1008. Dilute if necessary

For protein and glucose Uristix	Reagent strip	Dip in urine and remove	Protein portion turns green. Glucose portion turns purple, within 10 seconds

For blood Hemastix	Reagent strips	Dip in urine and remove. Compare with colour chart	Turns blue in 30 seconds
Microscopic examination			

Test	Reagent	Method	Reaction +
For glucose			
Clinistix	Reagent strips	Dip the test end of Clinistix in urine and remove	Turns purple in 10 seconds
N.B. If positive, use Clinitest to determine concentration of glucose			
Clinitest	Reagent tablets. These deteriorate with moisture and must not be used if blue in colour	1. With dropper provided, place 5 drops of urine in test tube. Rinse dropper, add 10 drops of water 2. Drop in 1 tablet and watch reaction 3. Do not shake till 15 seconds after reaction ceases	Colour change from blue-green to orange. Compare with colour chart provided. If during the test a bright orange colour appears and then changes to brown, more than 2 per cent of sugar is present
Benedict's	Benedict's solution (copper sulphate)	Place 5 ml of the solution in a test tube. Add 8 to 10 drops of urine with a pipette and boil for 2 minutes at least	Any change of colour within 15 minutes. This varies from a greenish-yellow to a deep orange precipitate
For acetone			
Acetest	Acetest tablets	Place tablet on clean surface. Add 1 drop of urine. Wait 30 seconds	Note colour change from lavender-mauve. Compare with chart provided
Rothera's	Ammonium sulphate crystals. Nitroprusside. Concentrated ammonia	Into half a test tube of urine put the ammonium sulphate crystals until the liquid is saturated. Dissolve 2 to 3 nitroprusside crystals in 8 ml of water and add 3 to 4 drops of this to the urine. Shake. Layer on top 2.5 cm of the ammonia	The urine has a sweet smell. Reddish-violet colour turning blue (in 15 minutes) throughout the fluid (turns yellow if acetic acid is added)
For diacetic acid			
Gerhardt's	Ferric choride solution	To half a test tube of urine add the solution drop by drop as long as a precipitate forms	The top of the urine shows a reddish-brown colour
N.B. Salicylates will also produce this reaction			

Test	Reagent	Method	Reaction+
For chlorides Quantitative test	Potassium chromate 20 per cent Silver nitrate 2.9 per cent	Rinse test tube with distilled water. Add 10 drops of urine. Rinse dropper with distilled water. Add 1 drop of potassium chromate. Rinse dropper. Add silver nitrate 1 drop at a time, until sharp colour change from yellow to red-brown. Shake between each drop	The number of drops of silver nitrate used indicates the number of grams of sodium chloride per litre of urine. 1 drop, chlorides absent. Normal 3 to 5 per litre
For bile pigments Ictotest	Reagent tablets Test mats	Place 5 drops of urine on a test mat. Put 1 tablet in the centre of the moist area and place 2 drops of water on the tablet	The mat around tablet turns bluish purple, within 30 seconds
Iodine	Tincture of iodine	To 5 ml of urine in a test tube add a few drops of iodine	Change of colour to green
For bile salts Hay's	Flowers of sulphur	Sprinkle on the surface of the urine	The sulphur sinks into the liquid due to lowered surface tension
For pus*	Solution of potassium hydroxide	Mix in a test tube equal parts of urine and the reagent and pour from one test tube to another	The fluid becomes ropy (mucus disappears)
	Hydrogen peroxide	Add the reagent to some urine in a test tube	Frothing occurs

*The best test for the presence of pus is microscopic examination for pus cells.

MEASUREMENT OF DRUGS

With the metric system now in common use the arithmetical problems likely to be encountered by the nurse are simple ones. However she will need to have reasonable working knowledge of the system. The following are suggestions.

Percentages, Fractions and Decimals

$$1 \text{ per cent equals 1 part in 100 or } \frac{1}{100}$$

$$5 \text{ per cent equals 5 parts in 100 or } \frac{5}{100} = \frac{1}{20}$$

Parts that are less than 1 can be written as fractions or decimals

$$1 \text{ divided by } 2 = \tfrac{1}{2} \text{ or } 0.5$$
$$1 \text{ divided by } 4 = \tfrac{1}{4} \text{ or } 0.25$$
$$\text{e.g. } 1 \text{ g} = 1000 \text{ mg}$$
$$\tfrac{1}{2} \text{ g or } 0.5 \text{ g} = 500 \text{ mg}$$
$$\tfrac{1}{4} \text{ g or } 0.25 \text{ g} = 250 \text{ mg}$$

Calculating Dosages

It frequently happens that the nurse has to calculate the dose of a drug because the required strength is not available. There is a formula for this which states quite simply the method to be used. It is as follows:

Divide the amount required by the amount already available and multiply this by the amount which is contained in the stock solution:

$$\frac{\text{Amount required}}{\text{Amount available}} \times \text{amount in stock}$$

This can be converted in the following manner. A dose of 100 mg of cortisone is required. The available solution is of 250 mg in 10 ml. Thus

$$\frac{100}{250} \times 10 = \frac{\overset{2}{\cancel{100}}}{\underset{5}{\cancel{250}}} \times \overset{2}{\cancel{10}} = 4 \text{ ml}$$

Or, as another example, 5000 units of heparin are required when the available solution is 25 000 units in 5 ml. Thus

$$\frac{5000}{25\ 000} \times 5 = \frac{5000}{25\ 000} \times \frac{1}{5} = 1 \text{ ml}$$

It is possible to calculate this by mental arithmetic as 5000 divides into 25 000 five times, and one-fifth of 5 equals 1. However the nurse should always write the problem down if she is in any doubt at all and if necessary have the result checked by a colleague.

Should it be necessary to divide one fraction by another, it can be done in a similar fashion by using the same formula. It should simply be remembered that the second of the two fractions must be inverted, as follows. To prepare chlorhexidine 1 in 2500 from a stock solution of 1 in 500 in 1 litre.

Strength required = 1 in 2500
Strength available = 1 in 500
Amount of solution = 1 litre

Thus

$$\frac{1}{2500} \div \frac{1}{500} = \frac{1}{2500} \times \frac{500}{1} = \frac{5}{25} = \frac{1}{5}$$

Therefore one-fifth of a litre is required. Since 1 litre = 1000 ml, one-fifth of a litre = 1000 ÷ 5 = 200 ml of solution required.

To divide decimals the decimal point may be moved, provided that it is moved the same number of places in each figure. Thus, to measure a dose of digoxin 0.125 mg from a stock solution of 0.5 mg in 2 ml, the formula is written in the following manner:

Strength required = 0.125 mg
Strength available = 0.5 mg
Amount of solution = 2 ml

$$\frac{0.125}{0.5} \times 2 = \frac{125}{500} \times 2 = \frac{1}{2} \text{ ml or 0.5 ml}$$

ABBREVIATIONS USED IN PRESCRIPTIONS

Abbreviations of Latin terms are being replaced by English versions which are considered safer. The nurse may still meet these terms.

Term	Latin	English
a.c.	*ante cibum*	before food
ad lib.	*ad libitum*	to the desired amount
b.d. or b.i.d.	*bis in die*	twice a day
c.	*cum*	with
o.m.	*omni mane*	every morning
o.n.	*omni nocte*	every night
p.c.	*post cibum*	after food
p.r.n.	*pro re nata*	whenever necessary
q.d.	*quaque die*	every day
q.i.d.	*quater in die*	four times a day
R̶	*recipe*	take
s.o.s.	*si opus sit*	if necessary
stat.	*statim*	at once
t.d.s.	*ter die sumendum*	three times a day
t.i.d.	*ter in die*	three times a day

DRUGS AND THEIR CONTROL

The two acts which control the use of poisons in medicine are: (1) The Misuse of Drugs Act 1971, which, with the Misuse of Drugs Regulations 1973, came into force on 1 July 1973. The Act combines and extends the Dangerous Drugs Acts 1965 and 1967 and the Drugs (Prevention of Misuse) Act 1964, which have been repealed; and (2) The Pharmacy and Poisons Act 1933 and the Poisons Rules (2). Additions are made to the drugs affected by these acts from time to time.

The Misuse of Drugs Act

This Act aims at checking the unlawful use of the drugs liable to produce dependence or cause harm if misused. Drugs affected by this Act are referred to as *Controlled Drugs* and are divided into 4 Schedules. Schedules 2 and 3 include those drugs which were previously controlled under the Dangerous Drugs Act and some additional ones. They include:

Cocaine	Amphetamine
Diamorphine (heroin)	Dexamphetamine
Levorphanol	Dihydrocodeine injection
Methadone	Mephentermine
Morphine	Methylphenidate
Opium	Methaqualone
Pethidine	Phenmetrazine

Medical practitioners and registered dentists may prescribe preparations containing these poisons. For exceptions see *The Misuse of Drugs (Notification of and Supply to Addicts) Regulations 1973.*

A prescription must bear:

(1) Patient's name and address
(2) Date
(3) Signature of prescriber (*not only initials*)
(4) Total quantity to be supplied, in words or figures

Every general practitioner is required to keep a record of all purchases of these drugs, and of the amounts issued to individual patients.

In hospitals the use of these drugs is under strict control, although minor variations in details may occur in individual institutions.*

(1) A special cupboard is used for storing such drugs, and this should be marked 'CD'.

* *See* Department of Health and Social Security report of joint sub-committee on the Control of Dangerous Drugs and Poisons in Hospital.

(2) The cupboard is kept locked, and the key carried on the person of the state registered nurse in charge.

(3) Renewal of supplies can only be obtained by an order signed by a medical officer; and the drugs can only be given under the written instructions of such.

(4) Each dose of these drugs administered must be entered into a special Register provided for the purpose, with the date, patient's name and time of giving. The persons giving and checking the drug must sign this entry.

In most hospitals it is a rule that each dose given must be checked by two persons, one of whom should be a state registered nurse. This person should see the bottle from which the drug is taken, and check the dose with the written prescription.

All bottles containing controlled drugs should be marked conspicuously with a special label.

The hospital pharmacist usually checks at intervals the contents of the C.D. cupboard and compares its contents with the records of the Register.

The Pharmacy and Poisons Act

Many substances are covered by this act and these are divided into 'Schedules', of which 1 and 4 are concerned with medicine.

In hospitals such drugs are kept under lock and key and they should be distinctively labelled and stored in bottles of special shape.

Schedule 1 lists all the preparations to which special restrictions apply under the Poisons Rules. These drugs may be sold only to persons known to the chemist, on a medical prescription or on a police order. The poisons book must be signed. The commoner ones, including their alkaloids or salts, which are used in hospitals are the following:

Apomorphine	Digitalis
Arsenic	Emetine
Atropine	Ergot
Belladonna	Hyoscine
Carbachol	Methylpentynol (Oblivon)
	Strychnine

Schedule 4 lists those substances to be sold by retailers only upon a prescription given by a duly qualified medical practitioner. These drugs are also included in Schedule 1. The group of drugs can be divided into Schedule 4A and 4B, the prescriptions for which must fulfil different requirements, Schedule 4A having rules similar to the Misuse of Drugs Act. This applies chiefly to pharmacists and doctors, but for nurses the same rules apply to all poisons.

Examples of Schedule 4A drugs:

Most barbiturate drugs	Cyclophosphamide
Gallamine injections	Mercaptopurine
Mustine injections	

Examples of Schedule 4B drugs:

Chlorpromazine	Sulphonamide drugs
Milder sedatives	Thiazide diuretics
Tranquillizers	Thyroid preparations

The Therapeutic Substances Act

This act controls the manufacture, supply and sale of certain drugs and preparations. The provisions of the Act are similar to those controlling the Poisons Schedules. The preparations controlled are:

Antibiotics	Heparin
Blood	Insulin
Corticosteroids and corticotrophin	Surgical ligatures
Curare	Vaccines and sera

The Misuse of Drugs (Notification of and Supply to Addicts) Regulations 1973

Medical practitioners may not prescribe, administer or supply cocaine or diamorphine, or their salts, to addicted persons, except for the purpose of treating organic disease or injury, unless they have obtained a special licence and work in a specially licensed NHS hospital or similar institution. Addicts will have to undergo treatment in such a hospital or clinic. For further information apply to the Department of Health and Social Security, Alexander Fleming House, London SE1 6BY.

THE NURSE AND THE LAW

The aim of this short appendix is to bring to the awareness of the nurse some legal aspects of nursing. Every student and nurse will do well to think seriously about the following points and to exert the utmost care both in carrying out all nursing procedures and in dealing with patients and their relatives since neglect may cause great distress to her patients and their families and damage the good name of the hospital. Carelessness or negligence may lead to an action in court and heavy damages could be awarded against the nurse or the hospital authority. A student nurse having a particular legal problem is advised to consult a senior trained nurse or her union representative. A trained nurse who is a member of her professional organization, the Royal College of Nursing and National Council of Nurses of the United Kingdom (the Rcn) or any other trade union, should without delay consult its legal department whether she is working in a hospital or in the community. Fully paid membership entitles her to free advice and representation at any inquiry or inquest, and the indemnity insurance will protect her should costs or damages be awarded against her.

Consent for Operation

A patient coming into hospital still retains his rights as a citizen and his entry only denotes his willingness to undergo an investigation or a course of treatment. Any investigation or treatment of a serious nature, or an operation in which an anaesthetic is used, requires the written consent of the patient. A patient may give his own consent if he is of full age, i.e. has attained the age of 18 years or is a minor who has attained the age of 16 years.

No one should be asked to sign an operation consent form before he has full understanding of the procedures involved. The proposed operation is described on the consent form in general terms only, leaving the exact extent of the surgery to the discretion of the surgeon, but a patient has the right to refuse surgery going beyond the extent to which he has agreed to submit. If he does so, or wishes further explanation, the nurse should refer the question to the surgeon before getting the form signed.

If a patient makes any reservations or conditions—even by word of mouth—when signing, the surgeon must be informed.

For patients under 16 years of age in England and Wales and for minors in Scotland (12 years for a girl and 14 years for a boy) the consent of the parent or guardian is normally obtained. In the event of any difficulty, the ward sister should inform the surgeon and the senior administrative officer. This also applies in those cases where the patient is unfit to give consent and no relative is available.

Correct Identity

The nurse or the midwife has the grave responsibility to make sure that all babies born in hospital are correctly labelled at birth and to ensure that at no time are they placed in the wrong cot or handed to the wrong mother.

All patients in general hospitals wear identity bands, in order that mistakes may be avoided. It is very important that the correct band is given to each patient and these are normally checked as part of the admission procedure. With young children or unconscious patients even greater care must be taken to ensure correct identity.

Every patient before being given premedication for an operation should be labelled in the manner approved by the hospital. The label should state the patient's name and hospital number. Moreover, a written request stating the same details should be brought to the ward by the theatre porters to ensure that the correct patient is taken to the right theatre. In the theatre it is the anaesthetist's and the surgeon's responsibility to see that they have received the proper patient and that the correct operation is carried out. It is not the nurses' duty to indicate the exact area of operation, which digit or whether the left or right side is to be operated on. But the ward sister or her deputy may be responsible for making sure that, before the patient is sent to the theatre, the medical staff have indicated clearly the site of operation, and for reporting to the surgeon if this has not been done.

In the Theatre

During operations the 'scrubbed' nurse must check the number of all instruments, needles, swabs and packs on her trolleys and, as the operation proceeds, check that each item used is returned to her. She will then have to carry out a final check before the body cavity is closed. If any doubt arises she must inform the surgeon, who should delay his final closure until a recount has taken place. At the conclusion the theatre nurse in charge and the surgeon sign the operation register stating that a correct final count was obtained.

Drugs

The legal requirements for the nurse in regard to the storage and administration of drugs are set out in Appendix 13.

Accidents or Injury

Should a patient sustain injury while in hospital he may bring an action against the hospital authority or against the person to whom he attributes the injury—this may be a member of the medical, nursing or ancillary staff. The hospital has a certain degree of responsibility for the actions of its staff, but a member of the staff who has been negligent or incompetent and has so caused loss or injury to a patient may be found guilty of culpable negligence and damages will then be awarded against her personally. In the case of a student nurse it may have to be shown that she has received proper instruction in the procedure undertaken, for example, where a burn has been received from an unprotected hot-water bottle.

Accidents can arise to visitors or employees of the hospital through negligence in such matters as cleaning equipment placed on stairways, polish or grease left on the floor, faulty electrical equipment or torn furnishings. Hospital staff should constantly be alert to the risks entailed and bring them to the notice of the persons concerned or the proper authority. In the case of a pure accident where no negligence or incompetence is involved there is no liability at law.

An action may be brought against the hospital several years after the accident has occurred. It is therefore necessary that at the time of the incident an accurate and full record should be made on the special form provided. This form should contain a complete factual statement of how the accident occurred, of the kind of steps taken, e.g. whether or not X-rays were made, and should list the names of witnesses and of the medical officer called to carry out an examination.

Self-discharge of Patient

When the patient demands to discharge himself the nurse on duty should try to dissuade him and should inform the medical officer concerned with his care. If the patient is adamant, each hospital will follow its own procedure. It is probable that a senior administrative officer will see the patient and ask him to sign a written statement to the effect that he is discharging himself against medical advice. Should he refuse to sign, a note to this effect will have to be made and signed by two witnesses, one of whom is usually the administrative officer concerned and the other the nurse in charge at the time. The patient must be allowed to leave, except in the case of a mentally disordered patient who is subject to a restriction order or where it is felt he may be a danger to himself or others, when he may be detained for three days to enable an order to be obtained.

Mentally Disordered Patients

The proper care and treatment of these patients which includes those with *mental illness, subnormality, severe subnormality* and *psychopathic disorder*, and the safeguarding of their property and affairs is laid down in the *Mental Health Act 1959*, and the rules made thereunder. Most of these patients are now admitted without legal formality (*informal admission*) provided that they are not unwilling to enter hospital. They may leave when they wish unless detained for three days.

A person may be liable to detention in hospital or guardianship under the Act only if he is suffering from one of the *named* forms of disorder and if, for his own health or safety or for the protection of others, he needs restraint or control.

Unless subject to a Court Order, subnormal or psychopathic patients can first be made subject to detention or guardianship only before the age of 21 years. This ceases at 25 years unless a report has been furnished by the responsible medical officer that they would be likely to act in a manner dangerous to themselves or others. Except in criminal cases and subject to the aforesaid, detention in hospital or guardianship is for two consecutive periods of 1 year and then for 2-yearly periods. Renewal of authority in each instance is on report by the responsible medical officer that continuance of the detention or guardianship is necessary for the patient's own health or safety or for the protection of others.

Professional Confidence

Guarding the confidences of the patient is an ethical duty of the medical and nursing professions and nurses must take care never to discuss personal information received by nature of their position, except with senior members of the staff when the knowledge may help in the patient's treatment. Even then it will in many cases be wise to ask the patient's permission to pass on the relevant information. No confidential information should be divulged to relatives or friends, nor should details of the patient's condition be passed on to his employer as this may cause loss to the patient for which the nurse may be legally liable. This does not mean that near relatives should not be informed of the patient's progress; but discretion must be exercised.

Patient's Property

The Department of Health and Social Security requires all hospitals under its care to inform patients that the hospital cannot accept responsibility for valuables or money unless these have been handed over for safe keeping. Where it is known that a patient has an excess of money he should be invited to hand it over against a signed receipt so that it may be placed in the hospital safe. The valuables and money of an unconscious patient admitted as an emergency should be listed, checked by two nurses and put in safe keeping.

While a patient is in hospital, the nurse has no right to go through his locker or personal property without his consent. Searching his possessions may be justified if it is suspected that the patient intends to injure himself or others and has the means to do so. Yet, even in such a case, the nurse will be wise to have a witness.

When a patient dies in hospital his possessions must be recorded in the property book, but money and valuables should be listed and packed separately. The property will then be checked and the book signed by two persons, usually a nurse and the sister or her deputy. Strictly speaking, the property should be handed over to the executors of the deceased, but unless property of considerable value is involved it is usual to hand it over, against a receipt, to the next of kin. This may be the responsibility of an administrative officer and in this case the nurse should on no account give property or valuables to relatives or friends of the deceased. Care must be taken in the descriptive terms used; for example, yellow metal is a safer term to use than gold and white metal than silver or platinum since the relatives may refuse to accept an article made of base metal that has been incorrectly described.

Making of Wills and Signing of Legal Documents

Most hospitals have a rule against or discourage nurses from signing legal documents or witnessing signatures during their professional duties. This is to protect the nurse should the document be challenged later on the ground of the unfitness of the patient. However the nurse has the duty to pass on immediately any request of this nature on the part of the patient so that the services of a solicitor may be obtained or those of a hospital administrative officer, who will assist the patient in every way, even in drawing up a simple will if so required.

Suspicion of Theft

The nurse is cautioned not to make accusations of theft against any hospital employee except to a senior trained colleague since without sufficient evidence she may easily lay herself open to an action for libel or slander. The nurse is also cautioned against the all too ready habit of borrowing as this could result in a charge of and conviction for theft. This refers to hospital property as well as borrowing from a private person. Conviction in turn leads to disciplinary action by the General Nursing Council, which means that her name may be removed from the Nurses Register.

Further Reading

Further information on the legal responsibilities of the nurse may be obtained from the following books and booklets, which are highly recommended to ward sisters and nursing administrators.

SPELLER, S. R. (1976) *Law Notes for Nurses*, 6th ed. London: Rcn.

WHINCUP, M. H. (1978) *Legal Aspects of Medical and Nursing Service*, 2nd ed. Ravenswood Publications.

Safeguards Against Failure to Remove Swabs and Instruments from Patients (1978) London: Medical Defence Council and Royal College of Nursing.

Safeguards Against Wrong Operations (1978) London: Medical Defence Council and Royal College of Nursing.

Watchdog: For the Record (1978) London: Royal College of Nursing.

THE REORGANIZED HEALTH SERVICE

For nurses, radical changes in the Health Service were prompted by the publication in 1966 of the report on senior nursing staff structure, which subsequently became known as the Salmon report. The committee which produced this considered carefully the nursing administration in British hospitals and recommended that extensive alterations be made. In order to assess the feasibility of these proposals, a number of pilot schemes were established, but unfortunately these had not been adequately assessed before many hospitals adopted the system. This led to much confusion and unrest amongst nurses and doctors, many of whom felt that the changes had been implemented too rapidly. The result of this was that the report became the subject of extremely severe criticism which has persisted to the present time.

Although the reorganization of the Health Service in 1974 brought even greater changes, some of the innovations which were introduced as a result of the Salmon report still remain. The following is a description of the nursing staff gradings from staff nurse to senior nursing officer, and a brief resumé of their responsibilities.

Staff Nurse

This is the first post to be held by a trained nurse and prepares her to take further responsibility. She normally takes charge of a ward in the absence of the ward sisters and by doing so learns the principles of ward management.

Ward Sister or Charge Nurse

From a staff nurse's post promotion can be gained to that of ward sister. A male nurse is known as a charge nurse.

This post carries considerable responsibility. The sister has a duty not only to her patients, but also to trainee nurses (she is a very important member of the teaching team), to other trained staff, and to the consultants and other doctors with whom she works. She is the one member of the ward staff who remains permanently, and so is the one who becomes most familiar with the nursing routines which are required. Because she is the stable element, great reliance is placed on her skill and knowledge.

Nursing Officer

This is the grade which has attracted the greatest criticism. The nursing officer usually has responsibility for several wards. The exception to this is in specialized units, where it is felt that the work is so demanding and complex that a nursing officer is required for a comparatively small number of patients. Her duties require her to ensure that ward management is undertaken efficiently and this she does through her ward sisters. She has to account to a senior nursing officer for the events which take place in her unit.

Senior Nursing Officer

A senior nursing officer has responsibility for a number of units or in some cases a small hospital. She has, in fact, replaced the matron of former times. She is responsible for all staff and patients in her area and she has to account to either a divisional or district nursing officer.

In schools of nursing, similar gradings have been established, in order that the 'service' and 'education' branches can be equated. This also facilitates the calculation of salary scales.

The Health Service Reorganization

In 1970 the Government planned to reorganize the structure of the Health Service, the purpose being described by Sir Keith Joseph in the foreword to the White Paper as 'to provide a better more sensitive service to the public.' From the time of the inauguration of the Health Service in 1948 until its reorganization, the administration had been on a tripartite basis, in the following manner:

(1) The hospital and specialist services.
(2) The family practitioner services.
(3) The personal health services, which included health visiting, home nursing and health centres amongst several others.

In order to effect the reorganization it was decided to unify these three aspects.

At the same time as these plans were being laid, there were radical changes being made in local government administration and it was felt that the fact that many county boundaries were to be altered should be considered when establishing the administrative areas for the Health Service.

The final arrangement was, briefly, as follows: there would be two levels apart from central government, namely regional and area.

The country was divided into fourteen regions, which comply with the new county boundaries, and each of these has its own administrative officers.

These regions are subdivided into areas, which also have their own administrative officers to cover the whole span of the health service commitments.

The day-to-day management is effected through the districts into which each area is subdivided, and once again each of these has its own officers. The districts are based on district hospitals serving a population of 200 000 to 500 000 people.

The White Paper stipulated that the districts would not form a separate tier, but they have in fact done so. The result has been much discussion regarding the necessity for three levels of administration and the costs involved in such a system.

The establishment of regional and area administration meant the abolition of hospital management committees and also, much to the chagrin of the teaching hospitals, of boards of governors. The only exception to this, being the post-graduate teaching hospitals, which were not to be incorporated into the system for five years. This was to allow suitable plans to be made for their future management.

Hospital boards of governors had for many years undertaken great responsibilities and their members gave their services voluntarily. It was not without sadness on the part of many that these philanthropic individuals were relieved of their duties.

The number of areas into which the country is divided is 72 outside the London area. The 32 London Boroughs are grouped to form a small number of areas. The grand total is now 89.

For nurses the reorganization meant yet another period of change. Further senior posts were established, the holders of which have had to create their own jobs. A description of the new grades is given below.

Divisional Nursing Officer

A divisional nursing officer takes responsibility for a large hospital or highly specialized unit. Frequently a group of hospitals is involved or, in the case of a community nurse, the services for a whole district. The equivalent grade in a school of nursing is a director of nurse education.

District Nursing Officer

This post includes its responsibilities the overseeing of management in a district hospital and its community. This means supervising the nursing service which is being provided for 200 000 to 500 000 people.

At both the area and regional levels there are nursing officers who are concerned with the wider concepts of administration. They have no clinical responsibility.

It is possible that further changes will be made in the future, as the effectiveness or otherwise of the reorganization becomes more apparent.

NURSING EDUCATION

Nurse education has in recent years experienced considerable change. This had been necessitated by a number of factors, not least of which is the progress of medical knowledge with which it is essential for nursing to keep abreast. Since the tuition of nurses both before and after qualification covers a very wide field, a brief resumé is given.

BASIC NURSE TRAINING

For nurses to become legally eligible to practice they are required to undertake a recognized period of training in accordance with the Nurses Act. The statutory body which is appointed to supervise nurse training is the General Nursing Council for England and Wales. Both Scotland and Northern Ireland have their own Councils and their own systems of training.

A trainee may follow a course of training which leads in three years to State Registration, or in two years to State Enrolment. These will be described separately. It is possible to specialize in mental or mental subnormality nursing (SRNs and SENs) or as a sick children's nurse.

Training for State Registration

In order to become a State Registered Nurse it is necessary to undertake a three-year period of basic training. During this time the student must receive a specified amount of theoretical instruction as well as adequate clinical experience. Hospitals must ensure that a training plan is followed and that this provides teaching and experience in logical sequence. Many hospitals have, with the approval of the General Nursing Council, introduced courses which either allow the student to attempt her final examination at an early date or combine the basic training with a degree or diploma. It is, however, required that she completes three years nursing before becoming eligible for registration.

Training schools are inspected regularly by the General Nursing Council and may not implement any major changes in their training plans without authorization. If the teaching is found to be inadequate, permission to train students is withdrawn.

In order to be accepted for student nurse training, applicants must have a minimum of two subjects at the Ordinary level of the General Certificate of Education or gain a satisfactory mark in a test set by the General Nursing Council. Individual hospitals, however, are permitted to stipulate their own entry requirements above the minimum.

Training for State Enrolment

In order to become State Enrolled it is necessary to undertake a course of two years' duration which is less academically demanding than the course for registration. The pupil does, however, have to receive both theoretical instruction and practical experience in accordance with the regulations of the General Nursing Council. The conditions are identical to those described above except that acceptance for training is not dependent on having acquired passes in the General Certificate of Education. Once qualified, the enrolled nurse works as a member of the trained staff, but her work is directed more towards direct patient care and she is less involved in administrative duties.

Once her name is on any one of the registers maintained by the General Nursing Council, the nurse may legally practice and accept the responsibilities of a fully trained nurse. In the event of her committing a crime, or being guilty of other misconduct, she may be required to appear before a disciplinary committee which is appointed by the Council. This may result in her name being removed from the register or roll.

As well as the general register and roll there are those which record the names of nurses who have undertaken training in highly specialized branches of nursing. Hospitals providing courses in these specialities have to conform to conditions similar to those previously quoted.

In order to comply with the regulations of the EEC, basic nurse training will undergo further changes. It is hoped that all the member countries of the community will be able to provide comparable training schemes, which will enable a trained nurse to work in any of the participant nations without having to undertake further examinations or apply for registration in the individual countries.

POST-BASIC TRAINING

Nowadays there is ample opportunity for nurses to undertake post-basic training in the clinical specialty of their choice. In 1970 the Joint Board of Clinical Nursing Studies was established with the prime function of coordinating and supervising the large number of courses which were being organized throughout the country. Many of these courses were utilized as a means of recruiting staff and had little or no educational content. This meant that a nurse could spend several months undertaking a course at the end of which she had a certificate but no specialized skill.

The Joint Board has been successful in rationalizing this situation. They appointed panels of nurses and doctors whose remit was to produce outline curricula for courses. Hospitals wishing to offer specialized training under the auspices of the Board have to apply for authorization to do so and provide teaching and experience in accordance with the conditions stipulated in the curricula. Nowadays applicants are reluctant to enrol for a course which is not approved by the Board, but those who have taken approved courses and have completed their training will be extremely competent to practice in their chosen field of nursing.

The publication of curricula is undertaken in accordance with the requirements of the nation for nurses who are skilled in specified clinical skills. In each instance, a new panel is elected and, having produced the curriculum, meets regularly to update it as necessary.

In order to obtain approval from the Board to organize a course, the hospitals have to conform to stringent conditions and undergo regular inspections. This has, however, ensured a marked improvement in the standards of post-basic education throughout the country.

THE DIPLOMA IN NURSING

The Diploma in Nursing is awarded by the University of London to those nurses who successfully undertake a course of academic study. The Diploma has two parts, the first of which is designed to give the student a deeper knowledge of basic science, psychology and the development of the profession. Success in the examination for these subjects must be achieved before the candidate goes on to the second part which concentrates on improving the student's knowledge of disease processes. As part of this the nurse is also examined in a specialty of her own choosing.

It is now essential to obtain the Diploma in Nursing before applying for most courses leading to registration as a nurse teacher.

NURSING DEGREES

Many nurses choose to study for a degree after completing their basic training and some, as described previously, obtain such a qualification in conjunction with their basic training.

It is possible to use the facilities offered by the Open University or those of colleges of further education. The degrees obtained are often not in nursing, but serve to improve the education of the student.

CLINICAL TEACHER TRAINING

Many nurses who train as nurse teachers undertake a course in which they learn the skills associated with teaching in clinical areas. It is possible to apply for either a full-time or a part-time course and once qualified the nurse teaches nurses at the bedside.

NURSE TUTOR TRAINING

In order to become a nurse tutor it is essential to undertake specialized training. Nowadays this may be done in one of two ways. The student may follow a course leading to the University of London's Sister Tutor's Diploma or she may train at a college of education, at the end of which course she becomes eligible for registration by the General Nursing Council as a nurse tutor.

MIDWIFERY TRAINING

Many nurses choose to become midwives after obtaining their initial qualification. At present, the course lasts for one year and can be undertaken at many hospitals in the country. The Central Midwives Board is the statutory controlling body, and has a function similar to that of the General Nursing Council.

PROFESSIONAL ORGANIZATIONS AND STATUTORY BODIES

ROYAL COLLEGE OF NURSING OF THE UNITED KINGDOM

Known as the Rcn, this is the professional organization in the United Kingdom for nurses holding a statutory qualification or in training for such a qualification. The Rcn is also a certificated independent trade union. While the Rcn's UK headquarters are in London, it has national headquarters in Scotland, Northern Ireland and Wales from which its National Boards operate; it also has various area offices in England. The Rcn is governed by a council elected by and from amongst its members.

The membership structure of the Rcn is based on some 200 local centres which relate to NHS areas or districts. The Rcn incorporates four associations, namely Associations of Nursing Education, Nursing Management, Nursing Practice and Nursing Students. It also incorporates the following six societies: Occupational Health Nursing, Oncology Nursing, Geriatric Nursing, Primary Health Care Nursing, Psychiatric Nursing and Research. Specialist forums, relating to more specific spheres of professional practice, are in being within the associations and societies.

The *Rcn Institute of Advanced Nursing Education* in London, Birmingham and Belfast offers a range of courses for qualified nurses, some of which prepare for an Rcn Certificate or for a University Diploma while any are short topic-centred or refresher courses. The Rcn Institute in London and Birmingham is recognized by the Department of Education and Science as an establishment of further education.

The *Professional Nursing Department* undertakes the work of the Rcn concerned with the advancement of nursing, the promotion of high standards of care and the formulation and presentation of the professional viewpoint on all matters relevant to professional practice in particular and to health service provision in general. The Rcn Centres, Associations, Societies and forums are staffed by expert nurse officers working within this department.

The *International Department* deals with the work arising from the Rcn's membership of the International Council of Nurses, the Commonwealth Nurses Federation and the European Nursing Group. The department is also much involved in activities within the EEC arising from the Rcn's role in representing the nurses of the UK on the Standing Committee of the EEC.

Programmes are arranged for nurses from overseas visiting this country on study tours on either an individual or a group basis; arrangements are also made for Rcn members wishing to study or work abroad.

The *Labour Relations and Legal Department* provides a comprehensive service to members in relation to matters arising in their employment situation. It is concerned with salaries and conditions of service and with the work of the Rcn as a nationally recognized negotiating body. It administers the Rcn Steward Scheme which provides members with a workplace representative; it also administers the Rcn Safety Representative Scheme and provides, or commissions, the necessary training programmes for both these schemes. The Rcn provides professional indemnity insurance for all its members.

The *Press and Public Relations Department* is concerned with communications to the membership, the profession and the general public. It maintains close links with the media. It is also responsible for the production of the Rcn's official newspaper—*The Nursing Standard*—which is delivered direct to every member. Since early 1979 this publication has been issued weekly and is free of charge. The department is also responsible for various other publications including a Series of research reports.

The Rcn offers a *Welfare Advisory Service* to all nurses experiencing personal problems.

GENERAL NURSING COUNCIL FOR ENGLAND AND WALES

Usually referred to as the General Nursing Council (GNC), it is the statutory body set up following the Nurses Registration Act of 1919. It is concerned with the training and registration of nurses. The same functions are fulfilled in Scotland by the General Nursing Council for Scotland and in Northern Ireland by the Joint Nursing and Midwives Council for Northern Ireland.

The General Nursing Council inspects and approves nurse training schools. It grants approval for combined training and experimental training schemes. The Council lays down a syllabus of training and conducts examinations for the State Registration of Nurses and maintains a register of successful candidates. Trained nurses from other countries who meet the requirements of the General Nursing Council are accepted for registration by the council.

The Council approves certain hospitals for training nurses in non-technical bedside care. It conducts ward assessments for these nurses and following a successful completion of the course their names are placed on the Roll and they become State Enrolled Nurses (SEN).

The General Nursing Council has a disciplinary function and has the power to remove nurses from the Register or the Roll for misdemeanour.

The allocation of money for nurse training made by the Department of Health and Social Security is disbursed by the Council's Finance Committee to the Area Nurse Training Committees.

REGIONAL NURSE TRAINING COMMITTEES

Members of a Regional Nurse Training Committee are appointed by the Department of Health and Social Security in each hospital region. The function of the committee is to supervise methods of training in its area and to advise Regional Boards and Boards of Governors on nurse training.

The committee also considers experimental schemes of training in the area and submits them to the General Nursing Council. It allocates the available money for nurse training to the nurse training schools within its region.

ROYAL COLLEGE OF MIDWIVES

The Royal College of Midwives is an educational and professional organization and trade union exclusively for midwives. The aim is to promote and advance the art and science of midwifery and to raise the efficiency of midwives. The College is the recognized negotiating body for midwives having representation on the Nurses and Midwives Whitley Council. Under the Midwives Act the College has representatives on statutory bodies for midwives of the United Kingdom and is approved by the Central Midwives Board for England and Wales to provide courses in preparation for the Midwife Teachers Diploma, Advanced Diploma in Midwifery and the majority of midwifery statutory refresher courses. Among other benefits of membership are a professional indemnity insurance scheme and a personal accident insurance scheme.

CENTRAL MIDWIVES BOARD

The Central Midwives Board is the statutory body set up by Act of Parliament to protect the public and to regulate the training and registration of midwives. It produces a handbook incorporating the rules of the Central Midwives Board for the guidance of midwives. These rules and amendments have been approved by the Department of Health and Social Security. There are separate subcommittees to deal with the approval of training schools, with examinations and with penal cases.

INTERNATIONAL COUNCIL OF NURSES (ICN)

Founded in 1899, the International Council of Nurses (ICN) is the oldest international professional organization in the health care field. ICN is a federation of national nurses associations representing nearly a million nurses.

ICN accepts into membership one association of nurses per country. There are 88 national nurses' organizations in membership. In addition, ICN works with approximately 50 other national associations or groups of nurses with a view to their future membership.

The governing body of the ICN is the Council of National Representatives (CNR), composed of the president of each of the member associations and operating on the principle of one country one vote. The CNR meets every two years to determine policy matters affecting the nursing profession. Every fourth year this meeting is held in conjunction with an ICN quadrennial Congress, open to nurses throughout the world.

ICN has one standing committee, the Professional Services Committee, which considers trends and problems in relation to nursing education, practice, service and the social and economic welfare of nurses. In addition there are frequent ad hoc committees.

The ICN Board of Directors consists of the President, three Vice-Presidents and 11 other members (seven area representatives and four members-at-large), elected by the CNR at the time of the ICN Congress. The area representatives on the Board are elected from the seven different ICN areas: Africa, the Eastern Mediterranean, Europe, North America, South an Central America, South-east Asia, and the Western Pacific.

ICN's objectives are:

1. To promote the development of strong national nurses associations.
2. To assist national nurses associations to improve the standards of nursing and the competence of nurses.
3. To assist national nurses associations to improve the status of nurses within their countries.
4. To serve as the authoritative voice for nurses and nursing internationally.

The activities of the ICN reflect the wide range of interests and needs of its international membership, focusing on such areas as nursing education, economic and general welfare of nurses, nursing practice and service, nursing legislation, nursing research, and cooperation with other helath professions.

ICN is in official relationship with the World Health Organization (WHO), is included on the special list of non-governmental organizations maintained by the International Labour Organization (ILO) for consultative purposes, is in relationship with the United Nations Educational, Scientific and Cultural Organization (UNESCO) and with the United Nations International Children's Emergency Fund (UNI-CEF), is on the Consultative Register of the Economic and Social Council (ECOSOC), is in relationship with the International Committee of the Red Cross, the League of Red Cross Societies, the World Medical Association, the International Hospital Federation and the Union of International Associations.

FLORENCE NIGHTINGALE INTERNATIONAL FOUNDATION (FNIF)

This educational trust in memory of Florence Nightingale was founded in 1934 by the International Council of Nurses and now forms the Educational Division, aimed at improving nursing service by the furthering of nursing education. It has established a centre of information on educational opportunities in nursing in all countries. The Foundation arranges study programmes, research projects and advices individual nurses on nursing education.

KING EDWARD'S HOSPITAL FUND FOR LONDON

This fund was founded by King Edward VII for the support, benefit or extension of the hospitals of London. It makes grants to hospitals and convalescent homes serving the London area. It maintains the Hospital

Centre for the dissemination of knowledge and improvements in design of hospital equipment. It has an extensive information and advisory service. The premises include a large reference library, a lecture hall, discussion rooms and a display area for hospital equipment.

The King Edward's Hospital Fund provides staff colleges for residential courses in preparation for senior positions in hospital. It also provides the Emergency Bed Service which in the London metropolitan regions aids doctors seeking a hospital bed for an acute case.

NUFFIELD FOUNDATION

The objects of the Nuffield Foundation are the advancement of health and the prevention and relief of sickness, particularly by medical research and teaching; the advancement of social well-being, particularly by scientific research; the care and comfort of the aged poor; and the advancement of education.

A subsidiary organization is the Nuffield Provincial Hospitals Trust, the aim of which is to improve the organization and the efficiency of hospital, medical and health services in the provinces. It finances the Nuffield Centre for Hospital and Health Service Studies of the University of Leeds. The centre provides residential courses in hospital administration and supports research.

WHITLEY COUNCILS FOR THE HEALTH SERVICES (GREAT BRITAIN)

The Whitley Councils are the national organizations set up to negotiate salaries and conditions of service for persons engaged in the National Health Service. It consists of a General Council that deals with matters common to all personnel, such as travelling and subsistence allowance, and of nine functional councils which deal with remuneration and conditions of service applying to a particular group. These comprise:

    Administrative and Clerical Staffs Council
    Ambulance Men's Council
    Ancillary Staffs Council
    Dental Whitley Council (Local Authorities)
    Medical and (Hospital) Dental Council
    Nurses and Midwives Council
    Optical Council
    Pharmaceutical Council
    Professional and Technical Staffs Council A and Council B

Each council has a management side and a staff side. In the case of the Nurses and Midwives Council the members of the management side are appointed by the Ministry of Health, regional boards and employing authorities. The staff side represents the employees, and the members are appointed by the participating organizations such as the Royal College of Nursing, Royal College of Midwives and National Unions of which nurses and midwives are members.

USEFUL ADDRESSES

Association of Nurse Administrators, 13 Grosvenor Place, London SW1X 7EN
   Tel. 01-235 5258

Association of Nursing Students, Royal College of Nursing, la Henrietta Place, Cavendish Square, London W1M 0AB
   Tel. 01-629 6441

British Association of Social Workers, 16 Kent Street, Birmingham B5 6RD
   Tel. 021-622 3911

British Diabetic Association, 10 Queen Anne Street, London W1M PBD
   Tel. 01-323 1531

British Red Cross, 9 Grosvenor Crescent, London SW1X YEJ
   Tel. 01-235 5454
   Telex 918657

Central Midwives Board for England and Wales, 39 Harrington Gardens, London SW7 4JY
   Tel. 01-373 4801

Central Midwives Board for Scotland, 24 Dublin Street, Edinburgh EH1 3PU
   Tel. 031-556 1671

Chartered Society of Physiotherapy, 14 Bedford Row, London WC1R 4ED
   Tel. 01-242 1941/7

Chest and Heart Association, Tavistock House North, Tavistock Square, London WC1H 9JE
   Tel. 01-387 3012

Department of Employment, St Martin's Place, London WC2N 4JH
   Tel. 01-930 7833

Department of Health and Social Security, Alexander Fleming House, Elephant and Castle, London SE1 6BY
   Tel. 01-407 5522

Emergency Bed Service, Fielden House, 28 London Bridge Street, London SE1 9SG
   Tel. 01-407 7181

Federated Superannuation Scheme for Nurses and Hospital Officers (Contributory), Rosehill, Park Rd, Banstead, Surrey
   Tel. 07373 57272

General Nursing Council for England and Wales, 23 Portland Place, London W1A 1BA
   Tel. 01-580 8334

General Nursing Council for Scotland, 5 Darnaway Street, Edinburgh EH3 6DP
   Tel. 031-225 6322-4

Health Services Superannuation Division, Department of Health and Social Security, North Fylde Central Offices, Hesketh House, 200–20 Broadway, Fleetwood, Lancs FY7 8LG
Tel. 039-17 77123

Hospital Savings Association, 30 Lancaster Gate, London W2 3LT
Tel. 01-723 7601

International Council of Nurses, 37 Rue Vermont, 1202 Geneva, Geneva 20.
Tel. Geneva 336400

Joint Nursing and Midwives Council of Northern Ireland, 5 Annadale Avenue, Belfast 7, Northern Ireland
Tel. 0232 644028

King Edward's Hospital Fund for London, 14A Palace Court, London W2 4HT
Tel. 01-727 0581

King's Fund Centre, 126 Albert Street, London NW1 7NF
Tel. 01-267 6111

King's Fund College, 2 Palace Court, London W2 4HS
Tel. 01-229 9361

National Association for the Welfare of Children in Hospital, 7 Exton Street, London SE1 8UE
Tel. 01-261 1738

National Staff Committee for Nurses and Midwives, 168 Blackfriars Road, London SE1 8EU
Tel. 01-703 6380

Nation's Fund for Nurses, 1 Henrietta Place, London W1M 0AB
Tel. 01-580 3965

Nuffield Foundation, Regent's Park, London NW1 4RS
Tel. 01-722 8871/9

Nurses and Midwives Council of the Royal College of Nursing (United Kingdom), Henrietta Place, London W1M 0AB
Tel. 01-636 3866

Nursing and Hospital Careers Information Centre, 121/123 Edgware Road, London W2 2HX
Tel. 01-402 5296

Princess Mary's Royal Air Force Nursing Service, Ministry of Defence, First Avenue House, High Holborn, London WC1V 6HE
Tel. 01-430 5639

Queen Alexandra's Royal Army Nursing Corps, Ministry of Defence, First Avenue House, High Holborn, London WC1V 6HD
Tel. 01-430 5555

Queen Alexandra's Royal Naval Nursing Service, Ministry of Defence, First Avenue House, High Holborn, London WC1V 6HD
Tel. 01-430 5555

Rcn Student Section, Henrietta Place, London W1M 0AB
Tel. 01-580 2646

Royal Association for Disability and Rehabilitation (RADAR), 25 Mortimer Street, London W1N 8AB
Tel. 01-637 5400

Royal British Nurses Association, 94 Upper Tollington Park, London N4 4NB
Tel. 01-272 6821

Royal College of Midwives, 15 Mansfield Street, London W1M 0BE
Tel. 01-580 6523/5

Royal College of Nursing of the United Kingdom, Henrietta Place, Cavendish Square, London W1M 0AB
Tel. 01-580 2646

Royal College of Nursing of the United Kingdom (Scottish Board), 44 Heriot Row, Edinburgh EH3 6EY.
Tel. 031-225 7231

Royal College of Nursing of the United Kingdom (Northern Ireland Board), 17 Windsor Avenue, Belfast BT9 6EE
Tel. 0232 668236/7

Royal College of Nursing of the United Kingdom (Welsh Board), Ty Maeth, King George V Drive East, Cardiff CF4 4XZ
Tel. 0222 751374/5

Royal National Institute for the Blind, 224 Great Portland Street, London W1N 6AA
Tel. 01-388 1266

Royal National Institute of the Deaf, 105 Gower Street, London WC1
Tel. 01-437 8030

Royal National Pension Fund for Nurses, Burdett House, 15 Buckingham Street, Strand, London WC2N 6ED
Tel. 01-839 6785

United Nursing Services Club, 40 South Street, London W1
Tel. Secretary 01-470 1564
Members 01-629 0896

Whitley Council for Nurses and Midwives, Staff Side Secretary, 1 Henrietta Place, London W1M 0AB
Tel. 01-636 3866

Women's Royal Voluntary Service Headquarters, 17 Old Park Lane, London W1Y 4AJ
Tel. 01-499 6040

DEGREES, DIPLOMAS, ORGANIZATIONS ETC.

ABPN	Association of British Paediatric Nurses
ADMS	Assistant Director of Medical Services
AIMSW	Associate of the Institute of Medical Social Workers
AHA	Area Health Authority
ARRC	Associate, Royal Red Cross
ASTMS	Association of Scientific Technical and Managerial Staffs
BA	Bachelor of Arts
BAO	Bachelor of the Art of Obstetrics
BC, BCh, BChir	Bachelor of Surgery
BChD, BDS	Bachelor of Dental Surgery
BDA	British Dental Association
BM	Bachelor of Medicine (Oxford University)
BMA	British Medical Association
BP	British Pharmacopoeia
BRCS	British Red Cross Society
BS	Bachelor of Surgery
BSc	Bachelor of Science
ChB	Bachelor of Surgery
CCD	Central Council for the Disabled
CCHE	Central Council for Health Education
CM, ChM	Master of Surgery
CMB	Central Midwives' Board
CNN	Certificated Nursery Nurse
COHSE	Confederation of Health Service Employees
CPH	Certificate of Public Health
CSP	Chartered Society of Physiotherapists
CU	Casualties Union
DA	Diploma of Anaesthetics
DCh	Doctor of Surgery
DCH	Diploma of Child Health
DCP	Diploma in Clinical Pathology
DDA	Dangerous Drugs Act
DDMS	Deputy Director of Medical Services
DDS	Doctor of Dental Surgery
DHyg	Doctor of Hygiene
DIH	Diploma in Industrial Health
DM	Doctor of Medicine (Oxford University)
DN	Diploma in Nursing
DNA	District Nursing Association
DO	Diploma in Ophthalmology
DObstRCOG	Diplomate of the Royal College of Obstetricians and Gynaecologists

DPH	Diploma in Public Health
DPhil	Doctor of Philosophy
DPM	Diploma in Psychological Medicine
DR	Diploma in Radiology
DSc	Doctor of Science
DTM&H	Diploma in Tropical Medicine and Hygiene
FACP	Fellow of the American College of Physicians
FACS	Fellow of the American College of Surgeons
FCSP	Fellow of the Chartered Society of Physiotherapists
FDS	Fellow in Dental Surgery
FFARCS	Fellow of the Faculty of Anaesthetists, Royal College of Surgeons
FNIF	Florence Nightingale International Foundation
FPS	Fellow of the Pharmaceutical Society
FRACP	Fellow of the Royal Australasian College of Physicians
FRACS	Fellow of the Royal Australasian College of Surgeons
FRCGP	Fellow of the Royal College of General Practitioners
FRCOG	Fellow of the Royal College of Obstetricians and Gynaecologists
FRCP	Fellow of the Royal College of Physicians
FRCPE	Fellow of the Royal College of Physicians, Edinburgh
FRCPI	Fellow of the Royal College of Physicians of Ireland
FRCPath	Fellow of the Royal College of Pathologists
FRCPsych	Fellow of the Royal College of Psychologists
FRCS	Fellow of the Royal College of Surgeons
FRCSE	Fellow of the Royal College of Surgeons, Edinburgh
FRCSI	Fellow of the Royal College of Surgeons of Ireland
FRFPS	Fellow of the Royal Faculty of Physicians and Surgeons
FRIPHH	Fellow of the Royal Institute of Public Health and Hygiene
FRS	Fellow of the Royal Society
FRSE	Fellow of the Royal Society of Edinburgh
FRSH	Fellow of the Royal Society of Health
FRSM	Fellow of the Royal Society of Medicine
FSR(R)	Fellow of the Society of Radiographers (Radiography)
FSR(T)	Fellow of the Society of Radiographers (Radiotherapy)
GMC	General Medical Council
GNC	General Nursing Council
HSA	Hospital Savings Association
HV	Health Visitor
ICN	International Council of Nurses
ICW	International Council of Women
IHF	International Hospitals Federation

LDS	Licentiate in Dental Surgery
LMRCP	Licenciate in Midwifery of the Royal College of Physicians
LMSSA	Licentiate in Medicine and Surgery of the Society of Apothecaries, London
LRCP	Licentiate of the Royal College of Physicians
LRCPE	Licentiate of the Royal College of Physicians of Edinburgh
LRFPS	Licentiate of the Royal Faculty of Physicians and Surgeons
LSA	Licentiate of the Society of Apothecaries
MA	Master of Arts
MAO	Master of the Art of Obstetrics
MAOT	Member of the Association of Occupational Therapists
MB	Bachelor of Medicine (other than from Oxford)
MC, MCh, MChir	Master of Surgery
MCSP	Member of the Chartered Society of Physiotherapists
MChOrth	Master of Orthopaedic Surgery
MChS	Member of the Society of Chiropodists
MD	Doctor of Medicine (other than from Oxford)
MIND	National Association for Mental Health
MRCOG	Member of the Royal College of Obstetricians and Gynaecologists
MRCP	Member of the Royal College of Physicians
MRCPath	Member of the Royal College of Pathologists
MRCPsych	Member of the Royal College of Psychiatrists
MRCS	Member of the Royal College of Surgeons
MRSH	Member of the Royal Society for the Promotion of Health
MS	Master of Surgery
MSA	Member of the Society of Apothecaries
MSR(R)	Member of the Society of Radiographers (Radiography)
MSR(T)	Member of the Society of Radiographers (Radiotherapy)
MSc	Master of Science
MTD	Midwife Teachers' Diploma
NALGO	National Association of Local Government Officers
NAMCW	National Association for Maternal and Child Welfare
NAMH	National Association for Mental Health
NAWCH	National Association for the Welfare of Children in Hospital
NHS	National Health Service
NHSR	National Hospital Service Reserve
NNEB	National Nursery Examination Board
NUPE	National Union of Public Employees
ONC	Orthopaedic Nursing Certificate
PMRAFNS	Princess Mary's Royal Air Force Nursing Service
PhD	Doctor of Philosophy

QARANC	Queen Alexandra's Royal Army Nursing Corps
QARNNS	Queen Alexandra's Royal Naval Nursing Service
QHP	Queen's Honorary Physician
QHNS	Queen's Honorary Nursing Sister
QHS	Queen's Honorary Surgeon
QIDN	Queen's Institute of District Nursing
RADC	Royal Army Dental Corps
RAMC	Royal Army Medical Corps
RCM	Royal College of Midwives
Rcn	Royal College of Nursing and National Council of Nurses of the United Kingdom
RFN	Registered Fever Nurse
RGN	Registered General Nurse
RHA	Regional Health Authority
RMO	Resident Medical Officer
RMN	Registered Mental Nurse
RN	Registered Nurse (USA and other overseas countries)
RNMD	Registered Nurse for Mental Defectives
RNMS	Registered Nurse for the Mentally Subnormal
RNT	Registered Nurse Tutor
RRC	Royal Red Cross
RSCN	Registered Sick Children's Nurse
StAAA	St. Andrew's Ambulance Association
StJAA	St. John Ambulance Association
StJAB	St. John Ambulance Brigade
SCM	State Certified Midwife
SEN	State Enrolled Nurse
SRN	State Registered Nurse
SSStJ	Serving Sister of the Order of St John of Jerusalem
VAD	Voluntary Aid Detachment
WHO	World Health Organization
WPHOA	Women Public Health Officers' Association
WRVS	Women's Royal Voluntary Service

PREFIXES AND SUFFIXES

Prefix	Meaning	Prefix	Meaning
a-	without	contra-	against, counter
ab-	away from	cost-	of the ribs
abdomin-	of the abdomen	crani-	of the skull
ad-	towards	crypt-	hidden, concealed
an-	without	cyst-	of the bladder
ana-	upwards	cyt-	of a cell
andr-	male	dacry-	of tears
angi-	of a blood vessel	dactyl-	of a finger
ante-	before, in front of	de-	down, from
anti-	against, counter	deci-	one-tenth
aort-	of the aorta	demi-	one-half
apo-	away from, back	dent-	of the teeth
arthr-	of the joints	derm-	of the skin
aut-	of self	dextr-	right
bi-, bis-	two	di-, diplo-	two, double
bili-	of bile, of the biliary tract	dis-	apart, away from
		dors-	of the back
bio-	of life	dys-	difficult, abnormal
blephar-	of the eyelid	ect-	outside
brachi-	of the arm	electr-	of electricity
brachy-	short	em-, en-,	in, inside, within
brady-	slow	end-,	
bronch-	of the bronchus	ent-	
cardi-	of the heart	enter-	of the intestines
carp-, kata-	of the wrist	epi-	above, over
cata-, kata-	down, negative	erythr-	red
centi-	one-hundredth	eu-	good, normal
cephal-	of the head	ex-, exo-	out of, outside
cerebr-	of the brain	extra-	outside, beyond
cervic-	of the neck	faci-	of the face
cheil-, chil-	of the lip	flav-	yellow
cheir-,	of the hand	galact-	of milk
chir-		gastr-	of the stomach
chem-	chemical	gen-	producing
chol-	of the bile, of the gall bladder	glyc-	of sugar
		gnath-	of the jaw
chondr-	of cartilage	haem-	of the blood
chrom-	colour	hemi-	a half
cine-, kine-	of motion	hepat-	of the liver
circum-	around	hex-	six
co-	together	hist-	of tissue
col-	of the colon	homeo-,	same, like
colp-	of the vagina	hom-	
con-	together	hydr-	of water

Prefix	Meaning	Prefix	Meaning
hyper-	above	ot-	of the ear
hypo-	below	pachy-	thick
hyster-	of the uterus	pan-	total, all
idi-	peculiar, distinct	para-	beside, beyond
ile-	of the ileum	path-	of disease, sickness
ili-	of the ilium	paed-	child
immun-	of immunity	pent-	five
in-	negative, without	per-	through
infra-	below	peri-	around
intra-	inside	pharyng-	of the pharynx
intro-	towards, inward	phleb-	of the veins
ischi-	of the ischium	phon-	of sound
iso-	equal	photo-	of light
kary-	of the nucleus	phren-	of the diaphragm, of the mind
kerat-	of the skin		
lact-	of milk	pleur-	of the pleura
laryng-	of the larynx	pneum-	of the lung
later-	side	pod-	of the foot
leuc-, leuk-	white	poly-	many
lymph-	of lymph	post-	after, behind
macr-	large	prae-, pre-, pro-	before in time or place
mal-	bad, abnormal		
medi-	middle	proct-	of the anus
mega-	large	pseud-	false
melan-	black	psych-	of the mind
meso-	middle	py-	of pus
meta-	between	pyr-	of fire, fever
micr-	small	quadr-	four
milli-	one thousandth	quint-	five
mono-	one, single	radi-	ray, radiation
multi-	many	re-	back, again
myc-	fungal	ren-	of the kidney
myel-	of the marrow	retro-	backwards
myo-	of the muscle	rhin-	of the nose
narc-	numb	rub-	red
neo-	new	salping-	of the (fallopian) tubes
nephr-	of the kidney		
neur-	of the nerves	sarc-	of flesh
norm-	of normality	semi-	one-half
nucle-	of nucleus	sept-	seven
ocul-	of the eye	splen-	of the spleen
oligo-	deficient, few	stear-	fat
onych-	of the nails	sub-	below
oo-	of an egg	super-, supra-	above
orchid-	of the testes		
or-	of the mouth	syn-	union with
orth-	straight	tachy-	fast
os-	of the mouth	tars-	foot, edge
os-, oste-	bone	tetra-	four

Prefix	Meaning	Prefix	Meaning
therm-	of heat	ultra-	beyond
thorac-	of the thorax	uni-	one
thromb-	of a clot	ureter-	of the ureter
tox-	poison	urethra-	of the urethra
trache-	of the trachea	vas-	of vessels (blood)
trans-	across, through	ven-	of veins
tri-	three	xanth-	yellow
trich-	of the hair	xiph-	of the cartilage of
troph-	of nourishment		the sternum

Suffix	Meaning	Suffix	Meaning
-aemia, -emia	of blood	-meter	measure
-aesthesia	of sensation	-odynia	pain in
-algia	pertaining to pain	-oid	having a likeness to
-blast	cell	-ology	study of
-caval	of the venae cavae	-oma	tumour
-cele	swelling, tumour	-osis	disease
-centesis	a puncturing	-ostomy	opening into
-coccus	spherical bacterium	-otomy	incision
		-pathy	disease of
-cyte	cell	-penia	lack of
-derm	skin	-pexy	fixing of
-desis	binding together	-phagia	swallowing
-ectasis	dilatation, extension	-phasia	of speech
		-phobia	fear
-ectomy	removal of	-phylaxis	prevention of, protection
-form	having the form of, like		
		-plasty	plastic surgery
-genesis, -genetic	origin, production	-plegia	paralysis
		-poiesis	formation of
-genic	causative	-rhoea	discharge
-gram	a tracing	-rhythmia	rhythm
-graph	description of, a tracing	-scope	instrument used for investigation by eye
-iasis	condition		
-itis	inflamation of	-scopy	visual examination
-kinesis, -kinetic	motion, energy	-somatic	of the body
		-somy	of chromosomes
-lith	stone	-sonic	sound
-lithiasis	presence of stones	-stasis	lack of movement, stagnation
-lysis	breaking down		
-malacia	softening of	-taxia, -taxis	arrangement, order
-megaly	enlargement of	-tome	cutting instrument

Nurses' Aids Series
Special Interest Texts

Special Interest Texts will enable the nurse to study a particular subject in greater detail during training or after basic studies have been completed.

ACCIDENT AND EMERGENCY NURSING/
Bradley *1980*

ANAESTHESIA & RECOVERY ROOM
TECHNIQUES/Wachstein and Smith *3rd edition 1981*

GASTROENTEROLOGICAL NURSING/Gribble
1977

NEUROMEDICAL AND NEUROSURGICAL
NURSING/Purchese *1977*

NUTRITION AND DIETETICS IN HEALTH
AND DISEASE/Huskisson *1981*

OPHTHALMIC NURSING/Darling and Thorpe
2nd edition 1981

ORTHOPAEDICS FOR NURSES/Pinney *6th edition*
1983

1. All the authors are nurses who know exactly what the student requires.
2. The books are frequently revised to ensure that advances in knowledge reach the student as soon as practicable.
3. The Aids are well printed and easy to read, clearly illustrated, and modestly priced.

Baillière Prize for Nursing Studies

In conjunction with the Royal College of Nursing, this annual prize is awarded for the best original paper incorporating the methods and principles of nursing care and/or education.

The closing date for receipt of essay is mid July. For full details apply in March to:

The Nursing Editor
Baillière Tindall
1 Vincent Square
London SW1P 2PN

BAILLIÈRE TINDALL

35 Red Lion Square
London, WC1R 4SG

BAILLIÈRE'S NURSING BOOKS

Basic Training

Hutton/BASIC NURSING CARE -
A Guide for Nursing Auxilliaries
Of value to every learner in the hospital ward. *2nd edition 1981*

Crispin/HANDBOOK OF PRACTICAL NURSING
A clear concise style giving the essential facts ...
a comprehensive textbook. *1976*

Atlas

Armstrong and Kidd/BAILLIÈRE'S ATLAS OF
FEMALE ANATOMY - Illustrating in full colour the relative
size, shape and position of every part of the human body.
7th edition 1969

Nurses' Aids Series

The complete nurses' library for your nursing training

ANATOMY AND PHYSIOLOGY FOR NURSES/ Jackson *9th edition 1979*

EAR, NOSE & THROAT NURSING/Marshall and Oxlade *5th edition 1979*

GERIATRIC NURSING/Storrs *2nd edition 1980*

MATHEMATICS IN NURSING/Jefferies *6th edition 1983*

MEDICAL NURSING/Chapman *9th edition 1977*

MICROBIOLOGY FOR NURSES/Parker and Stucke *6th edition 1982*

MULTIPLE CHOICE QUESTIONS BOOK 1 – Anatomy and Physiology, Medical, Surgical and Paediatric Nursing *1977*

MULTIPLE CHOICE QUESTIONS BOOK 2 – Practical Nursing and Personal and Community Health *1978*

MULTIPLE CHOICE QUESTIONS BOOK 3 – Psychology for Nurses and Pharmacology for Nurses *1980*

OBSTETRIC AND GYNAECOLOGICAL NURSING/Grayshon and Bailey *3rd edition 1982*

PAEDIATRIC NURSING/Duncombe and Weller *5th edition 1979*

PERSONAL AND COMMUNITY HEALTH/ Jackson and Lane *2nd edition 1981*

PHARMACOLOGY FOR NURSES/Connechen, Robson and Shanley *5th edition 1983*

PRACTICAL NURSING/Clarke *12th edition 1977*

PRACTICAL PROCEDURES FOR NURSES/Billing *3rd edition 1981*

PSYCHIATRIC NURSING/Altschul and Simpson *5th edition 1977*

PSYCHOLOGY FOR NURSES/Altschul and Sinclair *5th edition 1981*

SOCIOLOGY FOR NURSES/Chapman *1978*

SURGICAL NURSING/Fish *10th edition 1979*

THEATRE TECHNIQUE/Dixon *5th edition 1983*

Help For Your Examinations

DO-IT-YOURSELF REVISION FOR NURSES -
Books 1, 2, 3 & 4   E. J. Hull and B. J. Isaacs
The four books of this series provide a comprehensive
framework for revision of the GNC syllabus and develop-
ments made since to it. The student reviews a subject of
choice, answers questions selected from recent State Final
Examinations, and marks her replies against the model
answers provided.
Books 1-4 1982
'*Highly recommended to all student nurses as a planned guide
to revision*'. Nursing Times

MULTIPLE CHOICE QUESTIONS BOOK 1 - Anatomy
and Physiology, Medical, Surgical and Paediatric Nursing.
(NAS) *1977*

MULTIPLE CHOICE QUESTIONS BOOK 2 - Practical
Nursing and Personal and Community Health. (NAS) *1978*

MULTIPLE CHOICE QUESTIONS BOOK 3 - Psychology
for Nurses and Pharmacology for Nurses. (NAS) *1980*

QUIZZES AND QUESTIONS FOR NURSES/E.J. Hull &
B.J. Isaacs
Book A - Medical Nursing and Paediatric Nursing
Book B - Surgical Nursing and Geriatric Nursing

Key Facts — Baillière Tindall Nursing Cards

The Six Basic Subjects All Students Have To Learn

NURSING MEDICAL PATIENTS
NURSING IN THE COMMUNITY
NURSING ELDERLY PATIENTS
NURSING SURGICAL PATIENTS
NURSING MATERNITY PATIENTS
NURSING PSYCHIATRIC PATIENTS

* Assist students in the clinical areas to which they are allocated for experience.
* Invaluable reference proving information related to the care and treatment of patients.
* Based on the 'nursing process'
* Written by Nursing Tutors and Senior Nursing Officers with first-hand experience of the information required and problems encountered by students.
* A practical outline on which to base further reading, discussion and preparation of case histories.
* Invaluable at revision time.
* Pocket size for quick reference and learning in spare moments.

Ask for a Free Leaflet!

The Best Pocket Size Dictionaries

for students, nurses, midwives, medical secretaries and health workers

BAILLIÈRE'S NURSES' DICTIONARY
This world famous dictionary is a *must* for all nurses.
19th edition 1979

BAILLIÈRE'S MIDWIVES' DICTIONARY
Another invaluable book giving up-to-date definitions and factual statements for the midwife. *6th edition 1976*

BAILLIÈRE'S POCKET BOOK OF WARD INFORMATION
Concise, comprehensive and up-to-date. *13th edition 1980*

Champney and Smiddy/SYMPTOMS, SIGNS, AND SYNDROMES: A Medical Glossary
For rapid reference in the ward and clinic. *1979*

Steen/ABBREVIATIONS IN MEDICINE
Containing over 1300 medical abbreviations. *4th edition 1978*

The details and editions in this list are those current at the time of going to press but are liable to alteration without notice.

BAILLIÈRE TINDALL

Greycoat House, 10 Greycoat Place, London SW1P 1SB

THE NURSING PROCESS

Kratz

"Primarily intended for nurse learners, the book will make an excellent introductory reader for all British nurses." *Nursing Times*
1979 . 170 pp . 2 illus . Limp

COUNSELLING SKILLS FOR NURSES

Tschudin

A guide for ward sisters, community nurses and nursing officers which applies the principles of counselling to the clinical situation. Such nurses may not have had formal training in counselling skills but yet are asked to use and teach them. This book will help them, through its emphasis on awareness, to acquire the basic skills, and, through its learning models, to teach others.
1982 . 152 pp . 4 illus . Limp

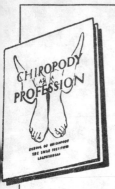